GESTATIONAL DIABETES

Edited by **Miroslav Radenković**

Gestational Diabetes
Edited by Miroslav Radenković

Published by InTech
Janeza Trdine 9, 51000 Rijeka, Croatia

Publishing Process Manager Romina Krebel

Technical Editor Teodora Smiljanic

Cover Designer InTech Design Team

Additional hard copies can be obtained from orders@intechopen.com

Gestational Diabetes, Edited by Miroslav Radenković
p. cm.
ISBN 978-953-307-581-5

For EU product safety concerns:
IN TECH d.o.o., Prolaz Marije Krucifikse Kozulić 3, 51000 Rijeka, Croatia,
info@intechopen.com or visit our website at intechopen.com.

Meet the editor

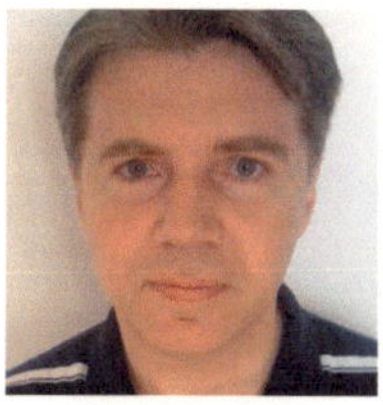

Dr. Miroslav Radenković was born in 1968. He graduated at the School of Medicine – University of Belgrade in 1995, and since 1996 he is working at the Department of Pharmacology, Clinical Pharmacology and Toxicology (School of Medicine – University of Belgrade), currently in the position of the associate professor. He received an MSc, board certified in clinical pharmacology and PhD in 1999, 2000 and 2004, respectively, from the School of Medicine – University of Belgrade. Since 2002 Dr. Radenković officially participates in research activities of several scientific projects supported by the Ministry of Science – Republic of Serbia. In 2007 he was a principal investigator in the scientific project financed by the Austrian Science Fund (Lise Meitner Program) and senior postdoc at the Medical University of Vienna. In the capacity of guest researcher he worked at the University Medical Center Hamburg – Eppendorf and the University of Graz. Dr. Radenković is a member of the Austrian Pharmacological Society, Austrian Atherosclerosis Society, German Atherosclerosis Society, European Atherosclerosis Society, Bioethical Society of Serbia, and Serbian Medical Society.

Contents

Preface

Gestational diabetes mellitus is generally defined as hyperglycemia with onset or first recognition during pregnancy. The incidence of gestational diabetes is still increasing and this pathological condition has strong association with adverse pregnancy outcomes. Given that gestational diabetes may have long-term pathological consequences for both mother and the child, it is important that it is promptly recognized and adequately managed. Preconceptional screening and medical informing of women with pre-existing diabetes, older age, family history of gestational diabetes, metabolic syndrome, obesity, polycystic ovary syndrome or hypertension would be significant in order to reduce the risk to the fetus and mother connected to gestational diabetes. Treatment of gestational diabetes is aimed to maintain euglycemia and it should involve regular glucose monitoring, dietary modifications, life style changes, exercise program, and when necessary, pharmacotherapy. In a long-term view, in order to prevent development of diabetes later in life, as well to avoid associated complications, an adequate education on lifestyle modifications should start in pregnancy and continue postpartum.

This book brings together 21 chapters of up-to-date information on gestational diabetes. The idea of this book is to direct the reader to comprehensively explore etiology and different aspects of prevention, screening, diagnosis, treatment, and postpartum follow-up in consideration to gestational diabetes. Furthermore, the presented facts provide a useful framework for both clinicians and basic investigators to further explore and update existing knowledge on diabetes related to pregnancy. We hope that this book will be used as a reference textbook for researchers, medical specialists, teachers and students.

We express sincere appreciation to all the authors of the chapters for their enthusiasm and expertise.

Miroslav Radenković, MD, PhD
Associate Professor
Department of Pharmacology, Clinical Pharmacology and Toxicology
School of Medicine, University of Belgrade
Serbia

1

Novel Screening Approaches for the Early Detection of Gestational Diabetes Mellitus

Harry M. Georgiou[1], Sebastián Illanes López[2] and Gregory E. Rice[3]
[1]Department of Obstetrics & Gynaecology, University of Melbourne, Victoria
[2]Departamento de Obstetricia & Ginecología y laboratorio de Biología de la Reproducción, Universidad de los Andes, Santiago
[3]University of Queensland Centre for Clinical Research, Queensland
[1,3]Australia
[2]Chile

1. Introduction

1.1 Complications of pregnancy

Within the discipline of clinical obstetrics, our understanding of the aetiology of complications of pregnancy is lacking. This lack of understanding limits our ability to identify and implement efficacious management and intervention strategies to ameliorate any adverse effects on both the mother and her baby. This situation is further confounded by the lack of reliable screening test(s) to identify pre-symptomatic women who subsequently develop complications of pregnancy. Gestational diabetes mellitus (GDM), extremes of birth weight (intrauterine growth restriction (IUGR) and fetal macrosomia (FM)), preeclampsia toxaemia (PET) and preterm labour ((PTL), including preterm rupture of membranes) are the most important complications of pregnancy that have no effective antenatal preventative treatment.

With an incidence each of about 5-10% of all pregnancies, these complications are common, responsible for the majority of obstetric and paediatric morbidity and mortality, and can permanently impact on lifelong health. For example, extreme preterm birth, whether spontaneous, or iatrogenic to protect the mother or fetus from progressive disease, can result in perinatal death or serious permanent disability such as blindness, deafness or neurological injury (Chandiramani, et al., 2007). Very low birth weight is not only an immediate threat to the fetus, but can programme adult onset hypertension, stroke and diabetes (Barker, 2006). Gestational diabetes is associated with a range of perinatal morbidities including fetal macrosomia, hyperinsulinaemia and hypoglycaemia, but may also programme childhood obesity and adult onset cardiovascular disease and diabetes (Moore, 2010, Nolan, 2011); diseases with the greatest impact on health economics. Moreover, women who develop gestational diabetes are at greatly increased risk of developing type 2 diabetes in later life (Henry and Beischer, 1991, Lee, et al., 2007).

Early detection of disease risk and onset is the first step in implementing efficacious treatment. If such early detection tests were available they would represent a major advance and contribution to the discipline and afford the opportunity to evaluate alternate treatment and clinical management strategies to improve health outcomes for both mother and baby. Based upon recent technological developments and studies, it is now realistic that clinically useful antenatal screening test(s) can be developed. Unlike diseases such as cancer where biomarkers need to be exquisitely specific, a useful antenatal screening test would ideally be highly sensitive, but not necessarily highly specific. The consequence of a false positive would be no worse than an erroneous triage to high-risk care.

1.2 The future of diagnostics

In the context of antenatal screening, the objective of proteomic approaches is to identify proteins or peptides that are informative of the risk of pre-symptomatic early pregnant women who subsequently develop complications of pregnancy. That is, how the antecedents of complications of pregnancy alter the expression of the genome and how this is manifested as altered protein and peptide expression. Informative proteins and peptides identified may be used to develop classification models (*e.g.* multiple biomarker diagnostic or prognostic tests) that assign the likelihood that an individual test sample came from a normal or "at-risk" group. Such tests (as with all *in vitro* diagnostic medical devices) inform clinical decision-making and provide an opportunity for timely and appropriate intervention. The performance of the test *(i.e.* its diagnostic efficiency) determines the quality of the information provided and ultimately patient management. The application of proteomics, thus, extends beyond mapping and comparing the protein complement of healthy and at-risk individuals and needs to be considered in the context of its contribution to the healthcare system.

Global health care is rapidly evolving, being driven by two processes - technological development and information management systems. Technological developments now provide opportunity to acquire complex information about patients. For example, rather than relying on a single measurement (*e.g.* a single biomarker diagnostic blood test) to detect disease, multiple disease markers may be simultaneously measured and combined to provide earlier and more accurate diagnosis. Information management systems are allowing such complex data to be ascribed to the individual over the course of their lifetime. The anticipated outcome of these forces is a move from the episodic, reactionary medicine of today to personalised medicine where pharmacogenetics and molecular medicine will afford the opportunity to identify predisposition to disease, risk assessment, and assign individuals to personalised, efficacious treatment/intervention groups. Both genomics and proteomics will be useful contributors to the evolving healthcare system by providing a better understanding of physiology, by defining disease risk, by enabling earlier diagnosis and by monitoring treatment responses (Figure 1).

It is now widely acknowledged that single biomarkers are unlikely to deliver the significant incremental gain in sensitivity and specificity required for the development of effective screening and classification tests requisite for the implementation of personalised medicine. New approaches based upon the measurement of multiple biomarkers of disease risk afford opportunity to increase diagnostic test sensitivity and specificity. Over the past decade, the advent and optimisation of new proteomic technologies has paved the way for new strategies for the development of such multiple biomarker diagnostic tests. Our research team has applied both candidate-based and discovery-based proteomic approaches to identify biomarkers that are informative of disease risk. The ultimate objective of these collective efforts is the generation of multivariate, classification models that, at the very least, will allow the triage of early pregnant, asymptomatic women into low- and high-risk cohorts (Figure 2).

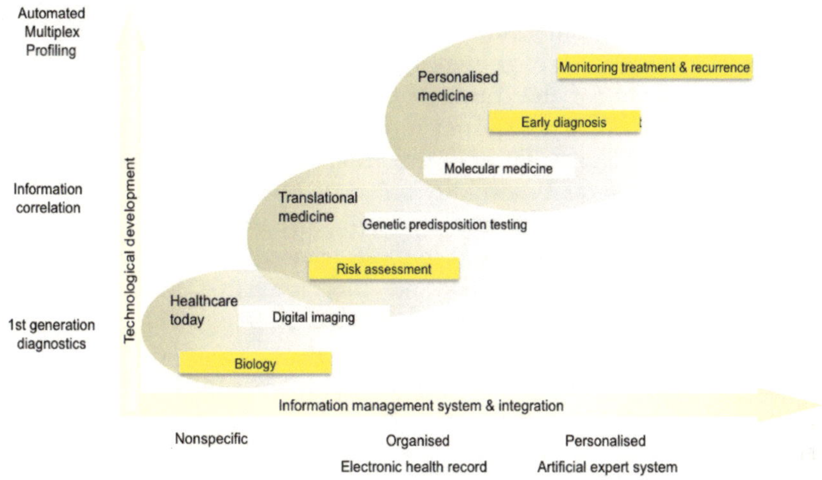

Fig. 1. The evolving healthcare system. The role of proteomics in the evolution of the healthcare system may be in the provision of multiple analyte protein and peptide profiles that facilitate risk assessment, earlier diagnosis and more effective treatment response monitoring. (Modified from *"Personalised Healthcare 2010", IBM Business Consulting Services*)

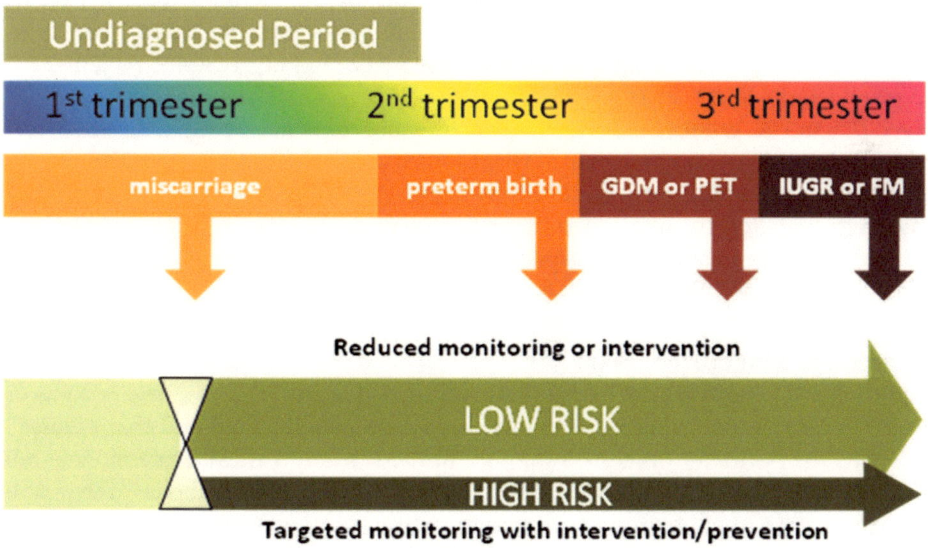

Fig. 2. Rationale for antenatal screening. The objective of implementing an antenatal screening test is to identify pre-symptomatic women who will subsequently develop complications of pregnancy and implement efficacious treatment to reduce morbidity and mortality. Currently, complications of pregnancy are not diagnosed until mid-late gestation.

2. Gestational diabetes mellitus

2.1 Current screening

Gestational diabetes mellitus (GDM) is defined as carbohydrate intolerance of varying severity with onset or first recognition during pregnancy (Metzger and Coustan, 1998). GDM usually manifests in the latter half of pregnancy and is typically diagnosed by an oral glucose tolerance test. If GDM is diagnosed, women will usually be counselled and advised to adopt a healthy lifestyle for the duration of their pregnancy and where it is deemed appropriate, women may also be required to undergo pharmacologic or insulin therapy. During this time, increased surveillance of the pregnancy is undertaken to help ameliorate the consequent maternal and fetal morbidity associated with GDM. The clinical importance of this surveillance is highlighted by recent published findings that demonstrate that even mild hyperglycaemia over a prolonged period is associated with numerous adverse perinatal outcomes (Schafer-Graf, 2009) and that intensive intervention therapy can significantly reduce maternal and fetal morbidity (Crowther, et al., 2005, Landon, et al., 2009). The effects of hyperglycaemia on pregnancy outcome are underpinned by experimental studies that identify putative effector pathways by which exposure to glucose concentrations may alter placental and maternal adipose tissue phenotype and responsiveness (Coughlan, et al., 2001, Coughlan, et al., 2004, Coughlan, et al., 2004, Lappas, et al., 2004).

The current 'gold standard' for the diagnosis of GDM is the oral glucose tolerance test (OGTT) and although there is no international consensus on the diagnostic methods or the blood glucose thresholds, it has become more widely accepted that the OGTT should be performed between 24-28 weeks' gestation using a 75 g glucose load with fasting, one-hour and two-hour venous glucose determinations (Coustan, et al., 2010, Metzger, et al., 2010). Universal screening and blood glucose thresholds remain contentious and may sometimes be based on resource availability and economic factors rather than clinical factors. Often, the more 'restrictive' blood glucose limits, leading to the diagnosis of the more severe hyperglycaemic patients, is all that can be provided in some instances. By contrast, professional associations advocate more 'inclusive' diagnostic criteria, and consequently more patients being diagnosed with less severe hyperglycaemia (Agarwal, et al., 2005, Lindsay, 2011, Metzger, et al., 2010, Ryan, 2011). With the obesity epidemic well entrenched in the Western world and with more women delaying pregnancy and the associated increase in pre-pregnancy body mass index (BMI), the incidence of GDM is increasing irrespective of the diagnostic criteria used (Kerrigan and Kingdon, 2010, Wein and Beischer, 2000).

2.2 The problem with current tests

It is important to recognise that by the time GDM is diagnosed in the late second or early third trimester of pregnancy, the 'pathology' is probably established and that reversal of the potential adverse perinatal outcomes may be limited. Many health professionals advocate the need for an earlier diagnostic/predictive test for GDM while at the same time acknowledging that avenues for preventative treatment may be limited (Guedj, 2010). In fact, it is the lack of a reliable early test for GDM that has hampered the development of useful intervention therapies. Although a direct clinical benefit of the early diagnosis of GDM remains to be established conclusively, identification of women at greatest risk would allow triage of patients to an appropriate model of care and identify those who are at greatest need of glucose tolerance assessment (Caliskan, et al., 2004, Shirazian, et al., 2009).

Numerous GDM risk-factor assessments have been attempted during first trimester pregnancy and include, but not limited to, family history of GDM and/or diabetes (Savvidou, et al., 2010), maternal demographics (Alanis, et al., 2010, Phaloprakarn, et al., 2009, Shirazian, et al., 2009, Wein, et al., 1995), maternal pregnancy weight gain (Morisset, et al., 2011), fasting plasma glucose (Riskin-Mashiah, et al., 2009, Riskin-Mashiah, et al., 2010), one-hour glucose challenge test (Maegawa, et al., 2003, Nahum, et al., 2002, Punthumapol and Tekasakul, 2008), oral glucose tolerance test (Bhattacharya, 2004, Phaloprakarn and Tangjitgamol, 2008, Sacks, et al., 2003) and haemoglobin A1c levels (Maegawa, et al., 2003). Although some tests have provided a good negative predictive measure for subsequent GDM, most tests suffer from poor positive predictive values and therefore are of limited efficacy. It is evident that other metabolic markers that precede hyperglycaemia would need to be identified if GDM were to be predicted from a test in early pregnancy.

3. Early screening of impending GDM

3.1 Single biomarker investigations

Recently, a number of first trimester studies have identified various biomarkers associated with subsequent development of GDM. In some cases these can be regarded as surrogate markers of inflammation such as C-reactive protein (Wolf, et al., 2003), of oxidative stress such as 8-iso$PGF_{2\alpha}$ (Rogers, et al., 2006) or of obesity such as serum triglycerides (Nolan, et al., 1995, Son, et al., 2010) and may not necessarily be specific for impending GDM. Perhaps the more exciting studies are those that have investigated serum or plasma protein biomarkers associated with early pregnancy placental function and carbohydrate/lipid metabolism. For example, it has been shown that lower sex hormone-binding globulin (Thadhani, et al., 2003), increased placental growth factor (Ong, et al., 2004), elevated leptin concentrations (Qiu, et al., 2004), reduced plasma adiponectin concentrations (Retnakaran, et al., 2004, Williams, et al., 2004) and lower follistatin-like-3 levels (Thadhani, et al., 2010) are all risk factors for subsequent development GDM. Although the associations are compelling further investigations are warranted as it appears that none of these markers alone provide adequate positive predictive values for subsequent GDM.

3.2 Multiple biomarker investigations

More recent studies have focused on multiple candidate-based profiling of blood-borne biomarkers to identify lead candidates for developing early pregnancy screening tests for gestational diabetes. For example, we measured multiple plasma biomarkers at 11 weeks' gestation in women who subsequently experienced a normal pregnancy outcome (n=14) and women who subsequently developed gestational diabetes (n=14) (Georgiou, et al., 2008). Of the biomarkers considered (insulin, adiponectin, leptin, resistin and glucose), receiver operator characteristic (ROC) curves for three biomarkers (adiponectin, insulin and random blood glucose) are presented together with a ROC curve based on the predicted posterior probability values (ppv) generated by a classification model that combined information from all three biomarkers (Figure 3). The combined model out performed individual biomarkers based upon the area under the ROC curve (combined model = 0.94; adiponectin = 0.867; insulin = 0.872 and glucose = 0.827). This simple example demonstrates the putative benefit of a multimarker approach for improving diagnostic efficiency. Similar multiple biomarker investigations in association with GDM early (Nanda, et al., 2011) or late (Bomba-Opon, et al., 2010, Lowe, et al., 2010) in pregnancy have been described.

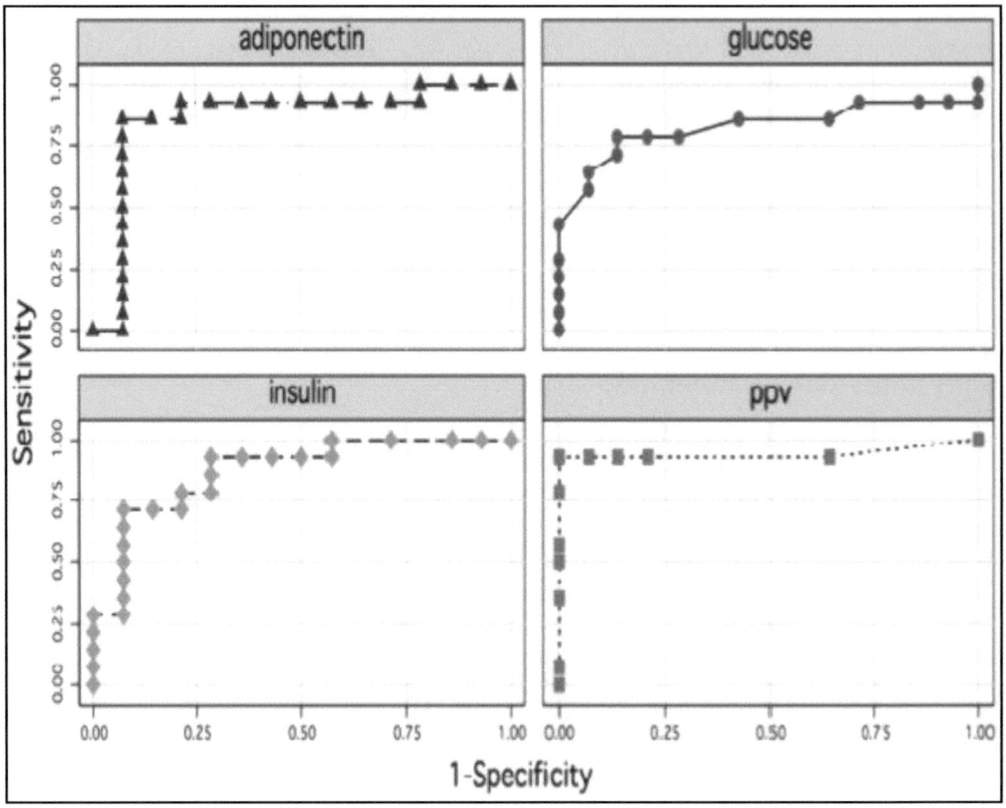

Fig. 3. The advantage of multiple biomarker screening. A comparison of ROC curves of the performance of individual biomarkers (adiponectin, insulin and glucose) and a combined model (ppv) to correctly classify women who subsequently developed gestational diabetes.

4. Proteomic approaches for early detection of GDM

4.1 Sample selection and processing

As with all analytical techniques, sample heterogeneity (*e.g.* variation from individual patients, sample collection and processing) needs to be minimised for proteomic analysis. This is particularly relevant to the collection of blood, where both the method of collection and processing may dramatically alter the peptide profile (*e.g.* clotting, temperature and time taken to process samples). For example, while the collection of serum may be suitable for some candidate-based approaches (*e.g.* protein solution array and immunoassay), the peptides generated during coagulation confound peptidomic analysis.

The impact of the method used to collect blood is demonstrated in Figure 4, in which paired plasma and serum samples were collected from pregnant women. Blood was either collected into EDTA or Serum Clot Activator tubes. The former was immediately centrifuged for 15 min at room temperature, while the latter was allowed to clot at room temperature for 60 min and then centrifuged for 15 min at room temperature. Following centrifugation, the resultant plasma or serum was stored at -80° C for mass spectrometry peptide profiling. Both plasma and serum samples were subjected to protein dye binding depletion (Affi-gel Blue™) as previously described (Ahmed, et al., 2003) followed by solid phase peptide enrichment using hydrophilic-lipophilic balanced solid phase extraction sorbent in 96-well micro-elution plates, eluted and analysed using matrix assisted laser desorption ionisation - time-of-flight (MALDI-ToF) mass spectrometry (AutoFlex II, Bruker Daltonics). The resultant peptide profiles of plasma and serum while showing some concordance at m/z >4000, exhibited dramatically different peptide ion profiles at m/z < 2000 (Figure 4). It is likely that these ions represent peptides generated during the coagulation process and/or by the action of peptidases during the 60 min incubation at room temperature. Thus, for the purpose of primary peptidomic profiling of blood peptides, serum presents significant methodological challenges. Indeed, even different anticoagulant methods (*e.g.* EDTA, heparin, citrate) have been found to alter peptide ion profiles (Banks, et al., 2005).

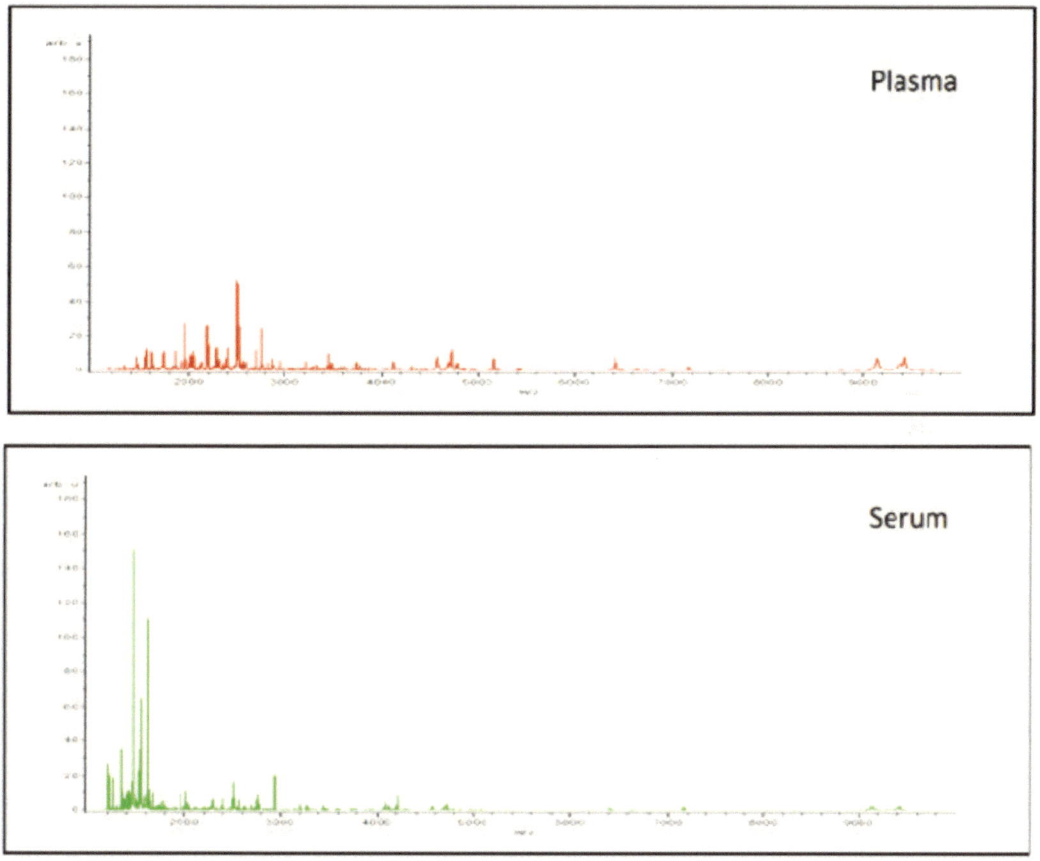

Fig. 4. Method of blood collection. Mass spectrometric peptidomic profiling of paired plasma and serum showing marked spectral differences.

4.2 Consideration of gestational change

Of particular relevance to any discussion of biomarkers for the development of antenatal screening tests is gestational variation. To be of clinical utility, any early pregnancy screening test would need to be independent of or well outside the normal early gestational changes in the subset of the proteome being interrogated. For example, in seeking to identify plasma protein biomarkers that may be of utility in identifying women at risk of developing a complication of pregnancy, it is critical to first establish the variation (both gestational and inter-patient) that occurs within the temporal window in which the test is to be applied. That is, if the objective is to identify plasma protein biomarkers using two-dimensional polyacrylamide gel electrophoresis (2D-PAGE) for a test that will be applied between 6-12 weeks of gestation then the variation that occurs in the subset of proteins being screened must be established.

To assess the early-pregnancy variation that plasma proteins display by 2D electrophoresis, we completed an initial study that begins to define the gestational variation in a subset of plasma proteins. Weekly peripheral blood samples were collected from women from 6-12 weeks of pregnancy. Plasma samples were immuno-depleted of high-abundance proteins (IgY14 column, Sigma) and then labelled with fluorescent CyDyes (Cy3, Cy5) for pair-wise comparison (GE Healthcare). A pooled plasma sample was labelled with Cy2 for normalisation across gels. Labelled proteins were pooled and then separated in the first dimension (24 cm Immobiline™ Dry- Strips, pH 3-11NL) and then in the second dimension (12.5% 24 cm hand-cast acrylamide gels with low fluorescent glass). Gel were imaged using a Typhoon Trio 9100 (GE Healthcare) and then analysed using Progenesis SameSpots software (v3.2.3107.24565, Nonlinear Dynamics). The analysis focussed on spots with a greater than 1.5 fold difference. Protein spots that were common to all gels (n=89) were further investigated. Figure 5 presents a box-plot summary of the gestational variation in these proteins for one patient. To identify protein spots that varied significantly across gestation and accounting for 'false discovery rates', the combined data set was subjected to nonparametric analysis methodology using Significance of Microarray (SAM) analysis. Using a false discovery rate of 1%, 5 protein spots were identified that varied significantly during 6-12 weeks of pregnancy (Figure 6).

4.3 Candidate-based profiling approaches (solution array workflow)

Protein and antibody arrays and multiple immunoassay methodologies represent examples of candidate or targeted proteomic approaches. The advantages of these approaches include: rapid, high throughput screening of known targets and quantitative endpoints. Multiplex protein solution array is one application that represents a generation of antibody-based detection technology that allows the simultaneous quantification of multiple analytes in a single, small volume sample. Multiplex protein solution array has a number of advantages over current analyte quantification technologies, including: measurement of many biomarkers (up to 100 different analytes) in a single sample; wider operational dynamic range; and increased sensitivity and specificity derived from multivariate modelling of combinations of biomarker analytes. This system utilises a sandwich ELISA-like protocol, in which capture antibodies are coupled to spectrally distinct polystyrene or metal beads (5-6 µm diameter). Biotinylated sandwich antibody and streptavidin-phycoerytherin (PE) fluorophore are used as a reporter complex. Assays are conducted in 96-well filter-bottom

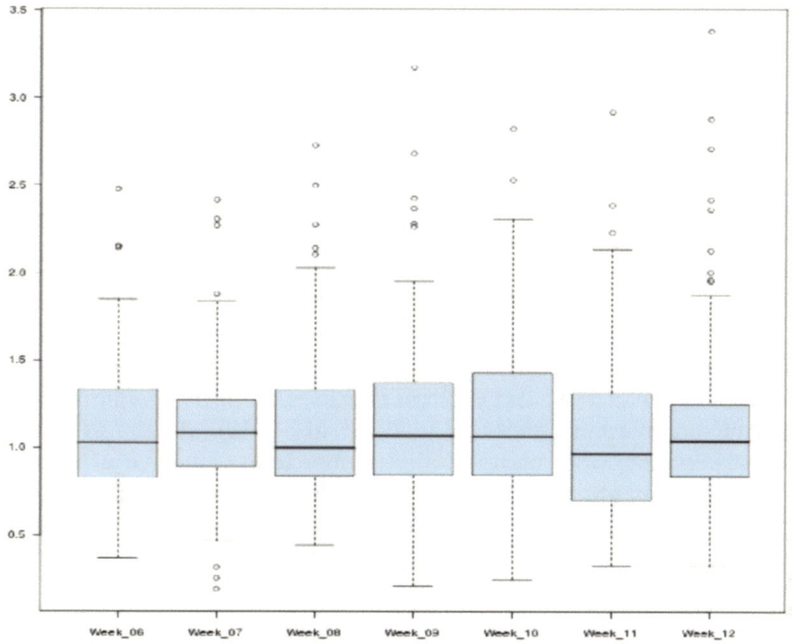

Fig. 5. Variation in plasma proteins displayed during early pregnancy (6-12 weeks of gestation). Serial peripheral blood samples were collected from women and displayed using 2D-DIGE. The data presented represent normalised spot volumes for 89 protein spot that were common to all gels.

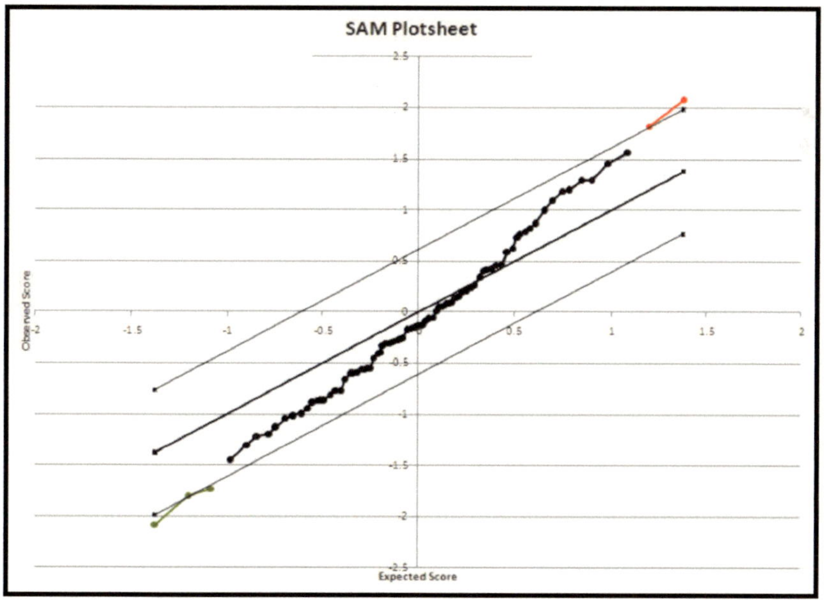

Fig. 6. Non-parametric, significance of microarray (SAM) analysis of the variation in normalised protein spot volumes during early pregnancy. Five protein spot (shown in colour) are identified as varying significantly.

plates and beads are washed by vacuum filtration. Bead identity and analyte-specific fluorescence are assessed using a flow cytometre (Luminex) fitted with dual lasers. Solution array offers excellent reproducibility (CV <10%) and analyte quantification and has the capacity to multiplex up to 100 different analytes in small sample volumes (*e.g.* 50-100 μl plasma).
Various manufacturers have now produced a myriad of multiplex assay kits consisting of premixed panels of biologically related biomarkers (*e.g.* cytokines/chemokines, endocrine hormones, matrix metalloproteinases, phosphoproteins etc) or disease-related panels (*e.g.* cancer markers, autoimmunity biomarkers and more recently, diabetes biomarkers). All suppliers also offer single-plex biomarkers that can be custom mixed to produce any panel of choice. We have previously used cytokine/chemokine multiplex panels to investigate pregnancy related complications such as GDM (Georgiou, et al., 2008), intrauterine growth restriction (Georgiou, et al., 2011) and preterm prelabour rupture of membranes (Hodges, et al., 2010) as well as ovarian cancer (Edgell, et al., 2010). Although the differentially expressed biomarkers may only be associative rather than causative of disease, these and other similar studies highlight the advantages of multiple biomarker screening for improved diagnostic/predictive modelling. An important consideration for any method that utilises multiple analyte determination is the appropriate control for the false discovery rate when multiple comparisons (hypotheses) are being tested.

4.4 Gel-based profiling approaches

Gel-based platforms such as 1-dimensional and 2-dimensional polyacrylamide gel electrophoresis (1D or 2D-PAGE) and fluorescence 2D difference gel electrophoresis (2D-DIGE) have been used in both expression and comparative studies to define plasma protein abundance and disease-associated or treatment-induced changes. The advantage of these approaches resides in their ability to identify post-translational modified protein isoforms. The limitation of gel-based systems is their relatively low throughput, the necessity for sample processing and fractionation prior to display and limited mass range (~10-200 kDa). In addition, procedural protein losses and the overall experimental variation in estimating endpoints by 2D-PAGE may be considerable. Procedural losses of proteins during 2D-PAGE display have been reported to be as high as 80% but this can vary depending on the starting protein load (Zhou, et al., 2005). As with any other technique, variation is apportioned between technical replication, both within assay and between assay, and biologic variation (*i.e.* sample-to-sample). Estimates of the variation attributable to technical replication average 25-40%. Biological variation has been estimated to be between 24 and 70% (Molloy, et al., 2003).

4.4.1 2-Dimensional Polyacrylamide Gel Electrophoresis (2D-PAGE)

Using a traditional 2D-PAGE approach, we analysed the maternal plasma proteome from women with a normal pregnancy and compared this with women who subsequently developed GDM. Plasma samples were obtained at approximately 12 weeks' (pre-GDM) and 28 weeks' gestation (overt GDM) and gestation-matched with an equal number of normal controls. Individual plasma samples were depleted of high abundance proteins (albumin and immunoglobulins) by matrix binding centrifugation (Affi-gel Blue and Affi-gel Protein A respectively), solubilised in a multiple chaotrope buffer and focused on 11 cm, pH4-7 immobilised pH gradient strips. Second dimension electrophoresis was performed on 10% polyacrylamide gels and proteins visualised with Sypro Ruby staining. Protein spots were matched and relative abundance was determined using PD-Quest software (v7.3.1,

Bio-Rad Laboratories). Using this approach more than 600 protein spots were visualised. Of these up to 20 proteins were significantly differentially expressed in pre-symptomatic women. Some of these protein spots are unique to pre-GDM (12 weeks' gestation) while others are also differentially expressed during overt disease (28 weeks' gestation). In some cases only specific isomers of a particular protein were differentially expressed (Figure 7).
The limitations of this methodology include (i) time consuming and sometimes unreliable matching of hundreds of spots in multiple gels, (ii) problems associated with spot normalisation, (iii) limited in-built statistical capacity of software to compare protein abundance, (iv) difficulty with excision of spots especially in small gel formats, and (v) the failure to reliably characterise proteins by MALDI-ToF mass spectrometry due to low protein abundance. This necessitates the need to scale-up methods for protein characterisation (orthogonal identification).

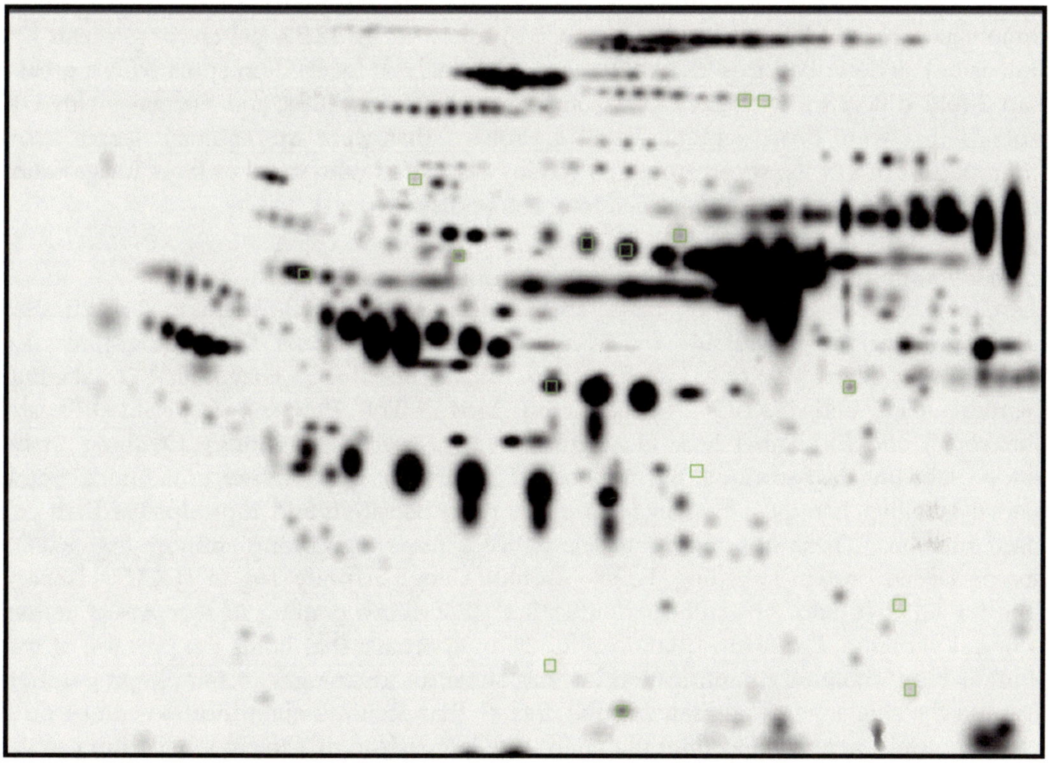

Fig. 7. 2D-PAGE Gaussian image of human plasma taken at approximately 12 weeks' gestation. Boxes indicate protein spots that were significantly differentially expressed in women who subsequently developed GDM compared to gestation-matched women who had a normal pregnancy.

4.4.2 2-Difference Gel Electrophoresis (2D-DIGE)

Some of the limitations of gel-based approaches have been overcome with the development of difference gel electrophoresis. This minimal labelling approach using fluorescent cyanine dyes increases throughput by reducing sample processing and both gel-to-gel and analytical variation by combining case and control samples into a single processing step, and by the use of an internal standard for normalisation of data across gels (as described in 4.2 above). 2D-DIGE also delivers useful relative quantification of protein expression profiles where the dyes are purported to have sub-nanogram sensitivity and a linear response to protein concentrations of over five orders of magnitude. The dyes are also compatible with mass spectrometric analysis. With respect to analysing the plasma proteome, 2D-DIGE is still limited by the compositional complexity of plasma and similarly benefits from sample fractionation and the removal of high-abundance proteins.

In these experiments, we collected plasma from asymptomatic pregnant women at 12-18 weeks' gestation. Pregnancies were retrospectively classified as normal (n = 10), GDM (n=5), small-for-gestational age (n=5) and large-for-gestational age (n=5). Plasma was pooled for each group and depleted of high abundance proteins (top 14) using the IgY14/Supermix system (Sigma). Samples were then concentrated and labelled with Cy2, Cy3 and Cy5 CyDye DIGE fluors (GE Healthcare) and subjected to 2D-PAGE using 13 cm, pH4-11 immobilised pH gradient strips (1st dimension) followed by 12.5% gel electrophoresis (2nd dimension) as described in section 4.2 above. The analysis focused on spots with a greater than 2-fold difference in expression. Comparison between GDM and normal yielded 10 proteins that were down-regulated and 4 proteins that were up-regulated (some being different isoforms of the same protein). Proteins associated with small or large for gestation fetal complications were also identified long before disease onset.

4.5 Mass-spectrometry based quantitative profiling approaches

There are now a number of mass spectrometry (MS)-based, relative quantification approaches currently available including: (i) Multidimensional Chromatography (*e.g.* MudPIT); (ii) Stable Isotope Labelling (*e.g.* metabolic-SILAC, enzymatic-^{18}O labelling, chemical ICPL and iTRAQ labelling); (iii) MALDI-ToF Profiling (*e.g.* SELDI™ and ClinProt™) and (iv) Label Free Quantification (*e.g.* spectral counting). Of these, stable isotope labelling is becoming the method of choice for quantitative proteomics. Stable isotope labelling has the advantages of being more sensitive and reproducible than gel-based methods. These approaches utilise either a mass tag coding strategy (*e.g.* ICPL - Isotope Coded Protein Labelling, ICAT - Isotope Coded Affinity Tag or iTRAQ - isobaric Tags for Relative and Absolute Quantification) that allow pooling of samples to reduce technical variation. Label-free quantification is an approach that holds the promise of true MudPIT-type 'shotgun' quantification but has some disadvantages in sample preparation, cost and the challenge of normalizing the data so that accurate quantification can be done across multiple samples and multiple analyses. Comparison of protein expression profiles between samples is based upon two metrics: ion peak intensities of extracted peptide signals from LC/MS profiles or spectral counting (number of times peptide precursor is selected for fragmentation) of identified proteins after MS/MS analysis (Zhu, et al., 2010).

In addition to its analytical applications, mass spectrometry affords opportunities to identify signature profiles contained within biological samples for the purpose of classification. The application of mass spectrometry is a burgeoning area within the domain of diagnostic and predictive medicine. This approach now affords the opportunity to develop disease-specific patterns or profiles based upon the presence of specific peptides in a patient sample. MS-based protein profiling relies on the presence and spatial relationships between peptide peaks to facilitate the classification of biological samples into different categories (*e.g.*

normal and disease). Based upon the analysis of a training sample set (*e.g.* disease-free patients), pattern recognition software and multivariate modelling are employed to build peptide profiles or motifs that characterise a disease-free condition. Once established, such reference profiles may be used as a template to detect variance and thus deliver a diagnosis or predictive capacity. Two of the mass spectrometry-based profiling approaches we have utilised to identify peptides that may be informative of disease risk are described.

4.5.1 MALDI-ToF peptide profiling (ClinProt™ workflow)

Matrix-affinity peptide capture coupled with mass spectrometry is a discovery-based tool for comparing peptide mass fingerprints between individual or groups of samples. Numerous 'magnetic bead capture' chemistries are available including metal affinity (Cu, Fe), cationic exchange and hydrophobic reverse phase. In a prospective study of GDM, plasma samples were collected from pregnant women at 10-14 weeks' and 26-30 weeks' gestation and retrospectively allocated to gestation-matched GDM and normal groups. Samples were analysed after removal of high abundance proteins (Affi-gel Blue/Affi-gel Protein A) following a single fractionation process. Processing of samples with magnetic beads was performed in quadruplicate using a robotic workstation. Samples were mixed with Copper Immobilised Metal Affinity Chromatography beads (IMAC-Cu, Bruker Daltonics) in 96-well plates. Unbound peptides in the supernatant were aspirated and discarded while magnetic beads were washed and bound peptides eluded. Extracted samples were then processed by traditional MALD-ToF methods and raw spectral files were analysed with ClinProTools software (v2.2, Bruker Daltonics). Based upon the analysis of peptide profiles, we were able to identify disease-specific differentially-detected peptide ion peaks (Figure 8) and to develop multivariate classification models (Support Vector Machine and Genetic Mutation Models) using ClinProtTools software that discriminated between women who subsequently experienced a normal or GDM pregnancy. For example, using a genetic mutation classification model, 5 peptides were selected that had the ability to correctly classify 100% of women to a low risk group (i.e. those women who subsequently experienced a normal pregnancy). Furthermore, the model correctly classified greater than 93% of those women who subsequently experienced a GDM pregnancy. An independent and larger cohort is now required to validate these observations.

4.5.2 Stable isotope labelling (iTRAQ workflow)

The other mass-spectrometry based approach we have used to identify disease-specific proteins is iTRAQ. This labelling method is arguably the benchmark for relative protein quantification. One significant benefit is that it allows sample multiplexing and hence the ability to perform comparative analyses of up to eight different samples. For example, seven disease conditions or treatment groups and a pooled internal control could be processed in tandem, allowing identification and quantification relative to control.

The same plasma samples described in section 4.4.2 above were subjected to iTRAQ analysis. Each pooled sample group was initially depleted of high abundance plasma proteins using the IgY14/Supermix system (Sigma). Depleted samples were digested with trypsin and each was labelled with one of four different iTRAQ reagents (ABSciex, normal - 114, IUGR - 116, GDM - 118 and FM - 121). After labelling, all 4 labelled reaction mixtures were combined and applied to a strong cation exchange (SCX) cartridge. A single fraction

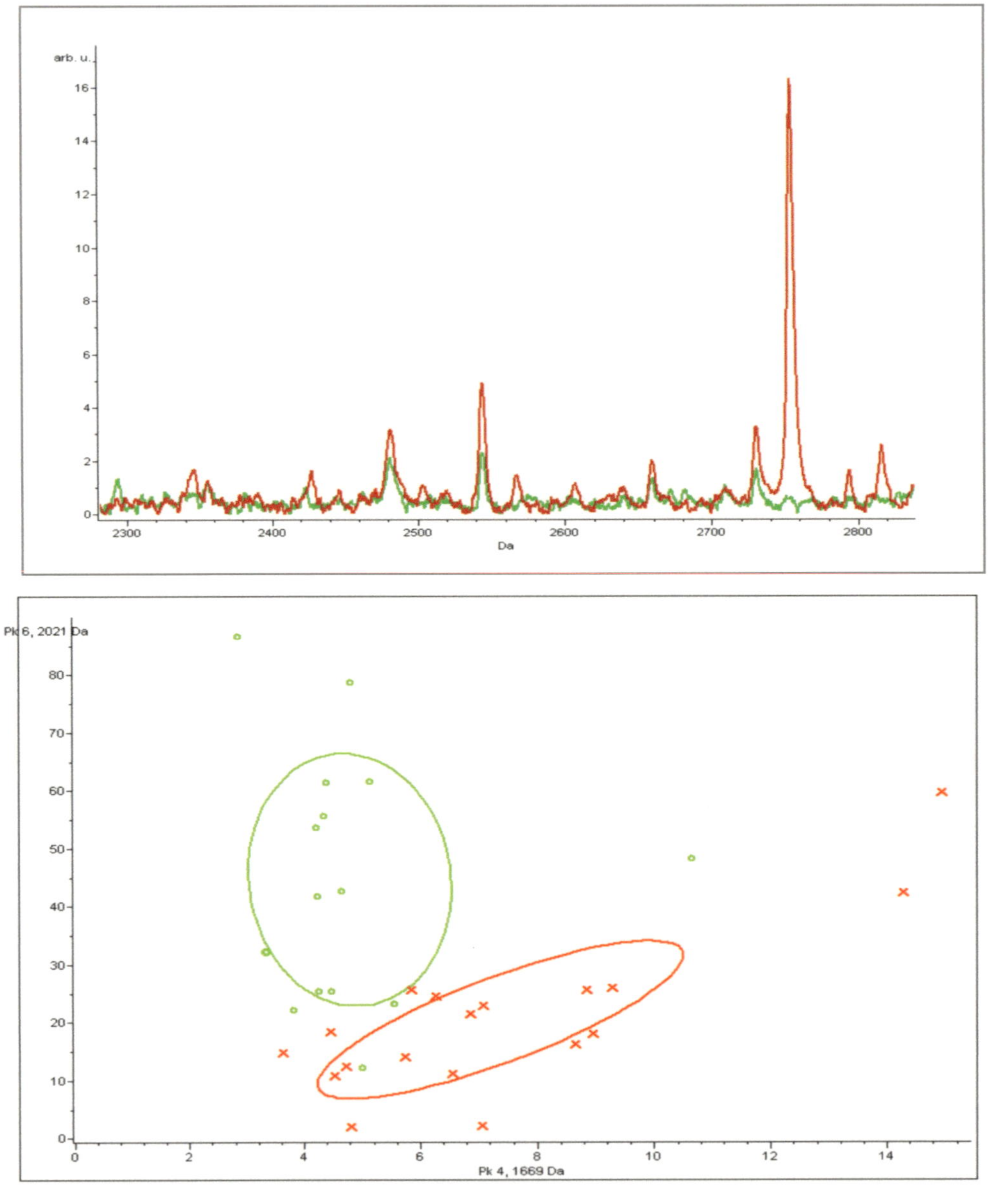

Fig. 8. MALDI-ToF peptide profile comparisons. **Top.** Example of the average peptide profiles over a limited spectral range (2300-2800 m/z) is presented to illustrate identified differences in peptide profiles between women with a normal pregnancy (red, n=19, 12 weeks) and women who subsequently developed GDM (green, n=16, 12 weeks). **Bottom.** A peptide peak cluster plot highlighting the potential for using differentially-expressed peptides to classify women into low- and high-risk groups for subsequent GDM. The plot presents the data (integrated area) of two peptide peaks (1669 vs 2021 m/z) observed in plasma obtained from women (12 weeks' gestation) who subsequently experienced a normal (red) or GDM pregnancy (green). Standard deviation envelopes are presented.

was eluted, collected, acidified and analysed by LC-MS/MS (QSTAR Elite, ABSciex) for simultaneous protein identification and peptide quantification (ProteinPilot ABSciex). Relative abundance of proteins in depleted plasma was determined by comparing the peak heights of reporter ions for each sample (m/z at 116, 118, 121) with those from the normal pregnancy (m/z at 114) pool. Using iTRAQ reagents and high resolution mass spectrometry, eight proteins that were differentially expressed (greater than 2-fold) in maternal plasma in association with GDM were unambiguously identified. Three of these proteins were up-regulated while five proteins were down-regulated. It is important to note that there was partial concordance between the identified proteins using iTRAQ and 2D-DIGE methods.

5. Conclusion

The methods we have described in this brief chapter provide proof-of-principle both technically and conceptually that biomarkers associated with disease can be reliably identified before the onset of overt disease. The challenge now remains to validate these findings in large independent cohorts to determine the predictive efficacy of these biomarkers. These emerging technologies and sophisticated modelling approaches now afford a realistic opportunity to develop and robustly evaluate the risk of asymptomatic early pregnant women developing complications of pregnancy such as GDM, IUGR, FM, PET and PTL. The development of such test(s) will provide data that better informs clinical decision-making and patient management that will not only directly benefit the immediate pregnancy, but will also help mitigate the longer-term ramifications of these conditions for both mother and baby.

6. Acknowledgement

All studies described above received prior approval from a relevant institutional human research ethics committee. The authors wish to acknowledge the invaluable help provided by research midwives from the Mercy Hospital for Women who have consented participants and processed blood samples. Technical assistance was provided by Gill Barker and Karen Oliva while mass spectrometry expertise was provided by Drs Mark Bailey, Alun Jones and Mustafa Ayhan. We acknowledge the expertise provided by representatives from Bruker Daltonics (Freemont, CA) and Bio-Rad Laboratories (Hercules, CA) for their platform technologies. This work was funded by the Medical Research Foundation for Women and Babies and grants from the National Health and Medical Research Council (NHMRC, Australia) 454451, 509127, 526686 and 586651. GER is in receipt of an NHMRC Principal Research Fellowship.

7. References

Agarwal, M. M., Dhatt, G. S., Punnose, J. & Koster, G. (2005). Gestational diabetes: dilemma caused by multiple international diagnostic criteria. *Diabet Med,* Vol.22, No.12, pp. 1731-1736, issn 0742-3071

Ahmed, N., Barker, G., Oliva, K., Garfin, D., Talmadge, K., Georgiou, H., Quinn, M. & Rice, G. (2003). An approach to remove albumin for the proteomic analysis of low abundance biomarkers in human serum. *Proteomics,* Vol.3, No.10, pp. 1980-1987, issn 1615-9853

Alanis, M. C., Goodnight, W. H., Hill, E. G., Robinson, C. J., Villers, M. S. & Johnson, D. D. (2010). Maternal super-obesity (body mass index > or = 50) and adverse pregnancy outcomes. *Acta Obstet Gynecol Scand,* Vol.89, No.7, pp. 924-930, issn 1600-0412

Banks, R. E., Stanley, A. J., Cairns, D. A., Barrett, J. H., Clarke, P., Thompson, D. & Selby, P. J. (2005). Influences of blood sample processing on low-molecular-weight proteome identified by surface-enhanced laser desorption/ionization mass spectrometry. *Clinical Chemistry,* Vol.51, No.9, pp. 1637-1649, issn 0009-9147

Barker, D. J. P. (2006). Adult consequences of fetal growth restriction. *Clin Obstet Gynecol,* Vol.49, No.2, pp. 270-283, issn 0009-9201

Bhattacharya, S. M. (2004). Fasting or two-hour postprandial plasma glucose levels in early months of pregnancy as screening tools for gestational diabetes mellitus developing in later months of pregnancy. *J Obstet Gynaecol Res,* Vol.30, No.4, pp. 333-336, issn 1341-8076

Bomba-Opon, D. A., Horosz, E., Szymanska, M. & Wielgos, M. (2010). Maternal plasma adipokines and insulin concentrations in relation to fetal biometry in the gestational diabetes. *Neuro Endocrinol Lett,* Vol.31, No.4, pp. 568-572, issn 0172-780X

Caliskan, E., Kayikcioglu, F., Ozturk, N., Koc, S. & Haberal, A. (2004). A population-based risk factor scoring will decrease unnecessary testing for the diagnosis of gestational diabetes mellitus. *Acta Obstet Gynecol Scand,* Vol.83, No.6, pp. 524-530, issn 0001-6349

Chandiramani, M., Tribe, R. M. & Sherman, A. H. (2007). Preterm labour and prematurity. *Obstetrics, Gynaecology and Reproductive Medicine,* Vol.17, No.8, pp. 232-237, issn

Coughlan, M. T., Oliva, K., Georgiou, H. M., Permezel, J. M. & Rice, G. E. (2001). Glucose-induced release of tumour necrosis factor-alpha from human placental and adipose tissues in gestational diabetes mellitus. *Diabet Med,* Vol.18, No.11, pp. 921-927, issn 0742-3071

Coughlan, M. T., Permezel, M., Georgiou, H. M. & Rice, G. E. (2004). Repression of oxidant-induced nuclear factor-kappa B activity mediates placental cytokine responses in gestational diabetes. *J Clin Endocrinol Metab,* Vol.89, No.7, pp. 3585-3594, issn 0021-972X

Coughlan, M. T., Vervaart, P. P., Permezel, M., Georgiou, H. M. & Rice, G. E. (2004). Altered placental oxidative stress status in gestational diabetes mellitus. *Placenta,* Vol.25, No.1, pp. 78-84, issn 0143-4004

Coustan, D. R., Lowe, L. P., Metzger, B. E., Dyer, A. R., International Association of the Diabetes and Pregnancy Study Groups. (2010). The Hyperglycemia and Adverse Pregnancy Outcome (HAPO) study: paving the way for new diagnostic criteria for gestational diabetes mellitus. *Am J Obstet Gynecol,* Vol.202, No.6, pp. 654.e651-656, issn 1097-6868

Crowther, C. A., Hiller, J. E., Moss, J. R., McPhee, A. J., Jeffries, W. S. & Robinson, J. S. (2005). Effect of treatment of gestational diabetes mellitus on pregnancy outcomes. *N Engl J Med,* Vol.352, No.24, pp. 2477-2486, issn 0028-4793

Edgell, T., Martin-Roussety, G., Barker, G., Autelitano, D. J., Allen, D., Grant, P. & Rice, G. E. (2010). Phase II biomarker trial of a multimarker diagnostic for ovarian cancer. *J Cancer Res Clin Oncology* Vol.136, No.7, pp. 1079-1088, pp. issn 0171-5216

Georgiou, H. M., Lappas, M., Georgiou, G. M., Marita, A., Bryant, V. J., Hiscock, R., Permezel, M., Khalil, Z. & Rice, G. E. (2008). Screening for biomarkers predictive of gestational diabetes mellitus. *Acta Diabetologica,* Vol.45, No.3, pp. 157-165, issn 0940-5429

Georgiou, H. M., Thio, Y. S., Russell, C., Permezel, M., Heng, Y. J., Lee, S. & Tong, S. (2011). Association between maternal serum cytokine profiles at 7-10 weeks' gestation and birthweight in small for gestational age infants. *Am J Obstet Gynecol,* pp. issn 1097-6868

Guedj, A. M. (2010). When should screening be performed for gestational diabetes? *Diabetes Metab,* Vol.36, No.6 Pt 2, Vol.204, No.5, pp. 415.e1-415.e12, 652-657, issn 1878-1780

Henry, O. A. & Beischer, N. A. (1991). Long-term implications of gestational diabetes for the mother. *Baillieres Clin Obstet Gynaecol,* Vol.5, No.2, pp. 461-483, issn 0950-3552

Hodges, R., Salvador, L., D'Antona, D., Georgiou, H. M. & Wallace, E. M. (2010). Activin A as a marker of intrauterine infection in women with preterm prelabour rupture of membranes. *J Perinatol,* Vol.30, No.1, pp. 22-26, issn 0743-8346

Kerrigan, A. M. & Kingdon, C. (2010). Maternal obesity and pregnancy: a retrospective study. *Midwifery,* Vol.26, No.1, pp. 138-146, issn 1532-3099

Landon, M. B., Spong, C. Y., Thom, E., Carpenter, M. W., Ramin, S. M., Casey, B., Wapner, R. J., Varner, M. W., Rouse, D. J., Thorp, J. M., Sciscione, A., Catalano, P., Harper, M., Saade, G., Lain, K. Y., Sorokin, Y., Peaceman, A. M., Tolosa, J. E., Anderson, G. B. & Eunice Kennedy Shriver, N. M. (2009). A Multicenter, Randomized Trial of Treatment for Mild Gestational Diabetes. *New Engl J Med,* Vol.361, No.14, pp. 1339-1348, issn 0028-4793

Lappas, M., Permezel, M. & Rice, G. E. (2004). Release of proinflammatory cytokines and 8-isoprostane from placenta, adipose tissue, and skeletal muscle from normal pregnant women and women with gestational diabetes mellitus. *J Clin Endocrinol Metab,* Vol.89, No.11, pp. 5627-5633, issn 0021-972X

Lee, A. J., Hiscock, R. J., Wein, P., Walker, S. P. & Permezel, M. (2007). Gestational diabetes mellitus: Clinical predictors and long-term risk of developing type 2 diabetes - A retrospective cohort study using survival analysis. *Diabetes Care,* Vol.30, No.4, pp. 878-883, issn 0149-5992

Lindsay, R. S. (2011). Gestational diabetes: costs and consequences. *Diabetologia,* Vol.54, No.2, pp. 227-229, issn 1432-0428

Lowe, L. P., Metzger, B. E., Lowe, W. L., Jr., Dyer, A. R., McDade, T. W., McIntyre, H. D. & Hapo Study Cooperative Research Group. (2010). Inflammatory mediators and glucose in pregnancy: results from a subset of the Hyperglycemia and Adverse Pregnancy Outcome (HAPO) Study. *J Clin Endocrinol Metab,* Vol.95, No.12, pp. 5427-5434, issn 1945-7197

Maegawa, Y., Sugiyama, T., Kusaka, H., Mitao, M. & Toyoda, N. (2003). Screening tests for gestational diabetes in Japan in the 1st and 2nd trimester of pregnancy. *Diabetes Res Clin Pract,* Vol.62, No.1, pp. 47-53, issn 0168-8227

Metzger, B. E. & Coustan, D. R. (1998). Summary and recommendations of the Fourth International Workshop-Conference on Gestational Diabetes Mellitus. The Organizing Committee. *Diabetes Care,* Vol.21 Suppl 2, pp. B161-167, issn 0149-5992

Metzger, B. E., Gabbe, S. G., Persson, B., Buchanan, T. A., Catalano, P. A., Damm, P., Dyer, A. R., Leiva, A. d., Hod, M., Kitzmiler, J. L., Lowe, L. P., McIntyre, H. D., Oats, J. J.

N., Omori, Y., Schmidt, M. I., International Association of Diabetes and Pregnancy Study Groups Consensus Panel. (2010). International association of diabetes and pregnancy study groups recommendations on the diagnosis and classification of hyperglycemia in pregnancy. *Diabetes Care,* Vol.33, No.3, pp. 676-682, issn 1935-5548

Molloy, M. P., Brzezinski, E. E., Hang, J., McDowell, M. T. & VanBogelen, R. A. (2003). Overcoming technical variation and biological variation in quantitative proteomics. *Proteomics,* Vol.3, No.10, pp. 1912-1919, issn 1615-9853

Moore, T. R. (2010). Fetal exposure to gestational diabetes contributes to subsequent adult metabolic syndrome. *Am J Obstet Gynecol,* Vol.202, No.6, pp. 643-649, issn 1097-6868

Morisset, A. S., Tchernof, A., Dube, M. C., Veillette, J., Weisnagel, S. J. & Robitaille, J. (2011). Weight Gain Measures in Women with Gestational Diabetes Mellitus. *J Womens Health,* Vol.20, No.3, pp. 375-380, issn 1540-9996

Nahum, G. G., Wilson, S. B. & Stanislaw, H. (2002). Early-pregnancy glucose screening for gestational diabetes mellitus. *J Reprod Med,* Vol.47, No.8, pp. 656-662, issn 0024-7758

Nanda, S., Savvidou, M., Syngelaki, A., Akolekar, R. & Nicolaides, K. H. (2011). Prediction of gestational diabetes mellitus by maternal factors and biomarkers at 11 to 13 weeks. *Prenatal Diagnosis,* Vol.31, No.2, pp. 135-141, issn 0197-3851

Nolan, C. J., Riley, S. F., Sheedy, M. T., Walstab, J. E. & Beischer, N. A. (1995). Maternal serum triglyceride, glucose tolerance, and neonatal birth weight ratio in pregnancy. *Diabetes Care,* Vol.18, No.12, pp. 1550-1556, issn 0149-5992

Nolan, C. J. (2011). Controversies in gestational diabetes. *Best Pract Res Clin Obstet Gynaecol,* Vol.25, No.1, pp. 37-49, issn 1532-1932

Ong, C. Y., Lao, T. T., Spencer, K. & Nicolaides, K. H. (2004). Maternal serum level of placental growth factor in diabetic pregnancies. *J Reprod Med,* Vol.49, No.6, pp. 477-480, issn 0024-7758

Phaloprakarn, C. & Tangjitgamol, S. (2008). Use of oral glucose tolerance test in early pregnancy to predict late-onset gestational diabetes mellitus in high-risk women. *J Obstet Gynaecol Res,* Vol.34, No.3, pp. 331-336, issn 1341-8076

Phaloprakarn, C., Tangjitgamol, S. & Manusirivithaya, S. (2009). A risk score for selective screening for gestational diabetes mellitus. *Eur J Obstet Gynecol Reprod Biol,* Vol.145, No.1, pp. 71-75, issn 0301-2115

Punthumapol, C. & Tekasakul, P. (2008). 50 grams glucose challenge test for screening of gestational diabetes mellitus in each trimester in potential diabetic pregnancy. *J Med Assoc Thailand,* Vol.91, No.6, pp. 787-793, issn 0125-2208

Qiu, C., Williams, M. A., Vadachkoria, S., Frederick, I. O. & Luthy, D. A. (2004). Increased maternal plasma leptin in early pregnancy and risk of gestational diabetes mellitus. *Obstet Gynecol,* Vol.103, No.3, pp. 519-525, issn 0029-7844

Retnakaran, R., Hanley, A. J., Raif, N., Connelly, P. W., Sermer, M. & Zinman, B. (2004). Reduced adiponectin concentration in women with gestational diabetes: a potential factor in progression to type 2 diabetes. *Diabetes Care,* Vol.27, No.3, pp. 799-800, issn 0149-5992

Riskin-Mashiah, S., Younes, G., Damti, A. & Auslender, R. (2009). First-trimester fasting hyperglycemia and adverse pregnancy outcomes. *Diabetes Care,* Vol.32, No.9, pp. 1639-1643, issn 1935-5548

Riskin-Mashiah, S., Damti, A., Younes, G. & Auslender, R. (2010). First trimester fasting hyperglycemia as a predictor for the development of gestational diabetes mellitus. *Eur J Obstet Gynecol Reprod Biol,* Vol.152, No.2, pp. 163-167, issn 1872-7654

Rogers, M. S., Wang, C. C. R., Tam, W. H., Li, C. Y., Chu, K. O. & Chu, C. Y. (2006). Oxidative stress in midpregnancy as a predictor of gestational hypertension and pre-eclampsia. *Bjog,* Vol.113, No.9, pp. 1053-1059, issn 1470-0328

Ryan, E. A. (2011). Diagnosing gestational diabetes. *Diabetologia,* Vol.54, No.3, pp. 480-486, issn 1432-0428

Sacks, D. A., Chen, W., Wolde-Tsadik, G. & Buchanan, T. A. (2003). Fasting plasma glucose test at the first prenatal visit as a screen for gestational diabetes. *Obstet Gynecol,* Vol.101, No.6, pp. 1197-1203, issn 0029-7844

Savvidou, M., Nelson, S. M., Makgoba, M., Messow, C. M., Sattar, N. & Nicolaides, K. (2010). First-Trimester Prediction of Gestational Diabetes Mellitus: Examining the Potential of Combining Maternal Characteristics and Laboratory Measures. *Diabetes,* Vol.59, No.12, pp. 3017-3022, issn 0012-1797

Schafer-Graf, U. (2009). Impact of HAPO study findings on future diagnostics and therapy of gestational diabetes. *Gynakol Geburtshilfliche Rundsch,* Vol.49, No.4, pp. 254-258, issn 1423-0011

Shirazian, N., Emdadi, R., Mahboubi, M., Motevallian, A., Fazel-Sarjuei, Z., Sedighpour, N., Fadaki, S.-F. & Shahmoradi, N. (2009). Screening for gestational diabetes: usefulness of clinical risk factors. *Arch Gynecol Obstet,* Vol.280, No.6, pp. 933-937, issn 1432-0711

Son, G. H., Kwon, J. Y., Kim, Y. H. & Park, Y. W. (2010). Maternal serum triglycerides as predictive factors for large-for-gestational age newborns in women with gestational diabetes mellitus. *Acta Obstet Gynecol Scand,* Vol.89, No.5, pp. 700-704, issn 1600-0412

Thadhani, R., Wolf, M., Hsu-Blatman, K., Sandler, L., Nathan, D. & Ecker, J. L. (2003). First-trimester sex hormone binding globulin and subsequent gestational diabetes mellitus. *Am J Obstet Gynecol,* Vol.189, No.1, pp. 171-176, issn 0002-9378

Thadhani, R., Powe, C. E., Tjoa, M. L., Khankin, E., Ye, J., Ecker, J., Schneyer, A. & Karumanchi, S. A. (2010). First-trimester follistatin-like-3 levels in pregnancies complicated by subsequent gestational diabetes mellitus. *Diabetes Care,* Vol.33, No.3, pp. 664-669, issn 1935-5548

Wein, P., Dong, Z. G., Beischer, N. A. & Sheedy, M. T. (1995). Factors predictive of recurrent gestational diabetes diagnosed before 24 weeks' gestation. *Am J Perinatol,* Vol.12, No.5, pp. 352-356, issn 0735-1631

Wein, P. & Beischer, N. A. (2000). Observed increase in prevalence of gestational diabetes is real. *Am J Obstet Gynecol,* Vol.182, No.4, pp. 992-993, issn 0002-9378

Williams, M. A., Qiu, C., Muy-Rivera, M., Vadachkoria, S., Song, T. & Luthy, D. A. (2004). Plasma adiponectin concentrations in early pregnancy and subsequent risk of gestational diabetes mellitus. *J Clin Endocrinol Metab,* Vol.89, No.5, pp. 2306-2311, issn 0021-972X

Wolf, M., Sandler, L., Hsu, K., Vossen-Smirnakis, K., Ecker, J. L. & Thadhani, R. (2003). First-trimester C-reactive protein and subsequent gestational diabetes. *Diabetes Care,* Vol.26, No.3, pp. 819-824, issn 0149-5992

Zhou, S., Bailey, M. J., Dunn, M. J., Preedy, V. R. & Emery, P. W. (2005). A quantitative investigation into the losses of proteins at different stages of a two-dimensional gel electrophoresis procedure. *Proteomics,* Vol.5, No.11, pp. 2739-2747, issn 1615-9853

Zhu, W., Smith, J. W. & Haung, C.-M. (2010). Mass Spectrometry-Based Label Free Quantitative Proteomics. *J Biomed BioTechnol,* Vol.2010, Article ID 840518, 6 pages, issn 1110-7243

2

Gestational Diabetes Mellitus - A Perspective

Veerasamy Seshiah[1], Vijayam Balaji[2] and Balaji Madhuri[2]
[1]*Diabetes Research Institute,*
[2]*Diabetes Care Centre*
India

1. Introduction

The prevalence of diabetes is increasing globally and the total number of people with this condition is projected to rise from 171 million in 2000 to 366 million in 2030 (Wild et al, 2004). India is no exception, with projected rates of 79.4 million in 2030—a 151% increase from 31.7 million in 2000 (Wild et al, 2004). The increased prevalence is attributed to the aging population structure, urbanization, the obesity epidemic, and physical inactivity (Hunt & Schuller, 2007). While all these factors contribute to the epidemic of diabetes, intrauterine exposures are emerging as potential risk factors (Barker, 1995). The "fetal origin of adult disease" hypothesis proposes that gestational programming may critically influence adult health and disease (Barker, 1995). Gestational programming is a process whereby stimuli or stresses occurring at critical or sensitive periods of fetal development, permanently change structure, physiology, and metabolism, which predisposes individuals to disease in adult life (Lucas, 1991). If the stimulus happens to be glucose intolerance in pregnancy, it predisposes the offspring to an increased risk of developing glucose intolerance in the future. This vicious cycle is likely to influence and perpetuate the incidence and prevalence of glucose intolerance in any population (Seshiah et al., 2004). Therefore, preventive measures against type 2 diabetes should start during the intrauterine period and continue from early childhood throughout life (Tuomilehto, 2005). In this respect, detection of gestational diabetes mellitus (GDM), defined as carbohydrate intolerance of variable severity with onset or first recognition during the present pregnancy (Metzger, 1991), becomes an important public health issue. The etiopathogenesis of glucose intolerance that develops in women with GDM could be the result of their inability to increase insulin secretion enough to overcome insulin resistance that occurs even in non diabetic pregnancy (Kuhl et al., 1985). The present concept is that GDM represents, detection of chronic β cell dysfunction, rather than development of relative insulin deficiency as insulin resistance increases during pregnancy (Buchanan et al., 2007).

2. Implications

The usual recommendation of lifestyle modifications or drug intervention for prevention of diabetes is likely to delay or postpone the development of overt diabetes in persons diagnosed with abnormal glucose tolerance. These measures essentially target only the post primary prevention of diabetes whereas the aim should be primary prevention of diabetes by keeping the genetically or otherwise susceptible individuals normoglycemic, apart from preventing them from developing type 2 DM (Tuomilehto, 2005). In this context, women with GDM become the ideal group for primary prevention of diabetes (Girling & Dornhorst, 2003), as women with GDM are at increased risk of developing diabetes predominantly type 2 DM as are their children (Dornhorst & Rossi, 1998). The diagnosis of GDM offers a unique opportunity in identifying individuals who will be benefited by early therapeutic intervention with diet and exercise, thus normalizing the weight to delay or even possibly prevent the onset of diabetes.

3. Prevalence

The epidemiology of GDM is subject to various factors such as the population to be screened, the screening methods, the gestational weeks for screening and the glycemic criteria for diagnosis. Screening recommendations range from inclusion of all pregnant women (universal) to the exclusion of all other women except those with very specific risk factors (selective): (e.g., age > 25 years, obesity: BMI > 30, ethnicity: Hispanic, Native American, Asian-American, African-American, family history: first degree relative, and previous GDM or large for gestational age infant) (Mazze, 2006). Different ethnic groups when exposed to the same environmental setting, experienced a widely variable risk. Among ethnic groups in South Asian countries, Indian women have the highest frequency of GDM (15%), followed by Chinese (13.9%), Vietnam-born (7.8%) and Australian-born (4.3%) (King, 1998).

For a given population and ethnicity, the risk of diabetes in pregnancy, mirrors that of the underlying frequency of type 2 DM in that population (King, 1998). Impaired Glucose Tolerance (IGT) is generally much more prevalent than diabetes in women of child bearing age (King, 1998). Among Indians, the prevalence of IGT in the age group of 20 to 29 years and 30 to 39 years was found to be 12.2% and 15.3% respectively. No gender difference was seen in the prevalence of IGT (Ramachandran et al., 2001). It was observed in a national survey performed in 2002, the frequency of the occurrence of GDM was 16.55% by the World Health Organization (WHO) criteria (Seshiah et al., 2004) which was closer to the prevalence of IGT in the child-bearing age group of women in India (Ramachandran et al., 2001). Parallel to the increased prevalence of IGT in the general population, the frequency of GDM had also increased. The prevalence of GDM was 2% in 1982 (Agarwal & Gupta, 1982) [IGT - 2% (Ramachandran et al., 1988)] which increased to 7.62% in 1991 (Narendra et al., 1991) [IGT – 8.2% (Ramachandran et al., 1992)], and doubled to 16.55% in 2002 (Seshiah et al., 2004) [IGT – 14.5% (Ramachandran et al., 2001)]. The prevalence data published (Seshiah et al., 2004) included pregnant women attending different health care providing centres spread in different parts of the country (Table – 1).

This phenomenal increase in the prevalence of GDM prompted the authors to initiate a project on 'Diabetes In Pregnancy Awareness and Prevention (DIPAP)', funded by the World Diabetes Foundation and supported by the government of Tamil Nadu, India. To have a community based prevalence data under the DIPAP project, the author's group screened a total of 4151, 3960 and 3945 pregnant women in the urban, semi urban and rural areas of Tamil Nadu, respectively (Seshiah et al., 2008a). This was the largest prospective study (N=12,056) other than Hyperglycemia and Adverse Pregnancy Outcome (HAPO) study. GDM diagnosis was based on the WHO criterion of 2-h plasma glucose (PG) ≥ 7.8 mmol/L with 75g oral glucose. WHO recommendation serves both as one step screening and diagnostic procedure, and is easy to perform besides being economical (Seshiah et al., 2004, 2005). WHO criterion of 2-h PG ≥ 7.8 mmol/L identifying a large number of cases may have a greater potential for prevention (Schmidt et al., 2001). In addition, a study performed by

	Centre	Number of pregnant women screened	Prevalence Rate
Dr. Balaji et al	North Chennai, Tamil Nadu	891	16.2%
Dr. Anjalakshi et al	South Chennai, Tamil Nadu	1002	15%
Dr. K. P. Paulose	Trivandrum, Kerala	750	15%
Dr. Mary John	Ludhiana, Punjab	220	17.5%
Dr. Prasanna Kumar	Bangalore, Karnataka	49	12%
Dr. Shyam Mukundan	Alwaye, Kerala	200	21%
Dr. Aruyerchelvan	Erode, Tamil Nadu	562	18.8%
	TOTAL	3674	16.55%

Table 1. Prevalence of GDM in different parts of India - 2002

Crowther et al found that treatment of GDM diagnosed by WHO criterion reduces serious perinatal morbidity and may also improve the women's health-related quality of life (Crowther at al., 2005). Similarly a long term outcome study conducted by Franks et al documented that when maternal 2-h PG was ≥ 7.8 mmol/L, the cumulative risk of offspring developing type 2 DM was 30% at the age 24 yrs (Franks et al., 2006). Both these short term and long term outcome studies validate the WHO criterion and hence the authors chose this criterion for the DIPAP project. In this project GDM was detected in 739 (17.8%) women in urban, 548 (13.8%) in semi urban and 392(9.9%) in rural areas. In this community based study, the overall prevalence of GDM was 13.9% (Seshiah et al., 2008a). The prevalence of GDM had increased from 16.55% to 17.8% in the urban areas in two years (Seshiah et al., 2004, 2008a). There is a definite divide between the rural and urban areas in the prevalence of GDM. The possible cause for the low prevalence in the rural settings may be due to the less mechanized, agriculture based lifestyle. In this population the risk factors for the development of GDM were: age ≥ 25 years, BMI ≥ 25 and family history of diabetes (Figure 1).

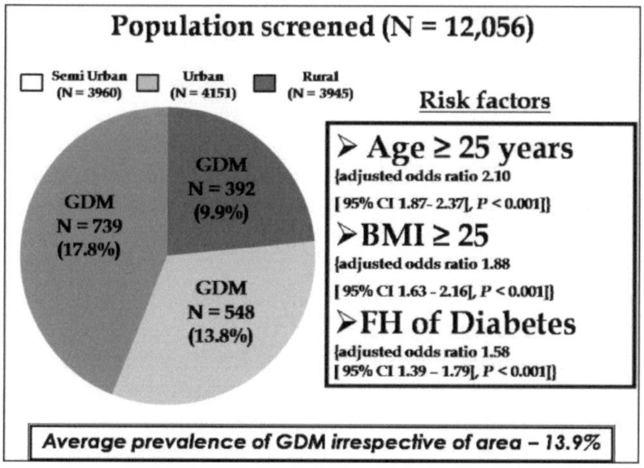

Fig. 1. Risk factors for the development of GDM

3.1 Geographical variations in the prevalence of GDM

Prevalence varies between 1% to 16% depending on the geographical variation and ethnicity and from one region to another in the same country (Yogev et al., 2003). The prevalence of GDM corresponds to the prevalence of IGT within a given population (King, 1998). The prevalence of GDM in India was 16.55% in the urban area and the frequency varied from 12% to 21% in different parts of the country (Seshiah et al., 2004) (Table 1). A low prevalence of GDM was observed in Kashmir (Zargar et al., 2004) (northern tip of India) 4.4% and a high prevalence of 16.55% in the southern part of India (Seshiah et al., 2004). The prevalence of GDM in other developing countries also showed regional variations. In Mexico, the prevalence of GDM varied from 4.3% to 11% when screening was done in different parts of the country (Forsbach et al., 1998). The rate of abnormal screening test results ranged from 8.0% to 20.7% for different regions of Poland (Wojcikowski et al, 2002). Among Pan Arab countries, Saudi Arabia (12.5%) and Bahrain (13.5%) had the highest prevalence of GDM (Al Mahroos et al, 2005; Ardawi et al, 2000). The frequency of GDM in Argentina was between 2% and 12% depending upon the population studied and geographical variations (Liliana et al, 2003).

4. Rationale for universal screening

Selective screening based on risk factors scored poorly in predicting GDM (Shamsuddin et al, 2001). If selective screening is employed, it is likely that 27% of GDM women will go undetected (Shamsuddin et al, 2001). GDM diagnosis is overlooked in about 1/3rd of the women, where selective rather than Universal screening is performed (Cosson et al., 2004a). Further selective screening recommended by American Diabetes Association (ADA) may be applicable for women belonging to the ethnic group with low prevalence of GDM. Risk factor screening does not take into account the inevitable difficulties in implementation, including the potential for substantial under-diagnosis of GDM (Simmons et al., 2009). Among ethnic groups in South Asian countries, Indian women have the highest frequency of GDM necessitating Universal Screening (Beischer et al., 1991). The recognition of glucose intolerance during pregnancy is more relevant as Indian women have 11 fold increased risk of developing GDM compared to Caucasians (Dornhorst et al., 1992).

Compared to selective screening, Universal screening for GDM detects more cases and improves maternal and offspring prognosis (Cosson, 2004b). Thus Universal screening appears to be the most reliable and desired method for the detection of GDM (Shamsuddin et al., 2001). For universal screening the test should be simple and cost effective. The two step procedure of screening with 50g Glucose challenge test (GCT) and then diagnosing GDM based on 75g OGTT is not feasible in a country like India, because the pregnant women may have to visit the antenatal clinic twice and at least 3 to 5 blood samples have to be drawn, which they resent. The scenario is likely to be the same in most of the developing countries.

5. Diagnosis of GDM

5.1 A single step procedure to diagnose GDM

All the diagnostic criteria require women to be in fasting, but most of the time pregnant women do not come in the fasting state because of commutation and belief not to fast for long hours. Attending the first prenatal visit in the fasting state is impractical in many settings (Metzger et al., 2010). The dropout rate is very high when a pregnant woman is asked to come again for the glucose tolerance test (Seshiah et al., 2004; Magee et al., 2001).

For the successful implementation of universal screening, a test has to be casual and reliable. A procedure that does not impose any restriction would be ideal for universal screening. The test performed should be able to diagnose GDM, as they walk into the prenatal clinic or clinical laboratory irrespective of their last meal timings. Hence the authors undertook a study to evaluate, whether a 2-h 75g oral glucose test performed in a non-fasting state, irrespective of last meal timing, is as efficacious as 2-h 75g oral glucose test done in the fasting state recommended by WHO in detecting GDM (Anjalakshi et al., 2009). A total of 862 consecutive pregnant women were subjected to 75g oral glucose test irrespective of time of the last meal. Venous samples were collected at 2-h after oral glucose administration. They were advised to follow a diet containing atleast 150g carbohydrate daily and usual activity for atleast 3 days and come to the prenatal clinic after an overnight fasting of 10-12 h. At the second visit 800 of them responded and underwent 2-h 75g oral glucose test in the fasting state recommended by WHO. The observation in this study was, all women diagnosed as GDM (N=87) by 75g glucose test irrespective of the last meal timings also satisfied the diagnostic criteria of 75-g oral glucose test performed in the fasting state recommended by WHO. It was also found that there was no statistically significant difference ($P > 0.05$) between the PG levels of the 75g glucose test in fasting and non fasting state, irrespective of last meal timing, performed in the GDM and in NGT pregnant women.
The rationale behind this study outcome is that, a normal glucose tolerant woman would be able to maintain euglycemia despite glucose challenge due to adequate insulin response, whereas in a woman with GDM who has impaired insulin secretion (Kuhl, 1991), her glycemic level increases with a meal and with glucose challenge, the glycemic excursion is expected to exaggerate. This cascading effect is advantageous as this would not result in false positive diagnosis of GDM. Performing this test procedure in the non-fasting state, irrespective of last meal timing, is prudent as glucose concentrations during the glucose tolerance are affected little by the time since the last meal (Gough et al., 1970).
Pettitt et al. observed that WHO criteria based on the glucose concentration 2-h after 75g oral glucose administered to non-fasting women correctly identified subjects with GDM (Pettitt et al., 1994). The non-fasting 2-h post 75g glucose concentration strongly predicts adverse outcome for the mother and her offspring (Pettitt et al., 1991). Philips et al also observed that plasma glucose value with a glucose challenge test was unaffected by the time after a meal or time of the day in Normal Glucose Tolerant non pregnant subjects (Philips et al., 2009). Thus, this single test procedure performed irrespective of the last meal timing is rational and a patient friendly approach, which causes least disturbance in her routine activities. This procedure is a modified version of WHO criteria in that, only 2-h PG is taken into consideration for the diagnosis of GDM and is being followed by the Diabetes In Pregnancy Study Group India (DIPSI) (Seshiah et al., 2009)

5.2 Comparison of WHO and IADPSG criteria

All the diagnostic criteria, except the existing diagnostic criterion of WHO 2-h plasma glucose (PG) ≥ 7.8 mmol/L with 75g oral glucose load (King, 1998), are country specific or recommended by various associations. Recently, based on the HAPO study, the International Association of Diabetes and Pregnancy Study Groups (IADPSG) consensus panel recommended that GDM can be diagnosed, if any one value of fasting plasma glucose (FPG), 1-h and 2-h PG concentrations meet or exceed 5.1 mmol/L, 10.0 mmol/L and 8.5 mmol/L respectively, with 75g oral glucose tolerance test (OGTT) (Metzger et al., 2010).
India one of the most populous countries in the world was not part of the HAPO study. Hence the authors group undertook a prospective, collaborative study to ascertain whether

the present practice of diagnosing GDM by the guidelines recommended by Diabetes In Pregnancy Study Group India (DIPSI) (Seshiah et al., 2009) based on WHO criterion of 2-h PG ≥ 7.8 mmol/L can still be followed in India or adopt IADPSG recommendations. A total of 1,463 consecutive pregnant women with no previous history of GDM/pre GDM underwent a 75g OGTT and fasting, 1-h and 2-h PG were measured. Using the DIPSI criterion, 196 (13.4%) women were diagnosed as GDM. By applying IADPSG recommendation the cumulative prevalence of GDM was 14.6% (n=214). There was no significant difference ($P > 0.05$) in the discordant pair of diagnosing GDM by the two criteria which in turn implies, that the disagreement in diagnosing GDM by both criteria was not significant ($P = 0.21$, by Mc Nemar test). The difference in the diagnostic capability between IADPSG and DIPSI was 1.2% which was not significant ($P>0.02$) (Seshiah et al., 2011). IADPSG recommendation necessarily requires estimation of PG in three blood samples after administrating 75g oral glucose load. Pregnant women despise this procedure, as venous blood is drawn three times and they feel too much of blood is drained. Whereas, DIPSI criterion requires one blood sample drawn at 2-h following a 75g glucose load for estimating the PG. The cost involved in performing IADPSG recommended procedure is high, as this procedure requires three blood tests compared to one blood test of DIPSI. The cost will escalate further, if IADPSG diagnostic procedure is performed in each trimester in high risk population in whom GDM manifests in all trimesters of pregnancy (Seshiah et al., 2007). Among women with normal OGTT results in the first visit when tested in the subsequent visits, 28% of them were detected to have GDM (Seshiah et al., 2007). Hence, DIPSI procedure based on WHO criterion is feasible, sustainable, cost-effective and best buy to diagnose GDM in any country and particularly in less resource nations. IADPSG recommendations are suitable in clinical settings where financial and technical supports are available. The performance of both IADPSG and WHO criteria are similar as per GRADE ratings.

5.3 Inadequacy of fasting plasma glucose to diagnose GDM

The IADPSG criteria suggests FPG ≥ 5.1 mmol/L but ≤ 7.0 mmol/L to diagnose GDM in the first prenatal visit (Metzger et al., 2010) whereas the authors observed in their study that by applying this criterion of FPG ≥ 5. 1 mmol/L, only 24% (3.2% of the total population) of those diagnosed as GDM using WHO criterion 2-h PG ≥ 7.8 mmol/L would have been classified as GDM (Balaji et al., 2011a). Further, FPG of 5.1 mmol/L was not able to diagnose GDM in comparison to 2-h PG ≥ 7.8 mmol/L (Table 2). This is due to the ethnicity of Asian Indians who have high insulin resistance (IR) and as a consequence, their postprandial plasma glucose is higher compared to Caucasians (Mohan et al., 2007; Snehalatha et al., 2009). Asian and South Asian ethnicity are both independently associated with increased IR in late pregnancy (Retnakaran et al., 2006). Siddhartha Das et al documented an increased IR during pregnancy in Asian Indian Women and IR escalates further in GDM (Das et al., 2010). These studies provide evidence that FPG may not be an appropriate option to diagnose GDM in Asian Indian women. Further, in all GDM, the FPG values do not reflect the postprandial hyperglycemia (Valensi et al., 2009), which is the hallmark of GDM (Weiss et al., 2000). In addition, there is a paucity of data regarding the reproducibility of the FPG test (Sacks et al., 2010). Hence, administering 75g oral glucose load and measuring 2-h PG serves as a one-step definitive procedure to diagnose GDM in less serviced regions. Perucchini et al also suggest one-step diagnostic procedure, though their observation was based on different ethnic population (Perucchini et al., 1999).

FPG (mmol/L)	Test positive	2- h PG value		Macrosomia	
		Sensitivity (95% CI)	Specificity (95% CI)	Sensitivity (95% CI)	Specificity (95% CI)
5.0	3.9	29.1 (22.9-36.1)	89.4 (87.6-91.0)	21.2 (12.5-33.3)	87.2 (85.0-89.2)
5.1	3.2	24.0 (18.3-30.7)	93.0 (91.4-94.3)	15.2 (7.9-26.6)	90.2 (88.2-91.9)
5.5	1.8	13.8 (9.4-19.6)	97.4 (96.3-98.2)	6.1 (2.0-15.6)	95.6 (94.1-96.7)
6.1	0.9	7.1 (4.1-11.9)	99.2 (98.5-99.6)	1.5 (0.1-9.3)	98.2 (97.1-98.9)
6.6	0.6	4.6 (2.3-8.8)	99.8 (99.4-100.0)	0.0 (0.0-6.9)	99.3 (98.6-99.7)
2- h PG 7.8	13.4			13.6 (6.8-24.8)	86.3 (84.0-88.3)

Table 2. Performance of FPG test for the predictor of gestational diabetes and macrosomia

5.4 The validation of WHO criterion (DIPSI criterion) based on the fetal outcome

The authors investigated whether the diagnosis of GDM by WHO criterion is rational based on the fetal outcome (N = 1463). Macrosomia was the end point of this study as this is the most common morbidity of GDM (Jovanovic, 2001). They observed that there was no statistically significant difference in the mean birth weight of neonates born to women in the normal glucose tolerance (NGT) and with intervention in GDM groups (P=0.705) (Balaji et al., 2011b). This was due to the medical nutrition therapy (MNT) and/or insulin in maintaining FPG ~ 5.0 mmol/L and 2-h post meal ~ 6.7 mmol/L in GDM women. Intervention helped in maintaining the pregnancy outcome in GDM women equivalent to that of NGT women. Gayle et al also observed that diagnosis of GDM with OGTT 2-h PG ≥ 7.8 mmol/L and treatment in a combined diabetes antenatal clinic is worthwhile with a decreased macrosomia rate and fewer emergency cesarean sections (Gayle et al., 2010). The distribution of birth weight of neonates born to GDM and NGT women were similar (Figure 2) in the study conducted by the authors, indicating that the intervention given to pregnant women with 2-h PG ≥ 7.8 mmol/L had a significant effect in obtaining neonatal birth weight appropriate for gestational age. The level of association between macrosomia and GDM status after controlling the factors: maternal age, gestational age, family history of diabetes and BMI was elucidated. It was found that, the GDM status (2-h PG ≥ 7.8 mmol/L) of the pregnant women after intervention was not associated with macrosomia (adjusted OR = 0.752; 95% CI (0.406-1.390); P=0.363). There are publications confirming that treatment of GDM women as defined by WHO criterion was associated with a reduced risk of pregnancy outcome (Crowther et al., 2005; Gayle et al., 2010). In pregnancy, the decision to perform a placebo controlled trial requires clinical equipoise (Gifford et al., 2001). Hence, in this study, the authors did not have a control group of untreated pregnant women with 2-h PG ≥ 7.8 mmol/L, as there are evidences confirming that the treatment of GDM women as defined by WHO criterion was associated with a reduced risk of pregnancy outcome (Crowther et al., 2005; Gayle et al., 2010). The policy of not treating women with 2-h PG ≥ 7.8 mmol/L amounts to deliberately exposing the pregnant mothers to unphysiological glycemic level despite our extensive knowledge of the benefits of treatment of mild hyperglycemia during pregnancy (Seshiah et al., 2008a; Landon et al., 2009; Bevier et al.,

1999; Negrato et al., 2008). Wahi et al observed in their prospective study, the advantage of adhering to a cut-off level of 2-h PG ≥ 7.8 mmol/L in diagnosis and management of GDM for a significantly positive effect on pregnancy outcomes (Wahi et al., 2011). Fetal exposure to high maternal glucose (1-h PG > 7.2 mmol/L with 50g GCT) in the absence of preexisting diabetes/GDM may contribute to the development of overweight/obesity in the offspring, independent of maternal pre-pregnancy BMI (Deierlein et al., 2011). All these studies validate WHO/DIPSI criterion for the diagnosis of GDM

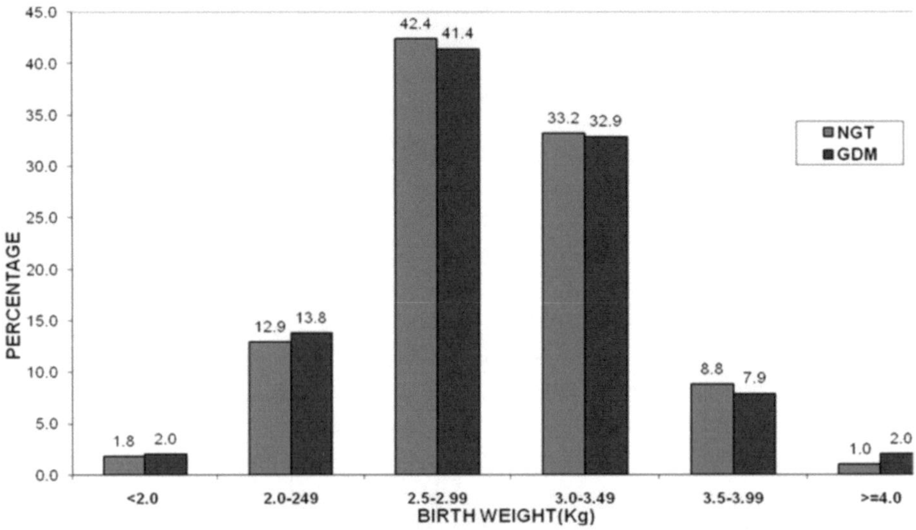

Fig. 2. Neonate Birth weight distribution of women with NGT and GDM

6. Gestational weeks for screening

The current recommendation is to perform screening test between 24 - 28 weeks of gestation, though there are reports that claim, about 40% to 66% of women with GDM can be detected early during pregnancy (Super et al., 1991; Nahum et al., 2002). Nahum et al also suggest that the ideal period to screen for GDM is around 16 weeks of gestation and even earlier in high-risk groups with a history of fetal wastage (Nahum et al., 2002). This is due to the embryological development of fetal β cells. Each islet cell functions as an endocrine organ and differentiates between 10th and 12th weeks of gestation. They recognize and respond to maternal glycemia before 15 weeks of gestation, suggesting that metabolic perturbations are underway before diagnosis and that earlier screening and intervention may be warranted (Tisi et al., 2011). The study performed by the present authors group in the DIPAP project revealed that, 16.3% had glucose intolerance within 16 weeks, 22.4% between 17 - 23 weeks and remaining 61.3% more than 24 weeks of gestation (Seshiah et., 2007). If a pregnant woman has an A1c level > 6%, she is more likely to be an overt diabetic (Balaji et al., 2007). These studies stress the need for screening for GDM during the early weeks of gestation. If the test is normal in the first visit, the test has to be repeated in the subsequent visits. GDM diagnosis may not be missed by screening around 24 -28 weeks of gestation, but a substantial number of pregnant women who develop GDM in the earlier weeks of pregnancy are likely to have delayed diagnosis and may not receive appropriate medical care. Further, early screening for glucose intolerance and care could avoid some diabetes related complications in women with gestational diabetes (Bartha et al., 2003). To substantiate the above observation the present author's group screened 207 pregnant women attending their referral centre for diabetes and pregnancy with a 75g OGTT (Seshiah et al., 2006). Among them, 87 (42.03%) were diagnosed with GDM. Women in whom GDM was detected between 0 - 23 weeks of gestation were classified as Group 1 [54 (62.7%)] and beyond 24 weeks of gestation as Group 2 [33 (37.93%)]. All of them were treated and followed till confinement. There was no statistically significant difference ($P < 0.05$) between the birth weight of the neonates born to Normal Glucose Tolerance (NGT) women (3.28 ± 0.50 kg) and GDM women in group 1 (3.13 ± 0.55 kg). In group 2, the neonatal birth weight was 3.42 ± 0.58 kg which is the upper limit of the normal range in Indian new born babies. In India, the normal birth weight varies between 2.5 to 3.5 kg (Paul et al., 2002). The observation of this study was that, by early detection of glucose intolerance during pregnancy and by giving adequate care to the antenatal women, a good fetal outcome can be achieved similar to that of NGT pregnant women (Seshiah et al., 2006, 2008b).

7. Management

The goal in the management is to avoid both low birth weight and macrosomic babies, as they are prone to develop diabetes in their adolescent and adult life (Jovanovic, 1998). In India, both under nutrition and over nutrition exists during pregnancy. There are two reported studies in India that relates size at birth to future risk of type 2 DM. In Mysore, low birth weight did not increase the risk of diabetes but babies who were short and fat at birth (higher BMI) were at increased risk (Fall et al., 1998). Fall et al speculate that the rise in type 2 DM in Indian urban populations would have been triggered by mild obesity in mothers, leading to glucose intolerance during pregnancy, macrosomic changes in the fetus and insulin deficiency in adult life (Fall et al., 1998). Yet another study attributes high prevalence of type 2 DM and IGT in Indian people linked to poor fetal growth (Yajnik et al., 1995) which is at variant to Fall *et al* observation (Fall et al., 1998).

7.1 Medical Nutrition Therapy (MNT)

The meal pattern should provide adequate calories and nutrients to meet the needs of pregnancy metabolism. The meal plan advised has to be simple and easy to practice. The MNT recommended is based on their routine diet habit and glycemic excursions that occur with the meal. In a normal person, the peaking of the plasma glucose is high after breakfast (due to 'Dawn phenomenon') than after lunch and dinner, and the insulin secretion also matches the glycemic excursions that occur with these three meals (Polonsky et al., 1988). Since GDM mothers have deficiency in first phase insulin secretion, the quantity of food at one time should also be less, to overcome this insulin deficiency, particularly after breakfast. To avoid the post prandial plasma glucose peaking with breakfast, the authors guide their women with GDM to distribute calorie consumption especially the breakfast into two portions 'Split Breakfast'. This implies splitting the usual breakfast into two halves and consuming these portions with a two-hour gap in between. By this, the undue peak in plasma glucose levels after ingestion of the total quantity of breakfast at one time is avoided.

7.2 Insulin therapy
7.2.1 Human insulin
The policy followed in India is to advise human insulin in women with GDM who failed to achieve FPG of ≤ 5.0 mmol/L and 2-h post meal plasma glucose level of ≤ 6.7 mmol/L with MNT. The aim is to maintain post meal peak plasma glucose level of ≤ 6.7 mmol/L. This time point is suggested as the diagnosis of GDM is made with 2-h PG and it is easy to remember the same timing. A number of studies have established the benefits of maintaining the plasma glucose at this level (Franks et al., 2006; de Sereday et al., 2003; Ben-Haroush et al., 2004). However whichever time is targeted for monitoring glycemic control and adjusting the insulin dose, the blood tests have to be done at the same time at each visit. GDM women usually have high post breakfast plasma glucose level compared to post lunch and post dinner. The period between breakfast and lunch are often problematical because of the physiological tendency to hyperglycemia at this time and may necessitate substantial increases in the morning dose of short acting insulin, together with careful adjustment of meal timing and snacks to avoid pre-lunch hypoglycemia (Langer et al., 2000).

7.2.2 Insulin analogues
Due to the pharmacokinetic action of human regular insulin, a considerable segment of pregnant women with GDM, fail to achieve optimum glycemic control, mostly the post prandial plasma glucose. In them, the best option is to administer ultra short acting analogues, insulin lispro (Humalog) or insulin aspart (Novo rapid). These analogues improve the post prandial glucose control in pregnant women with type 1, type 2 DM and GDM, and are also safe and effective (Hermansen et al., 2002; Jovanovic et al., 1999).
The authors group conducted an open label trial using a large independent cohort of GDM patients to evaluate the efficacy, safety and foetal outcome for Biphasic Insulin aspart (BIAsp 30) compared with biphasic human insulin (BHI 30) in the management of GDM (Balaji et al., 2010). GDM women (N = 323) who remained unable to maintain a FPG ≤ 5.0 mmol/L and 2-h PG ≤ 6.7 mmol/L with MNT were randomly allocated in a 1:1 ratio to receive either BIAsp 30 (Group A) or BHI 30 (Group B). There was no statistical significance in the levels of glycaemic control achieved by the groups by labour onset. However, the mean total insulin dose administered by the last visit was significantly lower for Group A [19.83±15.75 U compared with 26.34±23.15 U for Group B (p=0.006)], implying that those receiving BHI 30 required a higher dose to achieve a similar degree of glycaemic control. The frequency of macrosomia was 6.3% in Group A and 6.9% in Group B. Although the proportion of macrosomia was numerically higher for Group B than Group A, the difference was not statistically significant (p=0.819). It was found that BIAsp 30 was non-inferior to BHI 30 and was well tolerated during pregnancy. Yet in another study, the authors observed that pregnant women found BIAsp convenient as this preparation allows flexibility in the meal time insulin dosing and did not disturb their routine life pattern. Most importantly, BIAsp was found to be safe during pregnancy (Balaji et al., 2010).

7.3 Oral hypoglycemic agents
7.3.1 Glibenclamide
Glibenclamide (Glyburide) may be an alternative safe therapy for many GDM women who are hesitant to take insulin. This drug decreases the insulin resistance and improves insulin secretion, the pathogenic factors in the causation of hyperglycemia in GDM (Groop et al.,

1991; Rossetti et al., 1990). Another advantage is that, the human placental transfer of glibenclamide is negligible. Maternally administered glibenclamide in pharmacologic doses, and even doses greatly exceeding therapeutic levels, may not reach the fetus (Elliott et al., 1991). The landmark study of Langer et al concluded that glyburide was as effective as insulin in maintaining the desired glycemic levels and resulted in a comparable outcome (Langer et al., 2000). The author's group undertook a prospective study comparing insulin and glibenclamide in GDM. In this study, both Glibenclamide and insulin treatment achieved equally good glycemic control and the perinatal outcome was not different (Anjalakshi et al., 2007). The observation of this study was that the mean dose of glibenclamide required at term was 1.45 ± 0.57 mg/day and mean insulin requirement at term was 21.7 ± 13.55 units/day to achieve the same glycemic level (Anjalakshi et al., 2007). It is noteworthy that Glibenclamide is very much economical and cost effective compared to insulin, which is not only expensive but also inconvenient as it has to be taken parenterally. Yet an another observation was that in Indian population, the dose of glibenclamide required is very much less compared to the other published studies (Langer et al., 2005).

7.3.2 Metformin

Women with polycystic ovary syndrome (PCOS) are advised metformin to induce ovulation. The drug is not withdrawn if a woman conceives while on metformin therapy and the maximum dose prescribed in the author's clinical practice is 1500 mg. If the plasma glucose is not under control with metformin, insulin is always added. No adverse pregnancy outcome with metformin therapy was observed. A preliminary study showed that metformin was safe in pregnant, glucose intolerant women either as an adjunct to insulin treatment or even as a monotherapy (Ramachandran et al., 2005). A prospective study found no adverse influence on the pregnancy outcome in PCOS women treated throughout pregnancy with Metformin (Glueck et al., 2004).

Metformin in gestational diabetes (MiG) trial found that in women with gestational diabetes mellitus, metformin (alone or with supplemental insulin) was not associated with increased perinatal complications as compared with insulin (Rowan et al., 2008).

8. Monitoring glycemic control

The success of the treatment for a woman with GDM depends on the glycemic control maintained with meal plan or pharmacological intervention. To know the effectiveness of treatment, monitoring of glycemic control is essential.

- Once diagnosis is made, medical nutritional therapy (MNT) is advised initially for two weeks. If MNT fails to achieve control i.e., FPG ≥ 5.0 mmol/L and/or 2-h PG ≥ 6.7 mmol/L, insulin may be initiated.
- Once target blood glucose is achieved, woman with GDM till the 28th week of gestation require laboratory monitoring of both fasting and 2-h post breakfast once a month and at other time of the day as the clinician decides.
- After the 28th week of gestation, the laboratory monitoring should be more frequent atleast once in 2 weeks, if need be more frequently.
- After 32 weeks of gestation, laboratory monitoring should be done once a week till delivery
- In high risk pregnancies, frequency of monitoring may be intensified with self monitoring of blood glucose (SMBG).

- Continuous glucose monitoring devices are available but these equipments need special training and are expensive. These devices may be useful in high risk pregnancies to know the glycemic fluctuations and to plan proper insulin dosage.

8.1 Glycosylated haemoglobin – A1c levels

If the glucose intolerance is detected in the early pregnancy, A1c level will be helpful to differentiate between a pre gestational diabetic and GDM. If A1c level is more than 6% (Balaji et al., 2007), the chances are that she may be a pre GDM or GDM, in whom the glucose intolerance was detected in the early weeks of pregnancy; all the more validating that the screening needs to be performed in the early weeks of gestation. The estimation of A1c may help in distinguishing a pre GDM from an early onset GDM, but not essential, as this differentiation is of no consequence in clinical practice, as the treatment approach is going to be the same (Seshiah et al., 2007). Further, A1c is not estimated in the community health centres, barring a few tertiary care hospitals due to the difficulty in standardization, inadequate technical support and the cost.

8.2 Measuring other parameters

The blood pressure has to be monitored during every visit. Examination of the fundus and estimation of microalbuminuria, every trimester is recommended.

8.3 Ultrasound fetal measurement

The management of gestational diabetes, based on the foetal growth by ultrasonogram demands that the fetus at risk must first manifest overgrowth before treatment decisions are made. Further, the cost of performing a number of ultrasonograms to monitor the foetal growth and recommending therapy has to be kept in mind. Until there is evidence to absolutely prove that ignoring maternal hyperglycemia when the fetal growth patterns appear normal on the ultrasonogram, it is prudent to achieve and maintain normoglycemia in every pregnancy complicated by gestational diabetes.

9. Target glycemic level

Increased birth weight of neonates occurred even when the mother's glucose tolerance was less than the glycemic criteria recommended by WHO (2-h PG > 7.8 mmol/L) for diagnosis of GDM. Increasing carbohydrate intolerance in women without overt GDM was associated with graded increase in the incidence of macrosomia (Sermer et al., 1998). The author's group documented that the occurrence of macrosomia was continuum as the FPG increased > 5.0 mmol/L (Seshiah et al., 2008c) and the 2-h PG > 6.7 mmol/L (Balaji et al., 2006). Thus maintenance of mean plasma glucose level ~ 5.8 to 6.1 mmol/L is desirable for a good fetal outcome (Langer et al., 1989). This is possible if FPG and peak postprandial glucose levels are maintained ~ 5.0 mmol/L (4.4-5.0 mmol/L) and ~ 6.7 mmol/L (6.1 - 6.7 mmol/L, respectively)

10. Prevention of type 2 dm

The screening for glucose intolerance during pregnancy is not done routinely and probably the undiagnosed glucose intolerance that has been occurring in the past has resulted in the increased prevalence of diabetes in India. This is likely to be true as GDM has a far reaching consequence in predisposing their offsprings to glucose intolerance. This observation was substantiated and documented in Pima Indians (Dabelea et al., 2000). The children born in 1965 to women with GDM were followed up till 2000. By the time they reached 35 years, more than half of the group had diabetes (Dabelea et al., 2000). Hence as a policy to identify GDM and its consequences on the infant, a 75 g OGTT has been recommended to all women in the population during the third trimester of pregnancy (Dabelea et al., 2000). Now it is obvious that taking care of women with GDM is the first step in the primary prevention of diabetes.

The important aspect of diabetes and pregnancy is that, the intrauterine millieu interieur, whether one of nutritional deprivation or one of nutritional plenty, results in changes in fetal pancreatic development and peripheral response to insulin that may lead to adult-onset GDM and type 2 DM (Savona-Ventura & Chircop, 2003). Thus, the timely action taken now in screening all pregnant women for glucose intolerance, achieving euglycemia in them and ensuring adequate nutrition may prevent in all probability, the vicious cycle of transmitting glucose intolerance from one generation to another (Aerts, 2004). GDM offers an important opportunity for the development, testing and implementation of clinical strategies for diabetes prevention (Buchanan et al., 2007).

'No single period in human development provides a greater potential than pregnancy for a long range pay off via relatively short range period of enlightened metabolic manipulation' - Norbert Frienkel.

11. Summary

- GDM women are at increased risk of future diabetes as are their children and following generations.
- Prevalence of GDM varies from one region to another region in the same country.
- Compared with selective screening, Universal screening for GDM detects more cases and improves maternal and offspring prognosis.
- Asian women are ethnically more prone to develop glucose intolerance compared to other ethnic groups.
- GDM based on 2-h 75g OGTT defined by WHO predicts adverse pregnancy outcome and warrants treatment.
- A 2-h 75g post plasma glucose $\geq$ 7.8 mmol/L serves both as screening and diagnostic criteria which is a technically simple economical and evidence based one step procedure.
- IADPSG recommendations are suitable in clinical settings where technical and financial supports are available.
- Early screening for glucose intolerance and care could avoid some diabetes related complications in women with gestational diabetes
- Women with NGT in the first visit are advised to undergo glucose tolerance test in the subsequent trimesters.
- The meal pattern advised has to be simple, and easy to understand and follow.
- The goal is to maintain mean plasma glucose of 5.8 to 6.1 mmol/L
- Occurrence of macrosomia was continuum as the FPG increased from 5.0 mmol/L and 2-h PG increased from 6.7 mmol/L.

- At least one point testing in the third trimester of measuring haemoglobin, blood pressure and plasma glucose in pregnant women will go a long way in achieving safe maternal and fetal outcome.
- Taking care of women with gestational diabetes is envisaged as the first step in the primary prevention of diabetes.

12. References

Aerts, L. (2004). Intergenerative transmission of DM. Abstract volume of the 36th Annual Meeting of the DPSG, Luso - Portugal, September 2004.

Agarwal, S.; & Gupta, AN. (1982). Gestational Diabetes. *J Assoc Physicians India* Vol. 30, No.4, (April 1982): pp. 203 - 5, ISSN 0004-5772.

Al Mahroos, S.; Nagalla, DS.; Yousif, W.; et al (2005). A population - based screening for gestational diabetes mellitus in non-diabetic women in Bahrain. *Ann Saudi Med,* Vol. 25, No.2, (March-April 2005),129 - 33, ISSN 0256-4947.

Anjalakshi, C.; Balaji, V.; Balaji, MS.; et al (2007). A Prospective Study Comparing Insulin and Glibenclamide In Gestational Diabetes Mellitus In Asian Indian Women. *Dia Res Clin Pract,* Vol. 76, No. 3, (June 2007), pp. 474-5, ISSN 0168-8227.

Anjalakshi, C.; Balaji, V.; Balaji, MS.; et al (2009). A single test procedure to diagnose gestational diabetes mellitus. *Acta Diabetol,* Vol. 46, No.1, (March 2009), pp. 51-4, ISSN 0940-5429.

Ardawi, MS.; Nasrat, HA.; Jamal, HS.; et al (2000). Screening for gestational diabetes mellitus in pregnant females. *Saudi Med J.* Vol. 21, No. 2, (February 2000), pp. 155–60, ISSN 0379-5284.

Balaji, V.; Balaji, MS.; Seshiah, V.; et al (2006). Maternal glycemia and neonates birth weight in Asian Indian women. *Diabetes Res Clin Pract.* Vol. 73, No. 2, (August 2006), pp. 223-4, ISSN 0168-8227.

Balaji, V.; Madhuri, BS.; Ashalatha, S.; et al (2007). A1C in gestational diabetes mellitus in Asian Indian women. *Diabetes Care.* Vol. 30, No. 7, (July 2007), pp. 1865-7, ISSN 0149-5992.

Balaji, V.; Balaji, MS.; Alexander, C.; et al (2010). Premixed insulin aspart 30 (Biasp 30) vs. premixed human insulin 30 (BHI 30) in gestational diabetes mellitus-a pilot study. *J Assoc Physicians India.* Vol. 58, (February 2010), pp. 99-101, ISSN 0004-5772.

Balaji, V.; Madhuri, Balaji.; Anjalakshi, C.; et al. (2011). Inadequacy of fasting plasma glucose to diagnose gestational diabetes mellitus in Asian Indian women. *Dia Res Clin Pract.* In Press. ISSN 0168-8227.

Balaji, V.; Madhuri, Balaji.; Anjalakshi, C.; et al. (2011). Diagnosis of gestational diabetes mellitus in Asian-Indian women. *Indian J Endocrinol Metab.* In Press. ISSN 2230-8210.

Barker, DJ (1995). Fetal origins of coronary heart disease. *BMJ.* Vol. 311, No. 6998, (July 1995), pp. 171–4, ISSN 0959-8138.

Bartha, JL.; Martinez-Del-Fresno, P.; Comino-Delgado, R.; (2003). Early diagnosis of gestational diabetes mellitus and prevention of diabetes related complications. *Eur J Obstet Gynecol Reprod Biol.* Vol. 109, No. 1, (July 2003), pp. 41 - 4, ISSN 0301-2115.

Beischer, NA.; Oats, JN.; Henry, OA.; et al. (1991). Incidence and severity of gestational diabetes mellitus according to country of birth in women living in Australia. *Diabetes.* Vol. 40, Suppl. No. 2, (December 1991), pp. 35 - 8, ISSN 0012-1797.

Ben-Haroush, A.; Yogev, Y.; Chen R.; et al (2004). The post prandial glucose profile in the diabetic pregnancy. *Am J Obstet Gynecol*. Vol. 191, No. 2, (August 2004), pp. 576 - 81, ISSN 0002-9378.

Bevier, WC.; Fischer, R.; Jovanovic, L. (1999). Treatment of women with an abnormal glucose challenge test (but a normal oral glucose tolerance test) decreases the prevalence of macrosomia. Am J Perinatol. Vol. 16, No. 6, (1999), pp. 269-75, ISSN 0735-1631.

Buchanan, TA.; Xiang, A.; Kjos, SL.; et al. (2007). What is Gestational Diabetes.*Diabetes Care*. Vol. 30, Suppl No. 2, (July 2007), pp. S 105–11, ISSN: 0149-5992.

Cosson, E.; Benthimol, M.; Carbilon, L.; et al. (2004). Universal screening for gestational diabetes mellitus improves maternal and fetal outcomes compared with selective screening. In : Mateclinsky FM (ed). Abstract book of the 64th Scientific Sessions of the American Diabetes Association (ADA). Florida. American Diabetes Association 2004; A61.

Cosson, E. (2004). Screening and insulin sensitivity in gestational diabetes. Abstract volume of the 40th Annual Meeting of the European Association for the Study of Diabetes, September 2004: A 350.

Crowther, CA.; Hiller, JE.; Moss, JR.; et al. (2005). Effect of treatment of gestational diabetes mellitus. *N Engl J Med* 2005; Vol. 352, No. 24, (June 2005), pp. 2477-86, ISSN 0028-4793.

Dabelea, D.; Knowler, WC.; Pettitt, DJ. (2000). Effect of diabetes in pregnancy and offspring: follow up research in the Pima Indians. *J Matern Fetal Medicine*. Vol. 9, No. 1,(January - February 2000); 83–8, ISSN 1057-0802.

Das, S.; Behera, MK.; Misra, S.; et al. (2010). B-cell function and insulin resistance in pregnancy and their relation to fetal development. *Metab Syndr Relat disorder*. Vol. 8, No. 1, (February 2010), pp. 25-32. ISSN 1540-4196.

de Sereday, MS.; Damiano, MM.; Gonzalez, CD.; et al. (2003). Diagnostic criteria for gestational diabetes in relation to pregnancy outcome. *J Diabetes and complications*. Vol. 17, No. 3, (May-June 2003), pp. 115-119, ISSN 1056-8727.

Deierlein, AL.; Siega-Riz, AM.; Chantala, K.; et al. (2011). The association between maternal glucose concentration and child BMI at age 3 years. *Diabetes Care*. Vol. 34, No. 2, (February 2011), pp. 480-4, ISSN 0149-5992.

Dornhorst, A & Rossi, M. (1998). Risk and Prevention of Type 2 Diabetes in women with Gestational Diabetes. *Diabetes Care*. Vol. 21, Suppl No. 2, (August 1998), pp. B43-9, ISSN 0149-5992.

Dornhost, A.; Paterson, CM. ; Nicholls, JS. ; et al. (1992) High prevalence of GDM in women from ethnic minority groups. *Diabetic Med*. Vol. 9, No. 9, (November 1992), pp. 820-2, ISSN 0742-3071.

Elliott, BD.; Langer, O.; Schenker, S.; et al. (1991). Insignificant transfer of glyburide occurs across the human placenta. *Am J Obstet Gynecol*. Vol. 165, No. 4 pt 1, (October 1991), pp. 807 - 12, ISSN 0002-9378.

Fall, CH.; Stein, CE.; Kumaran, K.; et al. (1998). Size at birth, maternal weight, and type 2 diabetes in South India. *Diabet Med*. Vol. 15, No. 3, (March 1998), pp. 220-7, ISSN 0742-3071.

Forsbach, G.; Vazquez-Lara, J.; Alvarez-y-Garcia, C.; et al. (1998). Diabetes and pregnancy in Mexico. *Rev Invest Clin*. Vol. 50, No. 3, (May-June 1998), pp. 227-31, ISSN 0034-8376.

Franks, PW.; Looker, HC.; Kobes, S.; et al. (2006). Gestational Glucose tolerance and risk of type 2 diabetes in Young Pima Indian Offspring. *Diabetes*. Vol. 55, No. 2, (February 2006), pp. 460 – 5. ISSN 0012-1797.

Gayle, C.; Germain, S.; Marsh, MS.; et al. (2010). Comparing pregnancy outcomes for intensive versus routine antenatal treatment of GDM based on a 75 gm OGTT 2- h blood glucose (>140 mg/dl). *Diabetologia*. Vol. 53, Suppl. No. 1, (September 2010), pp. S435, ISSN 0012-186X.

Gifford F. (2001). Uncertainty about clinical equipoise. Clinical equipoise and the uncertainty principles both require further scrutiny. *BMJ*. Vol. 322, No. 7289, (March 2001), pp. 795. ISSN 0959-8138.

Girling, J. & Dornhorst, A. (2003). Pregnancy and diabetes mellitus. In: *Textbook of Diabetes 2*, John C Pick Up, Gareth Williams, editors. 3rd ed, pp. 65-66, Blackwell publishing company, ISBN 0-632-05915-X, United Kingdom.

Glueck, CJ.; Goldenberg, N.; Pranikoff, J.; et al. (2004). Height, weight and motor- social development during the first 18 months of life in 126 infants born to 109 mothers with polycystic ovary syndrome who conceived on and continued Metformin throughout pregnancy. *Hum Reprod*. Vol. 19, No. 6, (June 2004), pp. 1323-30. ISSN 0268-1161.

Gough, WW.; Shack, MJ.; Bennett, PH.; et al. (1970). Evaluation of glucose in the Pima Indians by longitudinal studies. *Diabetes*. Vol. 19, Suppl No. 1, (1970). pp. 388. ISSN 0012-1797.

Groop, LC.; Barzilai, N.; Ratheiser, K.; et al. (1991). Dose-dependent effects of Glyburide on insulin secretion and glucose uptake in humans. *Diabetes Care*. Vol. 14, No. 8, (August 1991), pp. 724-7. ISSN 0149-5992.

Hermansen, K.; Colombo, M.; Storgaard, H.; et al. (2002). Improved postprandial glycemic control with biphasic human insulin in patients with Type 2 diabetes. *Diabetes Care*. Vol. 25, No. 5, (May 2002), pp. 883-88. ISSN 0149-5992.

Hunt, KJ. & Schuller, KL. (2007). The increasing prevalence of diabetes in pregnancy. *Obstet Gynecol Clin North Am*. Vol 34, No. 2, (June 2007), pp. 173-99. ISSN 0889-8545.

Jovanovic, L. (1998). American Diabetes Association's Fourth International Workshop – Conference on Gestational Diabetes Mellitus: Summary and Discussion. Therapeutic interventions. *Diabetes Care*. Vol 21, Suppl No. 2, (August 1998), B131 - B137. ISSN 0149-5992.

Jovanovic, L. (2001). What is so bad about a big baby? *Diabetes Care*. Vol. 24, No. 8, (August 2001), pp. 1317-8. ISSN 0149-5992.

Jovanovic, L.; Ilic, S.; Pettitt, DJ.; et al. (1999). Metabolic and immunologic effects of insulin lispro in gestational diabetes. *Diabetes Care*. Vol. 22, No. 9, (September 1999), pp. 1422-27. ISSN 0149-5992.

King, H. (1998). Epidemiology of glucose intolerance and gestational diabetes in women of childbearing age. *Diabetes Care*. Vol. 21, Suppl No. 2, (August 1998), pp. B9 - B13. ISSN 0149-5992.

Kuhl, C.; Hornnes, PJ.; Andersen, O. (1985). Etiology and pathophysiology of gestational diabetes mellitus. *Diabetes*. Vol. 34, Suppl No. 2, (June 1985), pp. 66–70. ISSN 0012-1797.

Kuhl, C. (1991). Insulin Secretion and insulin resistance in pregnancy and GDM. Implications for diagnosis and management. *Diabetes.* Vol. 40, Suppl. 2, (December 1991), pp. 18-24. ISSN 0012-1797.

Landon, MB.; Spong, CY.; Thom, E.; et al. (2009). A multicenter, randomized trial of treatment for mild gestational diabetes. N Engl J Med. Vol. 361, No. 14, (October 2009), pp. 1339-48. ISSN 0028-4793.

Langer, O.; Levy, J.; Brustman, L.; et al. (1989). Glycemic control in gestational diabetes mellitus-how tight is tight enough: small for gestational age versus large for gestational age? *Am J Obstet Gynecol.* Vol. 161, No. 3, (September 1989), pp. 646-53. ISSN 0002-9378.

Langer, O.; Cornway, DL.; Berkus, MD.; et al. (2000). A comparison of glyburide and insulin in GDM. *N Engl J Med.* Vol. 343, No. 16, (October 2000), pp. 1134-8. ISSN 0028-4793.

Langer, O.; Yogev, Y.; Xenakis, EM.; et al. (2005). Insulin and glyburide therapy: dosage, severity level of gestational diabetes, and pregnancy outcome. *Am J Obstet Gynecol.* Vol. 192, No. 1, (January 2005), pp. 134-9. ISSN 0002-9378.

Lucas, A. (1991). Programming by early nutrition in man. In: *The childhood environment and adult disease.* Bock GR, Whelan J, editors. pp. 38-55. John Wiley and Sons, ISBN 0 471 92957 3, Chichester, UK.

Magee, S.; Walden, CE.; Benedetti, TJ.; et al. (1993). Influence of diagnostic criteria on the incidence of gestational diabetes and perinatal morbidity. *JAMA.* Vol. 269, No. 5, (February 1993), pp. 609-15. ISSN 0098-7484.

Mazze, R.; (2006). Epidemiology of Diabetes in Pregnancy. In: *The Diabetes In Pregnancy Dilemma, Leading change with Proven Solutions.* Langer, O.; pp. 13-22, University Press of America, ISBN 0-7618-3270X, Maryland, United States of America.

Metzger, BE.; (1991). Summary and recommendations of the Third International Workshop Conference on Gestational Diabetes Mellitus. *Diabetes.* Vol. 40, Suppl No. 2, pp. 197–201, ISSN 0012-1797.

Metzger, BE.; Gabbe, SG.; Persson, B.; et al. International Association of Diabetes and Pregnancy Study Groups Consensus Panel (2010). International association of diabetes and pregnancy study groups recommendations on the diagnosis and classification of hyperglycemia in pregnancy. *Diabetes Care.* Vol. 33, No. 3, (March 2010), pp. 676-82. ISSN 0149-5992.

Mohan, V.; Sandeep, S.; Deepa, R.; et al. (2007). Epidemiology of Type 2 diabetes: Indian Scenario. *Indian J Med Res.* Vol. 125, No. 3, (March 2007), pp. 217-30. ISSN 0971-5916.

Nahum, GG.; Wilson, SB.; Stanislaw, H.; (2002). Early pregnancy glucose screening for gestational diabetes mellitus. *J Reprod Med.* Vol. 47, No. 8, (August 2002), pp. 656-62. ISSN 0024-7758.

Narendra, J.; Munichoodappa, C.; Gurudas, A., et al. (1991). Prevalence of glucose intolerance during pregnancy. *Int J Diab Dev Countries.* Vol. 11, No. 2, (April – June 1991), pp. 2-4. ISSN 0973-3930.

Negrato, CA.; Jovanovic, L.; Tambascia, MA.; et al. (2008). Mild gestational hyperglycemia as a risk factor for metabolic syndrome in pregnancy and adverse perinatal outcomes. Diabetes Metab Res Rev. Vol. 24, No. 4, (May-June 2008), pp. 324-30. ISSN 1520-7552.

Paul, VK.; Deorari, AK.; Singh, M.;. (2002). Management of Low Birth Weight Babies. In: *IAP Textbook of Pediatrics*. Parthasarathy, A.; Menon, PSN.; Nair, MKC.; Lokeshwar, MR.; Srivastava, RN.; Bhave, SY.; editors., 2nd edition, pp. 60, Jaypee Brothers, New Delhi.

Perucchini, D.; Fischer, U.; Spinas, GA.; et al. (1999). Using fasting plasma glucose concentrations to screen for gestational diabetes mellitus: prospective population based study. BMJ. Vol. 319, No. 7213, (September 1999), pp. 812-15. ISSN 0959-8138.

Pettitt, DJ.; Bennett, PH.; Saad, MF.; et al. (1991). Abnormal glucose tolerance during pregnancy in Pima Indian women: Long term effects on the offspring. *Diabetes*. Vol. 40, Suppl. No. 2, (December 1991), pp. 126–130. ISSN 0012-1797.

Pettitt, DJ.; Bennett, PH.; Hanson, RL.; et al. (1994). Comparison of World Health Organization and National Diabetes Data Group procedures to detect abnormalities of glucose tolerance during pregnancy. *Diabetes Care*. Vol. 17, No. 11, (November 1994), pp. 1264-68. ISSN: 0149-5992.

Philips, LS.; Ziemer, DC.; Kolm, P.; et al. (2009). Glucose challenge test screening for prediabetes & undiagnosed diabetes. *Diabetologia*. Vol. 52, No. 9, (September 2009), pp. 1798 -1807. ISSN 0012-186X.

Polonsky, KS.; Given, BD.; Van Cauter, E.; (1988). Twenty four hour profiles and pulsatile patterns of insulin secretion in normal and obese subjects. *J Clin Invest*. Vol. 81, No. 2, (February 1988), pp. 442 – 8. ISSN 0021-9738.

Ramachandran, A.; Jali, MV.; Mohan, V.; et al. (1988). High prevalence of diabetes in an urban population in south India. *BMJ*. Vol. 297, No. 6648, (September 1988), pp. 587 –90. ISSN 0959-8138.

Ramachandran, A.; Snehalatha, C.; Dharmaraj, D.; et al. (1992). Prevalence of glucose intolerance in Asian Indians. *Diabetes Care*. Vol. 15, No. 10, (October 1992), pp. 1348-55. ISSN 0149-5992.

Ramachandran, A.; Snehalatha, C.; Kapur, A.; et al. For the Diabetes Epidemiology Study Group in India (DESI). (2001). High prevalence of diabetes and impaired glucose tolerance in India: National Urban Diabetes Survey. *Diabetologia*. Vol. 44, No. 9, (September 2001), pp. 1094-101. ISSN 0012-186X.

Ramachandran, A.; Snehalatha, C.; Vijayalakshmi, S.; et al. (2005). Use of metformin in pregnancies with diabetes: A Case series from India. *J Assoc Physicians India*. Vol. 53, No. 2, (February 2005), pp. 157 – 58. ISSN 0004-5772.

Retnakaran, R.; Hanley, AJ.; Connelly, PW.; et al. (2006). Ethnicity modifies the effect of obesity on insulin resistance in pregnancy: a comparison of Asian, South Asian and Caucasian women. *J Clin Endocrinol Metab* Vol. 91, No. 1, (January 2006), pp. 93-97. ISSN 0021-972X.

Rossetti, L.; Giaccari, A.; De Fronzo, RA.; (1990). Glucose toxicity. *Diabetes Care*. Vol. 13, No. 6, (June 1990), pp. 610-30. ISSN 0149-5992.

Rowan, JA.; Hague, WM.; Gao, W.; et al. MiG Trial Investigators. (2008). Metformin versus insulin for the treatment of gestational diabetes. *N Engl J Med*. Vol. 358, No. 19, (May 2008), pp. 2003-15. ISSN 0028-4793.

Sacks, DA.; (2010). Screening for hyperglycemia in pregnancy. In: *A practical Manual of Diabetes in Pregnancy*. Mc Cance DR, Maresh M, Sacks DA,. pp. 45-55, Blackwell Publishing Ltd, ISBN 978-1-4051-7904-1, United Kingdom.

Savona - Ventura C.; & Chircop, M.; (2003). Birth weight influence on the subsequent development of gestational diabetes mellitus. *Acta Diabetol.* Vol. 40, No. 2, (June 2003), pp. 101-4. ISSN 0940-5429.

Schmidt, MI.; Duncan, BB.; Reichelt, AJ.; et al. (2001). Gestational diabetes mellitus diagnosed with a 2-h 75-g oral glucose tolerance test and adverse pregnancy outcomes. *Diabetes Care.* Vol. 24, No. 7, (July 2001), pp. 1151–5. ISSN 0149-5992.

Sermer, M.; Naylor, CD.; Farine, D.; et al. (1998). The Toronto Tri Hospital Gestational diabetes project-A preliminary review. *Diabetes Care.* Vol. 21, Suppl. No. 2, (August 1998), pp. B33 - B42. ISSN 0149-5992.

Seshiah, V.; Balaji, V.; Balaji MS.; et al. (2004). Gestational diabetes mellitus in India.*J Assoc Physicians India.* Vol. 52, No. 9, (September 2004), pp. 707-11. ISSN 0004-5772.

Seshiah, V.; Balaji, V.; Balaji, MS.; et al. (2005). One step procedure for screening and diagnosis of gestational diabetes mellitus. *J Obstet Gynecol Ind.* Vol. 55, No. 6, (November/December 2005), pp. 525-29. ISSN: 0971-9202.

Seshiah, V.; Alexander, C.; Balaji, V.; et al. (2006). Glycemic control from early weeks of gestation and pregnancy outcome. *Diabetes.* Vol. 55, Suppl. No. 1, (June 2006), pp. A 604, ISSN 0012-1797.

Seshiah, V.; Balaji, V.; Balaji, MS,; et al. (2007). Gestational Diabetes Mellitus manifests in all trimesters of pregnancy. *Dia Res Clin Pract.* Vol. 77, No. 3, (September 2007), pp. 482-4. ISSN 0168-8227.

Seshiah, V.; Balaji, V.; Balaji, MS.; et al. (2008). Prevalence of gestational diabetes mellitus in South India (Tamil Nadu)-a community based study. *J Assoc Physicians India.* Vol. 56, No. 5, (May 2008), pp. 329-33. ISSN 0004-5772.

Seshiah, V.; Cynthia, A.; Balaji, V.; et al. (2008). Detection and care of women with gestational diabetes mellitus from early weeks of pregnancy results in birth weight of newborn babies appropriate for gestational age. *Dia Res Clin Pract.* Vol. 80, No. 2, (May 2008), pp. 199-202. ISSN 0168-8227.

Seshiah, V.; Balaji, V.; Panneerselvam, A.; et al. (2008). "Abnormal" fasting plasma glucose during pregnancy. *Diabetes Care.* Vol. 31, No. 12, (December 2008), pp. e92. ISSN. 1935-5548 (Electronic).

Seshiah, V.; Sahay, BK.; Das, AK.; et al. (2009). Gestational diabetes mellitus-Indianguidelines. *J Indian Med Assoc.* Vol. 107, No. 11, (Nov 2009), pp. 799-802, 804-6. ISSN 0019-5847.

Seshiah, V.; Balaji, V.; Siddharth, Shah,; et al. (2011). Diagnosis of Gestational Diabetes Mellitus in the Community. *J Assoc Physicians India.* In Press. ISSN 0004-5772.

Shamsuddin, K.; Mahdy, ZA.; Siti Rafiaah, I.; et al. (2001). Risk factor screening for abnormal glucose tolerance in pregnancy. *Int J Gynecol Obstet.* Vol. 75, No. 1, (October 2001), pp. 27-32. ISSN 0020-7292.

Simmons, D.; Devers, MC.; Wolmarans, L.; et al. (2009). Difficulties in the use of risk factors to screen for gestational diabetes mellitus. *Diabetes Care.* Vol. 32, No. 1, (January 2009), e8. ISSN 0149-5992.

Snehalatha C, Mary S, Selvam S, Sathish Kumar CK, Shetty SB, Nanditha A et al. (2009). Changes in insulin secretion and insulin sensitivity in relation to the glycemic outcomes in subjects with impaired glucose tolerance in the Indian Diabetes Prevention Programme - (IDPP- 1). *Diabetes Care.* Vol. 32, No. 10, (October 2009), pp. 1796-1801. ISSN 0149-5992.

Super, DM.; Edelberg, SC.; Philipson, EH.; et al. (1991). Diagnosis of gestational diabetes in early pregnancy. *Diabetes Care.* Vol. 14, No. 4, (April 1991), pp. 288-94. ISSN 0149-5992.

Tisi, DK.; Burns, DH.; Luskey, GW.; et al. (2011). Fetal exposure to altered amniotic fluid glucose, insulin, and insulin-like growth factor-binding protein 1 occurs before screening for gestational diabetes mellitus. *Diabetes Care.* Vol. 34, No. 1, (January 2011), pp. 139-44. ISSN 0149-5992.

Tuomilehto, J.; (2005). A paradigm shift is needed in the primary prevention of type 2 diabetes. In: *Prevention of type 2 diabetes.* Ganz M, pp. 153-65, John Willey & Sons Ltd, England, ISBN: 978-0-470-85734-2.

Valensi, P.; Benroubi, M.; Borzi, V.; et al. (2009). Initiating insulin therapy with, or switching existing insulin therapy to, biphasic insulin aspart 30/70 (NovoMix 30) in routine care: safety and effectiveness in patients with type 2 diabetes in the IMPROVE observational study. *Int J Clin Pract.* Vol. 63, No. 3, (March 2009), pp. 522–31. ISSN 1368-5031.

Voto, LS.; Uranga Imaz, M.; Margulies, M. (2003). Gestational diabetes in developing countries. In: *Textbook of Diabetes and Pregnancy.* Hod, M.; Jovanovic, L.; Di Renzo, GC.; de Leiva, A.; Langer, O.; 1st ed. pp. 183- 90. Martin Dunitz, Taylor & Francis Group plc, ISBN 1 84184 110 2, London.

Wahi, P.; Dogra, V.; Jandial, K.; et al. (2011). Prevalence of Gestational Diabetes
Mellitus (GDM) and its Outcomes in Jammu Region. *J Assoc Physicians India.* Vol. 59, No. 4, (April 2011), pp. 227-30. ISSN 0004-5772.

Weiss, PA.; Haeusler, M.; Tamussino, K.; et al. (2000). Can glucose tolerance test predict fetal hyperinsulinism?. *BJOG.* Vol. 107, No. 12, (December 2000), pp. 1480-5. ISSN 1470-0328.

Wild, S.; Roglic, G.; Green, A.; et al. (2004). Global prevalence of diabetes: estimates for the year 2000 and projections for 2030. *Diabetes Care.* Vol. 27, No. 5, (May 2004), pp. 1047-53. ISSN 0149-5992.

Wojcikowski, C.; Krolikowska, B.; Konarzewska, J.; et al. (2002). The prevalence of gestational diabetes mellitus in Polish population. *Ginekol Pol.* Vol. 73, No. 10, (October 2002), pp. 811-6. ISSN 0017-0011.

Yajnik, CS.; Fall, CH.; Vaidya, U.; et al. (1995). Fetal growth and glucose and insulin metabolism in four year old Indian children. *Diabetic Medicine.* Vol. 12, No. 4, (April 1995), pp. 330-6. ISSN 0742-3071.

Yogev, Y.; Avi Ben-Haroush, Moshe Hod: Pathogenesis of gestational diabetes mellitus; In: *Textbook of Diabetes and Pregnancy.* Hod, M.; Jovanovic, L.; Di Renzo, GC.; de Leiva, A.; Langer, O.; 1st ed. pp. 46. Martin Dunitz, Taylor & Francis Group plc, ISBN 1 84184 110 2, London.

Zargar, AH.; Sheikh, MI.; Bashir, MI.; et al. (2004). Prevalence of gestational diabetes mellitus in Kashmiri women from the Indian subcontinent. *Dia Res Clin Pract.* Vol. 66, No. 2, (November 2004), pp. 139-45. ISSN 0168-8227.

3

Gestational Diabetes: Evidence-Based Screening, Diagnosis and Treatment

Melania Maria Ramos Amorim and Leila Katz
Instituto de Medicina Integral Prof. Fernando Figueira (IMIP) – Recife, Pernambuco, Brazil

1. Introduction

Gestational diabetes (GD) is defined as carbohydrate intolerance that begins or is first diagnosed during pregnancy. Hyperglycemia is found only during pregnancy and diagnosis is confirmed when glucose tolerance test results return to normal levels in the postpartum (Metzger et al., 2007). GD occurs in around 4-10% of pregnancies; however, its incidence varies as a function of nutritional habits and differences in genetic patterns between populations (Metzger et al., 2007).

The importance of GD was first described around forty years ago when it was noticed that women with this disorder were more likely to develop diabetes mellitus later on in their lives. The original diagnostic criteria proposed by O'Sullivan and Mahan were in fact never validated for the development of gestational complications or adverse perinatal outcomes (O'Sullivan and Mahan, 1964). Throughout all this time, the importance of this diagnosis for the prognosis of the pregnancy has been the subject of debate (Holt et al., 2011). Whereas some specialists feared that even mild levels of hyperglycemia would negatively affect pregnancy outcome, others have questioned the very existence of GD as a disease (Buchanan and Kjos, 1999).

Recently, however, the harmful effects of hyperglycemia during pregnancy have been demonstrated (HAPO, 2008) and evidence is mounting on the risks of hyperglycemia during pregnancy, not only in terms of adverse perinatal outcome, but also for the future of the infant in adult life (Catalano, 2010; Chandler-Laney et al., 2011; Fall, 2010; Lawlor et al., 2011).

In this chapter, the rationale and current recommendations for the diagnosis and treatment of gestational diabetes will be evaluated based on the best scientific evidence currently available. The MEDLINE, EMBASE, SCOPUS and SciELO databases and the systematic reviews of the Cochrane Library were reassessed using the key words: gestational diabetes, screening, diagnosis and therapy. Preference was given to randomized clinical trials and meta-analyses, with observational studies and review articles being included only when studies with a better level of evidence were unavailable. Guidelines and recommendations established by medical societies for the screening, diagnosis and treatment of gestational diabetes were also consulted.

2. Physiopathology

As any carbohydrate metabolism disorder, GD is characterized by insufficient insulin levels for insulin demand (Metzger et al., 2007). The cause of this insulin insufficiency in pregnancy remains to be fully established; however, it is believed that the occurrence of this event during pregnancy reveals underlying maternal pancreatic disorders that would otherwise only become apparent later on in the woman's life (Metzger et al., 2007).

In a normal pregnancy, fetal and placental growth increases cortisol, growth hormone, human placental lactogen, progesterone, estrogen and prolactin levels. The presence of these stimuli triggers hyperinsulinemia, insulin resistance, fasting hypoglycemia and postprandial hyperglycemia. Consequently, there is a reduction in peripheral sensitivity to insulin and an increase in demand. As a compensatory mechanism, an increase occurs in pancreatic function at the cost of both hypertrophy and hyperplasia. Furthermore, in response to the high insulin levels, peripheral utilization of glucose by the muscles and peripheral glycogen storage increase in an attempt to maintain balance (Metzger et al., 2007; Pridjian and Benjamin, 2010).

As pregnancy advances, these compensatory mechanisms may be insufficient in susceptible women, resulting in an imbalance between insulin production and insulin requirements in pregnancy. Compared to a normal pregnant woman, a woman with GD has pancreatic β-cell dysfunction and a reduction in adaptive β-cell capacity. This results in insufficient insulin secretion and consequent hyperglycemia (Metzger et al., 2007; Pridjian and Benjamin, 2010).

3. Consequences for the mother and child

The consequences of gestational diabetes for the mother and child are summarized in Table 1.

Risks of Gestational Diabetes			
Mother	**Fetus**	**Newborn infant**	**Child/Adult**
Obstetric trauma	Hyperinsulinemia: • Large for gestational age • Macrosomia	Respiratory distress syndrome	Obesity
Higher rate of Cesarean sections	Cardiomyopathy	Hypoglycemia	Type 2 Diabetes Mellitus
Preeclampsia/ gestational hypertension	Obstetric trauma: • Shoulder dystocia • Fractures • Brachial plexus lesion	Hypocalcemia	Metabolic syndrome
Type 2 Diabetes mellitus	Stillbirth	Hypomagnesemia	
Metabolic syndrome		Polycythemia: • Hyperviscosity • Hyperbilirubinemia Cardiomyopathy	

Modified from Pridjian and Benjamin, 2010

Table 1. Risks of Gestational Diabetes

4. Screening and diagnosis of gestational diabetes

The screening and diagnosis of GD is the subject of intense debate and controversy worldwide (Holt et al., 2011; Leary et al., 2010). All aspects of diagnosis (who should be investigated, using which tests and what values are considered diagnostic) have been widely discussed over the past two decades (Holt et al., 2011). Consequently, the guidelines published by the major societies differ with respect to these aspects with the result that the practices of physicians worldwide differ to the same extent (Leary et al., 2010).

The World Health Organization (WHO) recommends screening high-risk women with a 75-gram oral glucose tolerance test in the first trimester of pregnancy and all other women at 24-28 weeks, with fasting glucose measurements of 126 mg/dl and two-hour glucose levels of 140 mg/dl being considered abnormal (WHO, 1999). However, until recently (up to autumn 2010), the American Diabetes Association (ADA) recommended screening only women with risk factors and advocated an oral load of 100 grams of anhydrous glucose (ADA, 2004). The values adopted in each one of the guidelines also differed greatly.

Recently, the International Association of Diabetes and Pregnancy Study Groups (IADPSG) assembled the evidence accumulated over recent years and published new criteria for the screening and diagnosis of GD (IADPSG, Metzger et al., 2010).

4.1 Screening

Screening is performed to select individuals to be investigated. Since 1999, the World Health Organization (WHO) has recommended the screening of all women or all women except those considered low-risk (WHO, 1999).

In 2003, a US taskforce was formed to evaluate screening for gestational diabetes. The authors' conclusion was that better-quality evidence was required to determine whether the benefits of screening are greater than the risks. They recommended that until such evidence was available, to screen or not to screen should be left to the discretion of each individual physician according to his/her own clinical judgment and that both options are reasonable (The US Preventive Services Task-Force - USPSTF, Brody et al., 2003-A).

The same taskforce evaluated the risk factors for gestational diabetes and found a strong association with: maternal obesity (body mass index > 25), age > 25 years, personal or family history of a carbohydrate metabolism disorder or a history of gestational diabetes in a previous pregnancy. Some ethnic groups such as Hispanics, Blacks, native American Indians and Asians are also at an increased risk of developing gestational diabetes. If all these criteria are taken into consideration, 90% of all women at risk of developing gestational diabetes will be identified (Brody et al., 2003-A).

A systematic review was conducted of observational studies published in the past thirty years to evaluate the presence and strength of the association between pre-gestational body mass index (BMI) and the presence of gestational diabetes. Seventy studies were included involving 671,945 women (59 cohort studies and 11 case-control studies). Compared to women with normal pregestational BMI, in accordance with the odds ratio (OR) the estimated risk of developing gestational diabetes was 1.97 [95% confidence interval (95%CI) 1.77 - 2.19], 3.01 [95%CI: 2.34 - 3.87] and 5.55 [95%CI: 4.27 - 7.21] for overweight, moderate obesity and severe obesity, respectively (Torloni et al., 2009).

In addition to the principal risk factors, Table 2 provides a detailed list of risk factors from previous pregnancies as well as risk factors that may appear during the course of pregnancy and may merit investigation.

Personal characteristics:
Age > 35 years
Obesity (BMI > 25)
Arterial hypertension
Family history of diabetes
Obstetric history:
Diabetes in previous pregnancy
Multiparity
Recurrent miscarriage
Prematurity
Recurrent preeclampsia
Fetal death, principally in the final weeks of pregnancy
Neonatal morbidity and mortality:
- Hypoglycemia
- Respiratory distress syndrome
- Hyperbilirubinemia
- Hypocalcemia
- Malformations
Complications in current pregnancy:
Excessive weight gain
Excessive growth of uterine fundal height
Polyhydramnios
Fetal macrosomia
Glycosuria
Use of hyperglycemic drugs (betamimetics, corticoids)

Amorim and Katz, 2011

Table 2. Risk factors for gestational diabetes

More recently, another systematic review evaluated the available literature, searching for further evidence on screening for gestational diabetes (Tieu et al.,2011). The authors searched for articles which evaluated any individual screening tool or screening program, protocol or guideline for gestational diabetes compared with the absence of screening; or any individual screening tool or screening program, protocol or guideline for gestational diabetes with another. Thirty-one trials were considered for inclusion into the review but after application of eligibility criteria, only four of these trials were included. After analysis the authors found that there was insufficient evidence to determine the effects of screening for gestational diabetes and its subsequent management, or the comparative effects of different protocols for screening. Although women who were routinely screened by 50 g glucose challenge testing were more likely to be diagnosed with gestational diabetes than those screened by their risk factors, effects of subsequent management on health outcome are unclear.

IADPSG recommends investigating "all women or all high-risk women" at their first prenatal consultation (IADPSG, Metzger et al., 2010). Universal investigation is justified by the increase in the prevalence of undiagnosed type 2 diabetes in young women (Leary et al.,

2010) and in the risk factors for the occurrence of GD such as, for example, obesity (Catalano, 2010). In addition, it ensures that cases of early-onset GD will be identified (Leary et al., 2010). Early screening reflects the preference for universal investigation.

In addition, IADPSG recommends **universal** investigation at 24-28 weeks of all women not previously diagnosed as having clinical or gestational diabetes (IADPSG et al., 2010).

The argument used by those who support universal screening is based on the randomized clinical trial entitled the *Australian Carbohydrate Intolerance Study in Pregnant Women* (ACHOIS) trial group (Crowther et al., 2005), which showed a reduction in healthcare costs with universal screening. Nevertheless, criticism to the use of these results for recommending IADPSG's proposal is based on the fact that the ACHOIS study used an oral glucose tolerance test of 75 grams, measuring fasting glucose levels and two-hour glucose levels alone, whereas the IADPSG recommendations also include measurement of glucose levels one hour after overload (Leary et al., 2010). Further studies should be conducted to evaluate the costs and benefits associated with this form of management.

4.2 Diagnosis

The origin of all this controversy surrounding the diagnosis of GD lies in the form in which testing was initially developed. The first authors to develop a diagnostic test for GD were John O'Sullivan and Clare Mahan in 1964 (O'Sullivan and Mahan, 1964). The test was developed to predict the risk of developing diabetes mellitus years after the pregnancy rather than the risk of an adverse perinatal outcome.

Although it constituted a watershed in the diagnosis of GD, faults were found in the study conducted by O'Sullivan and Mahan when analyzed from a methodological point of view, particularly with respect to the conclusions drawn and the validation of the test as a diagnostic technique, which was clearly demonstrated by Naylor in a study published in 1989 (Naylor, 1989). One of the questions raised was that gestational diabetes is more important as a predictor of a pregnancy with a higher maternal-fetal risk, whereas the end-point initially evaluated was the presence of carbohydrate intolerance after the end of pregnancy. Since the investigators' objective was to predict the development of diabetes mellitus over the long-term, this characteristic was taken into consideration to select the cut-off points. It was later shown that when pregnant women considered to be diabetic in accordance with the values selected were treated with insulin, the rate of macrosomia decreased when glucose levels returned to normal (O'Sullivan, 1996 and 1973). This is an indirect way of reaching conclusions that is, nonetheless, far from ideal and does not allow the diagnostic technique to be adequately validated. According to Naylor, it would have been more appropriate to try to record the immediate and long-term neonatal complications and test their association using an oral glucose tolerance test.

In the following years, changes were made to the diagnostic techniques used and glucose levels were no longer measured in full blood but rather in venous plasma. Furthermore, enzymatic methods began to be used to measure plasma glucose levels instead of the Somogyi-Nelson technique. These technical modifications led to the mathematical correction of the values initially proposed by O'Sullivan and Mahan with the appearance of different sets of values adopted by different organizations involved in the study of GD (National Diabetes Data Group [NDDG], 1979; Carpenter and Coustan, 1982).

Later, an intense debate ensued among investigators regarding the best form of diagnosing GD. Many investigators suggested the adoption of more rigid diagnostic criteria, including a reduction in blood glucose levels or the adoption of fewer points on the curve as being sufficient for diagnosis. It was even proposed that the presence of hyperglycemia below the levels established for diagnosis could be sufficient to lead to adverse maternal and perinatal outcomes, or that the hyperglycemia occurring irrespective of an overload should be taken into consideration (Aberg et al., 2001; Jensen et al., 2001; Langer et al., 1987; Rudge et al., 1990; Sermer et al., 1995).

If on the one hand evidence was accumulating to the effect that milder degrees of hyperglycemia, albeit below the levels established for a diagnosis of GD, could lead to unfavorable perinatal outcomes, on the other hand some authors questioned the very existence of this diagnosis as a valid entity and called attention to the possible negative effects of this diagnosis (Buchanan, 1999; Lucas et al., 1993). A diagnosis of GD may result in excessive medicalization of pregnancy, which in itself would be negative. Furthermore, this diagnosis may result in an increase in the number of interventions performed, including even Cesarean sections, in situations in which the need for this type of delivery is questionable, due to the mere presence of a diagnosis of diabetes. In addition, it is important to remember the psychological burden caused by a label of diabetes.

In 2005, an Australian group (ACHOIS) published the findings of a randomized clinical trial in which mild hyperglycemia was treated in women who did not fulfill the diagnostic criteria for GD, but who had measurements of 140 to 199 mg/dl in a 75-gram oral glucose tolerance test (OGTT) and were consequently considered to be carbohydrate intolerant (Crowther et al., 2005). These investigators found a reduction in composite final outcome (perinatal death, shoulder dystocia, fractures and brachial plexus palsy) compared with women managed in the usual manner.

In 2009, a clinical trial was conducted to treat women who were found not to fulfill the diagnostic criteria for GD after being submitted to an oral glucose tolerance test with 100 grams of carbohydrate, but whose glucose levels were not completely normal. Likewise, when this group was treated, a reduction was found in macrosomia, shoulder dystocia, Cesarean section and hypertensive diseases (Landon et al., 2009).

Finally, the HAPO (Hyperglycemia and Adverse Pregnancy Outcome) study was conducted to evaluate the risks of hyperglycemia during pregnancy for the mother, the fetus and the newborn infant (HAPO, 2008). A total of 25,505 women were included and followed up prospectively to evaluate a possible association between glucose levels and maternal and perinatal outcome. The women were submitted to an OGTT using 75 grams of anhydrous glucose.

The HAPO results were conclusive with respect to the existence of a linear association between elevated glucose levels in the pregnant woman and the rates of large-for-gestational-age infants, preeclampsia and Cesarean sections. Moreover, an association was found between maternal hyperglycemia and neonatal hypoglycemia, C-peptide in umbilical cord blood, premature delivery, admission to the neonatal intensive care unit (ICU) and hyperbilirubinemia. No association was found between maternal hyperglycemia and neonatal death; however, the sample size may have been insufficient to evaluate this particular outcome.

One of the most important findings of HAPO was the demonstration of an association that is continuous; hence no clear cut-off point can be defined above which adverse events occur (Leary et al., 2010).

The choice of the 75-gram curve to investigate these women has never been validated scientifically. The first glucose overload to be described in pregnancy was performed using

100 grams of anhydrous glucose (O'Sullivan and Mahan, 1964), a procedure that was also recommended by the American Diabetes Association in 2004 (ADA, 2004). Nonetheless, since the WHO proposal in 1980 to use a 75-gram overload, as used in non-pregnant women, this practice became more and more common and even the HAPO study used the 75-gram glucose overload. With the power obtained in the HAPO study showing the adverse perinatal effects of hyperglycemia associated with the levels obtained following a 75-gram overload of anhydrous glucose, this test will probably increase in popularity compared to the 100-gram overload (Leary et al., 2010).

Another interesting outcome of the HAPO study was the recommendation that a finding of only one abnormal value on the glucose curve should also be considered abnormal and diagnostic. This recommendation was made with the aim of increasing the likelihood of identifying milder degrees of hyperglycemia that had been associated with poorer maternal and perinatal prognosis in previous studies.

The cut-off points recommended by IADPSG are arbitrarily defined based on an odds ratio of 1.75 relative to the mean glucose levels at each time-point, i.e. those measurements that result in a 75% greater likelihood of adverse perinatal outcomes. The selection had to be made in this way, since, as previously mentioned, the association between glucose levels and adverse outcome is continuous. These values, however, are subject to criticism and the occurrence of adverse outcomes with glucose levels below the proposed values is to be expected. Nevertheless, use of a lower cut-off point would certainly result in a greater percentage of diagnosed cases and the impact of this excess number of diagnoses on perinatal outcomes has yet to be established (Leary et al., 2010).

The absence of any IADPSG recommendations regarding a category referred to as "carbohydrate intolerance" is noteworthy. According to current criteria, either a woman has normal glucose levels or she has gestational diabetes. However, cases need to be taken into consideration in which women have glucose levels outside the limits considered normal yet without reaching levels that would be considered diagnostic. The adoption of the term "carbohydrate intolerance" is suggested for such cases (Leary et al., 2010).

The findings of the HAPO study appear to indicate that only normal glucose levels would eliminate the risk of adverse perinatal outcome; therefore, it could be argued that any deviation above normal levels should be considered abnormal (Leary et al., 2010). However, the economic and even the psychological impact of so many diagnoses of an "abnormal pregnancy" needs to be taken into consideration and may be immense.

To determine the ideal cut-off point, a cost-benefit analysis has to be performed of different cut-off points. In addition to the cost of the diagnostic test itself, the financial burden caused by the additional cases diagnosed in terms of follow-up and treatment has to be taken into consideration. In addition, it has to be confirmed that treating these diagnosed cases will indeed lead to a reduction in the number of adverse outcomes (Leary et al., 2010) and, furthermore, that this reduction will cause a positive impact that will compensate for the costs of diagnosis and follow-up.

The change in the diagnostic criteria defined by IADPSG will certainly have significant clinical implications for women and for the healthcare system. The number of women diagnosed as having gestational diabetes will rise. This increase in the prevalence of GD may cause a significant impact on all the additional women who will be diagnosed (Holt et al., 2011). In addition to the greater volume of resources required to follow-up and treat these women, the effect on patients of the very existence of a diagnosis should be kept in mind.

Therefore, this change needs to be supported with convincing data showing beyond doubt that its adoption will improve pregnancy outcome. Since the HAPO study was merely observational, it is limited to associating adverse perinatal outcomes with higher glucose levels; however, it does not prove that normalizing glucose levels will necessarily result in any improvement in prognosis (Holt et al., 2011).
Two studies evaluated the benefits of treating milder degrees of hyperglycemia in pregnancy: the ACHOIS study (Crowther, 2005) and the US Multicenter Randomized Trial for Treatment of Mild GMD (Landon, 2009). Despite promising results, it should be remembered that these studies differed in relation to the glucose levels considered treatable and in the number of glucose measurements performed for diagnosis. This hampers extrapolation of these results to the findings of the IADPSG study (Holt et al., 2011).

4.3 Investigation

The IADPSG proposal for the screening and diagnosis of GD is shown in Table 3:

First prenatal consultation
Fasting glucose level or hemoglobin A1 (HgA1) or random measurement in women
• If clinical diabetes => treatment and follow-up for preexisting diabetes.
• If results are non-diagnostic for clinical diabetes:
• and fasting glucose level is > 92 and < 126 => diagnosis of GD
• and fasting glucose level is < 92 => test at 24-28 weeks with OGTT, 75 grams.
24 - 28 weeks of pregnancy
OGTT, 75 grams: fasting glucose measurement/1 hour/2 hours
• Consider clinical diabetes if fasting glucose > 126
• Consider GD if ONE or more measurements are above the cut-off points.
• Consider normal if all the values are below the cut-off points.

For a diagnosis of GD (OGTT, 75g)	
Fasting glucose	> 92 mg/dl
Glucose level at 1 hour after overload	>180 mg/dl
Glucose level at 2 hours after overload	>153 mg/dl
For a diagnosis of clinical diabetes during pregnancy (any one of these tests)	
Fasting glucose	> 126 mg/dl
Hemoglobin A1	> 6.5%
Random plasma glucose measurement	> 200 mg/dl

Table 3. Screening and diagnosis of GD according to the IADPSG

It is important, however, to call attention to the fact that controversies persist, despite the enormous number of studies conducted in this field. Analyzing the guidelines drawn up by

the different organizations, it is clear that there is no consensus with respect to the quantity of glucose that should be used in the oral glucose tolerance test (OGTT), to the glucose levels that should be considered abnormal, or to the number of abnormal measurements on the curve that would permit a diagnosis of GD to be made (Holt et al., 2011).
Table 4 shows the different criteria currently adopted for a diagnosis of gestational diabetes.

Organization	Glucose overload	Number of abnormal values required	Fasting glucose levels	Glucose levels after 1 hour	Glucose levels after 2 hours
IADPSG	75g	≥1	5.1mmol/l 92mg/dl	10.0mmol/l 180mg/dl	8.5mmol/l 153mg/dl
WHO	75g	≥1	7.0mmol/l 126mg/dl		7.8mmol/l 140mg/dl
ADA	100g	≥2	5.3mmol/l 95mg/dl	10.0mmol/l 180mg/dl	8.6mmol/l 155mg/dl
ADIPS	75g	≥1	5.5mmol/l 100mg/dl		8.0mmol/l 144mg/dl
CDA	75g	≥2	5.3mmol/l 95mg/dl	10.6mmol/l 190mg/dl	8.9mmol/l 160mg/dl
EASD	75g	≥1	6.0mmol/l 108mg/dl		9.0mmol/l 162mg/dl
NZSSD	75g	≥1	5.5mmol/l 100mg/dl		9.0mmol/l 162mg/dl
ADA: American Diabetes Association (until autumn 2010); ADIPS: Australasian Diabetes in Pregnancy Society; CDA: Canadian Diabetes Association; EASD: European Association for the Study of Diabetes; IADPSG: International Association of Diabetes and Pregnancy Study Groups; NZSSD: New Zealand Society for the Study of Diabetes; WHO: World Health Organization. *The ADA adopted the IAPDSG criteria in the autumn of 2010.					

Holt et al, 2011

Table 4. Comparison of diagnostic criteria for gestational diabetes

Until randomized clinical trials are conducted to compare the different strategies for screening and diagnosis and to define possible differences in maternal and perinatal outcome, the ideal test and the ideal criteria remain to be defined. The characteristics of each population should be evaluated, principally with respect to the frequency of gestational diabetes and macrosomia. In populations with a high risk for diabetes, we suggest that the IADPSG criteria be used; however, in low-risk populations in which there is no significant association between macrosomia and gestational diabetes, these criteria may not be applicable (Leary et al., 2010).

5. Treatment of gestational diabetes

5.1 Rationale for treatment

Normally, the proposal of any strategy for screening and diagnosis of gestational diabetes is aimed at establishing a therapeutic plan for diagnosed cases, since available evidence suggests that adequate treatment successfully reduces maternal and fetal morbidity, particularly macrosomia (Crowther et al., 2005; Langer et al., 2005; Landon et al., 2009).

Various therapeutic options are available such as diet, physical exercise, blood glucose monitoring and insulin therapy in cases in which diet alone fails to maintain adequate glucose levels (Pridjian and Benjamin, 2010). This chapter does not explore the details of each individual treatment, but simply reviews the available evidence regarding the need for treatment and its effectiveness.

A systematic review in the Cochrane Library specifically deals with the various alternative therapeutic options for gestational diabetes (Alwan et al., 2011). Eight randomized clinical trials involving a total of 1,418 women were included in which any form of treatment was compared with routine prenatal care or different treatments were compared with each other. Except for one large Australian study published in 2005 that included 1,000 women (ACHOIS trial) (Crowther et al., 2005), the sample sizes were small in all the other studies. When the treatment of mild hyperglycemia was compared with routine prenatal care, a significant reduction was found in the risk of preeclampsia and an increase in the risk of induced labor in the group that received treatment. There were no differences in Cesarean section rates, rates of hospital admission, instrumental delivery or postpartum hemorrhage or in the duration of hospital stay. With respect to perinatal outcome, the treatment of diabetes resulted in a significant reduction in composite perinatal morbidity (death, shoulder dystocia, bone fracture and nerve palsy), as well as in the frequency of macrosomia (birthweight > 4000 grams) and shoulder dystocia. Although in the ACHOIS study the rate of admittance to a neonatal intensive care unit was higher for the infants of mothers who received treatment for hyperglycemia, in the meta-analysis this difference was not found to be statistically significant. There were no significant differences between the two groups with respect to gestational age at delivery, incidence of bone fracture in newborn infants, incidence of nerve palsy in the newborn, perinatal death, neonatal hypoglycemia, incidence of respiratory distress syndrome in the newborn infant or in the need for mechanical ventilation. The conclusion reached by these reviewers was that specific treatment for mild gestational diabetes, including diet and insulin, reduces the risk of maternal and perinatal morbidity; however, the risk of labor induction increases. Further studies need to be conducted to evaluate the effect of the different therapeutic modalities, including oral hypoglycemic drugs and insulin, on infant short and long-term outcomes.

Specific analysis of the findings of the ACHOIS trial reveals a frequency of severe neonatal morbidity of 1% in the treated group compared to 4% in the group that received routine care. The incidence of neonatal admission to hospital was 71% versus 61%, respectively, whereas rates of labor induction were 39% in the treatment group versus 29% in the group receiving routine care. The rate of Cesarean sections was similar in both groups, 31% versus 32%. In addition, lower rates of depression and better quality of life scores were found in the treated women in the ACHOIS trial at three months postpartum (Crowther et al., 2005).

Another large randomized clinical trial conducted in the United States was published in 2009 and has yet to be included in the Cochrane systematic review (Landon et al., 2009). The study included 958 women. There was no statistically significant difference in composite outcome (32.4% in the treated group and 37% in the control group) and no perinatal deaths occurred in either group. Nevertheless, birthweight was significantly lower in the treated group (3302 grams versus 3408 grams), as was the frequency of large-for-gestational-age infants (7.1% versus 14.5%), fetal macrosomia (5.9% versus 4.0%), shoulder dystocia (1.5%

versus 4.0%) and Cesarean sections (26.9% versus 33.8%). The rates of preeclampsia and gestational hypertension were also lower in the treated group (8.6% versus 13.6%).

A more recent systematic review on the treatment of gestational diabetes included 18 studies, five of which compared the specific treatment of diabetes with routine treatment (including the 2009 US trial). Modest effects of treatment were found, including a reduction in the risk of fetal macrosomia and shoulder dystocia and a trend, albeit non-significant, towards a reduction in the rate of Cesarean sections. Different levels and intensity of treatment were compared in 13 trials, with findings showing a significant reduction in risk only with respect to shoulder dystocia in the group receiving intensive treatment (Horvath et al., 2010).

Based on the results of these more recent studies, we believe that it is important to diagnose and treat gestational diabetes in order to reduce maternal and neonatal morbidity. Data from the Hyperglycemia and Adverse Pregnancy Outcomes study (HAPO, 2008) reinforce this recommendation, since findings showed a significant association between increasing glucose levels and maternal complications such as preeclampsia, and neonatal complications such as macrosomia and metabolic alterations (Leary et al., 2010), leading, as previously discussed, to changes in the diagnostic criteria for gestational diabetes, as defined by the International Association of Diabetes and Pregnancy Study Groups (IADPSG) (Metzger et al., 2010). Nonetheless, some criticism remains with respect to the comparability of the HAPO study with the more recent clinical trials, since different screening strategies were used (Horvath et al., 2010).

5.2 Treatment strategies

5.2.1 Diet

The universal recommendation has been that all women with a confirmed diagnosis of gestational diabetes should receive dietary counseling and initiate an appropriate diet with the aim of normalizing glucose levels, preventing ketosis, ensuring adequate weight gain and contributing towards fetal well-being. The number of calories will depend on the woman's current weight, with an allowance of 30 kcal/kg of current weight for women with a normal body mass index (BMI), 24 kcal/kg for overweight women and 12-15 kcal/kg for obese women. Carbohydrates (preferably complex carbohydrates) should correspond to 33-40% of the total number of calories, with protein corresponding to 20% and fat to 40%, provided in the form of three main meals and three snacks. Moderate use of sweeteners such as aspartame is permitted. Following these dietary guidelines, glucose levels will normalize in around 75-80% of women with gestational diabetes (ADA, 2004).

Nevertheless, the most adequate strategy for the control of gestational diabetes still remains to be defined, since diet alone may fail to prevent macrosomia. A systematic review available in the Cochrane Library included four studies with 612 women with gestational diabetes and failed to find any differences in the rates of macrosomia (OR = 0.78; 95%CI: 0.45 - 1.35) or Cesarean section (Walkinshaw, 2011). However, the clinical trials included in this review were all small and old, with variations in quality and very wide confidence intervals that did not permit evaluation of the validity of dietetic therapy. The reviewers concluded that there is insufficient evidence to evaluate the use of primary dietetic therapy for women with impaired glucose metabolism in pregnancy. They recommended that larger studies should be conducted to evaluate the effects of diet on maternal outcome (particularly Cesarean sections) and perinatal outcome.

Compliance with treatment and weight gain constitute factors capable of modifying response to dietetic treatment. One large retrospective study including more than 30,000 women with gestational diabetes showed that in the women in whom weight gain was adequate maternal and perinatal outcomes were favorable, whereas those in whom weight gain was excessive had a higher risk of large-for-gestational-age infants, premature delivery and Cesarean sections (Cheng et al., 2008).

5.2.2 Physical exercise

Physical exercise has been proposed as part of the treatment for gestational diabetes based on the fact that, in adults, an improvement in physical fitness increases insulin sensitivity, improves glucose control and reduces the need for insulin (Colberg et al., 2010).
A systematic review available in the Cochrane Library evaluated the effects of exercise programs alone or in association with other therapies on maternal and perinatal morbidity in pregnant women with diabetes. The review included four small, randomized clinical trials involving 114 women with gestational diabetes recruited during the third trimester of pregnancy. The intervention (exercise) was performed over six weeks. There were no statistically significant differences between the group that performed exercise and the controls for any one of the endpoints evaluated. The authors' conclusion was that the evidence was insufficient to either recommend or contraindicate exercise for pregnant women with diabetes and that larger randomized clinical trials should be conducted to further evaluate this form of intervention (Ceysens et al., 2011).
Despite the consistent lack of evidence on the effects of exercise on maternal and perinatal prognosis in women with gestational diabetes, the American Association of Diabetes (ADA) suggests a program of moderate exercise as part of the therapeutic management of women with gestational diabetes as long as there are no medical or obstetrical contraindications to this level of physical activity (ADA, 2004).

5.2.3 Monitoring glucose levels

Monitoring glucose levels may also alter the progression of the condition in women with gestational diabetes. One study showed that daily monitoring of pregnant women treated with diet allows identification of those who could benefit from treatment with an anti-hyperglycemic agent, which may lead to a reduction in the rates of macrosomia (Hawkins et al., 2009; Hawkins, 2010). Nevertheless, the ideal frequency of self-monitoring in women with diet controlled gestational diabetes remains to be established and there is insufficient evidence regarding the ideal glucose levels and the duration of control that would allow longer intervals between capillary glucose measurements (Metzger, 2007).
With respect to the timing and frequency of capillary glucose monitoring, although there are still some controversies between investigators, most of them currently recommend measuring fasting levels immediately after waking and one hour after meals. The proposal for self-monitoring made by some specialists is to test capillary glucose levels four times a day in cases of diet controlled gestational diabetes (fasting and one hour after each meal) and six times a day in gestational diabetes requiring the use of insulin (fasting, one hour prior to and one hour after each meal) (Jovanovic, 2008).
A clinical trial comparing monitoring with schedules that involve either the measurement of pre-prandial glucose levels or fasting glucose and postprandial levels (one hour after meals) in patients with gestational diabetes using insulin therapy showed a better control of

glucose levels, a lower rate of large-for-gestational-age infants and a lower rate of Cesarean sections with the latter protocol (deVeciana et al., 1995). Comparing monitoring one hour postprandial with two hours postprandial, a prospective, observational study found less need for insulin therapy and a trend towards lower rates of fetal macrosomia and Cesarean sections with one-hour postprandial glucose measurements (Weisz et al., 2005). There is insufficient evidence to determine the role of continuous glucose monitoring in patients with gestational diabetes, although this may be useful in women who require insulin and who have difficulty in achieving adequate control of glucose levels (Hawkins, 2010).

5.2.4 Pharmacological treatment

5.2.4.1 Insulin therapy

With respect to insulin therapy, there is no consensus on the glucose levels that would indicate that insulin should be initiated after the implementation of dietetic therapy. The American College of Obstetricians and Gynecologists (ACOG) suggests that insulin should be administered to reduce the risk of macrosomia with fasting glucose levels ≥ 95 mg% OR one-hour postprandial glucose levels > 130-140 mg% OR two-hour postprandial glucose levels ≥ 120 mg% (ACOG, 2001). There are no randomized clinical trials available in which different glucose levels were compared with the objective of determining the cut-off point for the implementation of insulin therapy. Three randomized clinical trials suggest initiating insulin therapy irrespective of glucose levels if ultrasonographic measurement of fetal abdominal circumference exceeds the 75th percentile (Bonomo et al., 2004; Kjos et al., 2001; Rossi et al., 2000). The doses and types of insulin will not be discussed in this chapter.

5.2.4.2 Antihyperglycemic drugs

Oral hypoglycemic drugs are classically contraindicated in pregnancy. First generation drugs such as chlorpropamide and tolbutamide cross the placental barrier and may potentially cause prolonged and profound states of hypoglycemia, leading to fetal malformation. Nevertheless, the newer hypoglycemic drugs such as glibenclamide do not enter fetal circulation (Langer, 2007).

Furthermore, considering that in patients with gestational diabetes, the need for treatment initiates after embryogenesis (Langer, 2007), the newer oral hypoglycemic drugs were seen as a practical therapeutic option for this group of patients. Patient satisfaction with this route of administration may result in better compliance with treatment. Interest in evaluating these drugs as an option for the control of gestational diabetes has been intense and various randomized clinical trials using these agents have been published over the past ten years (Langer et al., 2000; Moore et al., 2010; Rowan et al., 2008).

In 2008, a systematic review was published that included a meta-analysis of all the clinical trials in which the use of insulin was compared with glibenclamide in women with gestational diabetes. Nine clinical trials were included involving 1,382 women with gestational diabetes. The use of glibenclamide was not found to be associated with any increased risk of macrosomia nor with differences in relation to fetal weight or the frequency of large-for-gestational-age infants, admission to the neonatal ICU or an increased risk of neonatal hypoglycemia. These findings suggest that there is no increased perinatal risk with the use of this drug; however, the effectiveness and safety of its use still need to be confirmed, since the majority of the studies included were not randomized (Moretti et al., 2008).

Another systematic review published by the Johns Hopkins University Evidence-Based Practice Center for the Agency for Healthcare Research and Quality evaluated oral hypoglycemic drugs in women with gestational diabetes. Nine studies were selected, four of which consisted of randomized clinical trials involving 1,229 participants, while five were observational studies involving 831 participants. Two clinical trials compared insulin with glibenclamide, while one compared glibenclamide with acarbose and another compared insulin with metformin. No statistically significant differences were found with respect to glycemic control, the weight of the newborn infant or in the rate of Cesarean sections when insulin was compared with glibenclamide. There was a greater proportion of newborn infants with hypoglycemia in the group that used insulin (8.1% versus 3.3%; $p = 0.008$). No statistically significant difference was found in the rate of congenital malformations when the pregnancies treated with insulin were compared with those treated with oral hypoglycemic drugs. The authors concluded that there are no substantial differences in maternal and neonatal outcomes between women with gestational diabetes using insulin and those using oral hypoglycemic drugs (glibenclamide and metformin) (Nicholson et al., 2009).

The most recent systematic review on oral hypoglycemic drugs for the treatment of gestational diabetes showed no difference either in glycemic control or in the outcome of pregnancy when insulin was compared with hypoglycemic drugs in six randomized clinical trials involving a total of 1,388 pregnant women. There was no increased risk of neonatal hypoglycemia, macrosomia or Cesarean section, and maternal glucose levels were similar (Dhulkotia et al., 2010).

Results with the use of glibenclamide for the treatment of gestational diabetes are encouraging and although the ADA and ACOG consensuses recommend not prescribing glibenclamide for women with gestational diabetes (ACOG, 2001; ADA 2004), it would appear that there is already sufficient and consistent evidence confirming its safety and effectiveness in this condition. Another issue to be evaluated with respect to glibenclamide is its cost, which is significantly lower compared to treatment with insulin (Melamed and Yogev, 2009). Nevertheless, the United States Food and Drug Administration (FDA) has not approved these drugs for this purpose.

5.2.5 Obstetric treatment

5.2.5.1 Evaluation of fetal vitality

Randomized clinical trials have yet to be conducted to evaluate the need for antenatal testing or the type of antenatal tests for the assessment of fetal well-being. Nonetheless, the fetuses of women with gestational diabetes, depending on glycemic control, may be at an increased risk of macrosomia (Durnwald et al., 2011) and intrauterine death (Yogev and Visser, 2009), and some observational studies have reported a reduction in the risk of fetal loss with various protocols for evaluating vitality (Graves, 2007; Kjos et al., 2005).

In 2001, the ACOG concluded that there is insufficient evidence to determine the ideal scheme for monitoring antepartum fetal vitality in women with gestational diabetes controlled by diet and in whom there are no additional perinatal risks (ACOG, 2001). The evaluation of fetal vitality in cases of gestational diabetes may include fetal biophysical profile and antepartum cardiotocography. Doppler blood flow measurement is not useful for evaluating fetal vitality in this context (Graves, 2007). The frequency with which these tests should be performed depends on the classification of diabetes and is not routinely recommended in cases controlled with diet (ACOG, 2001; Conway, 2007). In women who require insulin or antihyperglycemic drugs, it has been suggested that monitoring should be performed twice weekly beginning at 32 weeks (ACOG, 2001). The method of evaluating vitality and the periodicity of this evaluation, however, remains to be determined and varies in accordance with the protocol implemented in the service and the clinical situation (Conway, 2007).

5.2.5.2 Screening for fetal macrosomia

Macrosomia may be investigated by performing a single ultrasonography scan in the 36th week of pregnancy or by serial scans from 28 weeks onwards (Ben-Haroush et al., 2007). Nevertheless, the poor accuracy of ultrasonography for the prediction of fetal weight limits its use for this purpose (Wong et al., 2001). Based on specialist opinion, it has been suggested that fetal growth monitoring and the investigation of macrosomia is unnecessary in cases of gestational diabetes controlled by diet, principally because false-positive results may lead to unnecessary Cesarean sections (Melamed et al., 2010). Fetal weight estimated by ultrasonography would have to be ≥ 4,800 grams to have at least a 50% chance of predicting an infant being born with a birthweight of 4,500 kg or more (McLaren et al., 1995).

5.2.5.3 Anticipating delivery

Treatment of gestational diabetes may include anticipating delivery through induction or by elective Cesarean section. In a systematic review of the Cochrane Library, the policy of electively interrupting pregnancy by inducing labor in full-term diabetic women was evaluated (Boulvain et al., 2011). Only one study involving 200 women was included. Results showed that induction at 38 weeks reduced the frequency of newborn infants weighing > 4000 grams and above the 90th percentile, which is not surprising, since gestational age at delivery was lower in the induction group. This intervention, however, failed to reduce the risk of Cesarean section or of neonatal morbidities. Therefore, the authors concluded that further studies involving larger sample sizes are required in order to confirm the advantages of this intervention. Up to the present moment, there is insufficient evidence to enable this practice to be recommended.

More recently, a systematic review including five studies (the same clinical trial included in the Cochrane review plus four observational studies) compared active management at term (induction or Cesarean section) with expectant management. The results of the randomized clinical trial were similar to the findings of the previous systematic review. When the four observational studies were analyzed, however, a potential reduction was found in the rate of macrosomia, of shoulder dystocia in induced deliveries and in Cesarean sections indicated because of fetal macrosomia. The authors concluded that active management appears to reduce the rates of macrosomia and its complications; however, further clinical trials are clearly necessary to strengthen the evidence and support clinical practice (Witkop et al., 2009).

The ACOG suggests performing elective Cesarean sections as a means of reducing the risk of shoulder dystocia in cases of gestational diabetes when estimated fetal weight is ≥ 4,500 grams (ACOG, 2001). In diabetic pregnant women in whom estimated fetal weight is below 4,000 grams, Cesarean section is unjustified on the basis of fetal weight alone (Hawkins and Casey, 2007). On the other hand, the management of cases in which estimated fetal weight is between 4,000 and 4,500 grams remains controversial. In addition to estimated fetal weight, the size of the mother's pelvis and the progression of labor should also be taken into consideration when deciding on the type of delivery (Hawkins and Casey, 2007). It should also be noted that the limited accuracy of ultrasonography for adequately estimating fetal weight leads to unnecessary Cesarean sections because of the suspicion of macrosomia (Chauhan et al., 2005).

In the absence of macrosomia, specialists suggest that patients with gestational diabetes controlled by diet may be able to reach 40/41 weeks and recommend induction at this gestational age. In patients in use of insulin or oral antihyperglycemic drugs, labor should be induced at 39 weeks. In diabetic patients in use of insulin or those in whom glycemic control is poor, labor should be induced at 38 weeks and even prior to this gestational age if there are associated conditions such as severe preeclampsia, for example, or if fetal well-being is compromised. There is no need for amniocentesis to evaluate fetal lung maturity in patients after 38 weeks of pregnancy when gestational age is well documented (Conway et al., 2007; Nicholson et al., 2008).

6. Conclusions

The most recent evidence suggests that screening for gestational diabetes is beneficial; however, the best screening strategy remains to be defined. Clinical trials also need to be conducted to compare various diagnostic tests and glucose levels; however, until these studies are performed, clinicians and societies have to define their own protocols for screening and diagnosis taking the characteristics of the population to be screened into consideration. In populations with a high risk for diabetes and consequently for macrosomia, a universal screening policy leads to a significant reduction in perinatal morbidity.

With respect to treatment, although the Cochrane systematic review found only modest benefits with treatment, more recent randomized clinical trials suggest an improvement in perinatal outcome. Based on specialist opinion, initial dietetic therapy is recommended, with pharmacological treatment indicated when diet alone fails to control glucose levels. Despite recent evidence that treatment with antihyperglycemic drugs may represent a safe, reliable alternative for the pharmacological treatment of diabetes in pregnancy, the ADA and other guidelines continue recommending insulin therapy as standard treatment. There is insufficient evidence either to indicate or contraindicate exercise in women with gestational diabetes.

The types of tests and the ideal frequency at which fetal well-being should be monitored are factors that are yet to be determined; however, they are unnecessary in cases in which glucose levels are controlled by diet. In addition, there is insufficient evidence to recommend ultrasonography for the prediction of macrosomia and scans should not be performed routinely for this purpose in pregnant women on dietetic therapy in whom glucose levels are under control.

With respect to delivery, elective Cesarean sections are recommended by ACOG in the case of fetuses over 4,500 grams. In cases of gestational diabetes controlled by diet, it is possible to wait for spontaneous labor to occur up to a limit of 40/41 weeks. In patients in use of insulin or oral hypoglycemic drugs, labor should be induced at 39 weeks. In cases in which glucose control is poor, delivery should be anticipated at 38 weeks or earlier if fetal well-being is compromised or there are other associated morbid conditions.

7. References

Aberg, A., Rydhstroem, H., Frid, A. Impaired glucose tolerance associated with adverse pregnancy outcome: a population-based study in southern Sweden. *Am J Obstet Gynecol.* 2001 Jan; 184:77-83.

Alwan, N., Tuffnell, D.J., West, J. Treatments for gestational diabetes. Cochrane Database of Systematic Reviews. In: *The Cochrane Library,* Issue 04, 2011, Art. No. CD003395. DOI: 10.1002/14651858.CD003395.pub3

American College of Obstetricians and Gynecologists Committee on Practice Bulletins—Obstetrics. ACOG Practice Bulletin. Clinical management guidelines for obstetrician-gynecologists. Number 30, September 2001. Gestational diabetes. *Obstet Gynecol* 2001; 98: 525-38.

American Diabetes Association. Gestational diabetes mellitus. *Diabetes Care* 2004 Jan; 27 Suppl 1: S88-90.

Ben-Haroush, A., Chen, R., Hadar, E., Hod, M., Yogev, Y. Accuracy of a single fetal weight estimation at 29-34 weeks in diabetic pregnancies: can it predict large-for-gestational-age infants at term? *Am J Obstet Gynecol* 2007 Nov; 197:497.e1-6.

Bonomo, M., Cetin, I., Pisoni, M.P., Faden, D., Mion, E., Taricco, E., et al. Flexible treatment of gestational diabetes modulated on ultrasound evaluation of intrauterine growth: a controlled randomized clinical trial. *Diabetes Metab* 2004 Jun; 30: 237-44.

Boulvain, M., Stan, C.M., Irion, O. Elective delivery in diabetic pregnant women. Cochrane Database of Systematic Reviews. In: *The Cochrane Library,* Issue 04, 2011, Art. No. CD001997. DOI: 10.1002/14651858.CD001997.pub1

Brody, S.C., Harris, R., Lohr, K. Screening for gestational diabetes: a summary of the evidence for the U.S. Preventive Services Task Force. *Obstet Gynecol.* 2003 Feb; 101:380-92

Buchanan, A.T., Kjos, L.S.: Gestational diabetes: Risk or myth? *J Clin Endocrinol Metab* 1999 Jun; 84: 854-7.

Carpenter, M.W., Coustan, D.R.B. Criteria for screening tests for gestational diabetes. *Am J Obstet Gynecol* 1982 Jun; 144:768-73

Catalano, P.M. Obesity, insulin resistance, and pregnancy outcome. *Reproduction.* 2010 May; 140: 365-71.

Ceysens, G., Rouiller, D., Boulvain, M. Exercise for diabetic pregnant women. Cochrane Database of Systematic Reviews. In: *The Cochrane Library,* Issue 04, 2011, Art. No. CD004225. DOI: 10.1002/14651858.CD004225.pub3

Chandler-Laney, P.C., Bush, N.C., Rouse, D.J., Mancuso, M.S., Gower, B.A. Maternal glucose concentration during pregnancy predicts fat and lean mass of prepubertal offspring. *Diabetes Care.* 2011 Mar; 34:741-5.

Chauhan, S.P., Grobman, W.A., Gherman, R.A., Chauhan, V.B., Chang, G., Magann, E.F., Hendrix, N.W. Suspicion and treatment of the macrosomic fetus: a review. *Am J Obstet Gynecol* 2005 Aug; 193: 332-46.

Cheng, Y.W., Chung, J.H., Kurbisch-Block, I., Inturrisi, M., Shafer, S., Caughey, A.B. Gestational weight gain and gestational diabetes mellitus: perinatal outcomes. *Obstet Gynecol* 2008 Nov; 112: 1015-22.

Colberg, S.R., Sigal, R.J., Fernhall, B., Regensteiner, J.G., Blissmer, B.J., Rubin, R.R., Chasan-Taber, L., Albright, A.L., Braun, B.; American College of Sports Medicine; American Diabetes Association. Exercise and type 2 diabetes: the American College of Sports Medicine and the American Diabetes Association: Joint Position Statement. *Diabetes Care* 2010 Dec; 33: e147-67.

Conway, D.L. Obstetric management in gestational diabetes. *Diabetes Care* 2007 Jul; 30 Suppl 2: S175-9.

Crowther, C.A., Hiller, J.E., Moss , J.R., McPhee, A.J., Jeffries, W.S., Robinson, J.S.; Australian Carbohydrate Intolerance Study in Pregnant Women (ACHOIS) Trial Group. Effect of treatment of gestational diabetes mellitus on pregnancy outcomes. *N Engl J Med* 2005 Jun; 352: 2477-86.

de Veciana, M., Major, C.A., Morgan, M.A., Asrat, T., Toohey, J.S., Lien, J.M., Evans, A.T. Postprandial versus preprandial blood glucose monitoring in women with gestational diabetes mellitus requiring insulin therapy. *N Engl J Med* 1995 Nov; 333:1237-41.

Dhulkotia, J.S., Ola, B., Fraser, R., Farrell, T. Oral hypoglycemic agents vs insulin in management of gestational diabetes: a systematic review and metaanalysis. *Am J Obstet Gynecol* 2010 Nov; 203: 457.e1-9.

Durnwald, C.P., Mele, L., Spong, C.Y., Ramin, S.M., Varner, M.W., Rouse, D.J. et al. for the Eunice Kennedy Shriver National Institute of Child Health and Human Development (NICHD) Maternal-Fetal Medicine Units Network (MFMU). Glycemic Characteristics and Neonatal Outcomes of Women Treated for Mild Gestational Diabetes. *Obstet Gynecol* 2011 Apr; 117: 819-27.

Fall, C. Maternal nutrition: effects on health in the next generation. *Indian J Med Res.* 2009 Nov;130: 593-9.

Graves, C.R. Antepartum fetal surveillance and timing of delivery in the pregnancy complicated by diabetes mellitus. Clin *Obstet Gynecol* 2007 Dec; 50: 1007-13.

HAPO Study Cooperative Research Group. Hyperglycemia and adverse pregnancy outcomes. *N Engl J Med 2008* May; 358: 1991-2002.

Hawkins, J.S., Casey, B.M. Labor and delivery management for women with diabetes. *Obstet Gynecol Clin North Am* 2007 Jun; 34:323-34.

Hawkins, J.S., Casey, B.M., Lo, J.Y., Moss, K., McIntire, D.D., Leveno, K.J. Weekly compared with daily blood glucose monitoring in women with diet-treated gestational diabetes. *Obstet Gynecol* 2009 Jun; 113:1307-12.

Hawkins, J.S. Glucose Monitoring During Pregnancy. *Curr Diab Rep* 2010 Jun; 10: 229–34.

Holt, R.I., Coleman, M.A., McCance, D.R. The implications of the new International Association of Diabetes and Pregnancy Study Groups (IADPSG) diagnostic criteria for gestational diabetes. *Diabet Med.* 2011 Apr; 28: 382-5.

Horvath, K., Koch, K., Jeitler, K., Matyas, E., Bender, R., Bastian, H., Lange, S., Siebenhofer, A. Effects of treatment in women with gestational diabetes mellitus: systematic review and meta-analysis. *BMJ* 2010 Apr; 340: c1395.

International Association of Diabetes and Pregnancy Study Groups. International Association of Diabetes and Pregnancy Study Groups recommendations on the diagnosis and classification of hyperglycemia in pregnancy. *Diabetes Care* 2010 Mar; 33: 676–82.

Jensen, D.M., Damm, P., Sørensen, B., Mølsted-Pedersen, L., Westergaard, J.G., Klebe, J., Beck-Nielsen, H. Clinical impact of mild carbohydrate intolerance in pregnancy: a study of 2904 nondiabetic Danish women with risk factors for gestational diabetes mellitus. *Am J Obstet Gynecol*. 2001 Aug; 185:413-9.

Jovanovic, L.G. Using meal-based self-monitoring of blood glucose as a tool to improve outcomes in pregnancy complicated by diabetes. *Endocr Pract* 2008 Mar; 14: 239-47.

Kjos, S.L., Leung, A., Henry, O.A., Victor, M.R., Paul, R.H., Medearis, A.L. Antepartum surveillance in diabetic pregnancies: predictors of fetal distress in labor. *Am J Obstet Gynecol* 1995 Nov; 173: 1532-9.

Kjos, S.L., Schaefer-Graf, U., Sardesi, S., Peters, R.K., Buley, A., Xiang, A.H., et al. A randomized controlled trial using glycemic plus fetal ultrasound parameters versus glycemic parameters to determine insulin therapy in gestational diabetes with fasting hyperglycemia. *Diabetes Care* 2001 Nov; 24: 1904-10.

Langer, O., Brustman, L., Anyaegbunam, A., Mazze, R. The significance of one abnormal glucose tolerance test value on adverse outcome in pregnancy. *Am J Obstet Gynecol* 1987 Sep; 157:758-63.

Langer, O., Conway, D.L., Berkus, M.D., Xenakis, E.M., Gonzales, O. A comparison of glyburide and insulin in women with gestational diabetes mellitus. *N Engl J Med* 2000 Oct; 343: 1134-8.

Langer, O., Yogev, Y., Most, O., Xenakis, E.M. Gestational diabetes: the consequences of not treating. *Am J Obstet Gynecol* 2005 Apr; 192: 989-97.

Langer O. From educated guess to accepted practice: the use of oral antidiabetic agents in pregnancy. *Clin Obstet Gynecol* 2007 Dec; 50: 959-71.

Landon, M.B., Spong, C.Y., Thom, E., Carpenter, M.W., Ramin, S.M., Casey, B. et al. A multicenter, randomized trial of treatment for mild gestational diabetes. *N Engl J Med* 2009 Oct; 361: 1339-48.

Lawlor, D.A., Lichtenstein, P., Långström, N. Association of maternal diabetes mellitus in pregnancy with offspring adiposity into early adulthood: sibling study in a prospective cohort of 280,866 men from 248,293 families. *Circulation.* 2011 Jan;123:258-65.

Leary, J., Pettitt, D.J., Jovanovic, L. Gestational diabetes guidelines in a HAPO world. *Best Pract Res Clin Endocrinol Metab* 2010 Aug; 24: 673-85.

Lucas, M.J., Lowe, T.W., Bowe, L., McIntire, D.D. Class A1 gestational diabetes: a meaningful diagnosis? *Obstet Gynecol* 1993 Aug; 82:260-5.

Melamed, N., Yogev, Y. Can pregnant diabetics be treated with glyburide? *Womens Health* (Lond Engl) 2009 Nov; 5: 649-58.

Melamed, N., Yogev, Y., Meizner, I., Mashiach, R., Ben-Haroush, A. Sonographic prediction of fetal macrosomia: the consequences of false diagnosis. *J Ultrasound Med* 2010 Feb; 29: 225-30.

Metzger, B.E., Buchanan, T.A., Coustan, D.R., de Leiva, A., Dunger, D.B., Hadden, D.R., Hod, M., Kitzmiller, J.L., Kjos, S.L., Oats, J.N., Pettitt, D.J., Sacks, D.A., Zoupas, C. Summary and recommendations of the Fifth International Workshop-Conference on Gestational Diabetes Mellitus. *Diabetes Care.* 2007 Jul;30 Suppl 2:S251-60.

Metzger, B.E., Gabbe, S.G., Persson, B., Buchanan, T.A., Catalano, P.A., Damm, P. *et al.* International association of diabetes and pregnancy study groups recommendations on the diagnosis and classification of hyperglycemia in pregnancy. *Diabetes Care* 2010 Mar; 33: 676–82.

Moore, L.E., Clokey, D., Rappaport, V.J., Curet, L.B. Metformin compared with glyburide in gestational diabetes: a randomized controlled trial. *Obstet Gynecol* 2010 Jan; 115: 55-9.

Moretti, M.E., Rezvani, M., Koren, G. Safety of glyburide for gestational diabetes: a meta-analysis of pregnancy outcomes. *Ann Pharmacother* 2008 Apr; 42: 483-90.

National Diabetes Data Group: Classification and diagnosis of diabetes mellitus and other categories of glucose intolerance. *Diabetes* 1979; 28: 1039-1057,

Naylor, C.D. Diagnosing Gestational Diabetes mellitus. Is the Gold Standard Valid? *Diabetes Care* 1989 Sep; 12: 565-72.

Nicholson, W.K., Wilson, L.M., Witkop, C.T., Baptiste-Roberts, K., Bennett, W.L., Bolen, S. et al. Therapeutic management, delivery, and postpartum risk assessment and screening in gestational diabetes. *Evid Rep Technol Assess* (Full Rep) 2008 Mar; 162:1-96.

Nicholson, W., Bolen, S., Witkop, C.T., Neale, D., Wilson, L., Bass, E. Benefits and risks of oral diabetes agents compared with insulin in women with gestational diabetes: a systematic review. *Obstet Gynecol* 2009 Jan; 113: 193-205.

O'Sullivan, J.B., Mahan, C.M.: Criteria for the oral glucose tolerance test in pregnancy. *Diabetes* 1964 May-Jun; 13:278-85.
O'Sullivan, J.B., Gellis, S.S., Dandrow, R.V., Tenney, B.O. The potential diabetic and her treatment during pregnancy. *Obstet Gynecol* 1966 May; 27:683-9
O'Sullivan, J.B., Charles, D., Mahan, C.M., Dandrow, R.V. Gestational diabetes and perinatal mortality rates. *Am J Obstet Gynecol* 1973 Aug; 116:901-4
Pridjian, G., Benjamin, T.D. Update on gestational diabetes. *Obstet Gynecol Clin North Am* 2010 Jun; 37: 255-67.
Rossi, G., Somigliana, E., Moschetta, M., Bottani, B., Barbieri, M., Vignali, M. Adequate timing of fetal ultrasound to guide metabolic therapy in mild gestational diabetes mellitus. Results from a randomized study. *Acta Obstet Gynecol Scand* 2000 Aug; 79: 649-54.
Rowan, J.A., Hague, W.M., Gao, W., Battin, M.R., Moore, M.P; MiG Trial Investigators. Metformin versus insulin for the treatment of gestational diabetes. *N Engl J Med* 2008 May; 358: 2003-15.
Rudge, M.V.C., Peraçoli, J.C., Berezowski, A.T., Calderon, I.M., Brasil, M.A.M. The oral glucose tolerance test is a poor predictor of hyperglycemia during pregnancy. *Braz J Med Biol Res* 1990; 23:1079-89.
Sermer, M., Naylor, D.C., Gare, D.J., Kenshole, A.B., Ritchie, J.W.K., Farine, D., Cohen, H.R., McArthur, K., Holzapfel, S., Biringer, A., Chen, E. Impact of increasing carbohydrate intolerance on maternal-fetal outcomes in 3637 women without gestational diabetes. *Am J Obstet Gynecol* 1995 Jul; 173: 146-56.
Tieu, J., Middleton, P., McPhee, A.J., Crowther, C.A. Screening and subsequent management for gestational diabetes for improving maternal and infant health. Cochrane Database of Systematic Reviews. In: *The Cochrane Library*, Issue 04, 2011, Art. No. CD007222. DOI: 10.1002/14651858.CD007222.pub7
Torloni, M.R., Betrán, A.P., Horta, B.L., Nakamura, M.U., Atallah, A.N., Moron, A.F., Valente, O. Prepregnancy BMI and the risk of gestational diabetes: a systematic review of the literature with meta-analysis. *Obes Rev.* 2009 Mar; 10: 194-203.
Walkinshaw, S.A. Dietary regulation for 'gestational diabetes'. Cochrane Database of Systematic Reviews. In: *The Cochrane Library*, Issue 04, 2011, Art. No. CD000070. DOI: 10.1002/14651858.CD000070.pub3
Weisz, B., Shrim, A., Homko, C.J., Schiff, E., Epstein, G.S., Sivan, E. One hour versus two hours postprandial glucose measurement in gestational diabetes: a prospective study. *J Perinatol* 2005 Apr; 25: 241-4.
WHO Expert Committee on Diabetes Mellitus. second report. WHO Technical Report Series, 1980; 646: 1-80.
World Health Organization. Definition, diagnosis, and classification of diabetes mellitus and its complications: report of a WHO consultation. Geneva: WHO document Production Services, 1999. pp 19-20.
Witkop, C.T., Neale, D., Wilson, L.M., Bass, E.B., Nicholson, W.K. Active compared with expectant delivery management in women with gestational diabetes: a systematic review. *Obstet Gynecol* 2009 Jan; 113: 206-17.
Wong, S.F., Chan, F.Y., Cincotta, R.B., Oats, J.J., McIntyre, H.D. Sonographic estimation of fetal weight in macrosomic fetuses: diabetic versus non-diabetic pregnancies. *Aust N Z J Obstet Gynaecol* 2001 Nov; 41: 429-32.
Yogev, Y., Visser, G.H. Obesity, gestational diabetes and pregnancy outcome. *Semin Fetal Neonatal Med* 2009 Apr; 14:77-84.

4

Validity of Fasting Blood Glucose Test in Screening for the Pre-Diabetes State Among Pregnant Females

Mostafa A Abolfotouh and Mohammed A Al-Rowaily
King Saud Bin-Abdulaziz University for Health Sciences, Riyadh, Saudi Arabia

1. Introduction

Gestational diabetes mellitus (GDM) is defined as carbohydrate intolerance of varying degrees of severity with onset or first recognition during pregnancy (Metzer & Coustan, 1998). Glucose tolerance deteriorates in human pregnancy, but about 97% to 98% of all pregnant women retain a normal glucose tolerance and only 2% to 3% develops GDM (Kuhl, 1991). However, failure to diagnose and treat GDM will result in increased morbidity in some pregnancies, while an aggressive approach to diagnosis and treatment may result in unnecessary intervention in others (Kjos & Buchanan, 1999).

The prevalence of GDM ranges from 1% to 14% of all pregnancies, depending on the population studied and the diagnostic tests and criteria employed (World Health Organization [WHO], 1985). In a recent study by Al-Rowaily and Abolfotouh in Riyadh, Saudi Arabia, the prevalence of GDM was 12.5% and 3.8% by the WHO and American Diabetes Association criteria respectively (Al-Rowaily & Abolfotouh, 2010). The appropriateness of these different diagnostic criteria has been debated (Gabir et al., 2000); nevertheless women meeting the definition for GDM by either set of criteria are at greater risk of complications than women without the diagnosis.

The 75-g glucose load has been the international standard for the diagnosis of diabetes in nonpregnant adults for several decades. This oral glucose tolerance test (OGTT) identifies pregnant women who are at risk of pre-eclampsia and whose babies are at risk of macrosomia and perinatal mortality (Schmidt et al., 2001). Although the American Diabetes Association (ADA) still recommends a 3-h 100-g OGTT for the diagnosis of GDM, it has recently included in its recommendations the use of a 2-h 75-g OGTT (American Diabetes Association [ADA], 2000; Metzger & Coustan, 1998).

A recent WHO panel, although in general maintaining previous diagnostic recommendations, now characterizes GDM as the joint category of diabetes and impaired glucose tolerance (fasting glucose ≥ 7.0 mmol/L or 2-h glucose ≥ 7.8mmol/L (WHO, 1999).

At present, screening for gestational diabetes appears to be hampered by the lack of a clear definition, agreed diagnostic criteria and evidence to show that intervention and treatment for this condition leads to improved outcomes for the mother and fetus. Although fasting plasma glucose and Glucose Challenge Test (GCT) have the highest reported sensitivities and specificities in the literature, there also exists considerable debate about which screening test should be used if there is to be screening. A continuum of risk for GDM should be researched and risk of adverse pregnancy outcomes clarified on such a continuum. This would help to form the basis for diagnosis. The most appropriate strategies for screening, diagnosing and managing asymptomatic GDM remain controversial (Moody, 2003).

The pregnant females who attend the antenatal clinic of King Abdulaziz Medical City at the National Guard Health Affairs (usually between 24-28 weeks of gestation) are prepared for the test by fasting for a minimum of 8 hrs. After that, a fasting sample is analyzed for glucose. Then, every pregnant female is subjected to the Glucose Challenge Test (GCT) by being given 75-g Glucose solution [named *Glucola* which is a chilled glucose syrup with 75-g of glucose with orange flavor], and another blood sample is collected 2 hours after the drink (Berger et al., 2002). The diagnosis of GDM is based upon the results of both the fasting sample and the 2hr-glucose challenge test.

Although GCT showed good sensitivity and specificity in a previous study (79% and 87% respectively), yet it has been observed that with *Glucola* drink, there is always a tendency for the pregnant female to vomit (O'Sullivan et al., 1973). This usually leads to non-compliance with the glucose challenge test by most of the pregnant females. Thus, the aim of the present study was to determine the threshold value of fasting blood sugar that suggests the pre-diabetes status that needs further investigations including the GCT.

2. Methods

All pregnant females who attended the antenatal clinic of King Fahd Hospital at Riyadh National Guard Health Affairs during the period from July, 2005 to July, 2006 for the first time (n=769) constituted the target of the present study. For all respondents to the GCT (n=408,53.1%), all values of the fasting blood sugar were cross classified according to their status by the GCT, and by various cut-off points along the range of FBS values above which subjects may be considered having Impaired Glucose Tolerance (IGT) by the GCT(≥ 7.8mmol/L) result. From these tabulations, the sensitivity, specificity and positive predictive value were computed for Fasting Blood Sugar (FBS) at each cut of point.

The sensitivity of FBS diagnosis for the GCT diagnosis "gold standard" was determined by calculating how frequent the correct FBS diagnosis was made in each GCT diagnosis. The specificity of FBS diagnosis was determined by calculating how frequently the FBS diagnosis was not made when the corresponding GCT diagnosis was not present. Positive predictability indicated how frequently the FBS diagnosis was not made when the corresponding GCT diagnosis was not present. Positive predictability indicated how frequently the FBS diagnosis correctly reflected the GCT diagnosis. Also, the level of agreement between these two methods was determined at each cut-off point by the calculation of kappa coefficient (k).

The Receiver Operating Characteristic (ROC) curve of a diagnostic test is a graph of the pairs of sensitivity and 1 minus specificity that correspond to each possible cut-off for the diagnostic test result (Richardson et al., 1993). This curve was used to determine the threshold value of FBS that correspond to the value of 7.8mmol/L by the GCT. The Statistical Package for the Social Sciences (SPSS) software program version 17 was used for all statistical analyses.

3. Results

Based on the cut-off values recommended by the American Diabetic Association (ADA, 2010) for diagnosis of GDM, the results of fasting blood sugar for 769 pregnant females showed that 17.2% had Impaired Fasting Tolerance (IFT) and 1.4% had provisional diagnosis of GDM. The corresponding results for those who responded to the GCT, are 15.2% IGT and 1.2% provisional diagnosis of GDM (Table 1), although the results of these two tests were seen to be comparable, yet the agreement level, as tested by kappa, was low. (Table 2)

Category		No	%
Fasting Blood Glucose [N=769]			
Normal	[<100mg/dl(<5.6mmol/L)]	626	81.4
Impaired fasting tolerance	[100-125mg/dl(5.6-6.9mmol/L)]	133	17.2
Provisional diagnosis of GDM	[≥126mg/dl(7mmol/L)]	10	1.4
Glucose Challenge Test (2 hr after 75-g glucose drink) [N=408]			
Normal [<140mg/dl(<7.8mmol/L)]		341	83.6
Impaired glucose tolerance [140-199mg/dl (7.8-11mmol/L)]		62	15.2
Provisional diagnosis of GDM [≥ 200mg/dl (11.1mmol/L)]		5	1.2

Table 1. Distribution of pregnant females according to their results of fasting blood glucose and glucose challenge tests based on the ADA classification (ADA, 2010).

Fasting Blood Glucose	Glucose Challenge Test					
	Normal		IGT		Provisional GDM	
	No.	%	No.	%	No.	%
Normal	279	84.8	47	14.3	3	0.9
IFT	59	78.7	14	18.7	2	2.7
Provisional GDM	3	75.0	1	25.0	-	-

K = 0.054, p=0.25

Table 2. Association between the results of Fasting blood sugar and Glucose challenge test among pregnant females at the National Guard Hospital.

Figure 1 shows the scatter plot for the values and the correlation between the values obtained by the fasting blood glucose and those obtained by the 2hr-glucose challenge test. The correlation coefficient (*r*) was 0.25 (t-value = 5.24, p<0.0001) indicating a highly significant direct correlation between the values of blood sugar by the two methods. The linear regression equation was: y= 0.66 x + 2.98, where y is the result of the glucose challenge test, and x is the result of fasting blood sugar testing.

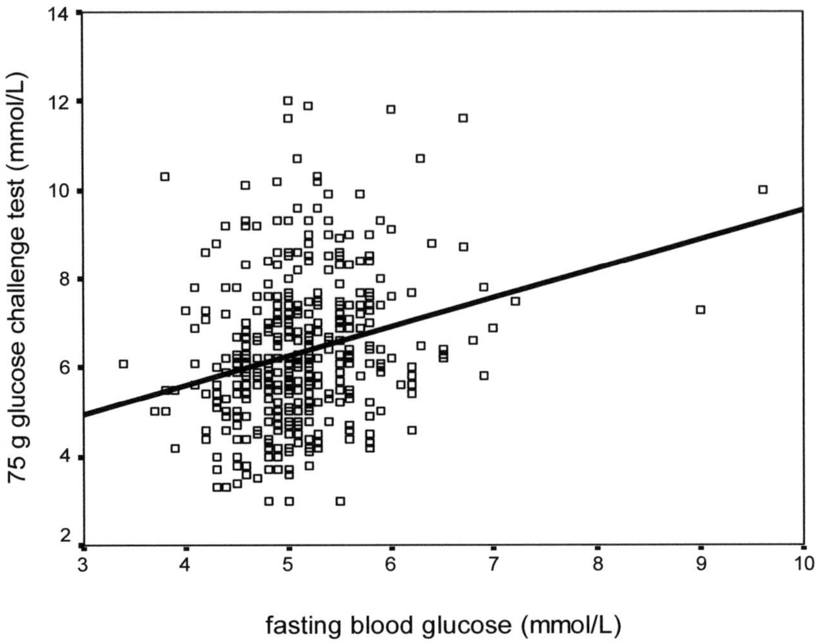

Fig. 1. Correlation between fasting blood glucose and 75g-2hr glucose challenge test. Solid line represents the linear regression line (y= 0.66 x + 2.98)

Table 3 shows an example for the measurements of all terms used in evaluating the fasting blood glucose test based on the studied data. In this example, a measurement of ≥5.1mmol/L by the fasting blood glucose test was considered a cut-off point at which subjects having that measurement or above was labeled to have pre-diabetes status by the FBS test result. At this particular cut-off level, it is noted that the sensitivity of the test was 0.64, specificity was 0.53 and the false positive rate (1- specificity) was 0.21.

True Pre-diabetic by GCT	FBS test result		Row total
	≥5.1 mmol/L (Pre-diabetic)	< 5.1 mmol/L (non-prediabetic)	
Pre-diabetic-yes (≥7.8mmol/L)	43	24	67
Pre-diabetic - no (<7.8mmol/L)	161	180	341
Column total	204	204	408

Sensitivity = 43/67 = 0.64
Specificity = 180/341 = 0.53
Positive predictive value = 43/204 = 0.21
False positive rate= 1 - specificity = 1 - 0.53 = 0.47

Table 3. 2x2 classification of 408 pregnant females by "true pre-diabetes" status and by a cut-off point ≥5.1 mmol/L for the fasting blood glucose test as one diagnostic criterion.

Computations for sensitivity and specificity were made for all cut-off levels along the range of values of the fasting blood glucose test. The resulting values for sensitivity were plotted against the corresponding values of (1 - specificity) to obtain the receiver operating characteristic curve as shown in. (Figure 2)

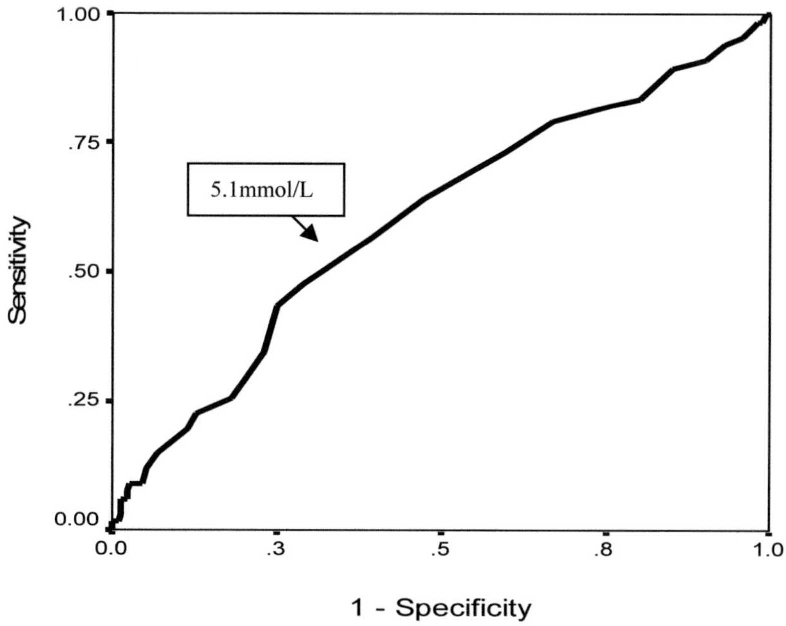

Fig. 2. Receiver operating characteristic curve of fasting blood glucose measurements at the value of 7.8mmol/L for the glucose challenge test. The optimal threshold value of 5.1mmol/L for fasting blood glucose test is marked with the arrow.

As mentioned earlier, the point on the curve that was closest to the upper left hand corner would be the optimum trade-off level for the test. The figure shows that point corresponding to ≥5.1 mmol/L. At this cut-off level, the test had a sensitivity = 0.64 and a specificity = 0.53. The computed positive predictive value was 0.21. Thus, at this cut-off level, the test correctly diagnosed 64% of the true pre-diabetics, missed 36% of these pre-diabetics, but misclassified 47% of normal (of low risk for GDM) pregnant females as pre-diabetics (false positives). The Area Under the Curve was reasonable (AUC=0.60). At this cut-off level, the level of agreement between the fasting blood glucose levels and those of glucose challenge test, as calculated by kappa coefficient is significant (k=0.093, p=0.011). If the sensitivity is to be increased, the cut-off level should be lowered, but it will be at the expense of specificity. For example, at a cut of 4.7 mmol/L (85mg/dl) only 16% of the true pre-diabetics would be misclassified as normal, but on the other hand, 80% of normal females would be misclassified as pre-diabetics(false positives).

4. Discussion

GDM is an asymptomatic condition most of the time, and effectiveness of its detection has not been adequately tested. Based on the American Diabetic Association criteria for

diagnosis of GDM, 17.2% of the studied pregnant females had impaired fasting tolerance (IFT) and 1.4% had provisional diagnosis of GDM. The corresponding results for those who responded to the GCT are 15.2% IGT and 1.2% provisional diagnosis of GDM. These figures are suggestive of the necessity for screening for GDM in our community. They are comparable with the figures of other nearby countries (Al-Mahroos et al., 2005), but still higher than those of the western countries (Naylor et al., 1996; Tsutomu et al., 2002).
Diagnostic levels for GDM remain uncertain. The guidelines present a confusing picture as regards screening tests for GDM. The use of a 4.7 mmol/L (85mg/dl) cut-off for fasting plasma glucose is suggested by some researchers, but others have suggested higher cut-offs (IDF, 2006). Fasting glucose may not be the most appropriate measure however, and the 75g glucose challenge test advocated by the WHO is increasingly used internationally (IDF, 2006).
The aim of the present study was to determine the threshold value of fasting blood glucose for which further testing by the 2hr-glucose challenge test is needed to confirm the pre-diabetic status among pregnant females attending the antenatal clinics of the King Fahd hospital at the National Guard in Riyadh city, Saudi Arabia.. Of all pregnant females subjected to the fasting blood glucose testing (n=769), only 408 subjects (53%) complied with the 2hr-glucose challenge test, a finding that may reflect the need for specifying the feasible indication for such GCT, so as not to subject all females for an unnecessary as well as unacceptable test.
The figures of the pre-diabetes by both the fasting blood glucose test (17.2%) and the GCT (15.2%) are nearly comparable, based on the cut-off points recommended by the American Diabetic Association (ADA, 2010). Correlation between the individual values of fasting blood glucose testing and those of 2hr-glucose challenge testing was highly significant ($r=0.25, p<0.0001$).However, the agreement between the categorical results of both tests (in terms of pre-diabetes, provisional GDM, and normal) was low as calculated by the kappa coefficient ($k=0.054, p=0.25$). This finding reflect the fact that the cut-off value of 5.6mmol/L for fasting blood glucose test is not the threshold value for the pre-diabetes status, especially when we see that out of those with impaired fasting test, only 18.7 were found with IGT by the GCT. (Table 2)
Thus, this suboptimal accuracy of the cut-off level of 5.6mmol/L will result in the misclassification of subjects. To overcome this problem to a great extent, the receiver operating characteristic curve analysis was used to determine the threshold value of fasting blood glucose. Based on the previously reported high sensitivity and specificity of the GCT (O'Sullivan et al., 1973), it was considered as a gold standard (in detection of the pre-diabetic status) against which to test the validity of different values of fasting blood glucose test. The levels of sensitivity and specificity found in this study for the cut-off value of 5.1mmol/L for fasting blood glucose (64% and 53%) might not suggest the use of this test, especially that in Brazil, examining a range of thresholds, maximum sensitivity (88%) and specificity (78%) was found at 4.9mmol/L (O'Sullivan et al., 1973).
However, in the present study, at this cut-off level of 4.9mmol/L, in spite of the high sensitivity (82%), very low and unacceptable specificity (24%) was attained. Thus, the cut-off level of 5.1mmol/L could be potentially useful. At this level, of all pregnant females subjected to the fasting blood glucose test, only 50% would be tested by the GCT. This may result in better compliance to the GCT. Moreover, if women with clinical characteristics consistent with a high risk of GDM (marked obesity, personal history of GDM, glycosuria, or a strong family history of diabetes) would be considered as the target group for screening (ADA, 2006 &

Dornhorst and Rossi, 1998), this perhaps will increase the validity of the fasting blood glucose threshold value of 5.1mmol/L.

5. Conclusion

From the collective findings of this study, and considering its limitations in terms of testing the validity of fasting blood glucose in defining the pre-diabetics and not the diabetics, it is concluded that the results may be considered preliminary and suggestive for potential validity of advantage of fasting blood glucose test at the specified cut-off point. This strategy allowed 50% of the study population to avoid the glucose challenge test altogether without compromising detection rates. Women with a cut-off value of fasting blood glucose below the threshold of 5.1mmol/L may not need to be subjected to further testing by the GCT. Also, a special consideration to women with high risk for GDM will improve the validity of this threshold, and thus, the unnecessary GCT will be avoided.

6. Acknowledgement

This project was approved by the institutional review board of King Abdulaziz Medical City, National Guard Health Affairs, Riyadh, Saudi Arabia. The authors would like to express their gratitude and thanks to the staff members of King Abdullah International Medical Research Center (KAIMRC) for their constructive support throughout the study. Special thanks to Mr. Mahmoud Salam, the research coordinator in the center, for his efforts in formatting the text in accordance with the requirements of the InTech -MS instructions.

7. References

Al-Mahroos, S., Nagalla, DS., Yousif, W., & Sanad, H. (2005). A population-based screening for gestational diabetes mellitus in non-diabetic women in Bahrain. *Ann Saudi Med,* Vol 25, pp. 29-33, ISSN 0256-4947

Al-Rowaily, MA. & Abolfotouh MA (2010). Predictors of gestational diabetes in a high-parity community in Saudi Arabia. *Eastern Mediterranean Health Journal.* Vol 16, pp. 636-641, PMID 20799591

American Diabetes Association (2000). *Gestational diabetes mellitus. Diabetes Care* 23 (Suppl.1) pp. S77–S79, PMID 12017686

American Diabetes Association (2010). *Diagnosis and classification of Diabetes Mellitus.* Retrieved from: http://care.diabetesjournals.org/content/29/suppl_1/s43.full

Berger, H., Crane, J. & Farine, D. (2002). Screening for gestational diabetes mellitus. *American Journal of Obstetrics and Gynecology,* Vol. 24(11), pp. 894-912, PMID 12417905

Dornhorst, A. & Rossi, M. (1998). Risk and prevention of type 2 diabetes in women with gestational diabetes. *Diabetes Care,* Vol. 21(2), pp. 43-49, ISSN 0149-5992

World Health Organization (1985). Diabetes mellitus report of a study group. *WHO Technical Report Series,* Geneva (No. 727), PMID 3934850

Gabir, MM. et al. (2000). The 1997 American Diabetes Association and 1999 World Health Organization criteria for hyperglycemia in the diagnosis and prediction of diabetes. *Diabetes care.* Vol. 23(8), pp. 1108-1112, ISSN 0149-5992

IDF (2006). A digest of the global guideline for type 2 diabetes. *Diabetes voice* (Supplement), Vol. 51, pp. 32-35, ISBN 2-930229-43-8

Kjos, SL. & Buchanan, TA. (1999). Gestational diabetes. *The New England Journal of Medicine*. Vol. 341, pp. 1749-1756, PMID 10580075

Kuhl, C. (1991). Aetiology of gestational diabetes. *Baillière's Clinical Obstetrics and Gynaecology*. Vo. 5(2), pp. 279-292, PMID 1954714

Metzger, BE. & Coustan, DR. (1998). The Organizing Committee: Summary and recommendations of the Fourth International Workshop-Conference on Gestational Diabetes Mellitus. *Diabetes Care*. Vol. 21, suppl. 1: pp. 161–167, PMID 9704245

Metzer, BE. & Coustan, DM. (1998). Organizing committee. Summary and recommendations of Fourth international Workshop. Conference on Gestational diabetes mellitus. *Diabetes Care*. Vol. 21, suppl 2: pp. 161-167, PMID 9704245

Moody, J. (Edi). (October 2003). *Antenatal care- routine care for the healthy pregnant woman : Clinical guideline*, RCOG press publisher, pp. 96-99, London, ISBN 1900364 913

Naylor, CD., Serner, M., Chen, E. & Sykora, K. (1996). Caesarian delivery in relation to birth weight and gestational glucose tolerance: pathophysiology or practice style. *The Journal of the American Medical Association*. Vol. 275, pp. 1165-1170, ISSN 0098-7484

O'Sullivan, JB., Mahan, CM., Charles, D. & Dandrow, RV. (1973). Screening criteria for high-risk gestational diabetic patients. *American Journal of Obstetrics and Gynecology*. Vol. 116, pp. 895–900, PMID 4718216

Richardson, DK., Schwartz, JS., Weinbaum, PJ., & Gabbe, SG. (1993). Diagnostic tests in Obstetrics: a method for improved evaluation. *American Journal of Obstetrics and Gynecology*. Vol. 152, pp. 613-618, PMID 4025419

Schmidt, MI. et al. (2001). Gestational Diabetes Mellitus Diagnosed with a 2-h 75-g Oral Glucose Tolerance Test and Adverse Pregnancy Outcomes. *Diabetes Care*. Vol. 24, pp. 1151–1155, ISSN 1935-5548

Tsutomu, K. et al. (2002). Young men with high normal blood pressure have lower serum adiponectin, smaller LDL, size and higher elevated heart rate than those optimal blood pressure. *Diabetes Care*. Vol. 25, pp. 971, PMID 12032101

WHO (1999). Consultation: Definition, Diagnosis and Classification of Diabetes Mellitus and Its Complications: Report of a WHO Consultation. Part 1. *Diagnosis and Classification of Diabetes Mellitus.*, WHO/NCD/NCS. Vol. 99.2, Geneva, ISSN 07423071

5

Prevalence and Risk Factors for the Development of GD in Some Eastern European Countries – Tendencies and Pharmacoeconomical Assessment for the Choice of Treatment

Valentina Petkova and Irina Nikolova
Medical University – Sofia, Faculty of Pharmacy
Bulgaria

1. Introduction

Diabetes is a metabolic disorder of fat, carbohydrate, and protein metabolism, characterized by resistance to the action of insulin, insufficient insulin secretion, or both. The two major classifications of diabetes mellitus (DM) are type 1 (insulin deficient) and type 2 (combined insulin resistance and relative deficiency in insulin secretion). They differ in clinical presentation, onset, etiology, and progression of disease. Two to five percent of pregnancies are complicated by diabetes, of which 90% are classified as gestational diabetes mellitus (GD) (Satman et al, 2002). GD is defined as glucose intolerance of variable severity which is first recognized during pregnancy, including individuals with previously undiagnosed diabetes as well as those in whom high glucose levels are provoked by pregnancy. This term should not be used for gravid women with previously diagnosed diabetes. GD has much in common with type 2 diabetes with similar genetic susceptibility, corresponding prevalence within a given population or ethnic group and similar risk factors. Both conditions can be considered as a mixture of insulin resistance (IR) and impaired insulin secretion. Indeed, GD is a predictor of future type 2 diabetes with a cumulative incidence of about 50% at 5 years. GD is also a predictor of the metabolic (resistance) syndrome and should probably be considered a cardiovascular risk factor for later life. Since its first description in the early 1950s, GD has been one of the most controversial syndromes in the field of diabetes. Pregnancy is a state of insulin resistance, characterized by raised circulating insulin concentrations as the maternal pancreas compensates for increased peripheral demands. If adequate compensation does not occur, GD develops. GD is a well-established risk factor for adverse infant health outcomes, including fetal macrosomia, birth trauma, neonatal hypoglycemia, and fetal death (Cetin et al., 1997). GD can predict that the children of women who have GD are at an increased risk for obesity, glucose intolerance, and diabetes during adulthood. There is still confusion about the type of diagnostic tests and diagnostic criteria for GD and a screening protocol (e.g. universal versus selective screening). Gestational diabetes complicates about 1-14% of all pregnancies, depending on the population and diagnostic tests that are used and ranges from mild degrees of hyperglycemia to insulin-dependent diabetes (Kim et al., 2007).

Gestational diabetes usually manifests in the latter half of pregnancy and is characterized by insulin levels that are insufficient to meet insulin demands.

2. Risk factors for GD

Risk factors for GD include obesity, family history of diabetes, age greater than 35 years of age, pre-diabetes detected before pregnancy, previous delivery of babies with birth weights greater than 4 kg, sedentary lifestyles and some ethnical groups. The frequency of GD significantly increases with increasing number of risk factors. However, even a combination of risk factors does not reliably predict the likelihood of developing GD, missing up to 50% of cases in population based studies (Fraser & Heller, 2007; Jang et al., 2003) estimates that if age > 30 years, obesity (BMI > 27.3), family history of diabetes mellitus and glycosuria in the present pregnancy were included as risk factors, 56.5% of the total population had risk factors for GD. However, in the stated report, the prevalence of GD in Korea was 2.0%, Thailand - 2.0% and U.S. Caucasians - 2.3%. One large study of women with GD showed that an increased incidence of GD was associated with age over 35, thin or obese prepregnancy weight, previous stillbirth, previous spontaneous or induced abortion, previous low- or high-birth-weight infant and chronic hypertension (Johnstone, 1999; Hossein-Nezhad et al., 2007) found the age distribution and GD prevalence in 15–24 age group was 0.39% and 2.68% in the 35–45 age group. The authors reported 33.33% of women with GD who had a positive family history of diabetes, compared with 10.3% of women in the normal group ($p < 0.0001$). It is now well established that women with a family history of diabetes had three times higher odds for GD than women without a family history of diabetes. Perhaps other maternal health and lifestyle behaviors, such as levels of physical activity, or selective immigration, could play an important role (Scholl et al., 2002).

Obesity in pregnancy is increasing worldwide and is associated with increased risk of adverse outcomes for both mother and child. Maternal obesity is also accompanied by alterations in glucose metabolism and by perturbations in inflammatory markers, adipokines and vascular dysfunction. The link between obesity and IR has been recognised for many years and much of this association has been attributed to disturbances in adipocyte function and metabolism (Huda et al. 2010). Obesity has considerable effects on glucose metabolism in pregnancy with a loss of the reduction in fasting glucose in early pregnancy and significant enhancement of peripheral and hepatic IR. All women increase maternal fat stores in early pregnancy irrespective of prepregnancy adiposity to meet the feto-placental and maternal demands of late gestation and lactation. Normal pregnancy is associated with marked changes in glucose metabolism and IR to facilitate provision of fuel substrate for the fetus. In early pregnancy insulin secretion increases, while insulin sensitivity is unchanged, or even slightly improved. However, as pregnancy progresses, insulin-mediated glucose utilization worsens by 40–60% and insulin secretion increases several fold in order to maintain euglycaemia in the mother. The mechanisms for this increased risk are multifactorial and include effects on insulin signalling similar to those seen in obese non-pregnant women. Women of normal weight gain around 3.8 kg of fat during pregnancy although there is substantial variation. In women of normal weight the majority of fat is accumulated centrally in the subcutaneous compartment of the trunk and upper thigh. A large population-based Swedish study highlighted that an increase in BMI of 3 kg/m^2 between two consecutive pregnancies resulted in an increased risk of pre-eclampsia, GD, gestational hypertension, caesarean delivery, stillbirth and large for gestation age births even if a woman has a healthy BMI during pregnancy. (Villamor & Cnattingius, 2006; Hossein-Nezhad et al, 2007) It reported 35% prevalence of obesity (BMI of more than 27) in women with GD, compared with 11.3% in normal women ($p < 0.0001$). Not only weight gained during pregnancy, but variations in body habitus or constitution, like high waist-hip ratios, short stature and higher body fat percentages at given BMI levels could contribute as a risk factors (Davis, 2008; Mensing et al., 2002; Scholl et al., 2002) Not surprisingly, obese women are 4 times more likely and severely obese women almost 9 times more likely to develop GD than lean women.

Pregnancy is also characterised by marked increases in plasma lipid concentrations as gestation advances. Plasma cholesterol and triglyceride concentrations rise by 25–50% and 200–400% respectively. The hyperlipidaemia of pregnancy is exaggerated further in obesity with higher serum triglyceride and very low density lipoprotein (LDL) cholesterol concentrations than those observed in lean women. This is seen together with lower high density lipoprotein (HDL) cholesterol, although LDL cholesterol and total cholesterol concentrations appear similar. This pattern of dyslipidaemia is similar to that of the metabolic syndrome in the non-pregnant population. Some of these pathways may well contribute to vascular and metabolic complications in obese pregnancy.

It is well established that people with high levels of visceral or intra-abdominal body fat are associated with increased risk for type 2 diabetes (Huxley et al., 2008) and impaired glucose tolerance even after adjustment for BMI. Recent evidence suggests that even modest fasting hyperglycaemia (between 4.2 and 5.6 mmol/L), currently thought to be within normal limits, is linearly associated with adverse pregnancy outcomes including increased birth weight, caesarean delivery and neonatal hypoglycaemia (Huda et al, 2010). Women with a history of GD are metabolically vulnerable with insufficient ß-cell reserve, and many are IR. Approximately 17-63% of women who are diagnosed with GD during pregnancy will develop it in future pregnancies, and are at a much greater risk of developing type 2 diabetes within 5-16 years. The risk varies with the magnitude of insulin resistance, for example, if the patient needed insulin in pregnancy or was noted to be obese, or developed GD before 24 weeks gestation, the risk is greater. There is also some evidence that further pregnancies accelerate the rate of decline of beta cell function in women with GD. Several studies have reported links between GD and the subsequent risk of type 2 diabetes. Recent meta-analysis reports that GD corresponds to a 7.4 fold increased risk for developing type 2 diabetes mellitus (Bellamy et al., 2009). In addition, numerous studies have reported an increased risk of GD in women who are overweight or obese compared with lean or normal-weight women (Chatzi et al., 2009). GD identifies pregnancies at increased risk for adverse perinatal outcome. It also identifies mothers who are at increased risk of developing type 2 DM in the future and offers the possibility of interventions and early detection. Severity of glucose intolerance during pregnancy, insulin requirement during pregnancy, earlier diagnosis during pregnancy, family history of diabetes, recurrence of GD, increasing parity, maternal age, prepregnancy obesity, weight gain during and after pregnancy, presence of islet cell antibodies, and delivery of a macrosomic infant were reportedly the key risk factors for type 2 DM in women with history of GD (Cho et al., 2006). One of the major determinants of the risk for the development of subsequent type 2 diabetes is ethnic origin. Ethnic group with high risk of developing diabetes are Hispanic, African, Native American,

South or East Asian, Pacific Islands or Indigenous Australian. Women with previous GD have a higher prevalence of polycystic ovary syndrome (PCOS), which is a condition associated with IR. Similarly in a study of women with PCOS, GD developed in 20% of these women compared with only 9% of controls with an odds ratio of 1.9. Women with PCOS often attend assisted fertility clinics and should be warned of the likelihood of developing GD if they become pregnant (Hyer & Shehata, 2005; Metzger et al., 2010).

Maternal diabetes during pregnancy exposes the fetus to hyperglycemia resulting in increased fetal insulin levels, which are associated with increased birth weight, increased childhood and adult obesity, and increased risk of GD and type-2 diabetes during childbearing age (Kim et al., 2007).

Perinatal and maternal morbidity can be reduced by maintaining normoglycaemia in GD. To achieve good glycaemic control, women diagnosed with GD should monitor their blood glucose levels, exercise, and undergo nutrition counselling. Besides, medical treatment options should be incorporated in care plans. However, despite intensive treatment aiming at near normoglycemia, a surprisingly high risk of macrosomia and birth trauma has been reported among the neonates of mothers with GD. It would seem that the prevention of macrosomia should be the primary goal of GD management. Several studies suggest an increased rate of preeclampsia among women with GD, and a combination of maternal diabetes and pre-eclampsia is associated with poor perinatal outcome (Fan et al., 2006).

Untreated or poorly controlled gestational diabetes can hurt the baby. It can raise the risk of certain pregnancy complications, like high blood pressure in the mother and having a larger-than-normal baby (macrosomia), which may require a C-section. Studies have shown that in GD the frequency of having an overweight baby is almost double, the frequency of having preeclampsia is almost double, and the frequency of early delivery is 40 percent greater. It was proven that the proper identification and management of GD are associated with a decrease in mortality and morbidity in infants.

3. Testing programs

GD is associated with maternal (pre-eclampsia, hypertension, caesarean section) and foetal morbidity (macrosomia, birth trauma, hypoglycaemia, hyperbilirubinemia, hypocalcemia, respiratory distress syndrome). Moreover, GD uncovers a pre-existing metabolic abnormality that may precede the development of overt diabetes mellitus. Therefore, prompt diagnosis of GD is essential to reduce maternal and foetal morbidity and to allow subsequent attempt at preventing or delaying the onset of Type 2 diabetes.

Whether or not to screen for gestational diabetes is an issue of significant controversy. The ADA favors screening a woman who has risk factors for developing GD (e.g., severe obesity, personal history of GD or previous delivery of large-for-gestational age infant, glycosuria, PCOS or a strong family history of diabetes) at her first prenatal visit (American Diabetes Association [ADA], 2011). If test is abnormal, these individuals should be considered to have "overt" (not gestational) diabetes (ADA, 2010). If this screen is normal, testing should be repeated between weeks 24 and 28 of gestation. Pregnant women without these risk factors should undergo screening for GD between weeks 24 and 28 of gestation unless they are considered low risk. To be low risk, a woman must fulfill all the following criteria:

- age younger than 25 years,
- normal prepregnancy weight,
- no known diabetes in first-degree relatives,

- not a member of an ethnic group with a high prevalence of GD,
- no history of abnormal glucose tolerance,
- no history of abnormal obstetric outcome.

Screening for GD utilizes the oral glucose challenge test. New ADA guidelines (ADA, 2011) and WHO guidelines stated to perform a 75 g oral glucose tolerance test (OGTT), with plasma glucose measurement fasting and at 1 and 2 h at 24-28 weeks. OGTT should be performed in the morning after an overnight fast of at least 10 hours and after at least 3 days of unrestricted diet and unlimited physical activity. The patient should remain seated and should not smoke during the test (Johnstone, 1999). Criteria for diagnosis of GD based on the OGTT are summarized in Table 1. Two or more values must be met or exceeded for a diagnosis of diabetes to be made.

Fasting	≥ 92 mg/dL (5.1 mmol/L)
1 hour	≥ 180 mg/dL (10.0 mmol/L)
2 hours	≥ 153 mg/dL (8.5 mmol/L)

Table 1. Diagnosis of GD with a 75 g Glucose Load

Results of the Hyperglycemia and Adverse Pregnancy Outcomes (HAPO) study (Metzger et al., 2008), a large-scale (~25,000 pregnant women) multinational epidemiologic study, demonstrated that risk of adverse maternal, fetal, and neonatal outcomes continuously increased as a function of maternal glycemia at 24–28 weeks, even within ranges previously considered normal for pregnancy. For most complications there was no threshold for risk. These results have led to careful reconsideration of the diagnostic criteria for GD. The International Association of Diabetes and Pregnancy Study Groups (IADPSG) recommended that all women not known to have prior diabetes undergo a 75 g OGTT at 24–28 weeks of gestation. This probably will significantly increase the prevalence of GD, however there is mounting evidence that treating even mild GD reduces morbidity for both mother and baby (International Diabetes Federation [IDF], 2004). Women at high risk should be screened as soon as feasible. If the initial screening is negative they should undergo retesting at 24 to 28 weeks' gestation.

There are two principles (selective and universal) in testing which need to be distinguished. First, there is selective (or at-risk) clinical need for high risk patient (obesity, a family history of diabetes, a history of macrosomic stillbirth, etc.). Second, there is universal screening, for women not clinically identified as being at particular risk. Universal screening is more sensitive, while selective screening is less costly. Unfortunately, the use of risk factors for individuals is not very effective, can result in great inconsistencies, and is a source of uncertainty for obstetricians and midwives. Universal screening should, at the moment, depend on the local prevalence of type 2 DM in the reproductive age group. Low-risk status requires no glucose testing, but this category is limited to those women meeting all of the following characteristics: age <25 years, normal weight before pregnancy, member of a population with a low prevalence of GD, no known diabetes in first-degree relatives, no history of abnormal glucose tolerance, no history of poor obstetric outcome. Where type 2 DM is common (for example many units in the USA, Saudi Arabia and the Gulf, and certain ethnic minorities), then a total population screen is justified (Forsbach et al., 1997). Universal screening is more sensitive and more practical when a family history of diabetes cannot be obtained reliably (Karcaaltincaba et al., 2009). The diagnosis of GD is associated with a risk of type 2 diabetes later in life, so it is unsurprising that the prevalence of GD in any population will be largely determined by those factors which predict such a risk (Fraser & Heller, 2007)

Any woman diagnosed with GD should be screened for diabetes 6–12 weeks postpartum and should be followed up with subsequent screening for the development of diabetes or pre-diabetes. If the fasting plasma glucose (FPG) level is normal, then reassessment for DM should occur every 3 years. Family planning for subsequent pregnancies should be discussed, and monitoring for the development of symptoms of DM should be undertaken.

The goal of treatment is to reduce the risks of GD for mother and child by keeping blood glucose levels equal to those of pregnant women who don't have such a disease. The highest risk of complications is established when there is an increase of the initial level of pre-prandial blood sugar and when there is an increase of the postprandial glucose.

Scientific evidences show that controlling glucose levels can result in less serious fetal complications and increased maternal quality of life and insulin administered twice daily during the third trimester to mothers who have even a mild degree of hyperglycemia will reduce fetal size, and in particular fetal adiposity. The proper management GD includes special meal plans and scheduled physical activity and of course - daily blood glucose testing. The further steps may require insulin injections.

4. Prevalence of GD

GD is the most common metabolic disease of pregnancy. The prevalence of GD varies across the globe, as well as between racial and ethnic groups within the same country. In recent years there has been a reported increased trend in the prevalence of GD throughout the world, with huge health-care and economic costs (Bellamy et al., 2009). This is particularly the case in developed countries, such as the USA, the UK, Australia, China and New Zealand (Sinha et al., 2003; Ferrara et al., 2004; Joshy & Simmons, 2006; Metzger & Counstan, 1998; Fan et al., 2006; Carolan et al., 2010). The increased prevalence has been recently disputed, suggesting that more cases were identified through more aggressive universal screening. For example, Lopez-de-Andres et al. (Lopez-de-Andres et al., 2011) did not found increase in the prevalence of GD is Spain from 2001 to 2008. This partly coud be explained with the fact that with the selective approach, women at low risk for GD do not need to be screened and some cases could be missed. Several teams have tried to improve the sensitivity of selective screening by making the relevant protocols more inclusive. Through this 'tinkering', age has emerged as the most important risk factor for type 2 DM and, by extension, gestational diabetes. Accordingly, the lower threshold for screening has decreased from 30 years in earlier studies to 25 years in more recent ones.

Approximately 8% of all pregnancies with wide-ranging differences between countries (ranging from 1 to 16% depending on the population studied, screening protocols and diagnostic criteria used) are complicated by GD (Hossein-Nezhad et al., 2007). Furthermore, within the same country, the prevalence of GD is strongly influenced by race and culture. High prevalence rates have been reported in studies from Australia (Indian-born 15%, Chinese 13.9%) and the United States (Zuni Indians 14.3%).

Increasing prevalence relates to a range of factors including advanced maternal age, obesity and migratory patterns (Ferrara et al., 2004; Joshy & Simmons, 2006). Of particular interest here is the increase seen among specific ethnic groups (Joshy & Simmons, 2006, Kim et al., 2007), which may relate to ethnic differences in maternal glucose concentrations (Scholl et al., 2002; Esakoff et al., 2005) and recent trends of obesity (Harris et al., 1997, Xiong et al.,

2001, Rosenberg et al., 2003; Ben-Haroush et al., 2004). Moreover, women of non-Caucasian ethnicity represent a considerable portion of childbearing populations in developed countries, and as rates of obesity and GD grow, there is a concordant increase in the risk of poorer pregnancy outcomes among these groups. GD is also associated with an increased maternal likelihood of developing diabetes type 2 in later life, and recent research postulates a link between GD, childhood obesity and later onset of diabetes in the offspring (Ferrara, 2007; Ricart et al., 2005; Carolan et al., 2010)

USA

In the USA more than 200,000 cases annually are complicated by GD (Bottalico, 2007). Only 1.5–2% of Midwestern white women develop GD, while up to 15% of Native American women from southwestern USA have been reported to develop GD. In the Hispanic, African-American and Asian populations of the USA, the incidence of GD is 5–8%. Most women will return to normoglycemia postpartum, but 30% to 50% will develop type 2 DM or glucose intolerance later in life. State-, city-, hospital-level GD prevalence estimates have consistently shown GD rates to be higher among Asian and Pacific Islander (API) mothers than among white, black, or Hispanic mothers (Lawrence et al., 2008; Chu et al., 2009) found that among 3,108,877 births, US APIs had a substantially higher age-adjusted prevalence of GD (6.3%) than whites (3.8%), blacks (3.5%), or Hispanics (3.6%).

Asia

Oriental populations have different demographic characteristics (maternal age, height, BMI and frequency of obesity) to other ethnic populations and it is not clear to what extent the effects of age and obesity are interrelated. In Korea the life styles have changed rapidly to a westernized pattern characterized by sedentary occupations and consumption of refined food and a high-fat diet. Therefore it is reasonable to predict that the prevalence of GD in Korean women will increase as the prevalence of type 2 DM increases in the developing countries (Jang et al., 1995; 2003). The overall prevalence of GD in Korean women was estimated as 2.2%. The patients with GD were older, shorter and had a higher prepregnancy weight, BMI and parity than normal controls. The prevalence of GD in women with a single risk factor was 1.3% higher than that in women without risk factors (0.6%, $p < 0.05$), but was lower than that in the population at large (2.2%). However the prevalence increased to 33.3% in patients with 4 risk factors.

The DECODA study showed that India has a higher prevalence of diabetes than China or Japan (Ferrara, 2007) reported 3.8% prevalence of GD in China (20512 women screened), however they could not determine if there is an increase in the incidence of GD, but state that it is possible that absolute rate of GD has increased in China, probably due to changes in the lifestyle, decreased physical activity and increased incidence of obesity. Shai et al. (Shai et al., 2006) found that Asian women had a higher risk of diabetes than White, Hispanic, or Black women. In addition, they found that weight gain increased risk of diabetes more for Asian than for other women. Hunsberger et al. (Hunsberger et al., 2010) found that, compared with women of other race/ethnicities, both high BMI and low BMI Asian women were at the greatest risk of having GD. Additionally, diabetes risk among Asians seems to increase with prolonged exposure to Western lifestyle. The Turkish Diabetes Epidemiology Study reported the highest prevalence of diabetes in southern Turkey compared with northern and central parts of Turkey (Satman et al., 2002). The approximately rate of GD in Turkey is 4% (Karcaaltincaba et al., 2009).

Europe

Di Cianni et al. (Di Cianni et al., 2003) performed a retrospective study to evaluate the prevalence of GD by using both the selective and the universal screening approach and the presence of risk factors for GD in a cohort of Italian women. From June 1st, 1995 to December 31st, 2001, universal screening for GD was performed in 3950 women. In this analysis GD was significantly and independently associated to age, pre-pregnancy BMI, weight gain, height and family history of diabetes. The generated figures indicate that GCT was positive in 35.2% of cases, while the true prevalence of GD was 8.7%. When the OGTT was performed in a random sample of women with negative GCT, about 6.5% were found to have GD. By extrapolation to the whole cohort, it was then calculated that the approximate true prevalence of GD in the general population can be as high as 12.3%.Lopez-de-Andres et al. (Lopez-de-Andres et al., 2011) reported the prevalence of GD is Spain from 2001 to 2008 to be 3.6%. In Sweden, 7817 infants (of total number 892084) were born of mothers with GD between 1992 and 2004. This represents an incidence of GD of 0.9% in the studied population (Ahlsson et al., 2010). The number of adults with diabetes in the European region is expected to reach 55.2 million. And 33.40% are from the eastern European region.

Eastern Europe

The prevalence of GD in Eastern Europe and especially in Bulgaria shows a very diverse prevalence. (IDF, 2011)

Country	percent with diabetes (20-79 years) 2010	number of people with diabetes 2010	percent with diabetes (20-79 years) 2030	population	GDP nominal total (USD)
1. Albania	4.8	102 800	5.1	2 986 952	12.224 billion
2. Belarus	9.1	661 100	9.0	9 648 533	52.887 billion
3. Bosnia and Herzegovina	9.1	271 100	8.6	3 842 566	16 631 billion
4. Bulgaria	9.0	519 500	7.8	7 351 234	44.843 billion
5. Croatia	9.2	315 900	8.0	4 486 881	59 917 billion
6. Estonia	9.9	97 900	9.0	1 340 021	19.123 billion
7. Greece	8.8	754 000	7.4	11 305 118	325 088 billion
8. Latvia	9.9	169 700	9.0	2 217 969	23 955 billion
9. Lithuania	9.7	239 800	9.0	3 244 000	35.152 billion
10. Macedonia	8.0	119 300	8.0	2 052 722	9470 billion
11. Moldova	8.7	233 500	9.0	3 567 500	5 403 billlion
12. Montenegro	8.4	35 700	8.0	620 000	
13. Romania	8.4	1 351 400	8.0	21 959 278	158 393 billion
14. Russia	9.0	9 624 900	9.0	142 905 200	1 477 trillion
15. Serbia	8.6	613 400	8.0	9 981 929	43.6 billion
16. Ukraine	9.6	3 328 400	9.0	49 100 000	37.6 billion

Table 2. The DM morbidity in Eastern European region.

According to the data, provided by the Diabetes Atlas, Estonia, Latvia and Ukraine are those eastern European countries with highest percentage of diabetes for 2010. Albania is the country with lowest percentage. Totally 18 438 400 is the number of the patients with diabetes in these sixteen countries. The mean percentage with diabetes for 2010 is 8.76. And the decrease for the next 20 years will be insignificant - 8.24. Of course all the eastern European countries are extremely diverse as the population and gross domestic product (GDP) are taken in mind. Russia is the richest, while Moldova, Macedonia and Albania are the poorest. The number of deaths attributable to diabetes (20-79 years) is 317 955. And there is no significant differentiation by sex 143 810 – males and 174 145 – females. A very interesting fact is that only five countries - Greece, Russia, Belarus, Ukraine and Romania have National Diabetes program according to a survey of International Diabetes Federation (IDF) member associations. Bulgaria for example is working in order to develop and implement a national diabetes program. The Bulgarian Diabetes Association (BDA) that is the only one national representative association for patients and diabetics in Bulgaria is working towards achieving this goal. It was created in 1990. On the initiative of the Group for parliamentary consensus to combat socially significant diseases in the 40th National Assembly of Bulgaria and under the auspices of the National Assembly on 2-3 February 2008 in Plovdiv, Bulgaria there was a consensus around three significant acts:

1. Restriction of diabetes in Bulgaria and particularly the preparation and implementation of diabetic register and national program to combat diabetes should be one of the priorities of all institutions in Bulgaria.
2. It is the creation of a working group of representatives of all stakeholders to draw up an action plan for prevention, early diagnosis and proper treatment of diabetes in Bulgaria. These documents must be submitted for consideration and adoption by the National Assembly during the autumn session of 2008.
3. After the program and action plan, responsible institutions is imperative to take all necessary actions to ensure adequate funding for their practical application in the country. So we can conclude that Bulgaria is working towards the development of a National program.

Of course not only the disease itself has to be assessed but also the complication that accelerates the mortality. Close to four million deaths in the 20-79 age group may be attributable to diabetes in 2010, accounting for 6.8% of global all-cause mortality in this age group. According to the literay sources - this number resembles the deaths in this age group from several infectious diseases. The highest number of deaths due to diabetes is expected to occur in countries with large populations as they have the largest numbers of people with diabetes like Russia.

Another very important aspect is the health expenditures per person with diabetes in 2010. As it can be seen there are very big fluctuations in the Eastern European region. For example Greece spent 2742 USD, while Moldova – only 76 USD. In order to be precise in the conclusions it has to be analyzed the GDP in order to compare these expenditures. For Greece it is 325 088 billion USD , while for Moldova – 5 403 billlion. For Greece these mean health expenditures per person with diabetes are 0.0084% from the GDP of the country, while for Moldova – 0.014%. Bulgaria spent 0.007% from the GDP of the country for treatment of a patient with diabetes. (IDF, 2011)

Country	Mean health expenditure per person with diabetes in 2010 (USD)
Albania	261
Belarus	238
Bosnia and Herzegovina	307
Bulgaria	301
Croatia	736
Estonia	584
Greece	2 742
Latvia	493
Lithuania	521
Macedonia	287
Moldova	76
Montenegro	14
Romania	145
Russia	261
Serbia	238
Ukraine	307

Table 3. Mean health expenditures per person with DM in 2010 for the Eastern European region.

The statistics by country for gestational diabetes shows that apporximatelly 1 in 2 014 or 0.05% or 135 000 women get GD every year in the USA. The analysis of the data for the eastern European region are shown in Table 4.

Country	Extrapolated Incidence	Population estimated used (US Census Bureau, International data base 2004)
Albania	1 759	3 544 808
Belarus	5 117	10 310 520
Bosnia and Herzegovina	202	407 608
Bulgaria	3 731	7 517 973
Croatia	2 231	4 496 869
Estonia	665	1 341 664
Greece	5 284	10 647 529
Latvia	1 144	2 306 306
Lithuania	1 790	3 607 899
Macedonia	1 012	2 040 085
Romania	11 095	22 355 551
Russia	71 457	143 974 059
Serbia and Montenegro	5 373	10 825 900
Ukraine	23 690	47 732 079

Table 4. Extrapolated incidence of GD (wrongdiagnosis.com, 2011)

These statistics are calculated extrapolations of various prevalence or incidence rates against the populations of a particular country or region. The statistics used for prevalence/incidence of GD are typically based on US, UK, Canadian or Australian prevalence or incidence statistics, which are then extrapolated using only the population of a given country. The base is that 0.05% from the population (women) will get GD annually. The literary data shows that the frequency of development of GD varies from 2 to 4-5 % from the pregnant women. Some authors even state that 9% from the pregnant women develop GD. In Bulgaria a pilot study shows that the frequency is even greater - 14%, but till today there was not perform a systematic screening. Unfortunatelly in Bulgaria there is a tendency for doubling the GD morbidity, because of the obesity and because of the increase survival rate of girls born with weight above 4 kg.

5. St. Vincent declaration – Review and principles

In 1989, in St. Vincent, Italy was signed the St. Vincent declaration, a joint initiative of the International Diabetes Federation European region and the WHO European regional office. It is a program for strategic action to reduce the human and economic burden of diabetes in Europe and has been adopted by most of the European governments. (IDF, 2004) The St. Vincent initiative has few target areas, which seek to improve the quality of life of people with diabetes and to promote education of patients so to prevent diabetes complications. Patient education is very important and a team approach, including physicians, pharmacists and nurses, is beneficial. Some of the main conclusions during the meeting were that "diabetes mellitus is a major and growing European health problem, a problem at all ages and in all countries. It currently threatens at least ten million European citizens. It is within the power of national governments and health departments to create conditions in which a major reduction in this heavy burden of disease and death can be achieved. Countries should give formal recognition to the diabetes problem and deploy resources for its solution. Plans for the prevention, identification and treatment of diabetes and particularly its complications should be formulated at local, national and European regional levels. General goals and five-year targets can be achieved by the organised activities of the medical services in active partnership with diabetic patients, their families, friends and workmates and organisations in:

- The management of their own diabetes and education for it.
- The planning, provision and quality audit of health care.
- National, regional and international organisations for disseminating information about health maintenance.
- Promoting and applying research. (IDF, 2004)

The St. Vincent's declaration outlined the following general goals for children and adults with diabetes:

- sustained improvement in health experience and a life experience approaching normal expectation in quality and quantity.
- prevention and cure of diabetes and its complications by intensifying research effort.

The five-year targets that are granted in the declaration are:

- elaboration, initiation and evaluation comprehensive programmes for the detection and control of diabetes and its complications with self-care and community support as major components.

- steps for raising the awareness in the population and amongst health care professionals of the present opportunities and the future needs for the prevention of diabetes and its complications.
- organisation training and teaching programs in diabetes management and care for people of all ages with diabetes, for their families, friends and working associates and for the health care team.
- ensuring that care for children with diabetes is provided by individuals and teams specialised in the management of both diabetes and children, and that families with a diabetic child get the necessary social, economic and emotional support.
- reinforcement of the existing centres of excellence in diabetes care, education and research.
- promotion of independence, equity and self-sufficiency for all people with diabetes, i.e. children, adolescents, those in the working years of life and the elderly.
- attempts for reducing the hindrances to the fullest possible integration of the diabetic citizen into society.
- implementation of effective measures for the prevention of costly complications:

a	reduce new blindness due to diabetes by one third or more.
b	reduce the number of people entering end-stage diabetic renal failure by at least one third.
c	reduce by one half the rate of limb amputations for diabetic gangrene.
d	cut morbidity and mortality from coronary heart disease in the diabetic by vigorous programmes of risk factor reduction.
e	achieve a pregnancy outcome in the diabetic woman that approximates that of the non-diabetic woman.

- establishment of monitoring and control systems, using new information technology for quality assurance of diabetes health care revision and for laboratory and technical procedures in diabetes diagnosis, treatment and self-management.
- promotion and granting of collaboration of European and international programmes of diabetes research and development through national, regional and World Health Organisation agencies and in active partnership with diabetes patients' organisations.
- taking urgent action in the spirit of the WHO programme 'Health for All' to establish joint initiative between the WHO and the International Diabetes Federation (European region) to initiate, accelerate and facilitate the implementation of these recommendations." (IDF, 2004)

Since 1989 further implementation and evaluation meetings have been held in Budapest (1992), Athens (1995), Lisbon (1997) and Istanbul (1999), where representatives of ISPAD have helped to formulate recommendations on behalf of children and adolescents.

6. Pharmacoeconomical assessment of GD drug treatment. The role of the pharmacist for GD management

The standard treatment of GD is insulin treatment. The metabolic control target in the GD treatment is blood sugar before meal under 5.8 mmo/l, postprandial blood sugar under 7.5 mmo/l and hemoglobin HbA_{1-c} under 6.5%. The postprandial blood glucose is of critical importance for the neonatal end of the pregnancy. That is why it is very important to determine the cost and effectiveness of the drug treatment for women with GD. It can be achieved by studying the clinical effectiveness of the treatment with diet and diet + insulin for pregnant women with GD and determination of the ratio treatment cost/effectiveness. A prospective study of 50 women with gestational diabetes from Sofia, Bulgaria were studied from pharmacoeconomical point of view. They were divided into 2 groups: Group I (n = 30) - pregnant women only on a diet and Group II (n = 20) - pregnant women treated by a diet and insulin. The following including criteria were applied: age above 18 years, one fetus pregnancy, insignificant additional disease without organ damages, without infectious diseases, without obesity and HbA_{1-c} under 7%. The key excluding criteria are the availability of diabetes before pregnancy, or prior insulin therapy, treatment with oral hypoglycemic drugs before pregnancy, income of drugs that have influence on the carbohydrate tolerance, existing obstetrics complications till the demonstration of the gestation diabetes. The diet treatment was with diet No 9 according to M.I. Pevzner. The diet satisfies the recommendations for feeding. Human insulin, in intensified insulin regimen type- bazal-prandial, including treatment with three doses rapid acting insulin and one or two doses intermediate acting insulin was applied. The total costs of the treatment of a patient, on a diet without complications in the peripartal period is 335.02 USD and is lower in comparison with the total cost of the treatment of a woman treated only with insulin that is 347.42 USD. (p=0.04). The difference in the treatment cost is 12.40 USD. The total treatment cost of a pregnant woman, treated with diet with complications in the peripartal period is 363.94 USD and is also lower in comparison with the total cost of the treatment of a woman treated with insulin and with complications that is 398.90 USD (p=0,03). (Todorova et al., 2007)

The cost-effectiveness coefficient is calculated based on the total direct medical costs, used for the reduction of the average 24-houred glucose under 5,8 mmol/l as for higher precision the calculations are proceeded with the received difference in the level of the glycated hemoglobin after the treatment. (Todorova et al., 2007) The over calculated CCE for 100 women is CCE is 5141.17 USD

CCE= 398.90 - 363.94/6,1 - 5,42 = 51.4117USD

51.4117x 100 = 5141.17 USD

The so calculated coefficient reflects the costs for complications that is saved by the insulin treatment and that should occur after an ineffective diet treatment. The interpretation of this coefficient shows that the spent 12.40 USD for insulin treatment for every woman in fact saves 51.41 USD that should be spent for the treatment of unfavorable peripartal maternal complications. Through the application of a model of mathematical modeling the total final cost for one beneficially treated woman with GD is calculated. The calculations for the two therapeutical alternatives are performed by the use of the probabilities for occurrence of effective treatment for each of them.

The total costs of the treatment with diet is 351.69 USD

(334.43 x 0,4) + (363.2x 0,6) = 351.69 USD

The total cost of the treatment with insulin is 349.35 USD.

(346.84x0,95) + (398.2x0,05) = 349.35 USD

The applied analytical model shows that on the base of the higher per cent successfully treated women, the spent final costs for successfully treated woman after the treatment with insulin are 388,13 USD (349.32/0,9), and the final costs after the treatment with diet are 879.1 USD (351.64/0,4). (Todorova et al., 2007)

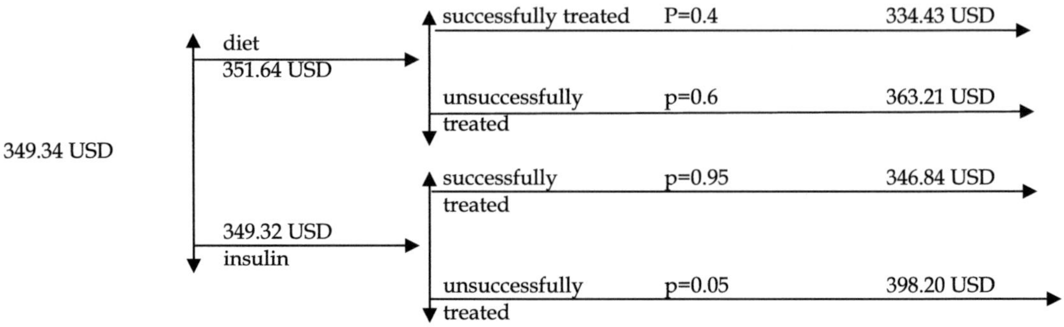

Table 5. "Three of decisions" of the alternatives for the treatment of GD.

There are four clinical paths, concerning diabetes that are included in the list of the Bulgarian Health Insurance fund. Unfortunatelly there is no clinical path concerning DM or the complications of this disease that decreases the accessibility towards proper management of this disease. And on this base it can be explained the prospective data about doubling the GD morbidity.

Clinical path No	disease	Hospital stay	Drug treatment	Prize (USD)/daily
8	Diabetes polineuropathia	3 days	• carbamazepine - 400-800 mg/daily. • gabapentin – from 3 times x 300 mg till 1500 mg daily; • pregabalin – up to 2 x 150 mg;	0.23-0.46 2.34 – 3.90 3.92
104	Decompensated DM for patients above 18 years	3 days	• Insulin • Electrolities	9.57 - once
105	Decompensated DM for patients bellow 18 years	3 days	• Insulin • Electrolities	9.57 - once
178	Surgical Intervention Of Diabetic Foot without vessel reconstruction	3 days		

Table 6. Clinical paths in Bulgaria, concerning diabetes.

Another aspect that is innovative in the Bulgarian pharmaceutical practice, concerning the management of GD is the role of the pharmacist as a health-care educator in order to be accomplished the St. Vincent declaration aims is demonstrated. Patient education is very important and a team approach, including physicians, pharmacists and nurses, is beneficial.(38). A study that included pregnant women attending antenatal clinic with GD January 2009 - December 2009 demonstrated the beneficial role of patients education. The following including criteria are used: age above 18 years, one-fetus pregnancy, GD, insignificant additional disease without organ damage, without infectious diseases. The study design is a pilot case-control study that includes 45 women with GD from city of Sofia, Bulgaria. The pregnant women were divided into two groups - Group I (n=22), that were educated on the proper management of their disease and were on a diet and treated with insulin, and Group II (n=23), that were not educated and on a diet, but treated with insulin on a regimen, prescribed by the physician. The assignment was based on the principle of random numbers through custom random number generator. The educational program continued 3 months. It was designed and adapted to the patients comfort, provided at the pharmacy they are attending. The course was presented to the 22 previously selected pregnant women with GD.

The educational course included the following teaching units:

- The essence of GD;
- The complication of improper disease management;
- Proper diet regimen (based on the Sample GD diet menu of the Endocrinology clinic of Minneapolis) and also proper drug treatment as well as hypo-and hyperglycaemia and physical activity for both of the groups.

The first unit acquainted each of the women with the aim of the educational program, provided general concept about GD and about self-monitoring and emphasized on the active patient participation in the treatment. The personal information of each of the patients was collected, concerning the duration of the disease, the prescribed drug treatment if any, the frequency of the hypoglycaemic and hyperglycaemic incidents. At the end of the first unit, each of the patients was supplied with written materials on the essence of GD. The goal was to learn the seriousness of GD.

The main topic discussed during the **second teaching unit** was complication of improper management. The educator explained the complications of GD. The educator discussed with every woman the effects on the fetus.

The main topic discussed during the **third teaching unit** was proper diet regimen (based on the GD diet menu of the Endocrinology clinic of Minneapolis, USA). At the end of the session the patients were supplied with the Sample GD diet menu. Each of the patients was supplied with written materials on proper nourishing for diabetic patients and physical activity.

The educational materials used during the program included:

- a set of one-page written materials that illustrate the most important aspects of every educational lecture, provided to the patient after every session;
- questionnaire cards for distribution among the participants as a standardized procedure for assessment of their knowledge acquired in the previous educational units;
- individual food and activity record for the self-monitored data (food, total grams of carbs, comments and activities, insulin treatment);

In the beginning and at the end of the educational process a patient satisfaction questionnaire was applied (Diabetes Questionnaire (IMG)). During the 3-months education and its end, the observed behavioural parameters performed changes. The results from the twice-applied questionnaire assessing the quality of life of the patients in the beginning and in the end of the educational programme show that the five main indices have been improved with on the average of 5% for the both groups, but greater for those included in Group I (Table 7). The greater increase was observed in the positive changes in the mood - 7,9% for Group I and 8,2% for Group II , followed by number of days "being easy" with 6.9 % for Group I and with 6,2% for Group II (6.7%) and possibility to perform physical activities 5.8 % for Group I and 5% for Group II. It could be considered that the educational process affects both the physical and the psychological well-being and thus it is beneficial for the global patient's quality of life.

	Time period			
Variable	0		3 month	
	Group I	Group II	Group I	Group II
QL-positive changes in the mood	10,8%	9,9%	18,7%	18,1%
QL-increase in days "being easy"	18,4%	17,9%	25,3%	24,1%
QL- increase in social activity	11,1%	12,2%	14%	15,1%
QL- increase in days being "rested"	15%	14,5%	17,4%	16,8%
QL- increase in physical activity	13,4%	14,0%	19,2%	19,0%
total	68,70%	68,50%	94,60%	93,10%
mean	13,74%	13,70%	18,92%	18,62%

Data are %. QL – "quality of life".

Table 7. Changes in the patients sample after the educational process

The advanced pharmacy practitioner in diabetes management is a relatively new approach. The role of the pharmacist in it, integrates drug management, patients' compliance assessment, blood glucose monitoring, skills training, prospective and retrospective drug utilization review, adverse drug reaction and toxicity screening and education of the patients.(Valentine et al, 2003). These skills in fact are not new for the pharmacist but their introduction, as systematized approach in everyday practice should correspond to the local circumstances. To match the context of the pharmaceutical care, defined by the APA as "Patient-centered, outcomes-oriented pharmacy practice that requires the pharmacist to work in concert with the patient to promote health, to prevent disease and to assess, monitor, initiate and modify medication use", is a real challenge for the management of diabetes, especially for Bulgaria.(American Pharmaceutical Association [APA], 2011). Despite the relatively small sample size, this study shows the role of education program for improvement of patient's outcomes. The results confirm the necessity of individual approach in the selection of therapeutic strategy for the women with GD. As the St. Vincent declaration assumed, the quality of life of people with diabetes has to be improved and to be promoted education of patients so to prevent diabetes complications. According to the St. Vincent declaration the aim of the treatment of GD is the achievement of child birth similar to the child birth by women without diabetes.(IDF, 2004) In this project are involved all healthcare givers, including the pharmacists in order to be achieved the goals. (Douglas et al., 2000; Dixon, 2002; Campbell et al., 1990; Mensing et al., 2002) The educational approach is a necessary step for better management of the disease in order to minimize the risk of maternal and fetal complications and the pharmacists are capable to perform it. The results obtained confirm the need for consistent patients' education, using variety of educational models, as an essential part of the diabetes care that will result in improvement of patient's quality of life.

7. Conclusion

Gestational diabetes is a subject of endless debate, uncertainty and confusion. Although it is a alteration during pregnancy, the true prevalence of GD remains a matter of discussion. The prevalence of GD in the general population is varied from 1% to 16% depending on both the country of origin and the nature of the indigenous population. The rate can vary due to differences in data collection methods, low response rates, non-random selection of the women, and lack of uniformity in the diagnostic criteria. More recently, the high rate of GD has been claimed to be an unrealistic estimation caused by universal screening, not carrying any specific benefit for pregnancy outcome.

GD is considered to be a state of prediabetes. The diagnosis of GD identifies women at high risk of diabetes after the pregnancy. Therefore, it is important for these women who may develop type 2 diabetes during their life to take preventive measures as well as to prevent pregnancy-related complications. It is well known that raised glucose levels in women with GD increase both morbidity and mortality among their offspring due mainly to an increased incidence of congenital abnormalities and excessive fetal growth in the third trimester. Women with a family history of diabetes had three times higher odds for GD than women without a family history of diabetes. With the prevalence of type 2 diabetes increasing across the world, and given that the prevalence of GD is thought to shadow that of type 2 diabetes, most populations will expect to see a rise in GD figures during the coming years. It is very important to establish clear policies to ensure that those at risk are reliably identified, appropriately treated during pregnancy and then equipped to make the necessary lifestyle changes to try and prevent them developing type 2 diabetes in later life.

8. References

ADA: American Diabetes Association. (2010). Standards of medical care in diabetes-2010. *Diabetes Care*, No 33, (Suppl 1):S11-61

ADA: American Diabetes Association. (2011). Standards of medical care in diabetes-2011. *Diabetes Care, No* 34(Suppl 1):S11-61

Ahlsson F, Lundgren M, Tuvemo T, Gustafsson J, Haglund B. (2010). Gestational diabetes and offspring body disproportion. *Acta Pediatrica*, No 99, pp.89-93

American College of Obstetricians and Gynaecologists Committee on Practice Bulletins - Obstetrics (2001) ACOG practice bulletin. Clinical management guidelines for obstetrician-gynecologists. No 30, September 2001 (replaces Technical Bulletin Number 200, December 1994). Gestational diabetes. *Obstet Gynecol* 98, pp.525-538

American Diabetes Association.(2008) Clinical Practice Recommendations - Diagnosis and Classification of Diabetes Mellitus. Diabetes Care; No 31(Suppl. 1), S55-S60

American Pharmaceutical Association. (2011). Principles of practice for pharmaceutical care. Available from: http://www.pharmacist.com/AM/Template.cfm?Section=Home2&CONTENTID=2906&TEMPLATE=/CM/HTMLDisplay.cfm)

Bellamy L, Casas JP, Hingorani AD, Williams D. (2009). Type 2 diabetes mellitus after gestational diabetes: a systematic review and meta-analysis. *Lancet.* May Vol. 23; No. 373(9677), pp.1773-9.

Ben-Haroush A, Yogev Y, Hod M. (2004) Epidemiology of gestational diabetes mellitus and its association with Type 2 diabetes. *Diabet Med.* Feb;Vol. 21, No2, pp.103-13.

Bottalico JN.(2007). Recurrent gestational diabetes: risk factors, diagnosis, management, and implications. *Semin Perinatol.* Jun;Vol. 31, No3, pp. 176-84.

Campbell LV, Barth R, Gosper JK, Jupp JJ, Simons LA, Chisholm DJ. (1990) Impact of intensive educational approach to dietary change in NIDDM. *Diabetes Care,* No13, pp.841-7

Carolan M, Steele C, Margetts H. (2010) Knowledge of gestational diabetes among a multi-ethnic cohort in Australia. *Midwifery,* December Vol. 26, No.6, pp. 579-88.

Cetin M, Cetin A. (1997). Time-dependent gestational diabetes screening values. *Int J Gynaecol Obstet.* Mar; Vol. 56, No.3,pp. 257-61.

Chatzi L, Plana E, Pappas A, Alegkakis D, Karakosta P, Daraki V, Vassilaki M, Tsatsanis C, Kafatos A, Koutis A, Kogevinas M. (2009). The metabolic syndrome in early pregnancy and risk of gestational diabetes mellitus. *Diabetes Metab.* Vol. 35, No.6, pp.490-4.

Cho NH, Jang HC, Park HK, Cho YW. (2006). Waist circumference is the key risk factor for diabetes in Korean women with history of gestational diabetes. *Diabetes Res Clin Pract,* February, Vol. 71, No. 2, pp. 177-83.

Chu SY, Abe K, Hall LR, Kim SY, Njoroge T, Qin C. (2009). Gestational diabetes mellitus: all Asians are not alike. *Prev Med.* Aug-Sep, Vol.49, No.2-3, pp. 265-8.

Crowther C. et al (2005) Effect of treatment of gestational diabetes mellitus on pregnancy outcome, *The New England Journal of Medicine,* Vol. 352, No. 24, pp. 2477-2486

Davis TM. (2008).Ethnic diversity in type 2 diabetes. *Diabet Med.* August, 25 Suppl 2, pp. 52-6

Di Cianni G, Volpe L, Lencioni C, Miccoli R, Cuccuru I, Ghio A, Chatzianagnostou K, Bottone P, Teti G, Del Prato S, Benzi L. (2003). Prevalence and risk factors for gestational diabetes assessed by universal screening. *Diabetes Res Clin Pract.* November, Vol.62, No.2, pp.131-7.

Dixon N (2002) Pharmacists as a part of an extended diabetes team, *Pharm J,* No. 268, pp.469-470

Douglas E, Hudson S, Bennie M, McGhee D, Dowers A, McShane C (2000) Pharmaceutical care needs in the primary care management of type 2 diabetes mellitus, *Pharm J,* No. 265, pp. 7114:R6, Available from http://www.pharmj.com/Editorial/20000916/practiceresearch/r6.html Accessed 11 February 2004

Esakoff TF, Cheng YW, Caughey AB. (2005). Screening for gestational diabetes: different cut-offs for different ethnicities? *Am J Obstet Gynecol.* Sep;No. 193, pp.1040-4.

Fan ZT, Yang HX, Gao XL, Lintu H, Sun WJ. (2006). Pregnancy outcome in gestational diabetes. *Int J Gynaecol Obstet.* Jul. Vol. 94, No. 1, pp.12-6.

Ferrara A, Kahn HS, Quesenberry CP, Riley C, Hedderson MM. (2004). An increase in the incidence of gestational diabetes mellitus: Northern California, 1991-2000. *Obstet Gynecol.* Mar; Vol. 103, No.3, pp. :526-33.

Ferrara A. (2007). Increasing prevalence of gestational diabetes mellitus: a public health perspective. *Diabetes Care.* Jul, Vol. 30 Suppl 2, pp.:S141-6.

Forsbach G, Cantú-Diaz C, Vázquez-Lara J, Villanueva-Cuellar MA, Alvarez y García C, Rodríguez-Ramírez E. (1997). Gestational diabetes mellitus and glucose intolerance in a Mexican population. *Int J Gynaecol Obstet,* Dec, Vol. 59, No. 3, pp.229-32.

Fraser R, Heller SR. (2007). Gestational diabetes: aetiology and management. *Obst Gin Rep Med,* Vol.17, No.12, pp.:345-348.

Georgiou H, Lappas M, Georgiou G, Marita A, Bryant V, Hiscock R, Permezel M, Khail Z, Rice G (2008) Screening for biomarkers predictive of gestational diabetes mellitus. *Acta Diabetologica,* No. 45, pp.157-165

Metzger BE, Lowe LP, Dyer AR, Trimble ER, Chaovarindr U, Coustan DR, Hadden DR, McCance DR, Hod M, McIntyre HD, Oats JJ, Persson B, Rogers MS, Sacks DA. (2008). Hyperglycemia and adverse pregnancy outcomes. *NEngl J Med.* No.358, pp.1991–2002

Harris SB, Caulfield LE, Sugamori ME, Whalen EA, Henning B. (1997). The epidemiology of diabetes in pregnant Native Canadians. A risk profile. *Diabetes Care,* September, Vol.20, No. 9, pp.1422-5.

Hillier TA, Pedula KL, Schmidt MM, Mullen JA, Charles MA, Pettitt DJ. (2007). Childhood obesity and metabolic imprinting: the ongoing effects of maternal hyperglycemia. *Diabetes Care,* September, Vol. 30, No. 9, pp.2287-92.

Hillier TA, Vesco KK, Pedula K,. Beil TL, Whitlock EP, Pettitt DJ. (2008). Screening for gestational diabetes mellitus: a systematic review for the US Preventive Services Task Force. *Ann Intern Med,* No 148, pp. 766-775.

Hossein-Nezhad A, Maghbooli Z, Vassigh AR, Larijani B. (2007). Prevalence of gestational diabetes mellitus and pregnancy outcomes in Iranian women. *Taiwan J Obstet Gynecol,* September, Vol. 46, No. 3, pp.:236-41.

Huda SS, Brodie LE, Sattar N. (2010). Obesity in pregnancy: prevalence and metabolic consequences. *Semin Fetal Neonatal Med,* Apr, Vol.15, No. 2, pp.70-6.

Hunsberger M, Rosenberg KD, Donatelle RJ. (2010). Racial/ethnic disparities in gestational diabetes mellitus: findings from a population-based survey. *Womens Health Issues,* September, Vol.20, No.5, pp.323-8.

Huxley R, James WP, Barzi F, Patel JV, Lear SA, Suriyawongpaisal P, Janus E, Caterson I, Zimmet P, Prabhakaran D, Reddy S, Woodward M. (2008). Obesity in Asia Collaboration. Ethnic comparisons of the cross-sectional relationships between measures of body size with diabetes and hypertension. *Obes Rev,* March, Vol. 9, Suppl 1, pp.53-61.

Hyer SL, Shehata HA. (2005). Gestational diabetes mellitus. *Curr Obstet Gynecol,* No. 15, pp.368-374

Metzger BE, Gabbe SG, Persson B, Buchanan TA, Catalano PA, Damm P, Dyer AR, Leiva A, Hod M, Kitzmiler JL, Lowe LP, McIntyre HD, Oats JJ, Omori Y, Schmidt MI. (2010). International association of diabetes and pregnancy study groups recommendations on the diagnosis and classification of hyperglycemia in pregnancy. *Diabetes Care, No.* 33, pp.676–682

International Diabetes Federation, (2011). Diabetes Atlas, http://www.diabetesatlas.org/

International Diabetes Federation, (2004). St Vincent Declaration, Available from http://www.idf.org/e-atlas/home/index.cfm?node=71, Accessed 17 February 2004

Jang HC, Cho NH, Jung KB, Oh KS, Dooley SL, Metzger BE. (1995). Screening for gestational diabetes mellitus in Korea. *Int J Gynaecol Obstet,* Nov, Vol.51, No.2, pp.115-22

Jang HC, Yim CH, Han KO, Yoon HK, Han IK, Kim MY, Yang JH, Cho NH. (2003). Gestational diabetes mellitus in Korea: prevalence and prediction of glucose intolerance at early postpartum. *Diabetes Res Clin Pract,* Aug, Vol.61, No.2, pp.117-24

Johnstone FD. (1999). Gestational diabetes. *Curr Obstet Gynecol, No.*9, pp.23-28

Joshy G, Simmons D. (2006). Epidemiology of diabetes in New Zealand: revisit to a changing landscape. *N Z Med J,* Jun Vol. 2. No.119(1235),U1999

Karcaaltincaba D, Kandemir O, Yalvac S, Güvendag-Guven S, Haberal A. (2009). Prevalence of gestational diabetes mellitus and gestational impaired glucose tolerance in pregnant women evaluated by National Diabetes Data Group and Carpenter and Coustan criteria. *Int J Gynaecol Obstet,* Sep, Vol.106, No.3, pp.246-9.

Kim C, Berger DK, Chamany S. (2007). Recurrence of gestational diabetes mellitus: a systematic review. *Diabetes Care,* May, Vol.30, No. 5, pp.1314-9

Kimmerle R, Zass RP, Cupisti S, Somville T, Bender R, Pawlowski B, Berger M (1995) Pregnancies in women with diabetic nephropathy: long-term outcome for mother and child. Diabetologia No. 38, pp.227-235

Lawrence JM, Contreras R, Chen W, Sacks DA. (2008). Trends in the prevalence of preexisting diabetes and gestational diabetes mellitus among a racially/ethnically diverse population of pregnant women, 1999–2005. *Diabetes Care,*. No.31, pp.899–904.

Lopez-de-Andres A, Carrasco-Garrido P, Gil-de-Miguel A, Hernandez-Barrera V, Jiménez-García R. (2011).Trends in deliveries in women with gestational diabetes in Spain, 2001-2008. *Diabetes Res Clin Pract,* Feb, Vol. 91, No.2, pp.27-9.

Madhavan A, Beena Kumari R, Sanal MG. (2008). A pilot study on the usefulness of body mass index and waist hip ratio as a predictive tool for gestational diabetes in Asian Indians. *Gynecol Endocrinol.* Dec, Vol.24, No.12, pp.701-7.

Mensing C, Boucher J, Cypress M, Weinger K, Mulcahy K, Barta P, et al. (2002) National standards for diabetes self-management education. *Diabetes Care,* No 25 (Suppl. 1):S140-7

Metzger B, Counstan DR (1998) Summary and recommendations of the fourth international workshop - conference on gestational diabetes mellitus. *Diabetes Care,* No. 21(Suppl 2):B161-B167

Metzger BE, Nelson L, Niznik C, Dooley SL. (2006) Update on gestational diabetes. Womens Health (Lond Engl). Mar;Vol. 2, No. 2, pp. 211-6

Ricart W, Lopez J, Mozas J, Pericot A, Sancho MA, González N, Balsells M, Luna R, Cortázar A, Navarro P, Ramírez O, Flández B, Pallardo LF, Hernández A, Ampudia J,

Fernández-Real JM, Corcoy R; (2005). Spanish Group for the Study of the Impact of Carpenter and Coustan GD thresholds. Potential impact of American Diabetes Association (2000) criteria for diagnosis of gestational diabetes mellitus in Spain. *Diabetologia,* Vol. 48, No.6, pp.1135–41

Rosenberg TJ, Garbers S, Chavkin W, Chiasson MA. (2003). Prepregnancy weight and adverse perinatal outcomes in an ethnically diverse population. *Obstet Gynecol.* Nov, No.102, pp.1022-7

Sahu L, satyakata R, Rani R. (2009). Comparison of the American Dia betes Association and World health Organisation criteria for gestational diabetes mellitus and the outcomes of pregnancy. *Obstet Med,* No.2, pp.149-153

Satman I, Yilmaz T, Sengul A, Salman S, Salman F, Uygur S, Bastar I, Tütüncü Y, Sargin M, Dinççag N, Karsidag K, Kalaça S, Ozcan C, King H. (2002).Population-based study of diabetes and risk characteristics in Turkey: results of the Turkish diabetes epidemiology study (TURDEP). *Diabetes Care, Vol.*25, No.9, pp.1551–6

Savitz DA, Janevic TM, Engel SM, Kaufman JS, Herring AH. (2008). Ethnicity and gestational diabetes in New York City, 1995-2003. *BJOG,* Jul, Vol.115, No.8, pp.969-78

Scholl TO, Chen X, Gaughan C, Smith WK. (2002). Influence of maternal glucose level on ethnic differences in birth weight and pregnancy outcome. *Am J Epidemiol,* Sep 15, Vol.156, No.6, pp.498-506

Shai I, Jiang R, Manson JE, Stampfer MJ, Willett WC, Colditz GA, Hu FB. (2006). Ethnicity, obesity, and risk of type 2 diabetes in women: a 20-year follow-up study. *Diabetes Care,*Vol.29, No.7, pp.1585-90

Sinha B, Brydon P, Taylor RS, Hollins A, Munro A, Jenkins D, Dunne F. (2003). Maternal ante-natal parameters as predictors of persistent postnatal glucose intolerance: a comparative study between Afro-Caribbeans, Asians and Caucasians. *Diabet Med,* Vol. 20, No.5, pp.382-6

The DECODA Study Group. Age- and sex-specific prevalence of diabetes and impaired glucose regulation in 11 Asian cohorts. Diabetes Care. 2003;26:1770–1780

The Diabetes Control and Complications Trial Research Group. (1996). Pregnancy outcomes in the Diabetes Control and Complications Trial (DCCT). *Am J Obstet Gynecol,* No.174, pp.1343-1353

Todorova K., Palaveev O, Petkova V., Stefanova M., Dimitrova Zl. (2007) A pharmcoeconomical model for choice of a treatment for pregnant women with gestational diabetes. *Acta Diabetologica,* Vol. 44, No.3, pp.144-148,

Valentine V, Kulkarni K, Hinnen D. (2003). Evolving roles: from diabetes educators to advanced diabetes managers. *Diabetes Spectrum,* Vol. 16,No. 1, pp.27-31

Villamor E, Cnattingius S. (2006). Interpregnancy weight change and risk of adverse pregnancy outcomes: a population-based study. *Lancet,* Sep 30;Vol. 368, No. 9542, pp.1164-70.

Wrongdiagnosis.com, Statistics by Country for Gestational diabetes http://www.wrongdiagnosis.com/g/gestdiab/stats-country.htm?ktrack=kcplink (2011)

Xiong X, Saunders LD, Wang FL, Demianczuk NN. (2001).Gestational diabetes mellitus: prevalence, risk factors, maternal and infant outcomes. *Int J Gynaecol Obstet*, Dec;Vol.75, No.3, pp.221-8.

6

Pathophysiology of Gestational Diabetes Mellitus: The Past, the Present and the Future

Mohammed Chyad Al-Noaemi[1] and
Mohammed Helmy Faris Shalayel[2]
[1]*Al-Yarmouk College, Khartoum,*
[2]*National College for Medical and Technical Studies, Khartoum,*
Sudan

1. Introduction

It is just to remember that "Pathophysiology" refers to the study of alterations in normal body function (physiology and biochemistry) which result in disease. E.g. changes in the normal thyroid hormone level causes either hyper or hypothyroidism. Changes in insulin level as a decrease in its blood level or a decrease in its action will cause hyperglycemia and finally diabetes mellitus.

Scientists agreed that gestational diabetes mellitus (GDM) is a condition in which women without previously diagnosed diabetes exhibit high blood glucose levels during pregnancy.

From our experience most women with GDM in the developing countries are not aware of the symptoms (i.e., the disease will be symptomless). While some of the women will have few symptoms and their GDM is most commonly diagnosed by routine blood examinations during pregnancy which detect inappropriate high level of glucose in their blood samples. GDM should be confirmed by doing fasting blood glucose and oral glucose tolerance test (OGTT), according to the WHO diagnostic criteria for diabetes.

A decrease in insulin sensitivity (i.e. an increase in insulin resistance) is normally seen during pregnancy to spare the glucose for the fetus. This is attributed to the effects of placental hormones. In a few women the physiological changes during pregnancy result in impaired glucose tolerance which might develop diabetes mellitus (GDM). The prevalence of GDM ranges from 1% to 14% of all pregnancies depending on the population studied and the diagnostic tests used. Although the majority of women with GDM return to normal glucose tolerance immediately after delivery, a significant number will remain diabetic or continue to have impaired glucose tolerance (IGT).

To understand how gestational diabetes occurs, it is necessary to understand the normal physiological metabolism of glucose during pregnancy and the physiological changes - mainly the endocrine changes during pregnancy in the feto-placental unit, which might explain the development of insulin resistance and GDM.

1.1 Insulin

Only about 1-2% of the pancreatic structure is endocrine tissues which are represented by the presence of 1-2 million islets of langerhans. These islets contain four main types of cells (A, B, D, and F cells). Insulin is secreted by B (beta) cells which constitute about 60-70% of the islets cells. Insulin is a 51-amino acid polypeptide (small protein) hormone consist of A and B-chains connected together by disulphide bridges (Ganong, 2003; Guyton & Hall, 2006).

1.2 Insulin Receptor (IR)

The IR is a large heterotetrameric, transmembrane glycoprotein, having a molecular weight of about 300,000. Each receptor consists of two alpha (α) subunit that lie outside the cell membrane and two beta (β) subunits that penetrate the cell membrane protruding into the cytoplasm connected together by disulphide bridges in a β-α- α-β configuration. IR is assembled from a single polypeptide pro-receptor, by dimerization, proteolytic cleavage, and glycosylation within the cytoplasm and Golgi apparatus, before trafficking of the mature receptor to the plasma membrane. These insulin receptors have also been designated recently as CD220 (cluster of differentiation 220) (Ganong, 2003; Guyton & Hall, 2006; Ward & Lawrence, 2009).

1.3 Insulin action

Insulin has many metabolic functions such as enhancing cellular uptake of glucose, fatty acids, amino acids, and potassium ions. It also has an anabolic action by increasing cellular formation of glycogen, lipids, and protein. These physiological functions will be reversed if insulin action is decreased as seen with the increase in insulin resistance during pregnancy.
The main function of insulin concerning gestational diabetes mellitus (GDM) is its action on glucose and lipid metabolism.

1.3.1 Insulin effect on lipid metabolism

Normally insulin stimulates the synthesis and release of lipoprotein lipase from the endothelial cells of blood vessels causing lipolysis of triglycerides in the blood and release of free fatty acids (FFA). Insulin enhances the transport of FFA to the fatty cells (adipocytes) to be stored as lipids. Furthermore, insulin inhibits lipoprotein lipase in adipose cells preventing lipolysis.

1.3.2 Insulin effect on glucose metabolism

Insulin enhances entrance of glucose to the cells through its action on the insulin receptors. Insulin receptor complex will stimulates mobilization of glucose carrier protein (GLUT- 4 transporter) from the interior of the cell to the plasma membrane which will transport glucose inside the cell by the process of facilitated diffusion. Furthermore, insulin-receptor complex will activates the storage of some glucose as glycogen while others will be metabolized into pyruvate and then fatty acids which are stored as triglycerides (fat) (Ganong, 2003; Guyton & Hall, 2006).

1.4 Insulin-receptor interaction

To initiate insulin effects on target cells, it first binds with and activates a membrane receptor protein. [4] It is the activated receptor, not the insulin that causes the subsequent effects. The combination of insulin with the alpha subunits will induce autophosphorylation of the beta subunits which will activates a local tyrosine kinase [(phosphatidylinositol 3-kinase (PI3-K)] , which in turn begins a cascade of cell phosphorylation that increase or decrease the activity of enzymes, including insulin receptor substrates (IRSs). There are different types of IRSs (IRS-1, IRS-2, and IRS-3) which are expressed in different tissues

which explain the diversity of insulin action, activating or inactivating certain enzymes to produce the desired effect on the cellular carbohydrate, fat, and protein metabolism (Zwick et al., 2001; Pawson, 1995; Hans-Georg,1995; Perz & Torlińska, 2001).
Within seconds after insulin binds with its membrane receptors, glucose transporters are moved to the cell membrane to facilitate glucose entry into the cell especially to the muscle and adipose tissues (Guyton & Hall, 2006; Sherwood, 2010).

2. Physiology of pregnancy

The endocrinology of human pregnancy involves endocrine and metabolic changes that result from physiological alterations at the boundary between mother and fetus, known as the feto-placental unit (FPU), this interface is a major site of protein and steroid hormone production and secretion. Many of the endocrine and metabolic changes that occur during pregnancy can be directly attributed to hormonal signals originating from the FPU (Ganong, 2003; Guyton & Hall, 2006; Monga & Baker, 2006).
During early pregnancy, glucose tolerance is normal or slightly improved and peripheral (muscle) sensitivity to insulin and hepatic basal glucose production is normal (Catalano et al., 1991; Catalano et al., 1992; Catalano et al., 1993). These could be caused by the increased maternal estrogen and progesterone in early pregnancy which increase and promote pancreatic ß-cell hyperplasia (Expansion of beta-cell mass in response to pregnancy) causing an increased insulin release (Carr & Gabbe, 1998; Rieck & Kaestner, 2010). This explains the rapid increase in insulin level in early pregnancy, in response to insulin resistance. In the second and third trimester, the continuous increase in the feto-placental factors will decrease maternal insulin sensitivity, and this will stimulate mother cells to use sources of fuels (energy) other than glucose as free fatty acids, and this will increase supply of glucose to the fetus (Catalano et al., 1991; Catalano et al., 1992; Ryan & Enns, 1988). In the normal physiological conditions, the fetal blood glucose is 10-20% less than maternal blood glucose allowing the transport of glucose in the placenta to the fetal blood by the process of simple diffusion and facilitated transport. Therefore, glucose is the main fuel required by the developing fetus, whether as a source of energy for cellular metabolism or to provide energy for the synthesis of protein, lipids, and glycogen.
During pregnancy, the insulin resistance of the whole body is increased to about three times the resistance in the non-pregnant state.
In general, the resistance to insulin can be characterized as pre-receptor (insulin antibodies) as in autoimmune diseases, receptor (decreased number of receptors on the cell surface) as in obesity, or post-receptor (defects in the intracellular insulin signaling pathway). In pregnancy, the decreased insulin sensitivity is best characterized by a post-receptor defect resulting in the decreased ability of insulin to bring about SLC2A4 (GLUT4) mobilization from the interior of the cell to the cell surface (Catalano, 2010). This could be due to increase in the plasma levels of one or more of the pregnancy-associated hormones (Kühl, 1991; Hornns, 1985).
Although, pregnancy is associated with increase in the beta-cell mass and increase in insulin level throughout pregnancy but certain pregnant women are unable to up-regulate insulin production relative to the degree of insulin resistance, and consequently become hyperglycemic, developing gestational diabetes (Kühl, 1991).

3. Diagnosis of gestational diabetes mellitus

Gestational diabetes mellitus (GDM) is defined as any degree of glucose intolerance resulting in hyperglycemia of variable severity, with onset or first recognition during pregnancy. It does not exclude the possibility that unrecognized glucose intolerance may have antedated but has been previously unrecognized (Metzger, 1991; Definition and Diagnosis of Diabetes Mellitus and Intermediate Hyperglycemia *World Health Organization* [WHO], 2006). Women who become pregnant and who are known to have diabetes mellitus which antedates pregnancy do not have gestational diabetes but have "diabetes mellitus and pregnancy" and should be treated accordingly before, during, and after the pregnancy (WHO, 2006).

Gestational diabetes generally has few symptoms and it is most commonly diagnosed by screening during pregnancy. Diagnostic tests detect inappropriately high levels of glucose in blood samples.

3.1 WHO diagnostic criteria for hyperglycemia and GDM (2006)

In the early part of pregnancy (e.g. first trimester and first half of second trimester) fasting and postprandial glucose concentrations are normally lower than in normal, non-pregnant women. Elevated fasting or postprandial plasma glucose levels at this time in pregnancy may well reflect the presence of diabetes which has antedated pregnancy. The occurrence of higher than usual plasma glucose levels at this time in pregnancy mandates careful management and may be an indication for carrying out an oral glucose tolerance test (OGTT). Nevertheless, normal glucose tolerance in the early part of pregnancy does not by itself establish that gestational diabetes will not develop later.

It may be appropriate to screen pregnant women belonging to high-risk populations during the first trimester of pregnancy in order to detect previously undiagnosed diabetes mellitus. Formal systematic testing for gestational diabetes is usually done between 24 and 28 weeks of gestation. To determine if gestational diabetes is present in pregnant women, a standard OGTT should be performed after overnight fasting (8-14 hours) by giving 75 g anhydrous glucose in 250-300 ml water. Plasma glucose is measured fasting and after 2 hours. Pregnant women who meet WHO criteria for diabetes mellitus or impaired glucose tolerance (IGT) are classified as having GDM. After the pregnancy ends, the woman should be re-classified as having either diabetes mellitus, or IGT, or normal glucose tolerance based on the results of a 75 g OGTT six weeks or more after delivery.

The following table (table 1) summarizes the 2006 WHO recommendations for the diagnostic criteria for diabetes and intermediate hyperglycemia (WHO, 2006).

Diabetes	
Fasting plasma glucose	≥7.0mmol/l (126mg/dl), or
2-h plasma glucose *	≥11.1mmol/l (200mg/dl)
Impaired Glucose Tolerance (IGT)	
Fasting plasma glucose	<7.0mmol/l (126mg/dl)
2-h plasma glucose*	≥7.8 and <11.1mmol/l (140mg/dl and 00mg/dl)
Impaired Fasting Glucose (IFG)	
Fasting plasma glucose	6.1 to 6.9 mmol/L (110mg/dl to 125 mg/dl)
2-h Plasma glucose*	< 7.8 mmol/dl (140mg/dl)

* Venous plasma 2-h after ingestion of 75gm oral glucose load (OGTT)

Table 1. Diagnostic criteria for diabetes and intermediate hyperglycemia

3.2 Glycosylated hemoglobin (HbA1c) as a diagnostic test for GDM

Since 1984, professor Alwan AAS and collaborators have adopted the measurement of HbA1c levels as another index for follow-up of pregnant diabetic patients, and reported a significant relationship between elevated levels of HbA1c late in the third trimester and feto-maternal complications (Al-Dahwi et al., 1986; Al- Dahwi et al., 1987; Al-Dahwi et al., 1988; Al-Dahwi et al., 1989). Recently, the American Diabetic Association (2009) added that HbA1c ≥ 6.5% is another criterion for the diagnosis of diabetes (Nathan, 2009). Therefore we highly recommend the measurement of HbA1c during pregnancy, as an additional diagnostic criteria and to anticipate the maternal and fetal complications if it is abnormally elevated.

4. Pathophysiology of GDM

In the pathophysiology of GDM we have to consider two main points.
4.1 Role of feto-placental unit in GDM.
4.2 Role of the adipose tissue in GDM.

4.1 The role of feto-placental unit in the development of GDM

The past; In the last century insulin resistance and the decrease in insulin sensitivity during pregnancy is mainly attributed to the increase in the levels of **pregnancy-associated hormones** as estrogen, progesterone, cortisol, and placental lactogen in the maternal circulation (Ryan, 1988; Hornns, 1985; Ahmed & Shalayel, 1999; Polderman et al., 1994; Barbour et al., 2002). Normally the insulin resistance of the whole body is increased to about three times that seen in the non-pregnant state (Kuhl, 1998; Catalano et al., 1999). The increased resistance is caused by post-insulin receptor events and is probably brought about by the cellular effects of the increased levels of one or all of the above hormones (Davis, 1990). As pregnancy progresses and the placenta grow larger, hormone production also increases and so does the level of insulin resistance. This process usually starts between 20 and 24 weeks of pregnancy. At birth, when the placenta is delivered, the hormone production stops and so does the condition, strongly suggesting that these hormones cause GDM (Ryan & Enns, 1988; Kuhl, 1975; Buchanan & Xiang, 2005).

4.1.1 Feto-placental unit

The placenta synthesizes pregnenolone and progesterone from cholesterol. Some of the progesterone enters the fetal circulation and provides the substrate for the formation of cortisol and corticosterone in the fetal adrenal glands. Some of the pregnenolone enters the fetus and, along with pregnenolone synthesized in the fetal liver, is the substrate for the formation of dehydroepiandrosterone sulfate (DHEAS) and 16-hydroxydehydroepiandrosterone sulfate (16-OHDHEAS) in the fetal adrenal. Some 16-hydroxylation also occurs in the fetal liver. DHEAS and 16-OHDHEAS are transported back to the placenta, where DHEAS forms estradiol and 16-OHDHEAS forms estriol. The principal estrogen formed is estriol, and since fetal 16-OHDHEAS is the principal substrate for the estrogens, the urinary estriol excretion of the mother can be monitored as an index of the state of the fetus (Ganong, 2003).

4.1.2 Diabetic action of steroid hormones (cortisol, estrogen, and progesterone)

These hormones are increased steadily with the advance of pregnancy. The anti-insulin action of these hormones is a well known fact since the last century (Ryan & Enns, 1988;

Barbour et al., 2002; Barbieri, 1999; Kirwan et al., 2002; Shalayel et al., 2010). The fetus and the placenta interact in the formation of these steroid hormones. It has been shown that the increase in **cortisol** level during pregnancy is considered as the main hormone which cause decrease in glucose tolerance in normal pregnancy (Hornns, 1985; Ahmed & Shalayel, 1999). While others considered that **estrogen** and **progesterone** which are elevated steadily during pregnancy are the main hormones which influence beta cell function in early pregnancy and insulin resistance especially in late pregnancy (Ryan & Enns, 1988; Polderman et al., 1994; Glass & Kase, 1984).

Although some scientists have considered that human chorionic gonadotropin (HCG) may participates in the development of insulin resistance during pregnancy as it shows higher level in women with GDM in comparison with normal pregnancies (Merviel et al., 2001). But, as we know from the normal changes during pregnancy, the main increase of HCG occurs during the first trimester, and this period is associated with an increase in insulin sensitivity and improvement of glucose tolerance. Therefore, we consider that HCG has no direct role as a cause of GDM.

4.1.3 Human placental lactogen (hPL), [human chorionic somatomammotropin (hCS)]

It is a single polypeptide chain held together by disulphide bonds. It is about 96% similar to human growth hormone (HGH), but has only 3% of HGH activity. Its half life is short (15minutes); hence its appeal as an index of placental problems (Glass & Kase, 1984). HPL, which is the product of the HPL-A and HPL-B genes, is secreted into both the maternal and fetal circulations after the sixth week of pregnancy (Handwerger & Freemark, 2000). The level of HPL in the maternal circulation is correlated with fetal and placental weight, plateauing in the last 4 weeks of pregnancy. Therefore, measurement of HPL levels is used as a screening test for fetal distress and neonatal asphyxia (Glass & Kase, 1984; Letchworth & Chard, 1972).

4.1.3.1 Physiologicalfunction of HPL

During pregnancy the maternal level of HPL can be altered by changing the circulating level of glucose. HPL is elevated with hypoglycemia and depressed with hyperglycemia (Barbour et al., 2002; Kuhl, 1998). The metabolic role of HPL is to mobilize lipids and free fatty acids. In the fed state, there is abundant glucose available, leading to increased insulin level, lipogenesis, and glucose utilization. This is associated with decreased gluconeogenesis, and a decrease in the circulating free fatty acid levels, as the free fatty acids are utilized in the process of lipogenesis to deposit storage packets of triglycerides (Glass & Kase, 1984; Kim & Feling, 1971).

4.1.3.2 Diabetogenic action of HPL

In the second half of pregnancy, HPL level rises approximately 10 folds. HPL stimulates lipolysis leading to an increase in circulating free fatty acids in order to provide a different fuel for the mother so that glucose and amino acids can be conserved for the fetus. The increase in free fatty acid levels, in turn directly interferes with insulin-directed entry of glucose into cells. Therefore, HPL is considered as a potent antagonist to insulin action during pregnancy (Glass & Kase, 1984; Mills et al., 1985). Furthermore, HPL and placental growth hormone act in concert in the mother to stimulate insulin-like growth factor (IGF) production and modulate intermediary metabolism, resulting in an increase in the availability of glucose and amino acids to the fetus (Handwerger & Freemark, 2000).

4.1.4 Placental growth hormone (PGH)

PGH is the product of the GH-V gene specifically expressed in the syncytiotrophoblast layer of the human placenta. PGH (20-kDa HGH-V) differs from pituitary growth hormone by 13 amino acids. It has high somatogenic and low lactogenic activities (Lacroix et al., 2002). PGH is produced by the placenta and found predominantly in the maternal circulation. It progressively replaces pituitary growth hormone (hGH) in the human maternal circulation from mid-gestation onwards, peaking towards term (Chellakooty et al., 2004). PGH appears to be an important potential regulator of maternal insulin resistance in human pregnancy and may influence fetal growth both by modifying substrate availability and through paracrine actions in the placental bed (McIntyre et al., 2009).

Barbour et al (2004) demonstrated a unique mechanism of insulin resistance in non-pregnant transgenic mice and suggested that human placental growth hormone (hPGH) may contribute to the insulin resistance of normal pregnancy secondary to its effect on p85α expression and its interference with PI 3-kinase activity in skeletal muscle.

Nevertheless, in a recent experimental study by Vickers and Gilmour (2009), it was demonstrated that rats treated with HGH enhanced insulin sensitivity and suggested that HGH have an antidiabetic action.

It seems that there is a controversy about the involvement of HGH with insulin resistance and GDM.

In conclusion, considering the previously discussed hormones, HPL is considered as the main diabetogenic hormone synthesized and released from the feto-placental unit. But during pregnancy, there is another maternal hormone which is involved in insulin resistance which is prolactin.

4.1.5 Prolactin

Prolactin level begins to rise at 5-8 weeks of gestation, followed by a progressively increase in its level as pregnancy advances (Shalayel et al., 2010; Glass & Kase, 1984). The increase in prolactin secretion is due the increase in the size and number of maternal pituitary lactotrophs (Kuhl et al., 1985) and its secretion from the uterine decidual cells seems to be stimulated by progesterone and insulin (Ahmed & Shalayel, 1999; Davis, 1990).

Shalayel et al (2010) revealed that prolactin increases progressively as pregnancy advances, reaching a peak in the third trimester when many pregnant ladies may develop gestational diabetes due to the state of insulin resistance which may occur although there is no evidence that prolactin may be directly incorporated with the pathogenesis of glucose intolerance in pregnancy. A decline in insulin secretion may lead to a decline in prolactin since insulin stimulates both acute secretion and de novo synthesis of decidual prolactin.

There were no significant differences in the level of plasma prolactin in normal or diabetic pregnancies; in fact its level might be lower in the pregnancies with GDM (Guyton & Hall, 2006). Therefore, prolactin might have no effect on glucose intolerance during pregnancy (Milasinovic et al., 1997).

4.2 The role of adipose tissue in the development of GDM

4.2.1 Adipocytokines

Historically, placental hormones have been considered as the primary mediators of insulin resistance during gestation. Over the past decade, adipose tissue has been shown to produce numerous factors (adipocytokines), most of them act as hormones. These adipocyte-derived hormones have been implicated in the regulation of maternal metabolism and gestational insulin resistance. Adipocytokines, including leptin, adiponectin, tumor necrosis factor alpha, interleukin-6, as well as the newly discovered resistin, visfatin, and apelin, are also known to be produced within the intrauterine environment (Catalano, 2010; Briana & Malamitsi-Puchner, 2009; Henry & Clarke, 2008).

Although human placental lactogen has often been cited as the cause of the decreased insulin sensitivity in pregnancy, because of its production from the placenta and increasing concentrations with advancing gestation as described previously (Ryan & Enns, 1988), more recently the role of adipocytokines and elevated lipid concentrations in pregnancy have been correlated with the longitudinal changes in insulin sensitivity in non-pregnant women (Hotamisligil et al., 1994) as well as in pregnant women (Kirwan et al., 2002; Hotamisligil et al., 1996). Evidence suggests that one or more of these adipokines (as TNF-α and leptin) could impair insulin signaling and cause insulin resistance (Briana & Malamitsi-Puchner, 2009; Xiang et al., 1999). TNF-α in specific has a potential effect in decreasing insulin sensitivity (Catalano, 2010). While other adipocytokines might increase insulin sensitivity as adiponectin which has been shown to be decreased especially in late pregnancy (Al-Noaemi & Shalayel, 2009).

4.2.1.1 Adiponectin

Adiponectin is a novel adipocyte secreting protein hormone discovered in 1995/1996 (Scherer et al., 1995; Nakano et al., 1996; Maeda et al., 1996; Hu et al., 1996; Tsao et al., 2002). Adiponectin is abundant in the circulation of humans, with plasma levels in the microgram per ml range, thus accounting for approximately 0.01% of total plasma protein.

Chen *et al.* (2006) reported that the human placenta produces and secretes adiponectin and that adiponectin and its receptors are differentially regulated by cytokines and their expression altered in women with gestational diabetes mellitus, suggesting that adiponectin may play a role in adapting energy metabolism at the materno-fetal interface.

4.2.1.1.1 Functions of Adiponectin

Although the physiological role of adiponectin is not yet fully determined, but it has been shown that there are a variety of physiological functions induced by adiponectin such as:

4.2.1.1.1.A General functions

i. Anti-atherosclerotic action: By inhibiting lipid-laden foam cell formation (Ouchi et al., 2001), and inhibiting the inflammatory adipokine, tumor necrosis factor-α (TNF-α) (Ouchi et al., 2000).
ii. Anti-inflammatory action: By inhibiting the phagocytic activity of macrophages and inhibiting the production of TNF-α by these macrophages (Yokota et al., 2000).
iii. Anti-oxidant action: By stimulating the endothelial cells to produce nitric oxide (NO) (Ouchi et al., 1999).
iv. Anti-tumor action: There is a significant inverse association of adiponectin with postmenopausal endometrial and breast cancer (Mantzoros et al., 2004; Petridou et al., 2003).

4.2.1.1.1.B Specific anti-diabetic functions such as its actions on glucose and lipid metabolism

i. Effects of adiponectin on insulin and glucose metabolism: Adiponectin has insulin-sensitizing effects. Replenishment of a physiological dose of recombinant adiponectin to lipoatrophic mice significantly ameliorated insulin resistance. Moreover, insulin resistance in lipoatrophic mice was completely reversed by the combination of physiological doses of adiponectin and leptin (Hotta et al., 2000; Berg et al., 2001). In addition to that, adiponectin has indirect insulin-sensitizing effect by decreasing tissue triglyceride (TG) content (Shulman, 2000). It is well known that tissue triglycerides interfere with insulin-stimulated phosphatidylinositol (PI) 3-kinase activation and subsequent glucose transporter 4 (GLUT-4) translocations and glucose uptake, leading to insulin resistance (Shulman, 2000; Godoy-Matos et al., 2010). Thus, decreased tissue TG content in muscle may contribute to the improved insulin signal transduction. Interestingly, in skeletal muscle, adiponectin increases expression of molecules involved in fatty acid transport such as CD36, in combustion of fatty-acid such as acyl-coenzyme-A oxidase, and in energy dissipation such as uncoupling protein 2. These changes led to decreased tissue TG content in skeletal muscle whether in experimental animals or in human (Godoy-Matos et al., 2010; Yamauchi et al., 2001; Thamer et al., 2002).

ii. Effect of adiponectin on glucose metabolism: It has been reported that an acute increase in circulating adiponectin levels triggers a transient decrease in basal glucose levels by inhibiting both the expression of hepatic gluconeogenic enzymes and the rate of endogenous glucose production in both wild-type mice and a type 2 diabetic mouse model (Berg et al., 2001; Combs et al., 2001). Furthermore, Kubota et al (2002) provided the first direct evidence that adiponectin plays a protective role against insulin resistance by generating adiponectin-deficient mice. Adiponectin improves insulin resistance and glucose tolerance in both heterozygous (+/-) and homozygous (-/-) adiponectin-deficient mice.

iii. Effects of adiponectin on lipid metabolism: Adiponectin activates AMP-Kinase (AMPK) and peroxisome proliferator-actvated receptor (PPAR α) in the liver and muscle, thereby stimulating fatty-acid oxidation and decreasing tissue TG content in the liver and muscle (Thamer et al., 2002; Fruebis et al., 2001; Yamauchi et al., 2003a). Furthermore, adiponectin decreases lipid synthesis and glucose production in the liver and causes a decrease in glucose and fatty acid concentration in the blood (Meier & Gressner, 2004; Yool et al., 2006).

4.2.1.1.2 Adiponectin and the pathophysiology of obesity and diabetes

Many studies have shown that plasma adiponectin concentration is negatively correlated with body mass index (BMI) and accordingly, lower in obese than in lean subjects (Ouchi et al., 1999; Hotta et al., 2000; Pena et al., 2009). Furthermore, scientists extended these finding by demonstrating that plasma adiponectin concentrations are inversely related to percentage of body fat, a direct measure of adiposity. And that is consistent across different ethnic groups. These results thus confirm that adiponectin is the main adipose-specific protein known to date that despite its excusive production in white adipose tissue, is negatively regulated in obesity (Hu et al., 1996; Weyer et al., 2001; Statnick et al., 2000). These scientific data suggest that adiponectin may have a role in the pathogenesis of obesity. As obesity is a predisposing factor for the development of diabetes mellitus in general and GDM in specific, this might explain the indirect involvement of a decreased adiponectin in the pathogenesis of diabetes mellitus. It has also been shown that in pregnant women there is a decrease in adiponectin which is associated with an increase in insulin resistance in the third trimester and a further decrease in women with IGT or GDM compared to pregnant women with normal glucose tolerance test, even after adjustment for varying degree of adiposity. Hypoadiponectinemia was also found in women with GDM independently of

their body fat mass compared to women with normal glucose tolerance during and after pregnancy (Yamauchi et al., 2003; Weyer et al., 2001; Kadowaki & Yamaushi, 2005).
On experimental animal studies, it was shown that adiponectin causes glucose-lowering effects and ameliorates insulin resistance in mice (Yamauchi et al., 2003b). Thus, decreased plasma adiponectin concentrations (hypoadiponectinemia) could be involved in the pathophysiology of pregnancy-driven insulin resistance and in the pathogenesis of GDM and Diabetes mellitus type 2 (DM2).
It is known that peroxisome proliferator-activated receptors (PPARs) are transcriptional factors involved in the regulation of insulin resistance, fat cell differentiation, and adipogenesis (*Joosen et al., 2006; Schoonjans et al., 1996; Zeghari et al., 2000)*. It has been shown that adiponectin activates AMP-kinase and PPARγ and α which improves insulin resistance and reduces fasting glucose level (Tsuchida et al., 2005; Kadowaki & Yamauchi, 2005). Low plasma adiponectin correlates highly with insulin resistance in obesity, type 2 DM and GDM (Weyer et al., 2001; *Worda* et al., 2004; *Cseh et al., 2004).*
Low adiponectin level in normal pregnancy and GDM could be due to the suppression effect of TNF-α and other inflammatory factors on adiponectin transcription in adipocytes (*Bruun* et al., 2003; *Fasshauer* et al., 2003). These data highly support the antidiabetic effect of adiponectin.

4.2.1.2 Tumor necrosis factor-α (TNF-α)

In 1975 Carswell et al discovered the so-called tumor necrosis factor (TNF) which is released from macrophages and induces tumor necrosis. Increased circulating TNF-α levels have been associated with insulin resistance in obesity, aging, sepsis, muscle damage, and burn patients (Hotamisligil et al., 1996; del Aguila et al., 2000; Kirwan et al., 2001; Ling et al., 1994; Conrad et al., 1998). Obese animals and humans show a positive correlation between TNF-α levels and BMI and hyperinsulinemia (Ling et al., 1994; Clapp & Kiess, 2000; Laham et al., 1994).
Kirwan et al (2001) reported that TNF-α is a significant predictor of insulin resistance during pregnancy. Together with a small additive contribution from leptin and cortisol, TNF-α exerted a significant influence on insulin-mediated glucose disposal. Circulating TNF-α showed a downward trend during early pregnancy and increased during the third trimester, thus mirroring insulin sensitivity changes during those periods. This observation is consistent with studies showing an increase in plasma TNF-α in late pregnancy (Kirwan et al., 2002; Clapp & Kiess, 2000; Boyd et al., 2007). TNF-α correlates inversely with insulin secretion in normal pregnancy and was significantly higher in GDM group (McLachlan et al., 2006).
TNF-alpha mRNA and protein are present in human placenta and uterine cells at both early and late stages of gestation (Chen et al., 1991). In maternal obesity, the level of TNF-α is increased in the placenta compared with the non-obese pregnant women (Denison et al., 2010). Furthermore, it has been shown that placenta and subcutaneous adipose tissues obtained from women with GDM release greater amount of TNF-α in response to high glucose compared with normal glucose. On the other hand, there was no stimulatory effect of high glucose on TNF-α release by tissues obtained from normal pregnant women which suggests that TNF-α might be involved in the pathogenesis and /or progression of GDM (Coughlan et al., 2001). These results could highly explain the increase in the level of TNF-α throughout pregnancy. The increased TNF-α levels in pregnancy fall rapidly after delivery (Kirwan et al., 2002; Uvena et al., 1999), which is consistent with the idea that the increase in

circulating TNF-α during late pregnancy is mainly due to placental secretion. These findings may also help to explain the rapid reversal of insulin resistance after delivery, since maternal levels of TNF-α decrease substantially after delivery of the placenta (Kirwan et al., 2002; Coughlan et al., 2001).

4.2.1.2.1 The Diabetogenic action of TNF-a

In-vitro studies have described a direct role for TNF-α in the pathophysiology of insulin resistance. TNF-α downregulates insulin receptor signaling in cultured adipocytes (Catalano, 2010), hepatocytes (Feinstein et al., 1993), and skeletal muscle (del Aguila et al., 1999). TNF-α activates a pathway that increases sphingomyelinase and ceramides and appears to interfere with insulin receptor autophosphorylation (Catalano, 2010). Also it has been shown that TNF-α promotes serine phosphorylation of insulin receptor substrate (IRS)-1, thus impairing its association with the insulin receptor (Rui et al., 2001). In pregnancy, there is an evidence that insulin receptor and IRS-1 tyrosine phosphorylation are impaired, and serine phosphorylation is increased in late gestation in skeletal muscle (Friedman et al., 1999; Shao et al., 2000). Therefore, it seems that elevated levels of TNF-α in late gestation could attenuate insulin signaling, thus causing the decreased insulin sensitivity observed in pregnancy.

Barbour et al (2007) demonstrated that in skeletal muscle there is 40% decrease in glucose entrance in normal pregnant women and 65% decrease in GDM compared with obese pregnant women. Although there is no decrease in GLUT4 protein transporter in skeletal muscle (Garvey et al., 1992), the GLUT4 transporters are decreased in adipose tissue (Garvey & Birnbaum, 1993). The increase in circulating TNF-α in women with GDM is also associated with an increased TNF-α in the skeletal muscle and the impaired insulin signaling persist in obese women with gestational diabetes mellitus up to one year postpartum (Kirwan et al., 2004).

TNF- α is considered as one of the factors which suppress PPAR-γ (Kirwan et al., 2002). Furthermore, it has been shown that TNF-α downregulates PPAR-γ expression in 3T3-L1 cells and can inhibit adipose differentiation (Zhang et al., 1996).

Catalano et al (2002) observed a decrease in steady-state PPARγ mRNA and protein concentration in normal and GDM subjects during late gestation. Furthermore, it has been demonstrated that TNF-α decreases adiponectin gene expression in human adipocytes (Kappes & Loffler, 2000), and 3t3-L1 adipocytes (Fasshauer et al., 2002). Whereas thiazolidinediones (synthetic PPAR-gamma ligand) significantly increases the plasma adiponectin concentrations in insulin resistant humans and rodents without affecting their body weight, suggesting that the anti TNF-α will restore the adiponectin and improve the insulin sensitivity (Maeda et al., 2005).

Thus the increase in TNF-α whether in subjects with normal pregnancy or with GDM might explain the lower level of adiponectin (insulin-sensitizing hormone). The above data highly suggest the involvement of TNF-α in the development of GDM.

4.2.1.3 Resistin

Steppan et al. (2001) showed that adipocytes secrete a unique signalling molecule, which is considered as a hormone and named 'resistin' (for resistance to insulin). Resistin is a 114-amino acid polypeptide hormone (Doshani & Konje, 2009).

There is a great argument about the involvement of resistin in the pathogenesis of diabetes mellitus. Some scientists reported the involvement of resistin in the pathogenesis of diabetes mellitus relying on their studies that revealed strong correlations between resistin and obesity as serum resistin levels increased with increased adiposity (Steppan et al., 2001; Vendrell et al.,

2004; Lee et al., 2005). Conversely, serum resistin levels have been found to decline with decreased adiposity following medical treatment (Valsamakis et al., 2004). This discovery is further authenticated by studies which confirmed a direct correlation between resistin levels and subjects with type 2DM (Steppan et al., 2001; Fujinami et al., 2004; McTernan et al., 2003). Nevertheless, this theory lacks support from the entire scientific community at large as an increasingly greater number of studies presenting contradictory evidences continue to emerge (Lee et al., 2003; Nagaev & Smith, 2001). Some studies found significant decreased serum concentrations of resistin with increased adiposity (Heilbronn et al., 2004; Way et al., 2001) suggesting that not only resistin is downregulated in obese subjects but that it also presents itself as an unlikely candidate for linking obesity to Type 2DM. Milan et al (2002) mentioned that a decrease of resistin mRNA after weight loss does not support the hypothesis that resistin may play a causative role in insulin resistance in obese rats.

Many studies reported that in patients with type 2 diabetes or obesity, both resistin levels and resistin expression in fat cells are increased, correlating with hepatic, but not muscle, insulin resistance. In humans, the major source of resistin is the immune cells rather than the adipocytes, resistin being a potent inflammatory agent. Insulin inhibits resistin expression in adipocytes. Therefore, the elevated basal plasma resistin levels found in patients with type 2 diabetes, despite increased insulin concentrations, may be the result of adipocyte insulin resistance. Resistin inhibits the phosphorylation of hepatic AMPK, decreasing β oxidation and increasing fatty acid esterification in triglycerides, and eventually leading to lipid accumulation (Maiorana et al., 2007).

4.2.1.4 Leptin

It was discovered as an antiobesity hormone in *ob/ob* mice (Zhang et al., 1994). In human adult, the white adipose tissue is the main source of leptin, and its circulating concentration is positively correlated with body mass index and fat mass (Maffei et al., 1995; Hellstrom et al., 2000).

Leptin has been detected in the placenta (Masuzaki et al., 1997), and shown to be increased in early pregnancy, remained elevated in late pregnancy (Kirwan et al., 2002; Highman et al., 1998), and was highest in the more obese GDM group (Kirwan et al., 2002). The increased leptin during pregnancy is not proportional with the change in adipose tissue mass, and it return to the normal level after delivery suggesting that leptin production by the placenta contributes to maternal leptinemia during pregnancy (Lepercq et al., 2001).

In vitro study on muscle, Muoio et al (1997) demonstrated that leptin attenuated both the antioxidative and the lipogenic effects of insulin by 50%. Cseh K et al (2002) suggested that the increased TNF-alpha and leptin levels may contribute to insulin resistance in GDM and in the third trimester of normal pregnancy. Furthermore, Qiu et al (2004) demonstrated that Hyperleptinemia, independent of maternal adiposity, in early pregnancy appears to be predictive of an increased risk of GDM later in pregnancy. Kirwan et al (2002) reported that leptin was increased in all women in early pregnancy, remained elevated in late pregnancy, and was highest in the more obese GDM group. But to adjust for the possible confounding effect of obesity and increased fat mass on the relationship between leptin and insulin sensitivity, they covaried for body fat and found that the correlation was no longer significant, because the increased leptin per se was not predictive of insulin sensitivity. They interpreted that, in addition to insulin resistance, leptin resistance may also develop in late pregnancy.

Chen et al (2010) carried out a study in which twenty women with normal pregnancy and 20 with GDM were recruited and blood samples were taken on the day of delivery and Days 1, 3 and 5 after delivery. Serum leptin levels were significantly higher in women with GDM than in the controls before delivery and decreased significantly after delivery ($p < 0.001$). After delivery there were no significant differences in serum leptin concentrations between women with GDM and the controls. Serum soluble leptin receptor concentrations did not differ neither between the two groups, nor before or after delivery. Thus, they concluded that Leptin may play a role in GDM through a positive correlation with insulin resistance.

4.2.1.5 Visfatin

Fukuhara et al (2005) isolated a newly adipocytokine, named as 'visfatin', which is highly enriched in the visceral fat of both humans and mice and whose expression level in plasma increases during the development of obesity. Visfatin exerted insulin-mimetic effects in cultured cells and lowered plasma glucose levels in mice by binding and activating the insulin receptors. Suggesting that visfatin's physiological role may lead to new insights into glucose homeostasis and/or new therapies for metabolic disorders such as diabetes.

According to some authors, plasma concentrations of visfatin are elevated in obesity (Berndt et al., 2005), type 2 diabetes (Chen et al., 2006) and the increase is typically observed in GDM (Krzyzanowska et al., 2006; Lewandowski et al., 2007), all of which are states characterized by insulin resistance. There are also, however, data pointing to possible lower visfatin levels in obese subjects (Pagano et al., 2006), similarly, Chan et al. (2006) have reported lower visfatin levels in women of Chinese origin with GDM. The precise reason for these differences is unclear.

Shali et al (2009) reported that maternal GDM, as well as delivery of a large-for-gestational-age (LGA) neonate were independently associated with higher maternal plasma visfatin concentrations. The linkage between increased maternal circulating visfatin and the presence of GDM or delivery of an LGA neonate supports the hypothesis that perturbation of adipokines homeostasis may play a role in the pathophysiology of GDM or excess fetal growth.

The current data regarding the relationship between visfatin and insulin sensitivity in humans are conflicting. Some authors report a lack of correlation (Berndt et al., 2005; Pagano et al., 2006; Zhang et al., 2010), while others observed a significant correlation (Chen et al., 2006; Lewandowski et al., 2007).

The role of visfatin in human physiology and pathophysiology remains to be elucidated and further work is needed to establish the exact function of visfatin and its mode of action on insulin resistance during normal pregnancy and GDM.

4.2.1.6 Apelin

Tatemoto et al (1998) isolated an APJ receptor ligand, designated apelin, from bovine stomach extracts. The preproproteins consisted of 77 amino acid residues, and the apelin sequence was encoded in the C-terminal regions indicating that apelin is an endogenous ligand for the APJ receptor.

Apelin has been described as an adipocyte-secreted factor (adipokine), that is up-regulated in obesity and the expression of apelin gene in adipose tissue is reported to increase by insulin and TNF-α (Carpéné et al., 2007). Apelin synthesis in adipocytes is stimulated by insulin, and plasma apelin level markedly increases in obesity associated with insulin resistance and hyperinsulinemia (Bełtowski, 2006).

Dray et al (2010) reported that apelin is increased in adipose tissue in different mice models of obesity and in the type2 diabetic patients. They reported that apelin plasma levels were significantly increased in type 2 diabetic patients. They suggested that apelin and APJ expression in mice and humans are regulated in a tissue dependent manner and according to the severity of insulin resistance. But, Meral et al (2010) reported that no significant relation was found between apelin and BMI, glucose, lipids levels, and also insulin sensitivity. In addition, Telejko et al (2010) reported that there is no associations between circulating apelin or apelin/APJ mRNA expression and GDM and no indices of insulin resistance were noted in their study. Furthermore, Tapan et al (2010) recently reported a significant decrease in plasma apelin and adiponectin levels in pubertal obese children.
More work is needed to establish the involvement/or not of apelin and insulin resistance in normal pregnancy and GDM.

5. The future

Every now and then, there will be a new factor, hormone, adipocytokine, etc. which is involved in the development of insulin resistance and GDM. But the precise pathophysiological mechanisms which make the women unable to balance insulin needs and develop GDM, remain unknown. However, a number of future studies could explain some of these mechanisms.

5.1 Genotyping

Genetic variants might be involved in the defect in B-cell function and/or subcellular insulin signaling which contribute to the development of GDM. Therefore, we suggest a screening genotyping test for a significant number of pregnant women, to identify any genetic variants in those who develop GDM. Extending this genotyping to involve familial studies, to demonstrate any involvement of these genetic variants and whether they run in families. Any positive result will help to give a special care to those women anticipated to develop GDM, and thus reducing the associated maternal or fetal complications.

5.2 Subcellular studies

Certain studies should be done to identify the exact subcellular reactions in the normal insulin resistance that develop during normal pregnancy compared with those subcellular changes that lead to glucose intolerance and GDM. The use of radioactive substances might help to identify the change in phosphorylation of serine instead of tyrosine residues, or in any other subcellular reaction change which occurs in GDM.

5.3 Autoimmunity

To study certain aspects of the immune system, which could demonstrate any B-cell dysfunction that develops GDM and is related to autoimmunity. Furthermore, if there is any interference of the immune system with insulin-receptor interaction, this might contribute to the development of GDM.

5.4 Environmental and diet factors

30-40 years ago or more, it has been reported that the percent of GDM range from 1-2%, 2-3% then the percent increased to 1-4%, 2-7%, 5-10%. Until recently using 1-hour glucose challenge OGTT had demonstrated that up to 17% of pregnant women develop GDM. That means there is a significant increase in the development of GDM in these days. Could there be more in future? Environmental factors, changes in life style, and change of diet, such as decrease in using fresh diet while increase in using canned food, in addition to the use of high caloric diet and food with high glycemic index. All these factors, could highly participate in the development of GDM whether directly or indirectly by increasing the incidence of obesity.

6. Conclusions

The precise mechanisms causing GDM remain unknown. All the previously described maternal and feto-placental factors interact in an integrated manner in the development of insulin resistance and GDM. The most prominent factors, which are involved in the pathogenesis of GDM, are the increase in HPL and TNF-α and the decrease in adiponectin during pregnancy.

Most of the women reverting to normal after delivery, will suggest that the placenta is the major contributing organ in the development of GDM.

The main cause of insulin resistance during GDM is post-cellular defect manifested by a decreased phosphorylation of tyrosine residues in insulin receptors and insulin receptor substrate-1, while serine phosphorylation is increased which inhibit insulin signaling from activating GLUT4 translocation.

Finally, GDM is probably produced by a complex and variable interaction of all the previously mentioned factors - pregnancy-induced factors, genetic, diet, environmental, autoimmunity, etc.

7. References

Ahmed SA, Shalayel MH. (1999). Role of cortisol in the deterioration of glucose tolerance in Sudanese pregnant women. *East Afr Med J*, 76(8):465-7.

Al- Dahwi AN, Al-Noaemi M, Alwan AAS, Al-Dahwi RN and Al-Taie ID. (1987) Glycosylated hemoglobin as an index for maternal and fetal complications. Abstract submitted in the first scientific congress of the Iraqi Society for obstetrics and gynecology. Baghdad, Iraq.

Al-Dahwi AN, Al-Noaemi M, Alwan AAS, et al. (1988). Glycosylated haemoglobin in normal and diabetic pregnancies. *Iraqi Medical Journal*, 37 (2): 68-371.

Al-Dahwi AN, Al-Noaemi M, Alwan AAS, et al. (1986). Glycosylated hemoglobin in diabetic Pergnancy. Abstract submitted in the first scientific congress of Al- Mustansiryah Medical College. Baghdad, Iraq.

Al-Dahwi RN, Alwan AAS, Al-Noaemi M and Al-Dahwi AN. (1989). Clinical experience with fifty pregnancies in diabetic patients Abstract submitted to the 4th congress of the Mediterranean Medical Association. Tunis 10-13th September 1989. Tunisia.

Al-Noaemi M and Shalayel MHF. (2009). Adiponectin (review article). *Sudan Journal of Medical Sciences*, 4 (30): 297-305.

Baker P N (2006) Physiology of pregnancy In: *Obstetrics by ten teachers* (18th Edition), pp 48-62. A Hodder Arnold Publication. ISBN: 0340816651.

Barbieri RL (1999) Endocrine disorders in pregnancy In: *Reproductive Endocrinology* (4th edition). Yen SSC, Jaffe RB, Barbieri RL, Eds. Philadelphia, W.B. Saunder.

Barbour LA, Carrie E. McCurdy, Teri L. Hernandez, John P. Kirwanet et al. (2007). Cellular Mechanisms for Insulin Resistance in Normal Pregnancy and Gestational Diabetes. *Diabetes Care,* 30 (2): S112-S119.

Barbour LA, Shao J, Qiao L, et al. (2002). Human placental growth hormone causes severe insulin resistance in transgenic mice. *Am J Obstet Gynecol,* 186: 512–517.

Barbour LA, Shao J, Qiao L, et al. (2004). Human Placental Growth Hormone Increases Expression of the P85 Regulatory Unit of Phosphatidylinositol 3-Kinase and Triggers Severe Insulin Resistance in Skeletal Muscle. *Endocrinology,* 145 (3): 1144-1150.

Bełtowski J. (2006). Apelin and visfatin: unique "beneficial" adipokines upregulated in obesity? *Med Sci Monit,* 12(6): RA112-9.

Berg AH, Combs TP, Du X et al. (2001). The adipocyte-secreted protein Acrp30 enhances hepatic insulin action. *Nat Med,* 7: 947-953.

Berndt J, Kloting N, Kralisch S et al. (2005). Plasma visfatin concentrations and fat-specific mRNA expression in humans. *Diabetes,* 54:2911–2916

Boyd E. Metzger, Thomas A. Buchanan, Donald R. Coustan, et al. (2007). Summary and Recommendations of the Fifth International Workshop-Conference on Gestational Diabetes Mellitus. *Diabetes Care,* 30 (2) S251-S260.

Briana DD, Malamitsi-Puchner A. (2009). Reviews: adipocytokines in normal and complicated pregnancies. *Reprod Sci.,* 16(10):921-37.

Bruun JM, Lihn AS, Verdich C, et al. (2003). Regulation of adiponectin by adipose tissue-derived cytokines: in vivo and in vitro investigations in humans. *Am J Physiol Endocrinol Metab.,* 285: E527–E533.

Buchanan TA, Xiang AH. (2005). Gestational diabetes mellitus. *J. Clin Invest.,* 115: 485-491.

Carpéné C, Dray C, Attané C, et al. (2007). Expanding role for the apelin/APJ system in physiopathology. *J Physiol Biochem.,* 63 (4): 359-73.

Carr DB, and Gabbe S. (1998). Gestational Diabetes: Detection, Management, and Implications. *Clinical diabetes,* 16: 5-19.

Carswell, E. A., Old, L. J., Kassel, R. L., et al. (1975). An endotoxin-induced serum factor that causes necrosis of tumors. *Proc. Natl. Acad. Sci. U. S. A.,* 72, 3666-3670.

Catalano PM, Huston L, Amini SB, Kalhan SC. (1999). Longitudinal changes in glucose metabolism during pregnancy in obese women with normal glucose tolerance and gestational diabetes mellitus. *Am J Obstet Gynecol.,* 180:903–916.

Catalano PM, Nizielski SE, Shao J, et al. (2002). Downregulated IRS-1 and PPARgamma in obese women with gestational diabetes: relationship to FFA during pregnancy. *Am J Physiol Endocrinol Metab.,* 282:E522–E533.

Catalano PM, Tyzbir ED, Roman NM, et al. (1991). Longitudinal changes in insulin release and insulin resistance in nonobese pregnant women. *Am J Obstet Gynecol.,* 165: 1667-1672.

Catalano PM, Tyzbir ED, Wolfe RR, et al. (1993). Carbohydrate metabolism during pregnancy in control subjects and women with gestational diabetes. *Am J Physiol Endocrinol Metab.,* 264: E60–E67.

Catalano PM, Tyzbir ED, Wolfe RR, et al. (1992). Longitudinal changes in basal hepatic glucose production and suppression during insulin infusion in normal pregnant women. *Am J Obstet Gynecol* , 167:913–9

Catalano PM. (2010). Obesity, insulin resistance, and pregnancy outcome. Focus Review on Obesity. *Reproduction*, 140: 365-371

Chan TF, Chen YL, Lee CH et al. (2006). Decreased plasma visfatin concentrations in women with gestational diabetes mellitus. *J Soc Gynecol Investig.*, 13: 364–367.

Chellakooty M, Vangsgaard K, Larsen T, et al. (2004). A longitudinal study of intrauterine growth and the placental growth hormone (GH)-insulin-like growth factor I axis in maternal circulation: association between placental GH and fetal growth. *J Clin Endocrinol Metab.*, 89: 384–391.

Chen D, Xia G, Xu P, Dong M. (2010). Peripartum serum leptin and soluble leptin receptor levels in women with gestational diabetes. *Acta Obstetrica et Gynecologica Scandinavica*, 89(12): 1595-1599.

Chen H, Yang Y, Hu X, et al. (1991). Tumor necrosis factor alpha mRNA and protein are present in human placental and uterine cells at early and late stages of gestation. *Am J Pathol.*, 139: 327–335.

Chen J, Tan B, Karteris E, et al. (2006). Secretion of adiponectin by human placenta: differential modulation of adiponectin and its receptors by cytokines. *Diabetologia*, 49(6): 1292-1302.

Chen MP, Chung FM, Chang DM et al. (2006). Elevated plasma level of visfatin/pre-B cell colony-enhancing factor in patients with type 2 diabetes mellitus. *J Clin Endocrinol Metab.*, 91:295–299.

Clapp JF, Kiess W. (2000). Effects of pregnancy and exercise on concentrations of the metabolic markers tumor necrosis α and leptin. *Am J Obstet Gynecol*, 182: 300–306.

Combs TP, Berg AH, Obici S et al. (2001). Endogenous glucose production is inhibited by the adipose-derived protein Acrp30. *J Clin Invest*, 108: 1875-1881.

Conrad KP, Miles TM, Fairchild Benyo D. (1998). Circulating levels of immunoreactive cytokines in women with preeclampsia. *AJRI*, 40:102–111.

Coughlan MT, K. Oliva, H. M. Georgiou, et al. (2001). Glucose-induced release of tumour necrosis factor-alpha from human placental and adipose tissues in gestational diabetes mellitus. *Diabetic Medicine*, 18 (11):921-927.

Cseh K, Baranyi E, Melczer Z, et al. (2002). The pathophysiological influence of leptin and the tumor necrosis factor system on maternal insulin resistance: negative correlation with anthropometric parameters of neonates in gestational diabetes. *Gynecol Endocrinol.*, 16 (6): 453-460.

Cseh K, Baranyi E, Melczer Z, et al. (2004). Plasma adiponectin and pregnancy-induced insulin resistance. *Diabetes Care*, 27:274–275.

Davis JRE. (1990). Prolactin and related peptides in pregnancy. *Bailliere's Clinical Endocrinology and Metabolism*, 4: 273-285.

Definition and Diagnosis of Diabetes Mellitus and Intermediate Hyperglycemia (2006). *World Health Organization*. www.who.int. http://www.who.int/diabetes/publications/Definition and diagnosis of diabetes_new.pdf. Retrieved 2011-02-20.

del Aguila LF, Claffey KP, Kirwan JP (1999). TNF-α impairs insulin signaling and insulin stimulation of glucose uptake in C2C12 muscle cells. *Am J Physiol*, 276: E849–E855.

del Aguila LF, Krishnan RK, Ulbrecht JS, et al. (2000). Muscle damage impairs insulin stimulation of IRS-1, PI3-kinase, and Akt-kinase in human skeletal muscle. *Am J Physiol.*, 279: E206–E212.

Denison FC, RobertsKA, Barr SM and Norman JE. (2010). Obesity, pregnancy, inflammation, and vascular function. *Reproduction*, 140: 373-385.

Doshani A and Konje JC. (2009). Review: Diabetes in pregnancy: insulin resistance, obesity and placental dysfunction. *British Journal of Diabetes & Vascular Disease*, 9(5): 208 - 212.

Dray C, Debard C, Jager J, et al. (2010). Apelin and APJ regulation in adipose tissue and skeletal muscle of type 2 diabetic mice and humans. *Am J Physiol Endocrinol Metab.*, 298(6): E1161-9.

Fasshauer M, Klein J, Neumann S, et al. (2002). Hormonal regulation of adiponectin gene expression in 3T3-L1 adipocytes. *Biochem Biophys Res Commun.*, 290: 1084-1089.

Fasshauer M, Kralisch S, Klier M, et al. (2003). Adiponectin gene expression and secretion is inhibited by interleukin-6 in 3T3–L1 adipocytes. *Biochem Biophys Res Commun.*, 301:1045–1050.

Feinstein R, Kanety H, Papa MZ, Lunefeld B, Karasik A. (1993). Tumor necrosis factor-alpha suppresses insulin-induced tyrosine phosphorylation of insulin receptor and its substrates. *J Biol Chem.*, 268:26055–26058.

Friedman JE, Ishizuka T, Shao J, et al. (1999). Impaired glucose transport and insulin receptor tyrosine phosphorylation in skeletal muscle from obese women with gestational diabetes. *Diabetes*, 49:1807–1814.

Fruebis J, Tsao TS, Javorschi S et al. (2001). Proteolytic cleavage product of 30-kDa adipocyte complement-related protein increases fatty acid oxidation in muscle and causes weight loss in mice. *Proc Natl Acad Sci U S A*, 98:2005-10.

Fujinami A, Obayashi H, Ohta K, et al. (2004). Enzyme-linked immunosorbent assay for circulating human resistin: resistin concentrations in normal subjects and patients with type 2 diabetes. *Clin. Chim. Acta.*, 339 (1-2): 57–63.

Fukuhara A, Matsuda M, Nishizawa M et al. (2005). Visfatin: a protein secreted by visceral fat that mimics the effects of insulin. *Science*, 307: 426–430.

Ganong WF (2003) Review of Medical Physiology (21st edition), pp 433-436. Lange Medical Books/McGraw-Hill Medical Publishing Division. ISBN: 0071402365.

Garvey WT, Birnbaum MJ. (1993). Cellular insulin action and insulin resistance. *Baillieres Clin Endocrinol Metab.*, 7:785–873.

Garvey WT, Maianu L, Hancock JA, et al. (1992). Gene expression of GLUT4 in skeletal muscle from insulin-resistant patients with obesity, IGT, GDM, and NIDDM. *Diabetes*, 41:465–475.

Glass R H, and Kase N G. (1984) Chapter 10: The endocrinology of pregnancy In: *Clinical Gynecology Endocrinology &Metabolism.* P271-305 (3rd edition), Leon Speroff. .

Godoy-Matos AF, Bahia LR, Dominhues RC et al. (2010). Adiponectin is related to intramyocellular lipid content in non-diabetic adults. *J Endocrinol Invest*, 33 (6): 382-7.

Guyton AC and Hall JE. (2006) Ch. 78: Insulin, Glucagon, and Diabetes, In: *Textbook of Medical Physiology* (11th edition), Guyton & Hall, pp.961-970, ELSEVIER SAUNDERS Publication. ISBN: 0-7216-0240-1.

Handwerger S, Freemark M. (2000). The roles of placental growth hormone and placental lactogen in the regulation of human fetal growth and development. *J Pediatr Endocrinol Metab.*, 13(4):343-56.

Hans-Georg Joost. (1995). Structural and functional heterogeneity of insulin receptors. *Cellular Signalling*, 7 (2): 85-91.

Heilbronn LK, Rood J, Janderova L, et al. (2004). Relationship between serum resistin concentrations and insulin resistance in nonobese, obese, and obese diabetic subjects. *J. Clin. Endocrinol. Metab.*, 89 (4): 1844–8.

Hellstrom L, Wahrenberg H, Hruska K, et al. Mechanisms behind (2000). Gender differences in circulating leptin levels. *J Intern Med.*, 247:457- 462.

Henry BA, Clarke IJ. (2008). Adipose tissue hormones and the regulation of food intake. *J. Neuroendocrinol.*, 2: 842-9.

Highman TJ, Friedman JE, Huston LP, et al. (1998). Longitudinal changes in maternal serum leptin concentrations, body composition, and resting metabolic rate in pregnancy. *Am J Obstet Gynecol.*, 178:1010–1015.

Hornns PJ. (1985). On the decrease of glucose tolerance in pregnancy. A review. *Diabet Metab.*, 11(5): 310-315.

Hotamisligil GS, Murray DL, Choy LN, Spiegelman BM. (1994). Tumor necrosis factor alpha inhibits signaling from the insulin receptor. *Proc Natl Acad Sci U S A.*, 91: 4854–4858.

Hotamisligil GS, Peraldi P, Budavari A, et al. (1996). IRS-1 mediated inhibition of insulin receptor tyrosine kinase activity in TNF-α and obesity-induced insulin resistance. *Science*, 271: 665–668.

Hotta K, Funahashi T, Arita Y et al. (2000). Plasma concentration of a novel, adipose-specific protein, adiponectin, in type2 diabetic patients. *Arteioscler Thromb Vasc Biol.* 20: 1595-9.

Hu E, Liang P, Spiegelman BM. (1996). Adipo1 is a novel adipose-specific gene dysregulated in obesity. *J Biol Chem.*, 271: 10697–10703

Joosen AM, Bakker AH, Zorenc AH, et al. (2006). PPARgamma activity in subcutaneous abdominal fat tissue and fat mass gain during short-term overfeeding. *Int J Obes (Lond)*, 30: 302–*307.*

Kadowaki T and Yamaushi T. (2005). Adiponectin and Adiponectin Reseptors. *Endocrine Reviews*, 26: 439-451.

Kappes A and Loffler G. (2000). Influences of ionomycin, dibutyrylcycloAMP and tumour necrosis factor-alpha on intracellular amount and secretion of apM1 in differentiating primary human preadipocytes. *Horm Metab Res.*, 32: 548-554.

Kim YJ, Feling P. (1971). Plasma chorionic somatomammotropin levels during starvation in mid-pregnancy. *J Clin Endocrinol Metab*, 32: 864-866.

Kirwan JP, Hauguel-De Mouzon S, Lepercq J, et al. (2002). TNF-α Is a Predictor of Insulin Resistance in Human Pregnancy. *Diabetes*, 51 (7): 2207-2213.

Kirwan JP, Krishnan RK, Weaver JA, et al. (2001). Human aging is associated with altered TNF-α production during hyperglycemia and hyperinsulinemia. *Am J Physiol.*, 281:E1137–E1143.

Kirwan JP, Varastehpour A, Jing M, et al. (2004). Reversal of Insulin Resistance Postpartum Is Linked to Enhanced Skeletal Muscle Insulin Signaling. *The Journal of Clinical Endocrinology & Metabolism*, 89(9): 4678-4684.

Krzyzanowska K, Krugluger W, Mittermayer F, et al. (2006). Increased visfatin concentrations in women with gestational diabetes mellitus. *Clin Sci.*, 110: 605-609.

Kubota N, Terauchi Y, Yamauchi T et al. (2002). Disruption of adiponectin causes insulin resistance and neointimal formation. *J Biol Chem.*, 277: 25863-6.

Kuhl C, HornnesPJ, Andersen O. (1985). Etiology and pathophysiology of gestational diabetes mellitus. *Diabetes*, 34 (2): 66-70.

Kühl C. (1991). Aetiology of gestational diabetes. *Baillieres Clin Obstet Gynaecol.*, 5: 279–92.
Kuhl C. (1998). Etiology and pathogenesis of gestational diabetes. *Diabetes Care,* 1 Suppl. 2:B19-26.
Kuhl C. (1975). Glucose metabolism during and after pregnancy in normal and gestational diabetic women. 1. Influence of normal pregnancy on serum glucose and insulin concentration during basal fasting conditions and after a challenge with glucose. *Acta Endocrinol (Copenh),* 79(4):709–719.
Lacroix MC, Guibourdenche J, Frendo JL, et al. (2002). Human placental growth hormone--a review. *Placenta,* 23 Suppl A: S87-94.
Laham N, Brennecke SP, Bendtzen K, Rice GE. (1994). Tumor necrosis factor α during human pregnancy and labor: maternal plasma and amniotic fluid concentration and release from intrauterine tissues. *Eur J Endocrinol.*, 131: 607–614.
Lee JH, Bullen JW, Stoyneva VL, Mantzoros CS. (2005). Circulating resistin in lean, obese, and insulin-resistant mouse models: lack of association with insulinemia and glycemia. *Am. J. Physiol. Endocrinol. Metab.*, 288 (3): E625–32.
Lee JH, Chan JL, Yiannakouris N, et al. (2003). Circulating resistin levels are not associated with obesity or insulin resistance in humans and are not regulated by fasting or leptin administration: cross-sectional and interventional studies in normal, insulin-resistant, and diabetic subjects. *J. Clin. Endocrinol. Metab.,* 88 (10): 4848–56.
Lepercq J, Challier JC, Guerre-Millo M, et al. (2001). Prenatal leptin production: evidence that fetal adipose tissue produces leptin. *J Clin Endocrin Metabol,* 86: 2409–2413.
Letchworth AT, Chard T. (1972). Placental lactogen levels as a screening test for fetal distress and neonatal asphyxia. *Lancet,* 1(7753):704-6.
Lewandowski KC, Stojanovic N, Press M et al. (2007). Elevated serum levels of visfatin in gestational diabetes: a comparative study across various degrees of glucose tolerance. *Diabetologia,* 50:1033–1037.
Ling PR, Bistrian BR, Mendez B, Istfan NW. (1994). Effects of systemic infusions of endotoxin, tumor necrosis factor, and interleukin-1 on glucose metabolism in the rat: relationship to endogenous glucose production and peripheral tissue glucose uptake. *Metabolism,* 43:279–284.
Maeda K, Okubo K, Shimomura I, et al. (1996). cDNA cloning and expression of a novel adipose specific collagen-like factor, apM1(AdiPose Most abundant Gene transcript 1). *Biochem Biophys Res Commun.*, 221(2):286-9.
Maeda N, Funahashi TTF, Kihara S, et al. (2005). PPARγ Ligands Increase Expression and Plasma Concentrations of Adiponectin, an Adipose-Derived Protein. *Diabetes,* 50(9): 2094-2099.
Maffei M, Halaas J, Ravussin E, et al. (1995). Leptin levels in human and rodent: measurement of plasma leptin and ob RNA in obese and weight-reduced subjects. *Nat Med.,* 1:1155–1161.
Maiorana A, Chiara Del Bianco, Cianfarani S. (2007). Adipose Tissue: A Metabolic Regulator. Potential Implications for the Metabolic Outcome of Subjects Born Small for Gestational Age (SGA). *Rev Diabet Stud,* 4(3): 134-146.
Mantzoros C, Petridou E, Dessypris N, et al. (2004). Adiponectin and Breast Cancer Risk. *The Journal of Clinical Endocrinology & Metabolism,* 89(3): 1102-1107.
Masuzaki H, Ogawa Y, Sagawa N, et al. (1997). Nonadipose tissue production of leptin: leptin as a novel placenta-derived hormone in humans. *Nat Med.,* 3:1029 –1113.

McIntyre HD, Zeck W, Russell A. (2009). Placental growth hormone, fetal growth and the IGF axis in normal and diabetic pregnancy. *Curr Diabetes Rev*, 5(3):185-9.

McLachlan KA, O'Neal D, Jenkins A, Alford FP. (2006). Do adiponectin, TNF alpha, leptin and CRP relate to insulin resistance in pregnancy? Studies in women with and without gestational diabetes, during and after pregnancy. *Diabetes Metab Res Rev.*, 22(2): 131-8.

McTernan PG, Fisher FM, Valsamakis G, et al. (2003). Resistin and type 2 diabetes: regulation of resistin expression by insulin and rosiglitazone and the effects of recombinant resistin on lipid and glucose metabolism in human differentiated adipocytes. *J. Clin. Endocrinol. Metab.*, 88 (12): 6098–106.

Meier U and Gressner AM. (2004). Endocrine Regulation of Energy Metabolism: Review of Pathobiochemical and Clinical Chemical Aspects of Leptin, Ghrelin, Adiponectin, and Resistin. *Clinical Chemistry*, 50: 1511-1525.

Meral C, Tascilar E, Karademir F, et al. (2010). Elevated plasma levels of apelin in children with type1 diabetes mellitus. *Journal of Pediatric Endocrinology and Metabolism*, 23(5): 497–502.

Merviel P, Muller F, Guibourdenche J, et al. (2001). Correlations between serum assays of human chorionic gonadotrophin (hCG) and human placental lactogen (hPL) and pre-eclampsia or intrauterine growth restriction (IUGR) among nulliparas younger than 38 years. *Eur J Obstet Gynecol Reprod Biol.*, 95(1): 59-67.

Metzger BE. (1991). Organizing Committee: Summary and recommendations of the Third International Workshop-Conference on Gestational Diabetes Mellitus. *Diabetes*, 40:197-201.

Milan G, Granzotto M, Scarda A, et al. (2002). Resistin and adiponectin expression in visceral fat of obese rats: effect of weight loss. *Obes. Res.*, 10 (11): 1095–103.

Milasinovic L, Djurdjevic J, Dokmanovic-Djordjevic M, et al. (1997). Prolactin levels in pregnant women with glucose intolerance at full-term delivery. *Med Pregl*, 50: 269-73.

Mills NC, Gyves MT, Ilan J. (1985). Comparisons of human placental lactogen mRNA levels from placentas of diabetics and normal term. *Mol Cell Endocrinol.*, 39(1):61-9.

Monga A and Baker P. (2006). Physiology of pregnancy, In: Obstetrics By Ten Teachers, Philip N Baker, pp 48-62, A Hodder Arnold Publication, ISBN-13: 978-0340816653.

Muoio DM, Dohm GL, Fiedorek FT, et al. (1997). Leptin directly alters lipid partitioning in skeletal muscle. *Diabetes*, 46 (8): 1360-1363.

Nagaev I, Smith U. (2001). Insulin resistance and type 2 diabetes are not related to resistin expression in human fat cells or skeletal muscle. *Biochem. Biophys. Res. Commun.*, 285 (2): 561–4.

Nakano Y, Tobe T, Choi-Miura NH, et al. (1996). Isolation and characterization of GBP28, a novel gelatin-binding protein purified from human plasma. *J Biochem.*, 120:803–812.

Nathan DM. (2009). International Expert Committee 'in the American Diabetes Association' Report on the Role of the A1C Assay in the Diagnosis of Diabetes. *Diabetes Care*, 32(7): 1327–1334.

Ouchi N, Kihara S, Arita Y et al. (2000). Adiponectin, an adipocyte-derived plasma protein, inhibit endothelial TNF-a signaling through a Camp-dependent pathway. *Circulation*, 102: 1296-1301.

Ouchi N, Kihara S, Arita Y et al. (1999). Novel modulator for endothelia adhesion molecules: adipocyte-derived plasma protein adiponectin. *Circulation*, 100: 2473-2476.

Ouchi N, Kihara S, Arita Y, et al. (2001). Adipocyte-derived plasma protein, suppresses lipid accumulation and class A scavenger receptor expression in human Monocyte-derived macrophages. *Circulation*, 103: 1057-1063.

Pagano C, Pilon C, Olivieri M et al. (2006). Reduced plasma visfatin/pre B-cell colony enhancing factor in obesity is not related to insulin resistance in humans. *J Clin Endocrinol Metab*, 91:3165–3170.

Pawson T. (1995). Protein modules and signalling networks. *Nature*, 373: 573–580.

Pena AS, Belobrajdic DP, Wiltshire E et al. (2009). Adiponectin relates to smooth muscle function and folate in obese children. *Int J Pediatr Obes.*, 15: 1-7.

Perz M, Torlińska T. (2001). Insulin receptor--structural and functional characteristics. *Med Sci Monit.*, 7(1): 169-77.

Petridou E, Mantzoros C, Dessypris N, et al. (2003). Plasma adiponectin concentrations in relation to endometrial cancer: a case control study in Greece. *J Clin Endocrinol Metab*, 88:993–997.

Polderman KH, Gooren LJ, Asscheman H, et al. (1994). Induction of insulin resistance by androgens and estrogens. *J Clin Endocrinol Meta,* 79: 265–271

Qiu C, Williams MA, Vadachkoria S, et al. (2004). Increased maternal plasma leptin in early pregnancy and risk of gestational diabetes mellitus. *Obstet Gynecol*, 103(3): 519-525.

Rieck S, Kaestner KH. (2010). Expansion of beta-cell mass in response to pregnancy. *Trends Endocrinol Metab.*, 21 (3): 151-8.

Rui L, Aguirre V, Kim JK, et al. (2001). Insulin/IGF-1 and TNF-α stimulate phosphorylation of IRS-1 at inhibitory Ser^{307} via distinct pathways. *J Clin Invest.*, 107:181–189.

Ryan EA and Enns L. (1988). Role of Gestational Hormones in the Induction of Insulin Resistance. *J Clin Endocrinol Metab.*, 67: 341-347

Scherer PE, Williams S, Fogliano M, et al. (1995). A novel serum protein similar to C1q, produced exclusively in adipocytes. *Biol Chem.*, 270(45):26746-9.

Schoonjans K, Staels B, Auwerx J. (1996). The peroxisome proliferator activated receptors (PPARs) and their effects on lipid metabolism and adipocyte differentiation. *Biochim Biophys Acta.*, 1302*: 93–109.*

Shalayel MH, Elrobh MS, Idris SA, Mohammed MS, and Ahmed SA. (2010). Prolactin and insulin estimates in pregnancy with glucose intolerance. Pak J Med Sci, 26 (1): 102-106.

Shali MT, Roberto R, Pedro K J, et al. (2009). Visfatin in human pregnancy: maternal gestational diabetes vis-à-vis neonatal birthweight. *Journal of perinatal medicine*, 37(3): 218-31.

Shao J, Catalano PM, Yamashita H, et al. (2000). Decreased insulin receptor tyrosine kinase activity and plasma cell membrane glycoprotein-1 overexpression in skeletal muscle from obese women with gestational diabetes mellitus (GDM): evidence for increased serine/threonine phosphorylation in pregnancy and GDM. *Diabetes*, 49: 603–610.

Sherwood L. (2010) The Peripheral endocrine glands In: *Human Physiology from Cells to Systems* (7th edition), Brooks/Cole. ISBN: 13:978-0-495-39184-5.

Shulman GI. (2000). Cellular mechanisms of insulin resistance. *J. Clin Invest.*, 106: 171-176.

Statnick MA, Beavers LS, Conner LJ, et al. (2000). Decreased expression of apM1 in omental and subcutaneous adipose tissue of humans with type 2 diabetes. *Int J Diabetes Res,* 1: 81-8.

Steppan CM, Bailey ST, Bhat S, et al. (2001). The hormone resistin links obesity to diabetes. *Nature,* 409(6818): 307-12.

Tapan S, Tascilar E, Abaci A, et al. (2010). Decreased plasma apelin levels in pubertal obese children. *Journal of Pediatric Endocrinology and Metabolism,* 23: 1039-1046.

Tatemoto K, Hosoya M, Habata Y, et al. (1998). Isolation and Characterization of a Novel Endogenous Peptide Ligand for the Human APJ Receptor. *Biochemical and Biophysical Research Communications,* 251: 471-476.

Telejko B, Kuzmicki M, Wawrusiewicz-Kurylonek N, et al. (2010). Plasma apelin levels and apelin/APJ mRNA expression in patients with gestational diabetes mellitus. *Diabetes Res Clin Pract.,* 87(2):176-83.

Thamer C, Machann J, Tschritter O et al. (2002). Relationship between serum adiponectin concentration and intramyocellular lipid stores in humans. *Horm Metab Res.,* 34: 646-9.

Tsao TS, Murrey HE, Hug C, et al. (2002). Oligomerization state-dependent activation of NF-kappa B signaling pathway by adipocyte complement-related protein of 30 kDa (Acrp30). *J Biol Chem.,* 16 (33): 29359-62.

Tsuchida A, Yamauchi T, Kadowaki T. (2005). Nuclear receptors as targets for drug development: molecular mechanisms for regulation of obesity and insulin resistance by peroxisome proliferator -activated receptor gamma, CREB-binding protein, and adiponectin. *J Pharmacol Sci.,* 97: 164-70.

Uvena J, Thomas A, Huston L, Highman T, Catalano PM. (1999). Umbilical cord leptin and neonatal body composition. *Am J Obstet Gynecol.,* 180:S41.

Valsamakis G, McTernan PG, Chetty R, et al. (2004). Modest weight loss and reduction in waist circumference after medical treatment are associated with favorable changes in serum adipocytokines. *Metab. Clin. Exp.,* 53 (4): 430–4.

Vendrell J, Broch M, Vilarrasa N, et al. (2004). Resistin, adiponectin, ghrelin, leptin, and proinflammatory cytokines: relationships in obesity. *Obes. Res.,* 12 (6): 962–71.

Vickers MH, Gilmour S. (2009). 20-kDa placental hGH-V has diminished diabetogenic and lactogenic activities compared with 22-kDa hGH-N while retaining antilipogenic activity. *AJP – Endo,* 297 (3): E629-E637.

Ward CW, Lawrence MC. (2009). Ligand-induced activation of the insulin receptor: a multi-step process involving structural changes in both the ligand and the receptor. *Bioessays,* 31 (4): 422–34.

Way JM, Görgün CZ, Tong Q, et al. (2001). Adipose tissue resistin expression is severely suppressed in obesity and stimulated by peroxisome proliferator-activated receptor gamma agonists. *J. Biol. Chem.,* 276 (28): 25651–3.

Weyer C, Funahashi T, Tanaka S, et al. (2001). Hypoadiponectinemia in Obesity and Type 2 Diabetes: Close association with Insulin Resistance and Hyperinsulinemia. *The journal of Clinical Endocrinology & Metabolism,* 86: 1930-1935.

Worda C, Leipold H, Gruber C, et al. (2004). Decreased plasma adiponectin concentrations in women with gestational diabetes mellitus. *Am J Obstet Gynecol,* 191*:* 2120–*2124.*

Xiang AH, Peters RK, Trigo E, et al. (1999). Multiple metabolic defects during late pregnancy in women at high risk for type 2 diabetes. *Diabetes,* 48: 848–854.

Yamauchi T, Hara K, Kubota N et al. (2003). Dual roles of adiponectin/ Acrp30 in vivo as an anti-diabetic and anti-atherogenic adipokines. Curr Drug Targets Immune Endocr *Metabol Disord*, 3: 243-254.

Yamauchi T, Kamon J, Ito Y, et al. (2003). Cloning of adiponectin receptors that mediate antidiabetic metabolic effects. *Nature*, 423(6941):762-9.

Yamauchi T, Kamon J, Waki H et al. (2001). The fat driven-hormone adiponectin reverses insulin resistance associated with both lipoatrophy and obesity. *Nat Med.*, 7: 941-946.

Yokota T, Oritani K, Takahashi I et al. (2000). Adiponectin, a new member of the family of soluble defense collagens, negatively regulates the growth of myelomonocytic progenitors and the functions of macrophages. *Blood*, 96: 1723-1732.

Yool MJ, Lee GY, Chung J et al. (2006). Adiponectin Increases Fatty Acid Oxidation in Skeletal Muscle Cell by Sequential Activation of AMP-Activated Protein Kinase, p38 Mitogene-Activated protein Kinase, and Peroxisome Proliferator- Activated Receptor a. *Diabetes*, 55: 2562-2570.

Zeghari N, Vidal H, Younsi M, et al. (2000). Adipocyte membrane phospholipids and PPAR-gamma expression in obese women: relationship to hyperinsulinemia. *Am J Physiol Endocrinol Metab.*, 279: E736–*E743.*

Zhang B, Berger J, Hu E, et al. (1996). Negative regulation of peroxisome proliferator-activated receptor-gamma gene expression contributes to the antiadipogenic effects of tumor necrosis factor-alpha. *Mol Endocrinol.*, 10: 1457–1466.

Zhang Y, Proenca R, Maffei M, et al. (1994). Positional cloning of the mouse ob gene and its human homologue. *Nature*. 372: 425– 432.

Zhang XJ, Wang Z, Li HH, Yu L, Gao S. (2010). Association between both resistin, visfatin and insulin resistance as well as β cell function in the first-degree relatives of type 2 diabetes mellitus. *Zhonghua Liu Xing Bing Xue Za Zhi*, 31(12):1393-1396.

Zwick E, Bange J, Ullrich A. (2001). Receptor tyrosine kinase signalling as a target for cancer intervention strategies. *Endocr. Relat. Cancer*, 8 (3): 161–173.

7

The Role of Adipocyte Mediators, Inflammatory Markers and Vitamin D in Gestational Diabetes

Sedigheh Soheilykhah
Shahid Sadoughi University of Medical Sciences
Iran

1. Introduction

Gestational diabetes mellitus (GDM) usually reveals itself in the latter half of pregnancy and it is identified by carbohydrate intolerance of variable severity.

The presence of GDM has implications for both the mother and the baby. Perinatal morbidity includes macrosomia, hypoglycemia, hyperbilirubinaemia and respiratory distress syndrome which lead to the subsequent complications (Hod et al., 1991). Long term outcomes for the offspring may include obesity and diabetes independent of genetic factors (Silverman et al., 1995; Van Assche et al., 1992, 2001). For the mother there is an increased risk of overt type 2 diabetes later in life (Mestman, 1987; O'Sullivan, 1989). Both type 2 diabetes and gestational diabetes have common pathogenic mechanisms where pregnancy tends to expose disease in those women who are at risk of developing type 2 diabetes later in life. Similar to all forms of hyperglycemia, GDM is characterized by insulin levels that are inadequate to proper insulin requirement (Metzger et al.,2007).The pathogenesis of GDM has not been clearly defined. The most common hypothesis is that GDM is caused by decreasing insulin sensitivity and increasing anti-insulin hormones that are secreted by the placenta during pregnancy, such as human placental lactogen, prolactin, glucocorticoid and progesterone (Xue-lian et al., 2008).

It has become increasingly evident that endocrine/metabolic hormones such as leptin, adiponectin, resistin, proinflammatory mediators including C-reactive protein (CRP) are strongly linked with abnormal carbohydrate metabolism.

In recent times a number of first trimester studies have shown association of different biomarkers with the development of GDM. These include elevated serum or plasma C-reactive protein (Wolf et al., 2003), lower sex hormone-binding globulin (Thadhani et al., 2003), increased placental growth factor (Ong et al., 2004) and elevated leptin (Qiu et al., 2004) and decreasing of adiponectin concentration.

Some studies have recommended that Vitamin D deficiency could play a role in pathogenesis of gestational diabetes.

This chapter will focus on the studies about the role of adipocytes mediators, proinflammatory factors and vitamin D in gestational diabetes.

2. Adipocyte mediators

It is becoming obvious that adipose tissue is not just a storage for extra energy but that it secretes a number of biologically active peptides as a group named adipocytokines that control glucose and fatty acid metabolism (Youn et al.,2004). These peptides have similar properties with cytokines, and so referred to as "adipocytokines", e.g. leptin, tumor necrosis factor-α(TNF-α), interleukin 6 (IL-6), adiponectin and resistin. These adipocytokines may influence activity of other tissues (Nedvidkova et al., 2005).

2.1 Adiponectin

2.1.1 Adiponectin structure

Adiponectin is a 244-amino-acid-long polypeptide that regulates a number of metabolic processes, including glucose regulation and fatty acid catabolism. Adiponectin is exclusively secreted from adipose tissue into the circulation and is very plentiful in plasma relative to other hormones. Adiponectin concentrations ranging from 5 to 30mg/ml and accounting for approximately 0.01% of total plasma protein . Females have higher levels of plasma concentration than males (Díez & Iglesias, 2003).

Adiponectin was first identified in mice as a transcript overexpressed in preadipocytes (Lara-Castro et al., 2007) differentiating into adipocyte (Matsuzawa et al., 2004). The human homologue was recognized as the most abundant transcript in adipose tissue. As opposed to anticipation, in spite of being produced in a fat tissue, adiponectin was found to decline in obesity (Díez & Iglesias, 2003; Nedvídková et al., 2005; Ukkola & Santaniemi, 2002). This down regulation has not been clearly described. The gene was localised to chromosome 3p27, a region highlighted as affecting genetic vulnerability to obesity and type 2 diabetes. Supplementation by varying forms of adiponectin improved control of insulin, blood glucose and triglyceride levels in mouse models.

Berbelin, a herbal folk medicine, has been shown to increase adiponectin expression which partly explains its advantageous effects on metabolic disturbances (Choi et al., 2009).

A reduction in adiponectin expression is associated with insulin resistance in animal models. Administration of adiponectin has been accompanied by a reduction in plasma glucose and an increase in insulin sensitivity. In addition, thiazolidinediones, drugs that increase insulin sensitivity by stimulation of the peroxisome proliferator-activated receptor-δ, increase plasma adiponectin and mRNA levels in mice.

A recent study has shown that phosphorylation and Levels of the hormone are conversely correlated with body fat proportion in adults although the association in infants and young children is less clear. The hormone plays a role in the inhibition of the metabolic disturbance that may end in type 2 diabetes (Ukkola & Santaniemi, 2002), obesity, atherosclerosis (Díez & Iglesias, 2003), non-alcoholic fatty liver diseases (NAFLD) and independent risk factors for metabolic syndrome (Renaldi et al., 2009)., Levels of adiponectin are decreased in diabetics compared to non-diabetics. Weight loss significantly increases circulating levels (Coppola et al., 2009).

Adiponectin automatically self-associates into larger structures. Initially, three adiponectin molecules bind together to form a homotrimer. The trimers continue to self-associate and form hexamers or dodecamers. Like the plasma concentration, the relative levels of the higher-order structures are sexually dimorphic, where females have increased proportions of the high-molecular weight forms.

Adiponectin exerts some of its weight reduction effects via the brain. This is similar to the action of leptin, but the two hormones perform complementary actions, and can have additive effects (Nedvídková et al., 2005).

2.1.2 Metabolic effect of adiponectin

Adiponectin affects glucose flux through decreasing gluconeogenesis and increasing glucose uptake (Díez & Iglesias, 2003; Nedvídková et al., 2005; Vasseur et al., 2003). Adiponectin has a role in lipid catabolism (Vasseur et al., 2003) by β-oxidation and triglyceride clearance (Nedvídková et al., 2005). The other metabolic effects of adiponectin are protection against endothelial dysfunction and improvement of insulin sensitivity and weight loss, and control of energy metabolism (Vasseur et al., 2006).Adiponectin has also another effects, including putative insulin-sensitising, anti-atherogenic and anti inflammatory characteristics (Berg et al., 2002; Ukkola & Santaniemi, 2002).

Consistent with the low circulating levels of adiponectin observed in type 2 diabetes, adiponectin concentration is contrarily related to both insulin resistance and central adiposity (Arita et al., 1999; Weyer et al., 2001). Low baseline adiponectin concentration can predict the subsequent development of insulin resistance although elevated baseline levels have been shown to be protective against the succeeding development of type 2 diabetes (Daimon et al., 2003; Lindsay et al., 2002; Snehalatha et al., 2003; Spranger et al. , 2003). Recognition of gestational diabetes mellitus helps in identification of populations of young women at high risk of developing type 2 diabetes. Therefore, reduction in serum adiponectin levels in GDM may be comparable to type 2 diabetes.

2.1.3 Adiponectin and GDM

Some studies exhibited hypoadiponectinemia in pregnant women with gestational diabetes. A cross sectional study of 180 women in their third trimesters illustrated gestational diabetic women had more hypoadiponectinemia compared with normoglycemic controls after adjustment for covariates including insulin resistance. This study showed adiponectin concentration is an independent correlate of beta cell function in late pregnancy. Adiponectin was correlated with insulin secretion-sensitivity index (ISSI). ISSI was positively correlated with adiponectin and negatively correlated with GDM and IGT. Therefore, adiponectin may play a principal role in mediating insulin resistance and beta cell malfunction in the development of diabetes (Rentakaran et al., 2005).To determine whether adiponectin relate to the postpartum metabolic disturbance linking GDM with type 2 diabetes a cohort study was done on 487 pregnant wemen in pregnancy and at 3 months post partum. This study demonstrated adiponectin was related to postpartum insulin sensitivity and hypoadiponectinemia in pregnancy predicts postpartum insulin resistance, beta cell dysfunction and fasting glycaemia, and hence may be relevant to the pathophysiology relating GDM with type 2 diabetes (Rentakaran et al., 2010). To investigate level of adiponectin and metabolic factors in women with gestational diabetes a cross sectional study was done . The result of this study showed the level of adiponectin was lower in gestational diabetes and adiponectin correlates negatively with insulin resistance in homeostasis model assessment-insulin resistance (HOMA-IR) (Altinova et al., 2007). To evaluate whether adiponectin is a predictive factor for gestational diabetes mellitus (GDM) and is appropriate as a screening test for GDM a study was done and the results demonstrated that adiponectin was an independent predictor for GDM. For GDM screening, adiponectin was not as strong a predictor as GCT. In any case, adiponectin could be used to rule out pregnant women at low risk of GDM (Weerakiet et al., 2006). In a cross sectional study serum level of adiponectin in GDM women and impaired glucose test and normal pregnant women was compared. This study showed the serum adiponectin level in gestational diabetes was significantly lower than the impaired glucose test and control groups and a negative correlation between prepregnancy BMI and adiponectin (Soheilykhah et al., 2009). In another study, class A2 and B gestational diabetes are associated with a suppressed level of adiponectin (Thyfault et al., 2005). To investigate changes in serum adiponectin during pregnancy and postpartum and assess its relationship with insulin resistance as measured by homeostasis model assessment (HOMA-IR) a study was done and revealed adiponectin was lower in gestational diabetes than in control groups during pregnancy and a significant post reduction in adiponectin was observed in maternal adiponectin after delivery indicating a significant placental contribution to adiponectin production (Vitoratos et al., 2008). The result of the another study identified weight gain as the strongest factor associated with declining β cell compensation for insulin resistance in Hispanic women at high risk for type 2 diabetes. Such effects may be mediated through at least two mechanisms: alteration in adipokine levels and increasing insulin resistance (Xiang et al., 2010). A prospective, nested case control study showed adiponectin concentration in early pregnancy was significantly lower in women with GDM than controls (4.4 vs. 8.1), approximately 73% of women with GDM, compared with 33% of controls, had adiponectin concentration less than 6.4μg/ml. After adjustment for confounding, women with adiponectin concentration in early pregnancy, less than 6.4μg/ml, experienced a 4.6-fold increased risk of GDM as compared with those with higher concentrations (Williams et al., 2004). Postpartum follow-up showed that women developing metabolic syndrome had significantly lower adiponectin and resistin concentration during pregnancy. Nonetheless, after adjustment for age, prepregnancy BMI, logistic regression analysis did not show independent relation between adiponectin and resistin with development of postpartum metabolic syndrome (Hossein-nezhad et al., 2010). To evaluate plasma adiponectin levels, insulin resistance and glucose tolerance in women with gestational diabetes mellitus and in normal pregnancies adiponectin measurement were performed two times as in 28–31 weeks of pregnancy and at 3 months after delivery. Insulin resistance was calculated by the homeostasis model assessment. This study demonstrated decreased adiponectin levels in GDM do not normalize instantaneously following the delivery. The difference is more apparent in adiponectin levels than in HOMA-IR (Cavit et al., 2007). Low plasma adiponectin concentration was associated with GDM in another study and adiponectin mRNA levels in adipose tissue biopsies from GDM subjects were reduced (Ranheim et al., 2004). Concentration of adiponectin may change before the appearance of the abnormal glucose level during pregnancy (Xue-lian et al., 2008). To identify potential biomarkers for impending gestational diabetes that appear in the plasma before impaired glucose tolerance a prospectively study was done and the results demonstrated a significant difference in insulin and adiponectin concentration at 11 weeks gestation and, compared to control groups, women with gestational diabetes exhibited elevated plasma insulin and reduced plasma adiponectin at 28 weeks gestation. Bivariate logistic regression analysis showed that both insulin and adiponectin were associated with subsequent development of gestational

diabetes. Based upon this study (Georgiou et al., 2008) the predictive threshold values for GDM at 11 weeks are >25μU/ml insulin and <3.5μg/ml adiponectin. This study confirmed the another survey (Wiliams et al., 2004) that a low blood concentration of adiponectin early in pregnancy is associated with increased risk of subsequent GDM.
In summary the results of case control and prospective studies demonstrated association of low adiponectin and GDM.

2.2 Leptin

2.2.1 Leptin structure

Leptin, a protein product of the obese (ob) gene with a 16 KDA molecular weight, is made of 167 amino acids (Hui-lan et al., 2004). It is a circulating hormone that is expressed plentifully in the adipose tissue. Leptin is also produced by non adipose tissue including the stomach, intestine and the placenta in humans (Masuzaki et al., 1997) and acts on the receptors of the hypothalamus to decrease food intake and increase energy consumption (Zhang et al., 1994). Leptin is encoded by the obesity gene. It signals to the brain when there has been enough eating to sustain body weight. It has been exhibited that laboratory mice have a mutation on the ob gene which inhibits the function of leptin causing the mice to become morbidly obese. In addition mutation in the gene that codes the leptin receptor causes obesity in the mice. Mutations in the ob gene affect expression of leptin, which in turn can cause obesity, infertility, and diabetes in lab mice (Zhang et al., 1997). It is hypothesized that alteration in the human ob gene causes some serious cases of early-onset obesity. Other less severe kinds of human obesity are considered not to be caused by mutation, but by changing in regulation or resistance to the action of leptin (Flier et al., 1995). Diminished production of leptin or fewer receptors may also be responsible for those who are overweight but not obese. It seems that the appropriate amount of leptin has to be present in the central nervous system to leptin act as weight lowering in human obesity (Zhang et al., 1997).

2.2.2 Leptin action

Homeostatic regulation of body weight depends on the capacity of the brain to sense and respond to changes in peripheral energy supplies. Insulin receptors were recognized in the brain and concentrated in the hypothalamus. These receptors have binding and signaling properties like peripheral insulin receptors. Leptin and insulin enter the brain and act on special hypothalamic neurons to prevent food intake and alter appetite. Leptin raise energy expenditure by regulating of neurotransmitters. (Porter et al., 2002). The evidence shows that insulin and leptin also act on the hypothalamus to control glucose production from the liver via stimulation of the autonomic nervous system. Thus, communication between leptin, insulin and significant hypothalamic neurons is necessary for normal energy balance and glucose homeostasis, deregulation of which will lead to obesity and type 2 diabetes. Indeed, in many forms of obesity, hypothalamic leptin and insulin resistance develops in which leptin and insulin are less effective in causing anorexia and decreased body weight. Some studies propose that leptin also has a specific effect on the regulation of whole body glucose homeostasis (Al-Dahhri et al., 2002; Ceddia et al., 2002). Numerous metabolic studies have shown a positive association between direct and indirect measures of adiposity with plasma leptin concentrations. Plasma leptin concentration correlated with BMI, percent of body fat and plasma insulin in both overweight/obese and normal weight and decreased after sustained weight loss (Havel et al., 1996).

2.2.3 Leptin and gestational diabetes

The increased risk of GDM with increasing maternal plasma concentration of leptin is biologically plausible and is likely accounted for by diverse molecular and biochemical pathways in multiple tissue. Leptin has been shown to regulate peripheral glucose homeostasis through its action in skeletal muscle and its effects on hepatic gene expression of the gluconeogenetic enzymes and phosphoenolpyruvate carboxykinase (Rossetti et al., 1997). In addition, leptin has been shown to directly modulate glucose handling in skeletal muscle by promoting fatty acid oxidation. Investigators have postulated that leptin induced insulin resistance may be secondary to glucose flux via the hexosamine pathway (Mueller et al., 1998). Although the pathophysiology of hyperleptinemia in GDM is unknown, it is clear that leptin has numerous actions on target tissues and is involved in regulation on several endocrine pathways. Although the biologic action of leptin primarily mediated through interactions with receptors expressed in the hypothalamus, leptin receptors are widely distributed across other tissues including the lungs, liver, kidney, pancreas, heart and the placenta (Chen et al., 1999; Hoggard et al., 1997; Kieffer et al., 1996; Schulz et al., 2000). This wide distribution of leptin receptors portends the peptide diverse influence on neuroendocrine, cardiovascular and reproductive functions. Leptin is correlated with a series of endocrine parameters including insulin, insulin-like growth factors, hemoglobin A1c and sex hormone-binding globulin

In pregnant women with changes in maternal fat stores and glucose metabolism, leptin increases (Schubring et al., 2000). Maternal leptin concentration increases 2 to 3 times above the non-pregnant concentration with the peak around 28 weeks of gestation (Schubring et al., 2000). The serum leptin level relates to body weight, body mass index, fat accumulation of the pregnant woman, fetal growth and development and fetal fat deposits. In recent years, it was considered that leptin is associated in pregnancy-induced hypertension syndrome, fetal intrauterine growth retardation and gestational diabetes. Increasing maternal plasma leptin levels may result from an upregulation of adipocyte leptin synthesis in the presence of increasing insulin resistance and hyperinsulinemia in the second half of pregnancy (Laivuori et al., 2000; Rossetti et al., 1997). Investigators have shown that leptin directly affects whole body insulin sensitivity through regulating the efficiency of insulin-mediated glucose metabolism by skeletal muscle (Cohen et al., 1996) and by hepatic regulation of gluconeogenesis (Rossetti et al., 1997). Some evidence suggests that leptin has an acute inhibitory effect on secretion of insulin (Ceddia et al., 2002). Large epidemiological studies have shown that plasma leptin concentrations were positively associated with insulin resistance in men and non-pregnant women (Donahue et al., 1999).

Available data suggest a complex relation between leptin and glucose homeostasis in humans. Two teams of investigators have studied maternal leptin concentrations in GDM women and the related published results are conflicting. On the other hand, the available data do not explain whether the alterations in leptin concentrations are the cause or result of the metabolic disturbances, such as hyperglycemia, that are essential to GDM. In addition, the severity of any possible association of GDM risk with different concentrations of leptin was not assessed in either study (Festa et al., 1999; Kautzky-Willer et al., 2001). In a case-control study reported that maternal third-trimester plasma leptin concentrations were higher in GDM women compared with the control group (24.9 versus 18.2 ng/mL; P=0.001) (Kautzky-Willer et al., 2001). Such a relation was also found in other study. (Vitoratus et al., 2000) Hyperleptinemia, independent of maternal adiposity, in early pregnancy appears to be predictive of an increased risk of GDM later in pregnancy. After adjusting for maternal prepregnancy adiposity and other confounders, women with leptin concentrations of 31ng/ml or higher experienced a 4.7-fold increased risk of GDM as compared with women who had concentrations of 14.3ng/ml or lower. Each 10-ng/ml increase in the leptin concentration was associated with a 20% increase in GDM risk (Qiu et al., 2004). Serum leptin level is correlated with glucose tolerance during pregnancy (Liu et al., 2003). In a case-control study, at 28 weeks of gestation, fasting serum concentration of leptin, insulin and homeostatic model assessment index were measured in three groups, GDM, IGT, and normal control, and compared them with each other. This study demonstrated that the serum leptin level was significantly higher in women with GDM than in the two other groups ($p = 0.03$). In women with GDM and IGT, leptin was significantly positively related with insulin and homeostatic model assessment index ($r = 0.221$, $p = 0.03$) and ($r = 0.246$, $p = 0.03$), respectively. (Soheilykhah et al., 2011)

In a case-control study, noted that maternal third trimester leptin concentrations were significantly lower in GDM cases as compared with controls after adjusting for possible confounding factors such as BMI and insulin concentrations (Festa et al., 1999). Concentration of leptin increased before the appearance of the abnormal glucose level during pregnancy (Xue-lian et al., 2008). Some studies evaluated the relationship between leptin concentration and insulin resistance. Leptin concentration was positively associated with insulin level and HOMA index (Maghbooli et al., 2007). A positive and significant correlation between the maternal leptin and fasting insulin levels (Liu et al., 2003) and also has shown that leptin predicts the development of GDM independent of maternal BMI and other risk factors. The findings of Kautzky-Willer et al are generally consistent with the Different reports. (Kautzky-Willer et al., 2001 ,Lappas et al., 2005 Qiu et al., 2004).

Several possible explanations are suggested for the disparities in the existing studies. The study design and the confounding factors such as the time of blood sampling (whether blood samples were collected before, after, or during labor) and maternal factors, including whether women were treated with medication or diet before blood was collected for leptin determination might account for differences. Moreover, variations in population characteristics and status of glycemic control could also account for some of the observed differences in the study results.

In summary, the results of different studies from experimental, clinical, and epidemiological investigations suggest that leptin is an important mediator of glucose homeostasis in pregnancy (Qiu et al., 2004) and measurement of leptin alone, or combined with the assessment of other risk factors, may help identify women at risk of developing GDM.

2.3 Resistin

2.3.1 Resistin structure

Insulin resistance is strongly associated with obesity, but even among obese subjects insulin sensitivity is different. Recently, a new adipocyte hormone, resistin, was identified, shown to decrease insulin-mediated glucose uptake, and shown to be increased in obese mice

Resistin, also known as adipose tissue-specific secretory factor , is a cystein-rich protein that in humans is encoded by the *RETN* gene (Wang et al., 2002). Resistin was discovered to be produced and released from adipose tissue to provide endocrine functions likely involved in insulin resistance. This thought initially developed from studies exhibiting that serum resistin levels increase with obesity in several species (humans, rats, and mice) . (Yamauchi et al., 2003; Gabriely et al., 2002; Steppan et al., 2001). Resistin is also produced by several

other tissues, including the hypothalamus, pituitary and adrenal glands, pancreas, gastrointestinal tract, myocytes, spleen and white blood cells
The role of resistin in obesity and insulin resistance in humans is controversial.

2.3.2 Resistin action

Resistin causes insulin resistance and glucose intolerance in mice. Serum resistin levels will rise with increased adiposity, particularly central obesity (Degawa-Yamauchi et al., 2003; Vendrell et al., 2004). Conversely, serum resistin levels decrease with lowering adiposity following medical treatment (Valsamakis et al., 2004). The level of tissue resistin is decreased by insulin, cytokines such as tumour necrosis factor, α endothelin-1 and increased by growth and gonadal hormones, hyperglycaemia, interleukin-6 and lipopolysaccharide (Adeghate, 2004). Animal study exhibited that resistin gene expression and protein levels are regulated in parallel with glucose and insulin during fasting and feeding Many researchers have shown positive correlations between resistin levels and insulin resistance.Thus resistin has been suggested to link obesity with type 2 diabetes (Hirosumi et al., 2002; Rajala et al., 2004; Silha et al., 2003; Smith et al., 2003). This discovery is further confirmed by studies which verified a direct correlation between resistin levels and subjects with type 2DM (Asensio et al., 2004; Fujinami et al., 2004; McTernan et al., 2003; Steppan et al., 2001). With the finding that resistin was at least in part a cause of the insulin resistance and T2DM, medications which specifically lead to decreased serum resistin in T2DM subjects were developed(Tjokroprawiro, 2006). The level of circulating resistin is decreased by the anti-diabetic drug such as rosiglitazone and increased by obesity. Administration of the anti resistin antibody decreases blood sugar and improve insulin action in mice with diet induced obesity. Treatment of normal mice with recombinant resistin impairs glucose tolerance and decreases insulin action. Insulin stimulated glucose uptake by adipocyte is increased by neutralization of resistin and is reduced by resistin treatment (Steppan et al., 2001). Because resistin is identical to a protein which had a role in allergic pulmonary infiltration, the effect of resistin in inflammation was studied and these researches demonstrated association of resistin with other physiological systems such as inflammation and energy homeostasis (Adeghate, 2004; Stumvoll & Häring, 2002; Vendrell et al., 2004).

2.3.3 Resistin and gestational diabetes

Resistin is expressed in human placenta and has been supposed to play a role in regulating energy metabolism in pregnancy. Resistin protein expression in placental tissue was much higher than that in subcutaneous adipose tissue in normal human abdomen, pregnant abdomen and thigh. It was indicated that resistin protein can be secreted from human placental tissue. Resistin might be one of the factors that lead to pregnant physiological insulin resistance and GDM (Yongming et al., 2006).Resistin is secreted by the placenta during human pregnancy (Sagawa et al., 2002) Serum resistin levels are not different among non-pregnant women and women in the first and second trimesters of pregnancy .Serum resistin increases by the third trimester (Chen et al., 2005). Resistin is detectable at 20 weeks of gestation. In newborns, resistin concentrations were two to three-fold higher than those reported in adults regardless of sex, birth weight, pattern of growth or metabolic state of the mother (Yongming et al., 2006). Resistin gene expression is found in placental tissues during pregnancy (Yura et al., 2003) and it has been supposed that it could be involved in the pathogenesis of the insulin resistance state found in the second half of pregnancy and in the development of gestational diabetes. Resistin levels were significantly higher in normal pregnant women than in nonpregnant controls and showed a negative correlation with gestational age. Resistin was detected in the umbilical venous blood in fetus from 20 to 41 weeks of gestation. Detection of high levels of resistin in cord blood during gestation is consistent with a regulatory action of these adipokines on tissue differentiation and foetal growth (Cortelazzi et al., 2007). Recent reports have measured the level of resistin during pregnancies complicated by gestational diabetes with inconsistent results (Cortelazzi et al., 2007, Chen et al., 2007). The result of a study showed resistin level in gestational diabetes was lower than normal pregnancy(Megia et al.,2008)This result inconsistent with other study that demonstrated serum resistin concentration was significantly higher in women with GDM than in controls before delivery and the serum levels of resistin significantly decreased after delivery in both the GDM group and controls.The serum level of resistin was different on days 1 and 3 but not by day 5 after delivery (Chen et al.,2007). The serum resistin levels were higher in the 1st, 2nd and 3rd trimesters of pregnancy and higher in GDM than in control groups and hyperresistinemia may also be associated with the pregnancy-induced insulin resistance (Palik et al., 2007). The discrepancy of these findings is unclear, but may be related to different populations of the studies, the type of study or the time of sampling during pregnancy.

3. Inflammatory mediators (C-reactive protein)

3.1 C-reactive structure and actions

C-reactive protein (CRP) is a sensitive marker of systemic infection and is widely used in clinical settings (Kushner I& Rzewnicki, 1994). CRP was first detected in 1930 by Tillet and Frances (Tillett & Francis, 1930), who identified a substance that formed a precipitate when combined with polysaccharide C of streptococcus pneumonia in the sera of patients acutely infected with pneumococcal pneumonia. Subsequently, it was found that this reaction was not unique to pneumococcal pneumonia but could be found with a variety of the other acute infections. This was early evidence of the body's chemical response to inflammatory states and led to characterization of other so called acute phase proteins (Abernathy & Avery, 1941). CRP is normally present in low levels in serum but increase rapidly and dramatically in response to a variety of infectious or inflammatory conditions (Ballou & Kushner, 1992).

Since its discovery, CRP has been studied as a screening device for occult inflammation, as a marker of disease activity and as a diagnostic tool (Pepys, 1981). Recently, more rapid and accurate methods of quantifying CRP have lead to a new interest in its value in clinical medicine (Palosuo et al., 1986) although low-grade inflammatory states not originated from infections and atherosclerosis have also been associated with an increase in CRP levels. For instance, obesity is linked to chronic subclinical inflammation as manifested by mild increases in CRP cytokines and adipocytokines and is the principal risk factor for type 2 diabetes. In addition, patients with increases in CRP are at risk of myocardial infarction and peripheral arterial disease (Engström et al., 2003; Ford, 1999; Ridker et al., 2000; Tracy et al., 1997; Yudkin et al., 1999). Elevated serum concentration of acute-phase proteins, exhibiting chronic subclinical inflammation, has been associated with insulin resistance syndrome in men and non-pregnant women (Festa et al., 2000; Han et al., 2002; Pradhan et al., 2002; Ridker et al., 2003). The molecular basis for the association between the inflammation and diabetes related to the action of cytokines such as interlukin-6 and tumor necrosis factor (TNF)-α which lead to insulin resistance and stimulate the acute phase inflammatory response (Fernandez-Real et al., 2001; Kern et al., 2001; Mohamed-Ali et al., 1998; Vozarova et al., 2001).

3.2 C-reactive protein and GDM

Some evidence supports the theory that chronic inflammation might be a risk factor for developing type 2 diabetes (Freeman et al., 2002; Pradhan et al., 2001; Taniguchi et al., 2002; Thorand et al., 2003). Inflammation may have a role in the pathogenesis of diabetes, suggesting that inflammatory markers may identify patients at risk of diabetes. The issue was investigated in a subset of women (1584 who developed diabetes and 2193 who were normal after 6 years. Women with diabetes had higher median baseline level of interleukin-6 (IL6), high sensitivity CRP and tumor necrosis factor alpha receptor 2 compared with control.Two markers (IL6 and CRP) were significantly associated with diabetes risk in all ethnic groups (Liu et al., 2007).Similar results were obtained in the women's health study (Pradhan et al., 2001) and the nurse health study (Hu et al., 2004). In a population -based study in Mexico City, serum CRP was a predictor of the metabolic syndrome and type 2 diabetes in women but not in men (Han et al., 2002). Among middle aged men in Germany those with a serum CRP in the highest quartile ≥2.91ng/ml had an increased risk of type 2 diabetes compared with men in the lowest quartile (≤0.67ng/ml) (RR 2.7,95%CI1.4-5.2) (Thorand et al., 2003). Epidemiological studies have shown that CRP predicts incident type 2 diabetes and increased cardiovascular disease. In healthy middle-aged women, or young men, CRP levels were associated with a three–fourfold increased risk of developing diabetes (Buchanan,2001; kjos &Buchanan,1999).

Very limited attention has been given to the role of inflammation in the etiology of gestational diabetes a condition that is biochemically and epidemiologically similar to type 2 diabetes (kjos & Buchanan,1999).The second and third trimesters of pregnancy represent a physiological type of insulin resistance (Kautzky-Willer et al., 1997). Insulin resistance is associated with dysfunction of endothelial and inflammation as well as increase production of cytokines by adipose tissue(Baalletshofer et al.,2000). Limited available data suggest that pro-inflammatory cytokines may be predictive of GDM(Winkler et al., 2002; Kirwan et al., 2002).

Some studies have measured CRP at various gestational ages in pregnant women and found inconsistent results regarding the association between inflammatory markers and the incidence of GDM and the interdependence with the degree of adiposity (Retnakaran et al., 2003; Wolf et al., 2003,2004). The interpretation of the results was influenced by coexistence of hypertension, preeclampsia, and different race groups or small sample size in some studies. The result of a study demonstrated women with GDM had significantly higher CRP serum levels than normal pregnant women at 37-38 weeks of gestation but at the time of OGTT (24-28 weeks of pregnancy) there was not any significant difference between the two groups (Leipold et al. , 2005). This report is inconsistent with the findings of the Massachusetts General Hospital obstetric maternal report, where increased CRP concentration was shown in the first trimester (10 weeks of gestation) and the association between GDM and CRP depended primarily on coexisting obesity (Wolf et al., 2004). The result of another study demonstrated that CRP concentration is not affected by GDM until the end of the second trimester of pregnancy (Retnakaran et al., 2003). In the third trimester, however, these results suggest an up-regulation of inflammatory markers by GDM resulting in elevation of CRP concentration at the end of pregnancy in women with GDM. In a prospective nested case control study Wolf et al found that CRP concentration in the first

trimester predicted the development of GDM in the pregnancy. In this study risk of developing GDM among women in the highest CRP tertile compared with the lowest tertile was 3.2 (95% CI 1.2-8.8), after adjusting for age, race, smoking, parity, blood pressure and gestational age at CRP sampling. The risk of developing GDM among women in the highest compared with the lowest tertile was 3.6 (95%CI 1.2-11.4), when BMI was included in the model; however, the association between increased CRP and GDM was reduced (odds ratio for the highest compared with the lowest tertile 1.5 (95% CI 0.4-5.51). Therefore, this association is mediated in part by increasing BMI (Wolf et al., 2003) and pregestational obesity as the most prominent risk factors of GDM (Wolf et al., 2003).
Another prospective study was done to examine the association between CRP and GDM risk. Women were recruited before 16 weeks gestation and were followed until delivery. This study demonstrated elevated CRP was associated with GDM risk. After adjustment of maternal prepregnancy BMI, family history of diabetes and nulliparity, women with CRP in the highest tertile experienced a 3.5-fold increased risk of GDM (95% CI 1.2-9.8) as compared with those in the lowest tertile. The association between CRP and GDM was evident when analyses were restricted to lean women (BMI<25kg/m2). Lean women with CRP ≥5.3mg/l had a 3.7-fold increased risk of GDM (95%CI 1.6-8.7) as compared with women with CRP < 5.3mg/l. This study concluded systemic inflammation is associated with an increased risk of GDM and this association is independent of maternal prepregnancy adiposity (Qiu et al., 2004). Serum CRP in gestational diabetes and pregnant control women was evaluated and showed CRP was positively related with fructose amine hemoglobin A1c, triglyceride and BMI. This study concluded CRP plays a role in pathogenesis of GDM (Li et al., 2010). The association of sex hormone-binding globulin, high sensitive C-reactive protein and fasting glucose and insulin in the late first trimester and early second trimester of pregnancy with the diagnosis of gestational diabetes were also evaluated. In this study sex hormone-binding globulin was lower and high-sensitive CRP was higher among women who subsequently developed gestational diabetes. Multivariate analysis suggested that sex hormone-binding globulin measurement was the best predictor of GDM (Smirnakis et al., 2007). A 180 healthy pregnant women undergoing oral glucose tolerance testing in the late second or early third trimester were evaluated . Based on OGTT and prepregnancy BMI, participants were divided to 4 groups: (1) normal OGTT and BMI<25kg/m2; (2) normal OGTT and BMI >25; (3) impaired glucose tolerance, and (4) GDM. This study showed CRP level was higher in overweight women with normal OGTT, followed by GDM, impaired OGTT groups and lean normal GTT. This study demonstrated that maternal CRP are not related to GDM, but rather correlate significantly with prepregnancy obesity (Rentakaran et al., 2003).

4. Vitamin D

4.1 Vitamin D structure and actions

Vitamin D, or calciferol, is a group of lipid soluble substance with a four-ringed cholesterol backbone. Human obtained Vitamin D from exposure to Sunlight, their diet and from dietary supplement. Ultraviolet light convert provitamin D to vitamin D3 (cholecalciferol) in the skin and afterwards Vitamin D3 was bounded by vitamin D binding proteins (DBP) and transported via blood to target organs for metabolism and activity. Vitamin D hydroxylate to form 25-hydroxy-vitamin-D (25OHD) in the liver. Hydroxylation of 25-hydroxy-vitamin-D to 1, 25-dihydroxy-vitamin D occurs in the mitochondria of the proximal tubules of the kidney.This form of vitamin D (1,25(OH)2-vitamin D) is the physiologically active form. The renal production of 1,25-dihydroxy-vitamin D is regulated by plasma parathyroid hormone and serum calcium and phosphorus levels.Vitamin D increases calcium and phosphorus absorption from the gut and reabsorption from the kidneys and increases plasma concentration of these elements. As such, the main effect of vitamin D is maintenance of mineral homeostasis and regulation of bone remodeling (Holick et al., 2006) .

Vitamin D deficiency is defined when the level of 25- Hydroxyvitamin D is less than 20 ng/ml(50 nmol/l). Level of 25-29 ng/ml can be considered to indicate a relative insufficiency of vitamin D and a level of 30 ng/ml or more indicate sufficient vitamin D.Vitamin D intoxication is observed when serum level of 25-hydroxyvitamin D are greater than 150 ng/ml(Dawson et al.,2005).

Vitamin D deficiency or resistance is caused by different mechanisms including reduced of vitamin D access due to insufficient dietary vitamin D, fat malabsorptive disorders, and/or lack of photoisomerization, Impaired hydroxylation of vitamin D by the liver and kidney to produce 25-OH vitamin and 1,25(OH)2-vitamin D respectively and end organ insensitivity to vitamin D metabolites.

4.2 Vitamin D deficiency and diabetes

Some human and animal studies have shown a relationship between diabetes type 1and vitamin D deficiency .Vitamin D deficiency make predispose subjects to type 1 and type 2 diabetes, and receptors for its activated form 1, 25-dihydroxy-vitamin D have been recognized in beta cells and immune cells. Vitamin D deficiency impairs insulin synthesis and secretion in humans and animal models of diabetes and some investigations suggested that vitamin D deficiency has a role in the development of type 2 diabetes. Epidemiological studies recommended a link between vitamin D deficiency in early life and the subsequently onset of type 1 diabetes. In some populations, type 1 diabetes is associated with certain polymorphisms within the vitamin D receptor gene. In studies in non obese diabetic mice, pharmacological doses of 1alpha,25-dihydroxyvitamin D3, or its structural analogues, have been shown to delay the onset of diabetes, mainly through immune modulation. Vitamin D deficiency may, therefore, be included in the pathogenesis of both types of diabetes.(Luong et al., 2005; Mathieu et al., 2005). Vitamin D supplementation could improve or prevent diabetes This effect may be due to immunomodulatory action of vitamin D. (Stene et al., 2000; Eva , 1999).

There was less data about the association between vitamin D and type 2 diabetes. Some evidences show the role of vitamin D in insulin secretion, for example the presence of vitamin D receptors in β cells and the vitamin D-binding proteins in pancreatic tissue and the association between specific allelic variations in the vitamin D receptor and vitamin D-binding protein genes with glucose tolerance and insulin secretion have further supported this hypothesis. The mechanism of action of vitamin D in type 2 diabetes is thought to be mediated not only through regulation of plasma calcium levels, which regulate insulin synthesis and secretion, but also through a direct action on pancreatic beta-cell function(Palomer et al.,2008).Vitamin D deficiency decreases insulin secretion without changing in glucagon secretion. The effects of a vitamin D deficiency on insulin and glucagon secretion was obtained in isolated perfused rat pancreas by radioimmunoassay of the secreted proteins. Throughout a 30-minute times of perfusion with glucose and arginine, pancreases from vitamin D-deficient rats showed a 48 percent reduction in insulin secretion compared to that for pancreases from vitamin D-deficient rats that had been resupplied with vitamin D. Vitamin D status had no effect on pancreatic glucagon secretion. This result, along with the previously demonstrated presence in the pancreas of a vitamin D-dependent calcium-binding protein and cytosol receptor for the hormonal form of vitamin D, 1,25-dihydroxyvitamin D3, indicates an important role for vitamin D in the endocrine functioning of the pancreas. The data demonstrated a positive correlation of 25(OH)D concentration with insulin sensitivity and a negative effect of hypovitaminosis D on function of ß cell. Subjects with hypovitaminosis D are at higher risk of insulin resistance and the metabolic syndrome.Vitamin D repletion in early stages of experimental dietary vitamin D deficiency and in vitamin D deficiency subjects improves glucose intolerance and increases insulin secretion. Some studies demonstrated that vitamin D supplementation increased insulin secretion in response to an oral glucose load in patients with type 2 diabetes but not in patients with established type 2 diabetes (Chiu et al., 2004; Inomata et al., 1986; Orwoll et al., 1994; Gedik & Akalin, 1986). Some evidence indicates that vitamin D increases insulin secretion from β cells by increasing intracellular calcium concentration through nonselective voltage-dependent calcium channels. The main effect of vitamin D on insulin secretion is acquired from conversion of proinsulin to insulin. Calcium is principal not only for insulin exocytosis but also for cell glycolysis (Boucher, 1998). Vitamin D also activates protein biosynthesis in pancreatic islets. Vitamin D deficiency reduces insulin secretion and action. Variation in the vitamin D receptor or vitamin D-binding protein causes glucose intolerance.

Vitamin D increases cellular glucose absorption either directly or by increasing insulin sensitivity. Vitamin D may directly or indirectly regulate β cell function and secretion by binding 1,25 dihydroxy vitamin D to β cell vitamin D receptors and controlling the balance between the extracellular and intracellular β cell calcium pools (Norman et al ., 1980).

Vitamin D can promote insulin sensitivity by stimulating the expression of insulin receptors and enhancing insulin responsiveness for glucose transport. It also regulates extracellular calcium and thus establishes normal calcium inflow through cell membranes and an adequate intracellular cytosolic calcium pool, which is necessary for the insulin-mediated intracellular process in insulin responsive tissues (Draznin et al.,1988).

4.3 Vitamin D deficiency and gestational diabetes

Data about vitamin D as a risk factor for GDM is spare. Pregnant women with diabetes are known to be more vitamin D deficient compared with normal pregnant women (Bikle, 1992). Intravenous administration of vitamin D to pregnant women with gestational diabetes transiently decreases fasting glucose; however, the level of insulin also decreases (Rudnicki & Molsted-Pedersen, 1997). Vitamin D deficiency was associated with a 2.66-fold increase in GDM risk and each 5 ng/ml decrease in 25-hydroxy D concentrations was related to a 1.29-fold increase in GDM risk (Zhang et al., 2008). Another study demonstrated that the serum concentration of vitamin D during 24-28 weeks of pregnancy in gestational diabetes was lower than normal groups (Maghbooli et al., 2007; Soheilykhah et al., 2009).Women with GDM had a 2.66 fold increased risk of vitamin D deficiency (25-hydroxy D<15ng/ml) compared with control group(Soheilykhah et al.,2009). Maternal hypovitaminosis was reported in diabetic pregnancies in Spain and fasting glycaemia decreased with vitamin D supplementation (Farrant et al., 2008). Vitamin D, insulin and proinsulin were measured at 30 weeks gestation in another study . This study demonstrated that vitamin D insufficiency is common in mothers but is not associated with gestational diabetes. There was no association between maternal 25(OH)D and gestational diabetes.In this study mothers with hypovitaminosis D, higher 25(OH)D concentrations were associated

with lower 30-min glucose concentrations and higher fasting proinsulin concentrations (Farrant et al., 2009). Clifton-Bligh et al. showed mean serum 25(OH)D concentration in pregnant women was negatively correlated with fasting plasma glucose, fasting insulin and insulin resistance as calculated by homeostasis model assessment. The association between fasting glucose and log-transformed 25OHD concentration was of borderline significance after accounting for ethnicity, age and body mass index in multivariate analyses. The odds ratio of gestational diabetes in women with 25OHD < 50 nmol/L did not reach statistical significance (1.92, 95% confidence interval 0.89-4.17) (Clifton-Bligh et al., 2008).
In another study total prevalence of vitamin D deficiency (<25 nmol/L) was 70.6% in pregnant women. Prevalence of severe vitamin D deficiency (<12.5) in GDM patients was higher than in normoglycaemic pregnancies. These results show that a positive correlation of 25(OH) vitamin D concentrations with insulin sensitivity and vitamin D deficiency could be a confirmative sign of insulin resistance (Maghbooli et al., 2007). Several studies suggest that vitamin D supplementation in children reduces the risk of type 1 diabetes. Increasing vitamin D intake during pregnancy reduces the development of islet autoantibodies in offspring (Chiu et al., 2003). In Finland, 10,366 children who were given 2000 IU of vitamin D_3 per day during their first year of life were followed for 31 years. The risk of type 1 diabetes was reduced by approximately 80% (relative risk, 0.22; 95% CI, 0.05 to 0.89) (Hypponen et al., 2001). Among children with vitamin D deficiency, the risk was increased by approximately 200% (relative risk, 3.0; 95% CI, 1.0 to 9.0). In another study, vitamin D deficiency increased insulin resistance, decreased insulin production, and was associated with the metabolic syndrome (Chiu et al., 2004). Another study demonstrated that a combined daily intake of 1200 mg of calcium and 800 IU of vitamin D lowered the risk of type 2 diabetes by 33% (relative risk, 0.67; 95% CI, 0.49 to 0.90) as compared with a daily intake of less than 600 mg of calcium and less than 400 IU of vitamin D (Pittas et al., 2006). 4000 IU vitamin D was administrated for 6 months to women with vitamin D less than 50 nm/Land median serum 25(OH)D3 increased significantly and insulin resistance and fasting insulin decreased (Von Hurst et al., 2010).In summary the result of different studies show high prevalence of vitamin D deficiency in pregnant women and most of these findings demonstrated the relationship between vitamin D status and glucose tolerance in pregnancy.

5. Conclusion

Early diagnosis of gestational diabetes prevents maternal and fetal complications . Recently a number of studies illustrated association of various biomarkers with subsequent development of GDM . These metabolic mediators are known to be produced in the intrauterine environment . Some studies demonstrated that decreased level of adiponectin and increased level of leptin and resistin preceded the onset of diabetes in pregnancy.
Some investigations also have been shown association between C-reactive protein and risk of GDM. Some researches exhibited maternal vitamin D concentration inversely related to fasting glucose and insulin concentration and vitamin D deficiency was associated with increasing risk of GDM.

6. Acknowledgement

The author would like to thank Dr Mahdieh Mojibian, Mrs Nahid Dara and Mrs Ashraf Ahmadi for their assistance.

7. References

Abernethy, T. J. and Avery, O. T. (1941). The occurrence during acute infections of a protein not normally present in the blood. *The Journal of experimental medicine*, Vol. 73, No.2, pp. 173, ISSN 0022-1007

Adeghate, E. (2004). An update on the biology and physiology of resistin. *Cellular and molecular life sciences*, Vol. 61, No.19, pp. 2485-2496, ISSN 1420-682X

Al Daghri, N., Bartlett, W. A., Jones, A. F., and Kumar, S. (2002). Role of leptin in glucose metabolism in type 2 diabetes. *Diabetes, Obesity and Metabolism*, Vol. 4, No.3, pp. 147-155, ISSN 1463-1326.

Altinova, A. E., Toruner, F., Bozkurt, N., Bukan, N., Karakoc, A., Yetkin, I., Ayvaz, G., Cakir, N., and Arslan, M. (2007). Circulating concentrations of adiponectin and tumor necrosis factor- in gestational diabetes mellitus. *Gynecological Endocrinology*, Vol. 23, No.3, pp. 161-165,ISSN 0951-3590.

Arita, Y., Kihara, S., Ouchi, N., Takahashi, M., Maeda, K., Miyagawa, J., Hotta, K., Shimomura, I., Nakamura, T., and Miyaoka, K. (1999). Paradoxical decrease of an adipose-specific protein, adiponectin, in obesity. *Biochemical and Biophysical Research Communications*, Vol. 257, No.1, pp. 79-83,ISSN 0006-291X

Asensio, C., Cettour-Rose, P., Theander-Carrillo, C., Rohner-Jeanrenaud, F., and Muzzin, P. (2004). Changes in glycemia by leptin administration or high-fat feeding in rodent models of obesity/type 2 diabetes suggest a link between resistin expression and control of glucose homeostasis. *Endocrinology*, Vol. 145, No.5, pp. 220.

Balletshofer, B. M., Rittig, K., Enderle, M. D., Volk, A., Maerker, E., Jacob, S., Matthaei, S., Rett, K., and Haring, H. U. (2000). Endothelial dysfunction is detectable in young normotensive first-degree relatives of subjects with type 2 diabetes in association with insulin resistance. *Circulation*, Vol. 101, No.15, pp. 1780,

Ballou, S. P. and Kushner, I. (1992). C-reactive protein and the acute phase response. *Advances in internal medicine*, Vol. 37, pp. 313,ISSN 0065-2822

Berg, A. H., Combs, T. P., and Scherer, P. E. (2002). ACRP30/adiponectin: an adipokine regulating glucose and lipid metabolism. *Trends in Endocrinology and Metabolism*, Vol .13 ,No.2, pp. 84-89, ISSN 1043-2760

Bikle, D. D. (1992). Clinical counterpoint: vitamin D: new actions, new analogs, new therapeutic potential. *Endocrine reviews*, Vol. 13, No.4, pp. 765,

Boucher, B. J. (1998). Inadequate vitamin D status: does it contribute to the disorders comprising syndrome X? *British Journal of Nutrition*, Vol. 79, No.04, pp. 315-327,ISSN 1475-2662.

Buchanan, T. A. (2001). Pancreatic B-cell defects in gestational diabetes: implications for the pathogenesis and prevention of type 2 diabetes. *Journal of Clinical Endocrinology & Metabolism*, Vol. 86, No.3, pp. 989.

Cavit, C., Suheyla, G., Rustu, S., Yavuz, D., Pinar, K., and Yalcin, A. (2007). Gestational diabetes mellitus and adiponectin levels. *Proceeding of European Congress of Endocrinology 2007*, pp.88, Budapest, Hungary, 28 April -2 May, 2007.

Ceddia, R. B., Koistinen, H. A., Zierath, J. R., and Sweeney, G. (2002). Analysis of paradoxical observations on the association between leptin and insulin resistance. *The FASEB journal*, Vol. 16, No.10, pp. 1163,ISSN 0892-6638

Chen, D., Dong, M., Fang, Q., He, J., Wang, Z., and Yang, X. (2005). Alterations of serum resistin in normal pregnancy and pre-eclampsia. *Clinical science*, Vol. 108, No.1, pp. 81-84,ISSN 0143-5221

Chen, D., Fang, Q., Chai, Y., Wang, H., Huang, H., and Dong, M. (2007). Serum resistin in gestational diabetes mellitus and early postpartum. *Clinical endocrinology*, Vol. 67, No.2, pp. 208-211,ISSN 1365-2265

Chen, S. C., Kochan, J. P., Campfield, L. A., Burn, P., and Smeyne, R. J. (1999). Splice variants of the OB receptor gene are differentially expressed in brain and peripheral tissues of mice. *Journal of Receptors and Signal Transduction*, Vol. 19, No.1-4, pp. 245-266,ISSN 1079-9893

Chiu, K. C., Chu, A., Go, V. L. W., and Saad, M. F. (2004). Hypovitaminosis D is associated with insulin resistance and _ cell dysfunction. *The American journal of clinical nutrition*, Vol. 79, No.5, pp. 820,ISSN 0002-9165

Choi, B. H., Kim, Y. H., Ahn, I. S., Ha, J. H., Byun, J. M., and Do, M. S. (2009). The inhibition of inflammatory molecule expression on 3T3-L1 adipocytes by berberine is not mediated by leptin signaling. *Nutrition research and practice*, Vol. 3, No.2, pp. 84,

Clifton Bligh, R. J., McElduff, P., and McElduff, A. (2008). Maternal vitamin D deficiency, ethnicity and gestational diabetes. *Diabetic medicine*, Vol. 25, No.6, pp. 678-684,ISSN 1464-5491

Cohen, B., Novick, D., and Rubinstein, M. (1996). Modulation of insulin activities by leptin. *Science*, Vol. 274, No.5290, pp. 1185,ISSN 0036-8075

Coppola, A., Marfella, R., Coppola, L., Tagliamonte, E., Fontana, D., Liguori, E., Cirillo, T., Cafiero, M., Natale, S., and Astarita, C. (2009). Effect of weight loss on coronary circulation and adiponectin levels in obese women. *International journal of cardiology*, Vol.134 ,No.3, pp. 414-416, ISSN 0167-5273

Cortelazzi, D., Corbetta, S., Ronzoni, S., Pelle, F., Marconi, A., Cozzi, V., Cetin, I., Cortelazzi, R., Beck Peccoz, P., and Spada, A. (2007). Maternal and foetal resistin and adiponectin concentrations in normal and complicated pregnancies. *Clinical endocrinology*, Vol. 66, No.3, pp. 447-453,ISSN 1365-2265

Dawson-Hughes.B., Heaney, R.p., Holick, M.F., lips,P.,Meunier,P.J.,Vieth.R.(2005). Estimates of optimal vitamin D status .Osteoporos Int,Vol .16,PP.713-6.

Daimon, M., Oizumi, T., Saitoh, T., Kameda, W., Hirata, A., Yamaguchi, H., Ohnuma, H., Igarashi, M., Tominaga, M., and Kato, T. (2003). Decreased serum levels of adiponectin are a risk factor for the progression to type 2 diabetes in the Japanese population. *Diabetes care*, Vol. 26, No.7, pp. 2015,ISSN 0149-5992.

Degawa-Yamauchi, M., Bovenkerk, J. E., Juliar, B. E., Watson, W., Kerr, K., Jones, R. M., Zhu, Q., and Considine, R. V. (2003). Serum resistin (FIZZ3) protein is increased in obese humans. *Journal of Clinical Endocrinology & Metabolism*, Vol. 88, No.11, pp. 5452,.

Diez, J. J. and Iglesias, P. (2003). The role of the novel adipocyte-derived hormone adiponectin in human disease. *European Journal of Endocrinology*, Vol. 148, No.3, pp. 293.

Donahue, R. P., Prineas, R. J., Donahue, R. D., Zimmet, P., Bean, J. A., De Court, Collier, G., Goldberg, R. B., Skyler, J. S., and Schneiderman, N. (1999). Is fasting leptin associated with insulin resistance among nondiabetic individuals? The Miami Community Health Study. *Diabetes care*, Vol. 22, No.7, pp. 1092,ISSN 0149-5992

Draznin,B., Sussman,K.E., Eckel, R.H., Kao, M., Yost,T.,Sherman, N. A. (1988). Possible role of cytosolic free calcium concentration in mediating insulin resistance of obesity and hyperinsulinemia. Clin Invest, Vol. 82, No.6,PP.1848-52

Engstrom, G., Stavenow, L., Hedblad, B., Lind, P., Eriksson, K. F., Janzon, L., and LindgSrde, F. (2003). Inflammation-sensitive plasma proteins, diabetes, and mortality and incidence of myocardial infarction and stroke. *Diabetes,* Vol. 52, No.2, pp. 442,ISSN 0012-1797

Eva, J. K. (1999). Vitamin D supplement in early childhood and risk for Type I (insulin-dependent) diabetes mellitus. The EURODIAB Substudy 2 Study Group. *Diabetologia,* Vol. 42, No.1, pp. 51-54,

Farrant, H. J. W., Krishnaveni, G. V., Hill, J. C., Boucher, B. J., Fisher, D. J., Noonan, K., Osmond, C., Veena, S. R., and Fall, C. H. D. (2008). Vitamin D insufficiency is common in Indian mothers but is not associated with gestational diabetes or variation in newborn size. *European journal of clinical nutrition,* Vol. 63, No.5, pp. 646-652,ISSN 0954-3007

Fernandez-Real, J. M., Vayreda, M., Richart, C., Gutierrez, C., Broch, M., Vendrell, J., and Ricart, W. (2001). Circulating interleukin 6 levels, blood pressure, and insulin sensitivity in apparently healthy men and women. *Journal of Clinical Endocrinology & Metabolism,* Vol. 86, No.3, pp. 1154.

Festa, A., Agostino Jr, R., Howard, G., Mykkanen, L., Tracy, R. P., and Haffner, S. M. (2000). Chronic subclinical inflammation as part of the insulin resistance syndrome: the Insulin Resistance Atherosclerosis Study (IRAS). *Circulation,* Vol. 102, No.1, pp. 42,

Festa, A., Shnawa, N., Krugluger, W., Hopmeier, P., Schernthaner, G., and Haffner, S. M. (1999). Relative hypoleptinaemia in women with mild gestational diabetes mellitus. *Diabetic medicine,* Vol. 16, No.8, pp. 656-662,ISSN 1464-5491

Flier, J. S. (1995). The adipocyte: storage depot or node on the energy information superhighway? *Cell,* Vol. 80, No.1, pp. 15,ISSN 0092-8674

Ford, E. S. (1999). Body mass index, diabetes, and C-reactive protein among US adults. *Diabetes care,* Vol. 22, No.12, pp. 1971,ISSN 0149-5992

Freeman, D. J., Norrie, J., Caslake, M. J., Gaw, A ,.Ford, I., Lowe, G., OőReilly, D. S. J., Packard, C. J., and Sattar, N. (2002). C-reactive protein is an independent predictor of risk for the development of diabetes in the West of Scotland Coronary Prevention Study. *Diabetes,* Vol. 51, No.5, pp. 1596,ISSN 0012-1797

Fujinami, A., Obayashi, H., Ohta, K., Ichimura, T., Nishimura, M., Matsui, H., Kawahara, Y., Yamazaki, M., Ogata, M., and Hasegawa, G. (2004). Enzyme-linked immunosorbent assay for circulating human resistin: resistin concentrations in normal subjects and patients with type 2 diabetes. *Clinica chimica acta,* Vol. 339, No.1-2, pp. 57-63,ISSN 0009-8981

Gabriely, I., Ma, X. H., Yang, X. M., Atzmon, G., Rajala, M. W., Berg, A. H., Scherer, P., Rossetti, L., and Barzilai, N. (2002). Removal of visceral fat prevents insulin resistance and glucose intolerance of aging. *Diabetes,* Vol. 51, No.10, pp. 2951,ISSN 0012-1797

Gedik, O. and Akahn, S. (1986). Effects of vitamin D deficiency and repletion on insulin and glucagon secretion in man. *Diabetologia,* Vol. 29, No.3, pp. 142-145,ISSN 0012-186X

Georgiou, H. M., Lappas, M., Georgiou, G. M., Marita, A., Bryant, V. J., Hiscock, R., Permezel, M., Khalil, Z., and Rice, G. E. (2008). Screening for biomarkers predictive of gestational diabetes mellitus. *Acta Diabetologica*, Vol. 45, No.3, pp. 157-165,ISSN 0940-5429

Han, T. S., Sattar, N., Williams, K., Gonzalez-Villalpando, C., Lean, M. E. J., and Haffner, S. M. (2002). Prospective study of C-reactive protein in relation to the development of diabetes and metabolic syndrome in the Mexico City Diabetes Study. *Diabetes care*, Vol. 25, No.11, pp. 2016,ISSN 0149-5992

Havel, P. J., Kasim-Karakas, S., Mueller, W., Johnson, P. R., Gingerich, R. L., and Stern, J. S. (1996). Relationship of plasma leptin to plasma insulin and adiposity in normal weight and overweight women: effects of dietary fat content and sustained weight loss. *Journal of Clinical Endocrinology & Metabolism*, Vol. 81, No.12, pp. 4406,

Hirosumi, J., Tuncman, G., Chang, L., G?rg_n, C. Z., Uysal, K. T., Maeda, K., Karin, M., and Hotamisligil, G. S. (2002 .(A central role for JNK in obesity and insulin resistance. *Nature*, Vol. 420, No.6913, pp. 333-336,ISSN 0028-0836

Hod, M., Merlob, P., Friedman, S., Schoenfeld, A., and Ovadia, J. (1991). Gestational diabetes mellitus. A survey of perinatal complications in the 1980s. *Diabetes*, Vol. 40, pp. 74, ISSN 0012-1797

Hoggard, N., Hunter, L., Duncan, J. S., Williams, L. M., Trayhurn, P., and Mercer, J. G. (1997). Leptin and leptin receptor mRNA and protein expression in the murine fetus and placenta. *Proceedings of the National Academy of Sciences of the United States of America*, Vol. 94, No.20, pp. 11073,

Holick, M.F. (2006). Resurrection of Vitamin D deficiency and rickets. J Clin Invest,Vol. 11,No. 6, pp2062-72

Hossein-nezhad, A., Kh, M., Zh, M., Rahmani, M., and Larijani, B. (2010). Resistin, adiponectin and visfatin; can adipocytokines predict gestational diabetes mellitus and early post partum metabolic syndrome? *Iranian Journal of Diabetes and Lipid Disorders*, Vol. 9, No.6.

Hu, F. B., Meigs, J. B., Li, T. Y., Rifai, N., and Manson, J. A. E. (2004). Inflammatory markers and risk of developing type 2 diabetes in women. *Diabetes*, Vol. 53, No.3, pp. 693,ISSN 0012-1797.

Hui-lan, P., Lai-ying, C. A. O., and Min, W. E. I. (2004). Development in study on Leptin in obstetrics [J]. *Foreign Medical Sciences Section of Maternal and Child Health*, Vol. 2.

Hypponen, E., Laara, E., Reunanen, A., Jarvelin, M. R., and Virtanen, S. M .(2001) . Intake of vitamin D and risk of type 1 diabetes: a birth-cohort study. *The Lancet*, Vol. 358, No.9292, pp. 1500-1503,ISSN 0140-6736

Inomata, S., Kadowaki, S., Yamatani, T., Fukase, M., and Fujita, T. (1986). Effect of 1 alpha (OH)-vitamin D3 on insulin secretion in diabetes mellitus. *Bone and mineral*, Vol. 1, No.3, pp. 187,ISSN 0169-6009

Kautzky-Willer, A., Pacini, G., Tura, A., Bieglmayer, C., Schneider, B., Ludvik, B., Prager, R., and WaldhSusl, W. (2001). Increased plasma leptin in gestational diabetes. *Diabetologia*, Vol. 44, No.2, pp. 164-172,ISSN 0012-186X.

Kautzky-Willer, A., Prager ,R., Waldhausl, W., Pacini, G., Thomaseth, K., Wagner, O. F., Ulm, M., Streli, C., and Ludvik, B. (1997). Pronounced insulin resistance and inadequate beta-cell secretion characterize lean gestational diabetes during and after pregnancy. *Diabetes care*, Vol. 20, No.11, pp. 1717,ISSN 0149-5992.

Kern, P. A., Ranganathan, S., Li, C., Wood, L., and Ranganathan, G. (2001). Adipose tissue tumor necrosis factor and interleukin-6 expression in human obesity and insulin resistance. *American Journal of Physiology-Endocrinology And Metabolism*, Vol. 280, No.5, pp. E745,ISSN 0193-1849

Kieffer, T. J., Heller, R. S., and Habener, J. F. (1996). Leptin Receptors Expressed on Pancreatic [beta]-Cells. *Biochemical and Biophysical Research Communications*, Vol. 224, No.2, pp. 522-527,ISSN 0006-291X.

Kirwan, J. P., Hauguel-De Mouzon, S., Lepercq, J., Challier, J. C., Huston-Presley, L., Friedman, J. E., Kalhan, S. C., and Catalano, P. M. (2002). TNF- is a predictor of insulin resistance in human pregnancy. *Diabetes*, Vol. 51, No.7, pp. 2207,ISSN 0012-1797.

Kjos, S. L. and Buchanan, T. A. (1999). Gestational diabetes mellitus. *New England journal of medicine*, Vol. 341, No.23, pp. 1749-1756,ISSN 0028-4793

Kushner, I. and Rzewnicki, D. L. (1994). The acute phase response: general aspects. *BailliFre's clinical rheumatology*, Vol. 8 ,No.3, pp. 513-530,ISSN 0950-3579

Laivuori, H., Kaaja, R., Koistinen, H., Karonen, S. L., Andersson, S., Koivisto, V., and Ylikorkala, O. (2000). Leptin during and after preeclamptic or normal pregnancy: its relation to serum insulin and insulin sensitivity. *Metabolism*, Vol. 49, No.2, pp. 259-263,ISSN 0026-0495

Lappas, M., Yee, K., Permezel, M., and Rice, G. E. (2005). Release and regulation of leptin, resistin and adiponectin from human placenta, fetal membranes, and maternal adipose tissue and skeletal muscle from normal and gestational diabetes mellitus-complicated pregnancies. *Journal of endocrinology*, Vol. 186, No.3, pp. 457,

Lara-Castro, C., Fu, Y., Chung, B. H., and Garvey, W. T. (2007). Adiponectin and the metabolic syndrome: mechanisms mediating risk for metabolic and cardiovascular disease. *Current opinion in lipidology*, Vol. 18, No.3, pp. 263,ISSN 0957-9672.

Leipold, H., Worda, C., Gruber, C. J., Prikoszovich, T., Wagner, O., and Kautzky Willer, A. (2005). Gestational diabetes mellitus is associated with increased C reactive protein concentrations in the third but not second trimester. *European journal of clinical investigation*, Vol. 35, No.12, pp. 752-ISSN 1365-2362.

Li, W. A. N., Jia-gui, J., and Fei, Y. (2010). Clinical significance of C-reactive protein in gestational diabetes mellitus. *Medical Journal of West China*,

Lindsay, R. S., Funahashi, T., Hanson, R. L., Matsuzawa, Y., Tanaka, S., Tataranni, P. A., Knowler, W. C., and Krakoff, J. (2002). Adiponectin and development of type 2 diabetes in the Pima Indian population. *The Lancet*, Vol. 360, No.9326, pp. 57-58,ISSN 0140-6736.

Liu, S., Tinker, L., Song, Y., Rifai, N., Bonds, D. E., Cook, N. R., Heiss, G., Howard, B. V., Hotamisligil, G. S., and Hu, F. B. (2007). A prospective study of inflammatory cytokines and diabetes mellitus in a multiethnic cohort of postmenopausal women . *Archives of internal medicine*, Vol. 167, No.15, pp. 167.

Liu, Z. J., Liu, P. Q., Ding, Y., Wang, A. M., Zhang, J. J., and Zhao, X. F. (2003). Maternal plasma leptin levels and their relationship to insulin and glucose in pregnant women with gestational diabetes mellitus and gestational impaired glucose tolerance. *Zhonghua fu chan ke za zhi*, Vol. 38, No.5, pp. 261,ISSN 0529-567X

Luong ,K., Nguyen,LTH,.Nguyenm ,D.N.P.(2005). The role of Vitamin D in protecting type 1 diabetes mellitus.Diabetes Metab Res Rev ,No.21,PP.338-346

Maghbooli, Z., Hossein nezhad, A., Karimi, F., Shafaei, A. R., and Larijani, B. (2008). Correlation between vitamin D3 deficiency and insulin resistance in pregnancy. *Diabetes/metabolism research and reviews*, Vol. 24, No.1, pp. 27-32,ISSN 1520-7560

Maghbooli, Z., Hossein-nezhad, A., Rahmani, M., Shafaei, A. R., and Larijani, B. (2007). Relationship between leptin concentration and insulin resistance. *Hormone and metabolic research*, Vol. 39, No.12, pp. 903-907,ISSN 0018-5043

Masuzaki, H., Ogawa, Y., Sagawa, N., Hosoda, K., Matsumoto, T., Mise, H., Nishimura, H., Yoshimasa, Y., Tanaka, I., and Mori, T. (1997). Nonadipose tissue production of leptin: leptin as a novel placenta-derived hormone in humans. *Nature Medicine*, Vol. 3, No.9, pp. 1029-1033,

Matheu,C.,Gysemans,C.,Guilietti,A.,Bouillon,R..(2005).VitaminDanddiabetes.Diabetologia, N0.48.PP.1247-57

Matsuzawa, Y., Funahashi, T., Kihara, S., and Shimomura, I. (2004). Adiponectin and metabolic syndrome. *Arteriosclerosis, thrombosis, and vascular biology*, Vol. 24, No.1, pp. 29,

McTernan, P. G., Fisher, F. F. M., Valsamakis, G., Chetty, R., Harte, A., McTernan, C. L., Clark, P., Smith, S. A., Barnett, A. H., and Kumar, S. (2003). Resistin and type 2 diabetes: regulation of resistin expression by insulin and rosiglitazone and the effects of recombinant resistin on lipid and glucose metabolism in human differentiated adipocytes. *Journal of Clinical Endocrinology & Metabolism*, Vol. 88, No.12, pp. 6098,

Megia, A., Vendrell, J., Gutierrez, C., Sabate ,M., Broch, M., Fernandez-Real, J. M., and Simon, I. (2008). Insulin sensitivity and resistin levels in gestational diabetes mellitus and after parturition. *European Journal of Endocrinology*, Vol. 158, No.2, pp. 173,

Mestman, J. H. (1987). Follow up studies in women with gestational diabetes mellitus. The experience at LAC/USC Medical Centre. *Gestational diabetes.New York: Springer-Verlag*, pp. 191-198,

Metzger, B. E., Buchanan, T. A., Coustan, D. R., de Leiva, A., Dunger, D. B., Hadden, D. R., Hod, M., Kitzmiller, J. L., Kjos, S. L., and Oats, J. N. (2007). Summary and recommendations of the fifth international workshop-conference on gestational diabetes mellitus. *Diabetes care*, Vol. 30, No.Supplement 2, pp. S251,ISSN 0149-5992

Mohamed-Ali, V., Pinkney ,J. H., and Coppack, S. W. (1998). Adipose tissue as an endocrine and paracrine organ. *International journal of obesity*, Vol. 22, pp. 1145-1158,ISSN 0307-0565

Mueller, W. M., Gregoire, F. M., Stanhope, K. L., Mobbs, C. V., Mizuno, T. M., Warden, C. H., Stern, J. S., and Havel, P. J. (1998). Evidence that glucose metabolism regulates leptin secretion from cultured rat adipocytes. *Endocrinology*, Vol. 139, No.2, pp. 551,

Nedvidkova, J., Smitka, K., Kopsky, V., and Hainer, V. (2005). Adiponectin, an adipocyte-derived protein. *Physiol Res*, Vol. 54, No.2, pp. 133-140,

Norman,A.W., Frankel,J.B., Heldt,A.M., Grodsky,G.M. (1980). Vitamin D deficiency inhibits pancreatic secretion of insulin . science, Vol. 209, pp. 823-825

O'Sullivan, J. B. (1989). The Boston gestational diabetes studies: review and perspectives. *Carbohydrate metabolism in pregnancy and the newborn.London: Springer-Verlag*, pp. 287-294,

Ong, C. Y .T., Lao, T. T., Spencer, K., and Nicolaides, K. H. (2004). Maternal serum level of placental growth factor in diabetic pregnancies. *JOURNAL OF REPRODUCTIVE MEDICINE-CHICAGO-*, Vol. 49, pp. 477-480,ISSN 0024-7758

Orwoll, E., Riddle, M., and Prince, M. (1994). Effects of vitamin D on insulin and glucagon secretion in non-insulin-dependent diabetes mellitus. *The American journal of clinical nutrition,* Vol. 59, No.5, pp. 1083,ISSN 0002-9165

Palik, E., Baranyi, E., Melczer, Z., Audikovszky, M., Szocs, A., Winkler, G., and Cseh, K. (2007). Elevated serum acylated (biologically active) ghrelin and resistin levels associate with pregnancy-induced weight gain and insulin resistance. *Diabetes research and clinical practice,* Vol. 76, No.3, pp. 351-357.

Palomer, X., Gonzblez Clemente, J. M., Blanco Vaca, F., and Mauricio, D. (2008). Role of vitamin D in the pathogenesis of type 2 diabetes mellitus. *Diabetes, Obesity and Metabolism,* Vol. 10, No.3, pp. 185-197,ISSN 1463-1326.

Palosuo, T., Husman, T ,.Koistinen, J., and Aho, K. (1986). C reactive Protein in Population Samples. *Acta Medica Scandinavica,* Vol. 220, No.2, pp. 175-179,ISSN 0954-6820.

Pepys, M. B. (1981). C-reactive protein fifty years on. *The Lancet,* Vol. 317, No.8221, pp. 653-657,ISSN 0140-6736.

Pittas, A. G., wson-Hughes, B., Li, T., Van Dam, R. M., Willett, W. C., Manson, J. E., and Hu, F. B. (2006). Vitamin D and calcium intake in relation to type 2 diabetes in women. *Diabetes care,* Vol. 29, No.3, pp. 650,ISSN 0149-5992.

Porte Jr, D., Baskin, D. G., and Schwartz, M. W. (2002). Leptin and insulin action in the central nervous system. *Nutrition reviews,* Vol. 60, pp. S20-S29,ISSN 1753-4887.

Pradhan, A. D ,.Manson, J. A. E., Rifai, N., Buring, J. E., and Ridker, P. M. (2001). C-reactive protein, interleukin 6, and risk of developing type 2 diabetes mellitus. *JAMA: The Journal of the American Medical Association,* Vol. 286, No.3, pp. 327,ISSN 0098-7484

Pradhan, A. D., Manson, J. A. E., Rossouw, J. E., Siscovick, D. S., Mouton, C. P., Rifai, N., Wallace, R. B., Jackson, R. D., Pettinger, M. B., and Ridker, P. M. (2002). Inflammatory biomarkers, hormone replacement therapy, and incident coronary heart disease *.JAMA: The Journal of the American Medical Association,* Vol. 288, No.8, pp. 980,ISSN 0098-7484

Qiu, C., Sorensen, T. K., Luthy, D. A., and Williams, M. A. (2004). A prospective study of maternal serum C reactive protein (CRP) concentrations and risk of gestational diabetes mellitus. *Paediatric and Perinatal Epidemiology,* Vol. 18, No.5, pp. 377-384,ISSN 1365-3016

Qiu, C., Williams, M. A., Vadachkoria, S., Frederick, I. O., and Luthy, D. A. (2004). Increased maternal plasma leptin in early pregnancy and risk of gestational diabetes mellitus. *Obstetrics & Gynecology,* Vol. 103, No.3, pp. 519,ISSN 0029-7844

Rajala, M. W., Qi, Y., Patel, H. R., Takahashi, N., Banerjee, R., Pajvani, U. B., Sinha, M. K., Gingerich, R. L., Scherer, P. E., and Ahima, R. S. (2004 .(Regulation of resistin expression and circulating levels in obesity, diabetes, and fasting. *Diabetes,* Vol. 53, No.7, pp. 1671,ISSN 0012-1797.

Ranheim, T., Haugen, F., Staff, A. C., Braekke, K., Harsem, N. K., and Drevon, C. A. (2004). Adiponectin is reduced in gestational diabetes mellitus in normal weight women. *Acta obstetricia et gynecologica Scandinavica,* Vol. 83, No.4, pp. 341-347,ISSN 1600-0412

Renaldi, O., Pramono, B., Sinorita, H., Purnomo, L. B., Asdie, R. H., and Asdie, A. H. (2009). Hypoadiponectinemia: a risk factor for metabolic syndrome. *Acta Med Indones,* Vol. 41, No.1, pp. 20-24,

Retnakaran, R., Hanley, A. J. G., Raif, N., Connelly, P. W., Sermer, M., and Zinman, B. (2003). C-reactive protein and gestational diabetes: the central role of maternal obesity. *Journal of Clinical Endocrinology & Metabolism,* Vol. 88, No.8, pp. 3507,

Retnakaran, R., Hanley, A. J. G., Raif, N., Hirning, C. R., Connelly, P. W., Sermer, M., Kahn, S. E., and Zinman, B. (2005). Adiponectin and beta cell dysfunction in gestational diabetes: pathophysiological implications. *Diabetologia,* Vol. 48, No.5, pp. 993-1001,ISSN 0012-186X

Retnakaran, R., Qi, Y., Connelly, P. W., Sermer, M., Hanley, A. J., and Zinman, B. (2010). Low adiponectin concentration during pregnancy predicts postpartum insulin resistance, beta cell dysfunction and fasting glycaemia. *Diabetologia,* Vol. 53, No.2, pp. 268-276,ISSN 0012-186X

Ridker, P. M., Buring, J. E., Cook, N. R., and Rifai, N. (2003). C-reactive protein, the metabolic syndrome, and risk of incident cardiovascular events: an 8-year follow-up of 14 719 initially healthy American women. *Circulation,* Vol. 107, No.3, pp. 391,

Ridker, P. M., Hennekens, C. H., Buring, J. E., and Rifai, N. (2000). C-reactive protein and other markers of inflammation in the prediction of cardiovascular disease in women. *New England journal of medicine,* Vol. 342, No.12, pp. 836-843,ISSN 0028-4793

Rossetti, L., Massillon, D., Barzilai, N., Vuguin, P., Chen, W., Hawkins, M., Wu, J., and Wang, J. (1997b). Short term effects of leptin on hepatic gluconeogenesis and in vivo insulin action. *Journal of Biological Chemistry,* Vol. 272, No.44, pp. 27758,ISSN 0021-9258

Rossetti, L., Massillon, D., Barzilai, N., Vuguin, P., Chen, W., Hawkins, M., Wu, J., and Wang, J. (1997). Short term effects of leptin on hepatic gluconeogenesis and in vivo insulin action. *Journal of Biological Chemistry,* Vol. 272, No.44, pp. 27758, ISSN 0021-9258

Rudnicki, P. M. and Molsted-Pedersen, L. (1997). Effect of 1, 25-dihydroxycholecalciferol on glucose metabolism in gestational diabetes mellitus. *Diabetologia,* Vol. 40, No.1, pp. 40-44,ISSN 0012-186X

Sagawa, N., Yura, S., Itoh, H., Mise, H., Kakui, K., Korita, D., Takemura, M., Nuamah ,M. A., Ogawa, Y., and Masuzaki, H. (2002). Role of leptin in pregnancy--a review. *Placenta,* Vol. 23, pp. S80-S86,ISSN 0143-4004

Schubring, C., Englaro, P., Siebler, T., Blum, W. F., Demirakca, T., Kratzsch, J., and Kiess, W. (2000). Longitudinal analysis of maternal serum leptin levels during pregnancy, at birth and up to six weeks after birth: relation to body mass index, skinfolds, sex steroids and umbilical cord blood leptin levels. *Hormone Research in Paediatrics,* Vol. 50, No.5, pp. 276-283,ISSN 12818-663

Schulz, S., HSckel, C., and Weise, W. (2000). Hormonal regulation of neonatal weight: placental leptin and leptin receptors. *BJOG: An International Journal of Obstetrics & Gynaecology,* Vol. 107, No.12, pp. 1486-1491,ISSN 1471-0528

Silha, J. V., Krsek, M., Skrha, J. V., Sucharda, P., Nyomba ,B. L., and Murphy, L. J. (2003). Plasma resistin, adiponectin and leptin levels in lean and obese subjects:

correlations with insulin resistance. *European Journal of Endocrinology*, Vol. 149, No.4, pp. 331,

Silverman, B. L., Metzger, B. E., Cho, N. H ,.and Loeb, C. A. (1995). Impaired glucose tolerance in adolescent offspring of diabetic mothers. Relationship to fetal hyperinsulinism. *Diabetes care*, Vol. 18, No.5, pp. 611,ISSN 0149-5992

Smirnakis, K. V., Plati, A., Wolf, M., Thadhani, R., and Ecker, J .L. (2007). Predicting gestational diabetes: choosing the optimal early serum marker. *American journal of obstetrics and gynecology*, Vol. 196, No.4, pp. 410-4e1,ISSN 0002-9378

Smith, S. R., Bai, F., Charbonneau, C., Janderovb, L., and Argyropoulos, G. (2003). A promoter genotype and oxidative stress potentially link resistin to human insulin resistance. *Diabetes*, Vol. 52, No.7, pp. 1611,ISSN 0012-1797

Snehalatha, C., Mukesh, B., Simon, M., Viswanathan, V., Haffner, S. M., and Ramachandran, A. (2003). Plasma adiponectin is an independent predictor of type 2 diabetes in Asian Indians. *Diabetes care*, Vol. 26, No.12, pp. 3226,ISSN 0149-5992

Soheilykhah, S., Mohammadi, M., Mojibian, M., Rahimi-Saghand, S., Rashidi, M., Hadinedoushan, H., and fkhami-Ardekani ,M. (2009). Maternal serum adiponectin concentration in gestational diabetes. *Gynecological Endocrinology*, Vol. 25, No.9, pp. 593-596,ISSN 0951-3590

Soheilykhah, S., Mojibian, M., Rashidi, M., Rahimi-Saghand, S., and Jafari, F. (2010). Maternal Vitamin D Status in Gestational Diabetes Mellitus. *Nutrition in Clinical Practice*, Vol. 25, No.5, pp. 524,ISSN 0884-5336

Soheilykhah, S., Mojibian, M., Rahimi-Saghand, S., Rashidi, M., Hadinedoushan, H. (2011). Maternal serum leptin concentration in gestational diabetes. *Taiwanese Journal of Obstetrics & Gynecology*, Vol. 50, No.2, pp.149-153, ISSN1028-4559.

Spranger, J., Kroke, A., Mohlig, M., Bergmann, M. M., Ristow, M., Boeing, H., and Pfeiffer, A. F. H. (2003). Adiponectin and protection against type 2 diabetes mellitus. *The Lancet*, Vol. 361, No.9353, pp. 226-228,ISSN 0140-6736

Stene, L. C., Ulriksen, J., Magnus, P., and Joner, G. (2000). Use of cod liver oil during pregnancy associated with lower risk of Type I diabetes in the offspring. *Diabetologia*, Vol. 43, No.9, pp. 1093-1098,ISSN 0012-186X.

Steppan, C. M., Bailey, S. T., Bhat, S., Brown, E. J., Banerjee, R. R., Wright, C. M., Patel, H. R., Ahima, R. S., and Lazar, M. A. (2001). The hormone resistin links obesity to diabetes. *Nature*, Vol. 409, No.6818, pp. 307-312,ISSN 0028-0836

Stumvoll, M. and HSring, H. (2002). Resistin and adiponectin--of mice and men. *Obesity research*, Vol. 10, No.11, pp. 1197,ISSN 1071-7323

Taniguchi, A., Nagasaka, S., Fukushima, M., Sakai, M., Okumura, T., Yoshii, S., Watanabe, T., Ogura, M., Yamadori, N., and Nin, K. (2002). C-reactive protein and insulin resistance in non-obese Japanese type 2 diabetic patients. *Metabolism*, Vol. 51, No.12, pp. 1578-1581,ISSN 0026-0495

Thadhani, R., Wolf, M., Hsu-Blatman, K., Sandler, L., Nathan, D., and Ecker, J. L. (2003). First-trimester sex hormone binding globulin and subsequent gestational diabetes mellitus. *American journal of obstetrics and gynecology*, Vol. 189 ,No.1, pp. 171-176,ISSN 0002-9378

Thorand, B., Lowel, H., Schneider, A., Kolb, H., Meisinger, C., Frohlich, M., and Koenig, W. (2003). C-reactive protein as a predictor for incident diabetes mellitus among middle-aged men: results from the MONICA Augsburg cohort study, 1984-1998. *Archives of internal medicine*, Vol. 163, No.1, pp. 93,

Thyfault, J. P., Hedberg, E. M., Anchan, R. M., Thorne, O. P., Isler, C. M., Newton, E. R., Dohm, G. L., and devente, J. E. (2005). Gestational diabetes is associated with depressed adiponectin levels. *Journal of the Society for Gynecologic Investigation*, Vol. 12, No.1, pp. 41,ISSN 1933-7191

Tillett, W. S. and Francis, T. (1930). Serological reactions in pneumonia with a non-protein somatic fraction of pneumococcus. *The Journal of experimental medicine*, Vol. 52, No.4, pp. 561,ISSN 0022-1007

Tjokroprawiro, A. (2006). New approach in the treatment of T2DM and metabolic syndrome (focus on a novel insulin sensitizer). *Acta medica Indonesiana*, Vol. 38, No.3, pp. 160,ISSN 0125-9326.

Tracy, R. P., Lemaitre, R. N., Psaty, B. M., Ives, D. G., Evans, R. W., Cushman, M., Meilahn, E. N., and Kuller, L. H. (1997). Relationship of C-reactive protein to risk of cardiovascular disease in the elderly: results from the Cardiovascular Health Study and the Rural Health Promotion Project. *Arteriosclerosis, thrombosis, and vascular biology*, Vol. 17, No.6, pp. 1121,

Ukkola, O. and Santaniemi, M. (2002). Adiponectin: a link between excess adiposity and associated comorbidities? *Journal of molecular medicine*, Vol. 80, No.11, pp. 696-702,ISSN 0946-2716.

Valsamakis, G., McTernan, P. G., Chetty, R., Al Daghri, N., Field, A., Hanif, W., Barnett, A. H., and Kumar, S. (2004). Modest weight loss and reduction in waist circumference after medical treatment are associated with favorable changes in serum adipocytokines .*Metabolism*, Vol. 53, No.4, pp. 430-434,ISSN 0026-0495

Van Assche, F. A., Aerts, L., and Holemans, K. (1992). Maternal diabetes and the effect for the offspring. *Verhandelingen-Koninklijke Academie voor Geneeskunde van Belgid*, Vol. 54, No.2, pp. 95,ISSN 6469-0302

Van Assche, F. A., Holemans, K., and Aerts, L. (2001). Long-term consequences for offspring of diabetes during pregnancy. *British medical bulletin*, Vol. 60, No.1, pp. 173,ISSN 0007-1420

Vasseur, F., LeprWtre, F., Lacquemant, C., and Froguel, P. (2003). The genetics of adiponectin. *Current Diabetes Reports*, Vol. 3, No.2, pp. 151-158,ISSN 1534-4827.

Vasseur, F., Meyre, D., and Froguel, P. (2006). Adiponectin, type 2 diabetes and the metabolic syndrome: lessons from human genetic studies. *Expert reviews in molecular medicine*, Vol. 8, No.27, pp. 1-12,ISSN 1462-3994

Vendrell, J., Broch, M., Vilarrasa, N., Molina, A., G£mez, J. M., Gutiqrrez, C., Sim£n, I., Soler, J., and Richart, C. (2004). Resistin, Adiponectin, Ghrelin, Leptin, and Proinflammatory Cytokines: Relationships in Obesity* &ast. *Obesity*, Vol. 12, No.6, pp. 962-971,ISSN 1930-7381

Vitoratos, N., Deliveliotou, A., Vlahos, N. F., Mastorakos, G., Papadias, K., Botsis, D., and Creatsas, G. K. (2008). Serum adiponectin during pregnancy and postpartum in women with gestational diabetes and normal controls. *Gynecological Endocrinology*, Vol. 24, No.11, pp. 614-619,ISSN 0951-3590

Vitoratos, N., Salamalekis, E., Kassanos, D., Loghis, C., Panayotopoulos, N., Kouskouni, E., and Creatsas, G . (2000) .(Maternal plasma leptin levels and their relationship to insulin and glucose in gestational-onset diabetes. *Gynecologic and obstetric investigation*, Vol. 51, No.1, pp. 17-21,ISSN 0378-7346

von Hurst, P. R., Stonehouse, W., and Coad, J. (2010). Vitamin D supplementation reduces insulin resistance in South Asian women living in New Zealand who are insulin resistant and vitamin D deficientûa randomised, placebo-controlled trial. *British Journal of Nutrition*, Vol. 103, No.04, pp. 549-555,ISSN 1475-2662

Vozarova, B., Weyer, C., Hanson, K., Tataranni, P. A., Bogardus, C., and Pratley, R. E. (2001). Circulating interleukin-6 in relation to adiposity, insulin action, and insulin secretion. *Obesity*, Vol. 9, No.7, pp. 414-417,ISSN 1930-7381

Wang, H., Chu ,W. S., Hemphill, C., and Elbein, S. C. (2002). Human resistin gene: molecular scanning and evaluation of association with insulin sensitivity and type 2 diabetes in Caucasians. *Journal of Clinical Endocrinology & Metabolism*, Vol. 87, No.6, pp. 2520,

Weerakiet, S., Lertnarkorn, K., Panburana, P., Pitakitronakorn, S., Vesathada, K., and Wansumrith, S. (2006). Can adiponectin predict gestational diabetes? *Gynecological Endocrinology*, Vol. 22, No.7, pp. 362-368,ISSN 0951-3590

Weyer, C., Funahashi, T., Tanaka, S., Hotta, K., Matsuzawa, Y., Pratley, R. E., and Tataranni, P. A. (2001). Hypoadiponectinemia in obesity and type 2 diabetes: close association with insulin resistance and hyperinsulinemia. *Journal of Clinical Endocrinology & Metabolism*, Vol. 86, No.5 ,pp. 1930,

Williams, M. A., Qiu, C., Muy-Rivera, M., Vadachkoria, S., Song, T., and Luthy, D. A. (2004). Plasma adiponectin concentrations in early pregnancy and subsequent risk of gestational diabetes mellitus. *Journal of Clinical Endocrinology & Metabolism*, Vol. 89, No.5, pp. 2306.

Winkler, G., Cseh, K., Baranyi, Melczer, Z., Speer, G ,.Hajos, P., Salamon, F., Turi, Z., Kovacs, M., and Vargha, P. (2002). Tumor necrosis factor system in insulin resistance in gestational diabetes. *Diabetes research and clinical practice*, Vol. 56, No.2, pp. 93-99,ISSN 0168-8227

Wolf, M., Sandler, L., Hsu, K., Vossen-Smirnakis, K., Ecker, J. L., and Thadhani, R. (2003). First-trimester C-reactive protein and subsequent gestational diabetes. *Diabetes care*, Vol. 26, No.3, pp. 819,ISSN 0149-5992.

Wolf, M., Sauk, J., Shah, A., Vossen Smirnakis, K., Jimenez-Kimble, R., Ecker, J. L., and Thadhani, R. (2004). Inflammation and glucose intolerance. *Diabetes care*, Vol. 27, No.1, pp. 21,ISSN 0149-5992.

Xiang, A. H., Kawakubo, M., Trigo, E., Kjos, S. L., and Buchanan, T. A. (2010). Declining-Cell Compensation for Insulin Resistance in Hispanic Women With Recent Gestational Diabetes Mellitus. *Diabetes care*, Vol. 33, No.2, pp. 396,ISSN 0149-5992

Xue-lian, G. A. O., Hui-xia, Y., and Yi, Z. (2008). Variations of tumor necrosis factor- , leptin and adiponectin in mid-trimester of gestational diabetes mellitus. *Chinese medical journal*, Vol. 121, No.8, pp. 701-705.

Yamauchi, T., Kamon, J., Ito, Y., Tsuchida, A., Yokomizo, T., Kita, S., Sugiyama, T., Miyagishi, M., Hara, K., and Tsunoda, M. (2003). Cloning of adiponectin receptors that mediate antidiabetic metabolic effects. *Nature*, Vol. 423, No.6941, pp. 762-769,ISSN 0028-0836

Yongming, Z., Muxun, Z., Wei, G., Meixia, Y., Keying, X., Shiang, H., Yanhong, C., Huanli, Z., Lijun, X., and Tiecheng, G. (2006). Expression of resistin protein in normal human subcutaneous adipose tissue and pregnant women subcutaneous adipose tissue and placenta. *Journal of Huazhong University of Science and Technology--Medical Sciences--*, Vol. 26, No.3, pp. 288-291,ISSN 1672-0733

Youn, B. S., Min, S. S., Park, K. S., Lee, H. W., Yu ,R., and Kwon, B. S. (2004). The role of adipocytokines in adipocyte-related pathological processes. *Drug News Perspect*, Vol. 17, No.5, pp. 293-298

Yudkin, J. S., Stehouwer, C. D. A., Emeis, J. J., and Coppack, S. W. (1999). C-reactive protein in healthy subjects: associations with obesity, insulin resistance, and endothelial dysfunction: a potential role for cytokines originating from adipose tissue? *Arteriosclerosis, thrombosis, and vascular biology*, Vol. 19, No.4, pp. 972,

Yura, S., Sagawa, N., Itoh ,H., Kakui, K., Nuamah, M. A., Korita, D., Takemura, M., and Fujii, S. (2003). Resistin is expressed in the human placenta. *Journal of Clinical Endocrinology & Metabolism*, Vol. 88, No.3, pp. 1394,

Zhang, C., Qiu, C., Hu, F. B., David, R. M., Van Dam, R .M., Bralley, A., and Williams, M. A. (2008). Maternal plasma 25-hydroxyvitamin D concentrations and the risk for gestational diabetes mellitus. *PLoS One*, Vol. 3, No.11, pp. e3753,

Zhang, F., Basinski, M. B., Beals, J. M., Briggs, S. L., Churgay, L. M., Clawson, D. K., DiMarchi, R. D., Furman, T. C., Hale, J. E., and Hsiung, H. M. (1997). Crystal structure of the obese protein Ieptin-E100. Nature , No.387, pp.206 - 209.

Zhang, Y., Proenca, R., Maffei, M., Barone, M., Leopold, L., and Friedman, J. M. (1994). Positional cloning of the mouse obese gene and its human homologue. Nature, Vol. 372, No.6505, pp. 425, ISSN 0028-0836.

8

Gestational Diabetes and the Metabolic Syndrome

Leanne R. De Souza[1], Joel G. Ray[1] and Ravi Retnakaran[2]
[1]*St. Michael's Hospital,*
[2]*Mount Sinai Hospital University of Toronto, Toronto, Ontario, Canada*

1. Introduction

The metabolic syndrome is a clustering of traditional cardiometabolic risk factors that include central obesity, dysglycemia, hypertension, hypertriglyceridemia, and reduced high-density lipoprotein (HDL) cholesterol. In recent years, its clinical utility, diagnostic criteria and underlying etiology have been the subject of continuous debate and controversy. While the debate continues, it remains incontrovertible that those identified with the metabolic syndrome are at high risk for the future development of type 2 diabetes (T2DM) and cardiovascular disease (CVD). In addition, an expanding body of evidence has linked the metabolic syndrome with several emerging non-traditional risk factors, including markers of hepatic fat, chronic inflammation (such as C-reactive protein (CRP)), and adipocyte dysregulation (such as low circulating levels of adiponectin). Interestingly, many of these features of the metabolic syndrome are also common to gestational diabetes mellitus (GDM). Indeed, GDM has also been the subject of longstanding debate throughout its history and it too identifies women who are at high risk of developing T2DM and CVD in the future. Moreover, in recent years, GDM has been similarly linked to an array of non-traditional cardiometabolic risk factors, including CRP and hypoadiponectinemia. A series of studies have demonstrated that women with GDM are at risk of developing the metabolic syndrome in the years following their index pregnancy. Furthermore, emerging evidence shows that components of the metabolic syndrome identified in early gestation and even prior to pregnancy can predict the subsequent development of GDM. Taken together, these findings have raised the intriguing possibility that women who develop GDM may have an underlying latent metabolic syndrome that warrants clinical evaluation and risk factor modification.

Though intricate and still incompletely understood, the gradual expansion of knowledge about inter-relationships between the metabolic syndrome, GDM and T2DM may provide us with opportunities to screen for and detect metabolic dysfunction at various stages of disease progression. In this way, GDM represents an important and early "metabolic flag" for an affected mother and, perhaps, her offspring. Thus, in this chapter, we explore the emerging relationship between GDM and the metabolic syndrome. We review the definitions of each condition, their limitations and controversies, and their utility and predictive value in identifying T2DM and CVD risk. The clinical evidence for metabolic syndrome as a precursor to the development of GDM and, in turn, T2DM is also discussed.

Emerging non-traditional risk factors for both metabolic syndrome and GDM will be described, alongside the evidence for metabolic syndrome as a consequence of GDM and as a potential predictive tool to detect risk for GDM before and during early pregnancy. Finally, we consider the concept that women who develop GDM may have a latent metabolic syndrome.

2. Metabolic syndrome

2.1 General definition and varying sets of diagnostic criteria

The metabolic syndrome, also referred to as the insulin resistance syndrome, was initially proposed as a model for understanding the underlying biology and risk factors for CVD. In his Banting award lecture, Gerald Reaven first described 'Syndrome X' as the clustering of abnormalities related to insulin resistance (Reaven, 1988). The World Health Organization formally proposed the term 'metabolic syndrome' in 1998 (Alberti et al., 1998; DeFronzo & Ferrannini, 1991) to identify those at high risk for metabolic disorders and CVD. Though the syndrome was originally intended to identify individuals at risk for CVD, it has since expanded to capture those at high risk for T2DM, with which it is thought to have a stronger association (Ford et al., 2008). The definition of metabolic syndrome continues to evolve today, and is widely studied as a promising marker of cardiovascular risk.

The syndrome is characterized by a clustering of central abdominal (visceral) obesity, glucose intolerance, insulin resistance, dyslipidemia and hypertension (Reaven, 1988). The presence of any one risk factor implies the existence of others, such that their concomitant occurrence collectively describes a positive dysmetabolic risk profile for CVD, or 'cardiometabolic risk' (Despres et al., 2008).

While several organizations and authoritative bodies have proposed diagnostic criteria for the metabolic syndrome, the most cited working definitions are those of the International Diabetes Federation (IDF), the World Health Organization (WHO), and the National Cholesterol Education Program - Adult Treatment Panel III (NCEP-ATP III) (Alberti et al., 2005; WHO Expert Consultation, 2004; Alexander et al., 2003). These authorities have synthesized, analyzed and translated information gathered from a vast, globally representative body of research studies, in order to provide a set of diagnostic criteria with clinically relevant thresholds and measurements that can identify the metabolic syndrome and hence the risk of diabetes and CVD. Despite continued efforts, there are variations in the definitions, which have prompted international debate about the actual utility and strength of the metabolic syndrome as a diagnostic tool. Table 1 lists the criteria and diagnostic thresholds defined by the IDF, WHO, NCEP ATP-III, and, lastly, the recently published harmonized criteria (discussed in section 2.2).

Although the ATP III and IDF definitions differ in their diagnostic threshold criteria for metabolic syndrome, both include the same 5 components: increased adiposity, hypertriglyceridemia, low levels of high density lipoprotein cholesterol (HDL-C), hypertension and dysglycemia. The WHO definition also includes a urine albumin to creatinine ratio. Meeting the dichotomous cut-off points for an abnormality in 3 or more of the 5 components fulfills the requirements for diagnosis according to the ATP III definition (Hunt et al., 2004). Though all definitions include an obesity criterion, the IDF definition provides ethnicity-specific values for diagnosing abdominal obesity (Reaven, 2009). Moreover, for diagnosing metabolic syndrome, the IDF definition requires the presence of increased waist circumference (WC) as a necessary prerequisite along with any 2 of the other criteria. Elevated triglycerides and/or low HDL-C must fall within the prescribed threshold or can be applied if a person is being treated specifically for the lipid abnormality. In addition, the defining criteria consider those with T2DM, an elevated WC and at least 1 other risk factor as having metabolic syndrome. The WHO requires the presence of diabetes, impaired fasting glucose (IFG), impaired glucose tolerance (IGT) or insulin resistance and at least 2 other criteria. Among the 3 definitions, the IDF and ATP III are more commonly cited within the recent literature. The prevalence of metabolic syndrome in U.S. adults is estimated to be approximately 22% to 34% using the ATP III definition and 39% when the IDF criteria are applied (Ford, 2005).

	NCEP-ATP III	IDF	WHO	Harmonized IDF/AHA
Central obesity	WC >102 cm- (M) WC >88 cm- (F)	WC >94 cm- White (M) WC >80 cm- White (F) WC >90cm- Asian (M) WC >80cm- Asian (F)	Waist-to-hip ratio: >0.90- (M) >0.85- (F)	Same as IDF cut points for non-Europeans & either IDF or AHA criteria for Europeans
Elevated triglycerides	≥1.7 mmol/L	>1.7 mmol/L	≥1.7 mmol/L	≥1.7 mmol/L
Reduced HDL-C	<1.0 mmol/L- (M) <1.3 mmol/L- (F)	<1.03 mmol/L- (M) <1.29 mmol/L- (F)	<0.9 mmol/L- (M) <1.0 mmol/L- (F)	<1.0 mmol/L- (M) <1.3 mmol/L- (F)
Elevated blood pressure	≥130/85 mm Hg	>130/85 mm Hg	≥140/90 mm Hg	Systolic ≥130 and/or diastolic ≥85 mmHg
Fasting hyperglycemia	≥6.1 mmol/L	>5.6 mmol/L or diabetes or IGT	Diabetes, IFG, IGT	≥5.6 mmol/L
Urine albumin: creatinine ratio	-	-	≥ 3.4 mg/mmol	-

Table 1. Various diagnostic criteria for the metabolic syndrome

2.2 Controversy regarding the metabolic syndrome

The debate surrounding the metabolic syndrome stems from disagreement about its definition and diagnostic criteria, alongside questions related to its pathogenesis, origins, and applicability across populations. However, despite this ongoing debate, central obesity and insulin resistance have been widely postulated (Lann & LeRoith, 2007) as comprising the fundamental basis of the metabolic syndrome. Categorically, the syndrome is influenced by the complex genetic, hormonal and nutritional origins of its individual component risk factors. Discrepancies among the commonly used NCEP-ATP III, IDF and WHO definitions of the metabolic syndrome, have contributed substantially to this debate. For example, ATP III and WHO differ in their criteria for blood pressure, and neither definition provides specific guidance on how to implement these diagnostic thresholds (i.e., whether to use abnormal systolic vs. diastolic or both; whether to obtain measures in a particular body position; or whether to calculate an averaged measure). Recently, the American Heart Association/National Heart, Lung and Blood Institute (AHA/NHLBI) and IDF attempted to resolve such discrepancies with new harmonized criteria. These criteria, shown in Table 1, include (i) clarification of the blood pressure measurement to specify elevated levels of systolic and/or diastolic pressure and (ii) elimination of abdominal obesity as a mandatory prerequisite, such that the presence of any 3 of the 5 criteria is sufficient for diagnosis of metabolic syndrome (Alberti et al., 2010). The ATP III and IDF definitions differ in their criteria for increased fasting glucose and central obesity (using WC) (Alberti et al., 2006; NCEP 2001) and while obesity is measured by WC according to the ATP III and IDF definitions, waist-to-hip ratio is used in the WHO definition. Furthermore, urine albumin-creatinine ratio is a criterion in the WHO definition, but is not found in the ATP III and IDF definitions, while several risk factors associated with insulin resistance are not considered in any of the definitions, including physical inactivity, family history, sex and age (Kahn et al., 2005).

Further complicating the controversy is the practical observation that, despite its centrality to the metabolic syndrome, contrasting evidence suggests that many overweight or obese individuals may, by any guideline, have normal metabolic profiles (Wildman et al., 2008), and are not prone to future development of metabolic syndrome. Similarly, among those who display metabolic syndrome, not all are obese (Bruce & Hanson, 2010). Some lean individuals are insulin resistant and exhibit increased cardiometabolic risk. In a study of otherwise healthy obese individuals and insulin resistant lean individuals with a family history of T2DM, obesity was associated with higher insulin resistance and diastolic blood pressure, but conveyed no difference in other metabolic markers. In addition, within each BMI category, insulin resistance independently predicted metabolic syndrome, while WC did not. Only when age was combined with WC (but not BMI) did obesity independently predict metabolic syndrome, and, even so, WC was less predictive of insulin resistance at higher WC values (Utzschneider et al., 2010). The authors concluded that insulin sensitivity is a stronger predictor of metabolic syndrome than obesity, and is better than WC at identifying obese individuals with an otherwise healthy metabolic profile. They also recommended employing metabolic testing among lean individuals with a first-degree relative with T2DM (Utzschneider et al., 2010). Nevertheless, even when weight is considered, cut-points used to define obesity are not universally agreed upon and may vary by ethnicity (Despres et al., 2008).

The use of different definitions of the metabolic syndrome has clouded our ability to compare findings across research studies. In addition, there is the question of whether the diagnostic criteria are too restrictive, missing those at highest risk, or, conversely, are too broad, resulting in an overestimation of the prevalence of metabolic syndrome. Considering its inherently chronic and progressive nature, it is reasonable to infer that indicators of dysmetabolism, especially in younger adults, underestimate its consequences for predicting T2DM and CVD. Indeed, manifestation may even occur at different time-points in the disease trajectory, such that risk factor assessment necessitates systematic evaluation across a spectrum of sub-diagnostic and diagnostic ranges standardized for age.

Another criticism of the metabolic syndrome is whether its value extends beyond that of its individual components. The criticism highlights both the redundancy of the classification as a 'syndrome' and the inadvertent undermining of the importance of the individual components. The diagnosis of metabolic syndrome, by any definition, has been studied in relation to the predictive value of the individual criteria. The Framingham study (Wilson et al., 2005) demonstrated no substantial increase in risk associated with clusters of 3 of the 5 metabolic syndrome criteria compared with clusters of only 2 traits. In contrast, data from the Third National Health and Nutrition Examination Survey (Ninomiya et al., 2004) indicated that each of the 5 components of metabolic syndrome was an independent predictor of CVD. These studies illustrate the controversy over whether a diagnosis of metabolic syndrome provides more useful information about CVD risk than any of its individual components (Reaven, 2009). Furthermore, by the current definitions, it is unclear whether any one risk factor is more predictive than the other, in the form of a weighted hierarchy.

To address these criticisms, the American Diabetes Association (ADA) and European Association for the Study of Diabetes (EASD) issued a joint statement about the clinical utility of the metabolic syndrome; they recommended that clinicians evaluate and treat discrete risk factors, without diagnosing the metabolic syndrome, per se (Kahn et al., 2005). Specifically, rather than solely relying on diagnosis of metabolic syndrome, identification of one or more of its component features should prompt investigation for the presence of the other features. For the latter, one may also consider specific emerging risk factors not included in the existing definition, as outlined below.

2.3 Metabolic syndrome and the identification of future risk of T2DM and CVD

The IDF recommends screening for metabolic syndrome features in those with T2DM (Alberti et al., 2006, Alberti et al., 2005). While current recommendations are subject to criticism and controversy, they nevertheless provide a practical basis upon which to adopt management strategies. Individuals with metabolic syndrome have a 5-fold higher risk of developing T2DM (Alberti et al., 2010). Similarly, in a study from the UK that examined the prognostic impact of metabolic syndrome in T2DM, the investigators modified the ATP III definition to include BMI instead of WC, and found that the metabolic syndrome further predicted CVD incidence five years after the diagnosis of T2DM (Guzder et al., 2006).

Showing that dysglycemia predicts metabolic syndrome necessarily identifies a predictive potential for T2DM as well. This is so given that metabolic syndrome -- and especially glucose intolerance -- is central to the development of T2DM. In the GENFIEV study, metabolic syndrome prevalence was 42% in those with IFG, 34% in IGT, and 74% in IFG + IGT (Bianchi et al., 2010). In addition, the prevalence of insulin resistance was higher in those with metabolic syndrome than in its absence. Hypertriglyceridemia (odds ratio [OR] 3.38; 95% confidence interval [CI] 2.29-4.99), abdominal obesity (3.26; 95% CI 2.18-4.89), hyperglycemia (3.02; 95% CI 1.80-5.07) and hypertension (1.69; 95% CI 1.12-2.55) were all associated with insulin resistance. These findings suggest that the prevalence of the metabolic syndrome is high in individuals with dysglycemia, and is generally associated with insulin resistance (Bianchi et al., 2010). Moreover, dysglycemia and insulin resistance are highly predictive of T2DM. Similarly, long-term glycemic excursions will identify those at high risk for metabolic syndrome and T2DM. In their exploratory study, Giuffrida et al. (2010) investigated the relation between glycated hemoglobin (GHb), an indicator of long-term glycemic control, and metabolic syndrome with T2DM. Each 1% increase in GHb was associated with metabolic syndrome (OR 1.31, 95% CI 1.18–1.45), demonstrating a strong relation between chronic hyperglycemia and metabolic syndrome (Giuffrida et al., 2010).

Aboriginal Canadians have a 5-fold higher risk of T2DM compared to non-Aboriginals. Among the former, the metabolic syndrome can be readily identified using available clinical measures, and thus, may be a useful clinical tool (Reaven, 2009; Ley et al., 2009). In a prospective study, Ley and colleagues (2009) found that the 10-year cumulative incidence of T2DM in the Aboriginal Canadian population was 17.5%, with an age-dependent gradient ranging from 10.5% among those aged 10–19 years, to 43.3% among those aged 40–49 years.

The authors reported that, at baseline, metabolic syndrome had a low positive predictive value for future diabetes; however, the syndrome predicted incident diabetes to the same degree as IGT, while its high negative predictive value identified disease-free individuals at follow-up (Ley et al., 2009).

In addition to identifying those at risk of T2DM, metabolic syndrome also independently predicts risk of CVD. In the joint statement from the ADA and the EASD (2005), the authors emphasized the practical use of the metabolic syndrome, focusing on its predictive value for CVD (Kahn et al., 2005). A meta-analysis of a series of European trials reported that metabolic syndrome raises the hazard ratio for CVD in women from 0.6 to 2.8 (Hu et al., 2004). Moreover, patients with metabolic syndrome are at twice the risk of developing CVD over a 5-10 year period than those without the syndrome (Alberti et al., 2010). Several population studies have described an increased cardiovascular risk in the presence of metabolic syndrome (Alexander et al., 2003; Ford, 2004, 2005; Hunt et al., 2004; Isomaa et al., 2001; McNeill et al., 2005). Alexander and colleagues (2003) used the ATP III criteria to assess the prevalence of coronary heart disease (CHD) among patients with the metabolic syndrome. They reported that those without metabolic syndrome, regardless of diabetes status, had a low CHD prevalence (less than 10%), while those with diabetes but not the metabolic syndrome exhibited no increased risk of CHD (Alexander et al., 2003). Otherwise, metabolic syndrome was a significant predictor of CHD (OR 2.07, 95% CI 1.66-2.59) and conferred a risk beyond that of diabetes alone (Alexander et al., 2003).

In the San Antonio Heart Study, metabolic syndrome at baseline was a significant predictor of cardiovascular mortality over a mean follow-up of 13 years (Hunt et al., 2004). Similarly, using the WHO definition, Isomaa and colleagues (2001) found that the risk for CHD and stroke was increased 3-fold in those with the metabolic syndrome ($P < 0.001$), as was cardiovascular mortality ($P < 0.001$) (Isomaa et al., 2001). In a study of individuals without diabetes or CVD at baseline, the ATP III- defined metabolic syndrome had an adjusted hazard ratio of CHD of 1.46 (95% CI, 1.23–1.74) for men and 2.05 (95% CI, 1.59–2.64) for women (McNeill et al., 2005).

Ford and colleagues (2004) showed a linear association between ATP III-based metabolic syndrome and CVD-related mortality as well as all-cause mortality (Ford et al., 2004). A meta-analysis of worldwide data from studies published between 1998 and 2005, showed pooled relative risks (RR) of 1.27 (95% CI, 0.90–1.78) for all-cause mortality, 1.65 (95% CI, 1.38–1.99) for CVD and 2.99 (95% CI, 1.96–4.57) for T2DM using ATP III-defined metabolic syndrome; in the fewer studies that used the most exact WHO definition, the pooled RRs were 1.37 (95% CI, 1.09–1.74) for all-cause mortality and 1.93 (95% CI, 1.39–2.67) for CVD (Ford, 2005). Thus, there is considerable evidence for the predictive value of the metabolic syndrome for identifying risk of T2DM and CVD.

2.4 Metabolic syndrome and emerging non-traditional risk factors

As the components of metabolic syndrome continue to be better understood, the syndrome appears to be a promising diagnostic and screening tool. Recent studies have identified chronic low-grade inflammation as a systemic consequence of obesity that is related to both metabolic and vascular disease. For example, the inflammatory nature of atherosclerosis prompted the study of inflammatory proteins, such as high-sensitivity C-reactive protein (CRP), as potential predictors of CVD. Indeed, epidemiological studies have shown the independent relation between CRP and CHD (Ridker, 1997, 1998).

Nakano et al, (2010) investigated the clinical significance of LDL and CRP in coronary artery disease (CAD) risk (Nakano et al., 2010). Among those without the metabolic syndrome, high CRP was not associated with a higher risk of CAD; however, those with both high CRP and metabolic syndrome had a doubling in their risk of CAD (Ridker et al., 2003; Sattar et al., 2003). Despite uncertainty regarding the utility of adding CRP to the metabolic syndrome definition, investigation of its potential as a predictive tool and meaningful addition to metabolic syndrome is advocated (Ridker et al., 2004).

Previous studies have also examined the use of adipose tissue biomarkers, including adiponectin, in predicting CVD risk. Adiponectin is an adipocyte-derived polypeptide -- an adipokine -- that is inversely associated with obesity, insulin resistance and T2DM. As a protective adipokine, it inhibits gluconeogenesis and suppresses lipogenesis. Low levels of adiponectin result in reduced fatty acid oxidation and increased fat accumulation in the liver. Adipose tissue plays a central role to metabolic syndrome, and low adiponectin levels are associated with metabolic syndrome. In addition, the strong association between hypoadiponectinemia and CVD risk implicates adiponectin in the disease trajectory. Compared with lean controls, patients with metabolic syndrome and T2DM have lower circulating levels of total and high molecular weight (HMW) adiponectin, and higher levels of leptin and interleukin-6 (IL-6). Decreased total and HMW adiponectin, and increased levels of leptin and IL-6, are characteristic of patients with metabolic syndrome and T2DM (Lee et al., 2009). There may also be a link between low adiponectin and fatty liver disease (Matsubara et al., 2004).

Hepatic dysregulation is characterized by insulin resistance -related steatosis and oxidative stress (Kim & Younossi, 2008). Non-alcoholic fatty liver disease (NAFLD) -- ranging from simple steatosis (fatty infiltration) to inflammatory steatohepatitis (NASH), to long-term injury (fibrosis) -- is a strong indicator of insulin resistance in non-pregnant adults (Youssef & McCullough, 2002). The process of NAFLD development is in itself an extension of insulin resistance that reduces free fatty esterification and triglyceride storage in adipose tissue, subsequently resulting in the deposition of free fatty acids in non-adipose tissues, especially the liver (Utzschneider & Kahn, 2006). Hence, NAFLD is considered to be the principal liver manifestation of the metabolic syndrome (Kim & Younossi, 2008), as it requires the presence of insulin resistance and is closely associated with T2DM (Targher et al., 2005). In a recent study of adults with newly diagnosed T2DM, there was significant interplay between T2DM and liver injury, likely explained by NAFLD (Porepa et al., 2010). NAFLD may also be detected with the novel serum marker, Fetuin-A, an endogenous inhibitor of insulin receptor tyrosine-kinase, and a recognized "hepatokine". Elevated plasma Fetuin-A levels positively predict the incidence of T2DM independent of other established risk factors (Ix et al., 2008; Stefan et al., 2008). In a study of 330 adults at risk for T2DM, liver fat was the strongest predictor of prediabetes (Kantartzis et al., 2010) (Kantartzis et al., 2010). Among studied biochemical measures, serum Fetuin-A was a more significant predictor of fasting hyperglycemia than serum adiponectin (Kantartzis et al., 2010). In addition, individual liver enzymes, such as alanine aminotransferase, have varying positive associations with the components of the metabolic syndrome (Zhang et al., 2010).

While hyperuricemia is prevalent among those with metabolic syndrome, its clinical utility remains controversial. Nonetheless, it appears to be a predictor of metabolic syndrome. One hypothesis is that enhanced insulin resistance due to fatty acid synthesis in the liver may be linked to additional purine synthesis, thereby accelerating production of uric acid. Since insulin resistance is considered an underlying mechanism connecting visceral obesity and metabolic syndrome (Matsuura et al., 1998), it follows that insulin resistance is related to elevated serum uric acid levels in those with metabolic syndrome (Borges et al., 2010). While a sex-dependent association between hyperuricemia and metabolic syndrome is apparent, there is no current evidence for its association with sex hormones. Sex hormone binding globulin (SHBG) is a liver-derived glycoprotein regulated by insulin, which inhibits its production in hepatocytes. Low serum SHBG levels are associated with increased insulin resistance and hyperinsulinemia. In a recent review Brand et al. (2011) examined 52 observational studies and found that, for both sexes, metabolic syndrome was associated with low levels of SHBG (Brand et al., 2011).

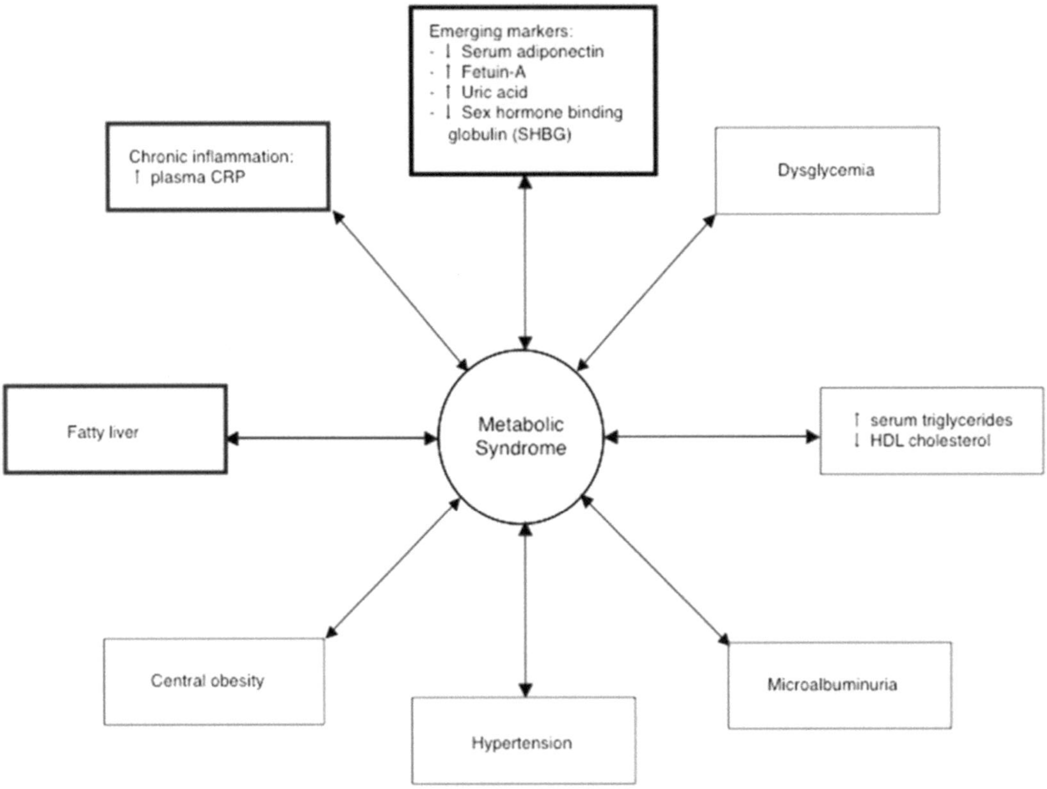

Fig. 1. Traditional & non-traditional (bolded) cardiometabolic risk factors associated with metabolic syndrome.

3. Gestational Diabetes Mellitus (GDM)

3.1 General definition and varying sets of diagnostic criteria

GDM, defined as glucose intolerance of varying severity with first onset in late pregnancy, bears many of the same risk factors as T2DM, including: older maternal age, a family history of T2DM, non-White ethnicity, obesity, sedentary lifestyle, and previous GDM (Dornhorst et al., 1992; Hedderson & Ferrera, 2008; Hillier et al., 2008; Ray et al., 2001). GDM has both short and long-term risks for a mother and her child. Acute maternal effects include pregnancy-induced hypertension and increased risk of Caesarian-section, while long-term consequences include increased risks of T2DM and CVD. Neonatal complications include fetal macrosomia and the associated risk of shoulder dystocia (Athukorala et al., 2007) which in turn can lead to neonatal musculoskeletal and brachial plexus injury (Christoffersson & Rydhstroem, 2002), while long-term sequelae are childhood obesity (Metzger, 2007), metabolic syndrome, and higher risk of T2DM and hypertension (Athukorala et al., 2007; Boney et al., 2005; Joffe et al., 1998; Leon, 1998; Metzger, 2007; Reece et al., 2009).

Though practices vary, many countries recommend that all pregnant women be screened at 24 to 28 weeks' gestation with a 1- hour 50-g glucose challenge test (GCT), followed by a confirmatory 2-hour 75-g, or 3-hour 100-g oral glucose tolerance test (OGTT). While a strategy of selectively screening only women at high risk of GDM may improve the true positive detection rates, some women without classical risk factors for GDM will be missed, accordingly. Table 2 outlines some commonly used diagnostic criteria for GDM.

	NDDG (National Diabetes Data Group)	**ADA 2003**	**WHO 1999**	**IADPSG 2010 (Harmonized)**
Diagnostic OGTT	3-h, 100-g	3-h, 100-g	2-h, 75-g	2-h, 75-g
OGTT-Fasting	5.8 mmol/L	5.3 mmol/L	7.0 mmol/L	5.1 mmol/L
OGTT-1 h	10.5 mmol/L	10.0 mmol/L	-	10.0 mmol/L
OGTT-2 h	9.2 mmol/L	8.6 mmol/L	7.8 mmol/L	8.5 mmol/L
OGTT-3 h	8.0 mmol/L	7.8 mmol/L	-	-
Abnormal values needed for diagnosis	≥2	≥2	≥1	≥1

Table 2. Diagnostic criteria for GDM according to commonly used definitions.

Despite variations in diagnostic criteria, the utility of these definitions for predicting clinical outcomes has been demonstrated. As an example, while the ADA and WHO diagnostic criteria for GDM differ slightly (International Association of Diabetes and Pregnancy Study Group [IADPSG], 2010), the antepartum 2-hour 75g OGTT predicts adverse pregnancy outcomes based on both criteria: the ADA criteria resulted in an increased risk of macrosomia (RR 1.29, 95% CI 0.73-2.18), preeclampsia (RR 2.28, 95% CI 1.22-4.16) and perinatal death (RR 3.10, 95% CI 1.42-6.47) (Schmidt et al., 2001) and similar results were observed using the WHO criteria. Some speculate that the restrictive diagnostic criteria for GDM may overlook the risks faced by women with lesser degrees of dysglycemia (Ferrara et al., 2007; Vambergue et al., 2000). Others assert that lack of international uniformity and agreement of diagnostic thresholds for GDM limits their utility within clinical settings (Metzger & Coustan, 1998). For example, the UK guidelines recommend that only high-risk groups be screened (IADPSG, 2010). In Canada, screening for GDM is routinely done, but not in a universal manner (Wen et al., 2000). Furthermore, current guidelines do not account for the variable risk attributed to ethnicity, in which there are considerable differences in the prevalence of GDM. In a study of ethnicity and postpartum metabolism in women with prior GDM, South Asian Indian women had higher serum triglycerides and lower HDL-C levels, while African-Caribbean women had a higher WC, blood pressure, and insulin levels (Savitz et al., 2008).

3.2 Controversy regarding GDM

Like the metabolic syndrome, GDM has also been the subject of controversy, especially surrounding the timing of screening, the choice of diagnostic test, and the defining thresholds on these tests for its identification. Existing guidelines used to identify GDM, and hence the high risk of T2DM following pregnancy, were initially adapted from criteria that were applied to the non-pregnant population; they were not designed to identify those at risk for adverse perinatal outcomes (IADPSG, 2010). Extensive research has led to modifications of the definition (Cutchie et al., 2006) following the original publication of the criteria (O'Sullivan & Mahan, 1964). Of note, these original criteria were based on the identification of those women at risk of developing diabetes in the years after the index pregnancy (O'Sullivan & Mahan, 1964).

The clinical justification for screening for GDM currently focuses on the prevention of fetal macrosomia and associated obstetrical complications (Retnakaran et al., 2009c). Notably, this focus has resulted in a single set of diagnostic criteria used to identify women at risk for two different adverse outcomes (Retnakaran et al., 2009c), which effectively leads to the assumption that a diagnosis of GDM optimally identifies the risks of both macrosomia and postpartum prediabetes/diabetes. In a study designed to test this assumption, subjects representing the full spectrum of antepartum glucose tolerance underwent a 3-hour OGTT, and the results showed that only fasting glucose emerged as a significant predictor for delivery of a large-for-gestational-age (LGA) infant, with an OR of 2.0 (95% CI 1.20-3.34) per 1 mmol/L incremental increase (Retnakaran et al., 2009c). However, all three post-load measures were significant predictors of postpartum prediabetes/diabetes (1-h glucose: OR 1.37, 95% CI 1.17-1.61; 2-h glucose: OR 1.55, 95% CI 1.32-1.83; 3-h glucose: OR 1.30, 95% CI 1.10-1.53). Thus, fasting glucose values may better predict LGA risk, but post-load values better predict postpartum glucose intolerance (Retnakaran et al., 2009c). Clearly, an additional challenge to the GDM diagnostic definition includes how the results are applied.

The prevailing consensus within the existing framework for diagnosing GDM is that hyperglycemia, including levels below those for overt diabetes, is associated with the adverse pregnancy outcomes common to GDM. In addition, most agree that screening for GDM at 24-28 weeks' gestation identifies individuals in whom effective management can reduce glycemic excursions and minimize adverse perinatal outcomes. It remains to be determined, however, whether these current strategies can effectively reduce long-term risks of metabolic syndrome, T2DM and CVD in affected women (Nolan, 2011). Indeed, women who do not meet the prescribed thresholds for GDM may incur glucose-mediated fetal macrosomia (Mello et al., 1997; Rudge et al., 2000; Scholl et al., 2001; Sermer, et al., 1995), and may be at risk for T2DM and CVD (Retnakaran et al., 2008a, 2008b, 2009a, 2009b, 2009c, 2009d, 2009e, 2010c; Shah et al., 2008).

The Hyperglycemia and Adverse Pregnancy Outcome (HAPO) study was undertaken to examine the risks associated with glucose values below traditional thresholds used to diagnose GDM. The study findings were translated by the IADPSG, in order to harmonize the existing diagnostic criteria (Table 2). The practical implications of these revised criteria includes the universal adoption of a 2-hour, 75-g OGTT. In doing so, these recommendations may identify an increased number of women at lower risk for complications. How the IADPSG recommendations will impact the risk of long-term development of metabolic disease remains unknown at this time (IADPSG, 2010).

3.3 GDM and the Identification of future risk of T2DM and CVD

It is estimated that 20 to 60% of women with a history of GDM will eventually develop T2DM. Indeed, the relation between GDM and T2DM is well described, and the two conditions share a similar pathophysiology, characterized by insulin resistance of peripheral tissues and insufficient secretion of insulin by the pancreatic beta cells to compensate for this resistance (Buchanan, 2001; Buchanan & Xiang, 2005; Retnakaran et al., 2010a). Pregnancy itself has been described as a "stress test" for T2DM and CVD (Reece et al., 2009). It necessarily involves a state of severe acquired insulin resistance that is comparable to that of a non-pregnant person with T2DM (Bergman, 1989). Furthermore, adult offspring with prediabetes, born to women with previous GDM, display an 8-times higher risk of T2DM (Clausen et al., 2008), demonstrating the cyclical nature of diabetes (Damm, 2009) and the compounding effects of dysmetabolism in pregnancy.

Since O'Sullivan's early research illustrating high rates of IGT in the years following GDM (O'Sullivan, 1991), many studies have investigated the phenomena of elevated risk of T2DM attributed to previous GDM. In their systematic review and meta-analysis to quantify the risk of T2DM following GDM, Bellamy and colleagues (2009) found that women with GDM had an increased risk of developing T2DM compared to those women who had normoglycemic pregnancies (RR 7.43, 95% CI 4.79-11.51 (Bellamy et al., 2009). Epidemiological evidence shows that, for all populations and ethnic groups, GDM increases the risk of T2DM (Ben-Haroush et al., 2004). While the shared risk factors between GDM and T2DM imply a common etiology, the salient message is that women with a history of GDM represent a highly vulnerable group for the development of T2DM. This is readily evident in the 2% prevalence of T2DM following GDM as early as 6 weeks postpartum, with reported rates of 50-60% at 5-10 years postpartum, and 70% by 28 years postpartum (Kim et al, 2002; Lauenborg et al., 2004). Furthermore, at the population level, the health significance of GDM is apparent in the number of individuals with diabetes preceded by GDM. In their meta-analysis of follow-up studies of women with previous GDM, Cheung and Byth (2003) calculated the population-attributable risk percent (PAR%) for the proportion of cases of T2DM associated with prior GDM. The PAR% ranged from 10-31% (Cheung & Byth, 2003). These data suggest that up to one third of parous women with T2DM have a history of GDM.

In addition to identifying women at risk for T2DM, GDM also has implications for future risk of CVD. Indeed, women with a history of GDM are at risk for sub-clinical atherosclerosis (Tarim et al., 2006). Studies also show an increased prevalence of cardiovascular risk factors in women with previous GDM (Carr et al., 2006; Lauenborg et al., 2005; Verma et al., 2002). Shah and colleagues (2008) used large population-based administrative databases to examine the CVD risk in women with a history of GDM. They found that, by 11.5 years after delivery, the hazard ratio for CVD in women with GDM was 1.71 (95% CI 1.08-2.69)(Shah et al., 2008). Moreover, even mild glucose intolerance in pregnancy is associated with an increased risk of CVD. Compared with normoglycemic women who did not receive an OGTT, those who had an abnormal GCT followed by an OGTT that was not diagnostic of GDM still had an increased risk of CVD within 12 years of the index pregnancy (Retnakaran & Shah, 2009b).

GDM likely increases the risk for developing cardiometabolic dysfunction after an affected pregnancy. In a longitudinal study comprising 12-18 years of follow-up, 45% of women with previous GDM went on to develop hypertension compared to only 4% in the control group (Mestman, 1972). Another study demonstrated significantly higher rates of dyslipidemia, hypertension and mortality 26 years after GDM (O'Sullivan, 1991). Further exacerbating the burden of disease is family history of T2DM, which adds to the elevated risk associated with GDM. Carr and colleagues (2006) quantified the increased risk of CVD in women with GDM and a family history of T2DM, compared to women without a history of GDM (OR 1.85, 95% CI: 1.21-2.82) (Carr et al., 2006). It is generally recommended that women with GDM undergo a postpartum OGTT to detect ongoing dysglycemia. If lower thresholds for GDM are adopted, then more women are likely to be screened for T2DM postpartum. One hopes that this will offer a preventive opportunity that would otherwise be missed in these women.

3.4 GDM and emerging non-traditional risk factors

CVD is described as an inflammatory disease, with analogous findings in diabetes and obesity (Stern, 1995). Studies have also demonstrated the presence of inflammation in GDM, with high concentrations of serum CRP associated with GDM, but which are attenuated by further adjustment for BMI (Winzer et al., 2004; Wolf et al., 2003). In a cross-sectional study examining the role of maternal obesity in the association between CRP and GDM, pre-pregnancy BMI emerged as the most important determinant of serum CRP concentration, independent of GDM (Retnakaran et al., 2003). It thus emerges that obesity may mediate a systemic inflammatory response that underlies the relation between CRP and GDM.

Similar to its potential as a metabolic syndrome risk factor, adiponectin is also a promising marker of GDM. Compared to unaffected women, those with GDM have lower levels in pregnancy of both total and HMW adiponectin (Retnakaran et al., 2004; Retnakaran et al., 2007). These lower levels of total and HMW adiponectin are associated with both insulin resistance and pancreatic beta-cell dysfunction (Retnakaran et al., 2005; Retnakaran et al., 2007). Furthermore, hypoadiponectinemia in pregnancy independently predicts postpartum metabolic dysfunction, including fasting glycemia, insulin resistance and beta-cell dysfunction (Retnakaran et al., 2010d). Thus, hypoadiponectinemia may play a role in the development of T2DM in women with a history of GDM.

Another novel marker potentially associated with GDM is the presence of a fatty liver. In non-pregnant women with previous GDM who underwent MRI of the liver, those with high liver fat had elevated fasting serum triglyceride and insulin concentrations and lower whole-body insulin sensitivity than those with low liver fat on MRI (Tiikkainen et al., 2002). Given that NAFLD is common in T2DM, Forbes and colleagues (2011) investigated the prevalence and risk for NAFLD among European women with previous GDM. The prevalence of NAFLD was much higher in women with previous GDM (38%, 95% CI 28-47) than in those without GDM (17%, 95% CI 10-24)(Forbes et al., 2011).

Limited evidence exists for the association between uric acid and GDM, although its predictive value in T2DM makes it a promising candidate for studies of GDM. High uric acid levels have been detected in women with GDM (Seghieri et al., 2003), and are considered a marker of preeclampsia (Barden et al., 2004).

SHBG (Smirnakis et al., 2007) is another biochemical marker of much interest. Bartha et al. (2000) compared serum SHBG levels between women with and without GDM, and found that SHBG levels were lower in the GDM group (Bartha et al., 2000). Similarly, SHBG, in addition to adiponectin, was shown to be lower in women with GDM than unaffected controls (Nanda et al., 2011). Even when measured in early pregnancy, first-trimester SHBG

levels were lower among women who went on to develop GDM compared to their peers (187 nmol/L vs 233 nmol/L) (Thadhani et al., 2003).
In addition to traditional measures for GDM, these emerging risk factors are the same as those described for metabolic syndrome arising outside of pregnancy (Figure 2). Accordingly, they raise the question of whether the metabolic syndrome relates to GDM.

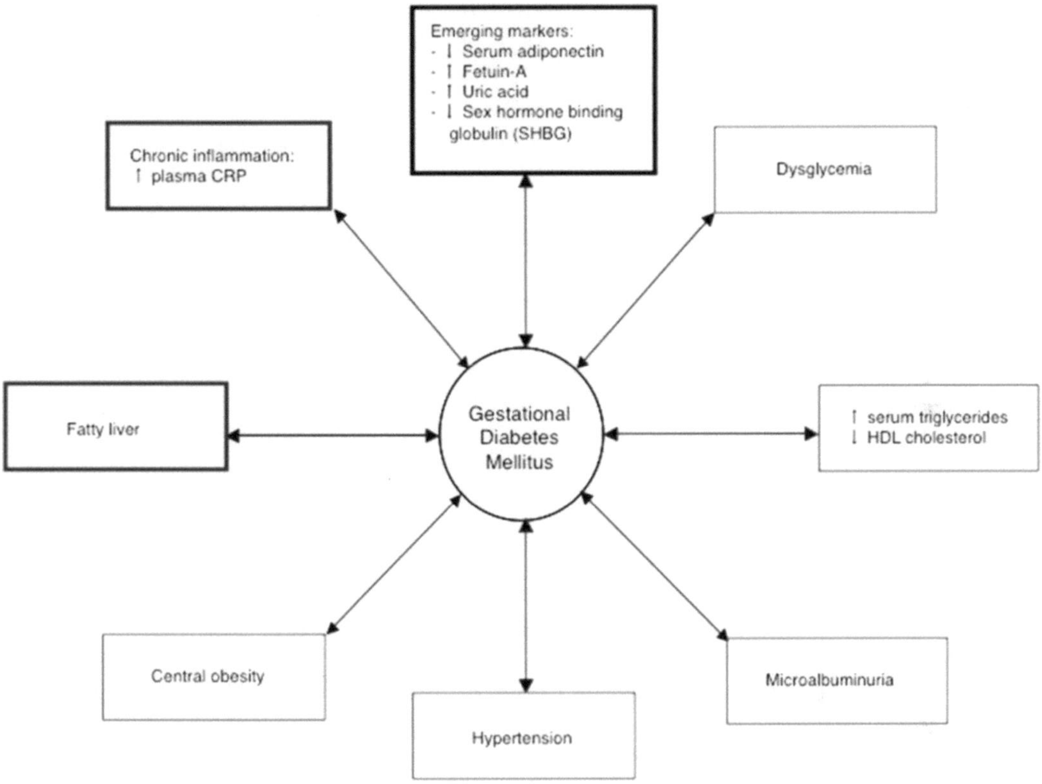

Fig. 2. Traditional and non-traditional (bolded boxes) cardiometabolic risk factors associated with GDM.

4. Risk of metabolic syndrome and its sequelae following GDM

4.1 Development of metabolic syndrome after GDM

Evidence that the metabolic syndrome both precedes and follows GDM suggests an increased lifetime risk of T2DM in women with prior GDM. In addition to chronic beta-cell dysfunction, women with GDM have chronic insulin resistance that is apparent after delivery. Indeed, in the decade after pregnancy, many women with previous GDM exhibit features of the metabolic syndrome. Considering the shared risk factors of metabolic syndrome and T2DM, and the similarities between GDM and T2DM, it is not surprising that GDM is likewise associated with metabolic syndrome. Akinci and colleagues (2010) collected antepartum characteristics of women who developed metabolic syndrome in their later years. Using the ATP III and IDF definitions for metabolic syndrome, pre-pregnancy obesity, weight gain, and OGTT fasting glucose levels each predicted the development of metabolic syndrome. Moreover, even a fasting glucose concentration above 5.5 mmol/L at the antepartum OGTT was an independent predictor of metabolic syndrome (Akinci et al., 2010). Indeed, many studies have demonstrated an increased prevalence of features of the metabolic syndrome following GDM.

Egeland and Meltzer (2010) investigated the effects of GDM on future risk of metabolic and cardiovascular abnormalities. The prevalence of glucose intolerance at 15 years follow-up was 44.4% among women with prior GDM, vs. only 13.1% in those without GDM. WC at 15-year follow-up was the strongest predictor of this difference (Egeland & Meltzer, 2010). Similarly, in a U.S. study, the prevalence of the metabolic syndrome was 27.2% 11 years after pregnancy in women with previous GDM, compared to only 8.2% in unaffected controls (Verma et al., 2002). Lauenborg et al. (2005) estimated the risk of metabolic syndrome in a Danish cohort of women 9.8 years after delivery. Women with previous GDM had a 3-fold higher risk of metabolic syndrome compared to non-GDM controls (Lauenborg et al., 2005). A similar study in Europe reported prevalences of metabolic syndrome of 21% and 4.6%, respectively, 8.5 years' postpartum (Bo et al., 2004b). Indeed, prior gestational hyperglycemia in the absence of fulfilling the overt criteria for GDM results in a future risk of metabolic syndrome 2-4 times that of those with normoglycemia in pregnancy. This risk is 10 times higher in women with concomitant pre-pregnancy obesity (Bo et al., 2004a). Thus, even mild gestational hyperglycemia predicts metabolic syndrome (Bo et al., 2004b), and metabolic syndrome is increasingly more likely to develop over time following the index pregnancy (Bo et al., 2006). These studies highlight the chronic nature of the metabolic dysfunction associated with GDM. Furthermore, they raise the possibility that a diagnosis of GDM may indicate the presence of an underlying latent metabolic syndrome (Retnakaran et al., 2010b).

4.2 Development of metabolic syndrome in the early postpartum after GDM

Recent evidence implicates GDM as an early expression of metabolic syndrome (Haffner & Taegtmeyer, 2003). Indeed, it was recently reported that both GDM (OR 2.05, 95% CI 1.07-3.94) and the milder state of gestational impaired glucose tolerance (GIGT) (OR 2.16, 95% CI 1.05-4.42) independently predict postpartum metabolic syndrome by 3 months postpartum, even after adjustment for covariates (Retnakaran et al., 2010d). Furthermore, by 3 months postpartum women with GDM and GIGT also exhibit non-traditional risk factors associated with metabolic syndrome, including low levels of adiponectin and increased serum CRP (Retnakaran et al., 2010c). While many of the metabolic disturbances of pregnancy resolve after delivery, growing evidence supports the concept that pregnancy provides an opportunity to observe a pronounced expression of an otherwise subclinical metabolic disorder. Such metabolic disturbances, which include the metabolic syndrome component disorders, may indeed be apparent prior to the diagnosis of GDM.

5. Prediction of GDM by metabolic syndrome components and associated risk factors

5.1 Prediction of GDM by metabolic syndrome components in early pregnancy

It is quite likely that the metabolic syndrome exists prior to the development of GDM. Indeed, GDM has even been proposed to be a component of the metabolic syndrome (Clark et al. 1997). In their study, Clark et al. (1997) showed that, at the time of their antepartum OGTT, women with GDM expressed markers of the metabolic syndrome, including low serum HDL cholesterol and higher fasting plasma insulin, triglycerides, free fatty acids and pre-pregnancy BMI. These common features of the metabolic syndrome were each individually predictive of GDM, and persisted after adjustment for differences in BMI (Clark et al., 1997).

In addition to conventional measures of metabolic syndrome, several non-traditional biomarkers have also emerged as possible predictors of GDM. As discussed earlier, low adiponectin is a risk factor for T2DM and an emerging risk factor for metabolic syndrome and GDM. Using a prospective nested case-control study design, Williams et al. (2004) determined whether first trimester hypoadiponectinemia predicts GDM. They found that 73% of those with GDM had a low adiponectin level compared to 33% of controls (adjusted OR 4.6, 95% CI 1.8-11.6) (Williams et al., 2004). Similarly, Lain and colleagues (2008) found that women with low adiponectin concentrations in the first trimester were much more likely to be diagnosed with GDM (OR 10.2, 95% CI 1.3, 78.7) (Lain et al., 2008).

In choosing an optimal early serum marker to predict GDM, Smirnakis and colleagues (2007) compared SHBG, high-sensitive CRP, and the homeostasis model of assessment of insulin resistance (HOMA-IR) in late first trimester and early second trimester of pregnancy (Smirnakis et al., 2007). Serum SHBG was lower, and serum CRP higher, in women who went on to develop GDM, who also had elevated HOMA-IR in the second trimester. After multivariate analysis, SHBG emerged as the best predictor of GDM (Smirnakis et al., 2007). Alternately, Wolf et al. (2003) found that the risk of developing GDM was higher in women in the upper vs. lower tertiles of first-trimester CRP, after adjusting for confounders (OR 3.6, 95% CI 1.2-11.4). Importantly, the association was attenuated when BMI was included in the analysis (OR 1.5, 95% CI 0.4-5.5) (Wolf et al., 2003), suggesting that obesity confounds the relation between inflammation and GDM.

Qiu and colleagues (2004) found that, even after adjusting for maternal pre-pregnancy BMI and other confounders, women with CRP in the highest vs. lowest tertiles experienced a 3.5-times increased risk of GDM (95% CI 1.2-9.8) (Qiu et al., 2004). Moreover, even lean women had an OR for GDM of 3.7 (95% CI 1.6-8.7), suggesting that the association between elevated CRP and GDM may not solely depend on the presence of maternal obesity (Qiu et al., 2004). However, Savvidou and colleagues (2010) evaluated various first-trimester conventional and novel biomarkers, including adiponectin and CRP, and found only a low HDL-C and a high tissue plasminogen activator were significant independent predictors of GDM (Savvidou et al., 2010). Laughon et al (2009) reported that a first trimester concentration of uric acid in the highest quartile had an OR for GDM of 3.25 (95% CI 1.35-7.83), after adjusting for BMI and age (Laughon et al., 2009). Together, these emerging risk factors present an opportunity for early detection of GDM, and possibly, the identification of an effective tool for long-term prevention of metabolic syndrome.

It is likely that components of metabolic syndrome exist before and after GDM. Similar to T2DM, where persons with IGT and IFG are at significant risk of T2DM, so too may be the case for metabolic syndrome in early pregnancy. Ray and colleagues (2010) coined the term "gestational prediabetes" to describe the absence of diabetes before pregnancy, and the presence of a blood glucose level (or a related marker) in early pregnancy that is higher than normal, but not yet high enough to meet the diagnostic criteria for GDM (Ray et al., 2010). Given the promising findings of using emerging biomarkers to detect dysmetabolism in early pregnancy and predict GDM, the next step is to identify a robust biomarker that can be assayed at a low cost in early pregnancy. Since they are chronic in nature, metabolic abnormalities likely precede pregnancy, which means that they should be detectable in early pregnancy as well.

5.2 Prediction of GDM by metabolic syndrome components prior to pregnancy

A modest body of literature exists about the existence of metabolic syndrome prior to the detection of GDM. Gunderson and colleagues (2009) examined pre-pregnancy cardiometabolic risk factors and the risk of GDM in subsequent pregnancies. They found that metabolic impairment often predated the onset of GDM, and that 27% of overweight women with one or more cardiometabolic risk factors developed GDM (Gunderson et al., 2009). Normoglycemia with at least one metabolic risk factor (i.e., low plasma HDL-C and/or hyperinsulinemia) was present before pregnancy in 34% of those who developed GDM; among overweight women, the presence of any cardiometabolic feature was associated with an almost 4 times higher risk of GDM. Hedderson and Ferrara (2008) measured blood pressure before pregnancy and in early pregnancy, and found that women with mild hypertension in early pregnancy had a small increased risk of GDM (OR 1.56, 95% CI 1.16-2.10). Those with frank hypertension had a 2-fold increased risk of GDM (OR 2.04, 95% CI 1.14-3.65) compared to normotensive women, even after adjusting for confounders. These findings were paralleled by mild (OR 1.44, 95 CI 0.95-2.19) and frank (OR 2.01, 95% CI 1.01-3.99) hypertension detected before pregnancy (Hedderson & Ferrara, 2008).

6. Conclusions

We have reviewed the parallels and associations between the metabolic syndrome and GDM. Both conditions have had multiple sets of diagnostic criteria and a history marked by controversies about their definition, clinical utility and significance. Both conditions identify a patient population that has an increased future risk of T2DM and CVD. Furthermore, both conditions have been associated with a similar set of emerging non-traditional risk factors. Consistent with these parallels, GDM predicts an increased risk of metabolic syndrome both in the early postpartum and in the years thereafter. Moreover, it is now becoming apparent that the metabolic syndrome and its associated risk factors may precede the diagnosis of GDM, both in early gestation and prior to the pregnancy. Taken together, these data suggest that GDM may represent a transient 'unmasking' of a latent metabolic syndrome, which may extend in both directions through (i) the pre-gravid state and early pregnancy, and (ii) the early and late postpartum. Figure 3 illustrates this lifetime continuum that may link metabolic syndrome, GDM, T2DM, and CVD. The chronic nature of the features of metabolic syndrome suggests that what we know about the temporal relation between metabolic syndrome, GDM, T2DM, and CVD is limited. The global burden of diabetes has been estimated at more than 171 million individuals with an expected increase to 366 million by 2030 (Wild et al., 2004). The prevalence of obesity and related metabolic dysfunction worldwide is a vivid demonstration of the undiscriminating potential of cardio-metabolic diseases across ethnicities and age groups. In this context, the emerging relation between metabolic syndrome and GDM may offer the opportunity for early detection of at-risk individuals, long before the manifestation of overt disease. Ideally, this opportunity may lead to new strategies for early risk modification and ultimately disease prevention. As such, the emerging relation between metabolic syndrome and GDM represents an important area of research that may hold both clinical and public health implications.

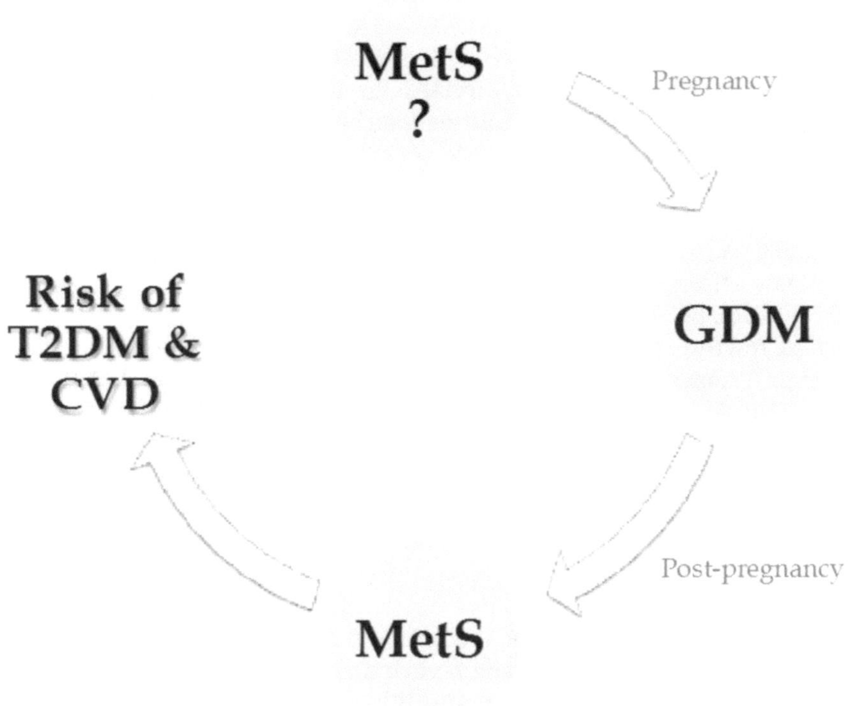

Fig. 3. Theoretical framework and conceptual model for latent metabolic syndrome preceding GDM.

7. References

Alberti, KG. & Zimmet, PZ. (1998). Definition, diagnosis and classification of diabetes mellitus and its complications. Part 1: Diagnosis and classification of diabetes mellitus provisional report of a WHO consultation. *Diabetic Medicine*, Vol. 15, No. 7, (July 1998), pp. 539-553, doi:10.1002/(SICI)1096-9136(199807)15:7<539::AID-DIA668>3.0.CO;2-S

Alberti, KG.; Zimmet, PZ. & Shaw, J. IDF Epidemiology Task Force Consensus Group. (2005). The metabolic syndrome--a new worldwide definition. *Lancet*, Vol. 366, No. 9491, (Sept. 2005), pp. 1059-1062, doi:10.1016/S0140-6736(05)67402-8

Alberti, KG.; Zimmet, PZ. & Shaw, J. (2006). Metabolic syndrome--a new world-wide definition. A Consensus Statement from the International Diabetes Federation. *Diabetic Medicine*, Vol. 23, No. 5, (May 2006), pp. 469-480, doi:10.1111/j.1464-5491.2006.01858.x

Alberti, KG.; Eckel, RH., Grundy, SM., Zimmet, PZ., Cleeman, JI., Donato, KA., et al. (2010). Harmonizing the metabolic syndrome: A joint interim statement of the international Diabetes Federation Task Force on Epidemiology and Prevention; National Heart, Lung, and Blood Institute; American Heart Association; World Heart Federation; International Atherosclerosis Society; and International

Association for the Study of Obesity. *Circulation*, Vol. 120, No. 16, (Oct. 2009), pp. 1640-1645, doi:10.1161/CIRCULATIONAHA.109.192644

Alexander, CM.; Landsman, PB., Teutsch, SM. & Haffner, SM. Third National Health and Nutrition Examination Survey (NHANES III), National Cholesterol Education Program (NCEP). (2003). NCEP-defined metabolic syndrome, diabetes, and prevalence of coronary heart disease among NHANES III participants age 50 years and older. *Diabetes*, Vol. 52, No. 5, (May 2003), pp. 1210-1214, doi:10.2337/diabetes.52.5.1210

Akinci, B.; Celtik, A., Yener, S. & Yesil, S. (2010). Prediction of developing metabolic syndrome after gestational diabetes mellitus. *Fertility and Sterility*, Vol. 93, No. 4, (March 2010), pp. 1248-1254, doi:10.1016/j.fertnstert.2008.12.007

Athukorala, C.; Crowther, CA., Willson, K. & Austrailian Carbohydrate Intolerance Study in Pregnant Women ACHOIS Trial Group. (2007). Women with gestational diabetes mellitus in the ACHOIS trial: Risk factors for shoulder dystocia. *The Australian & New Zealand Journal of Obstetrics & Gynaecology*, Vol. 47, No. 1, (Feb. 2007), pp. 37-41, doi:10.1111/j.1479-828X.2006.00676.x

Bartha, JL.; Comino-Delgado, R., Romero-Carmona, R. & Del Carmen, M. (2000). Sex hormone-binding globulin in gestational diabetes. *Acta Obstetricia et Gynecologica Scandinavica*, Vol. 79, No. 10, (Oct. 2000), pp. 839-845, doi:10.1080/00016340009169212

Bellamy, L.; Casas, J., Hingorani, AD. & Williams, D. (2009). Type 2 diabetes mellitus after gestational diabetes: A systematic review and meta-analysis. *Lancet*, Vol. 373, No. 9677, (May 2009), pp. 1773-1779, doi:10.1016/S0140-6736(09)60731-5

Ben-Haroush, A.; Yogev, Y., & Hod, M. (2004). Epidemiology of gestational diabetes mellitus and its association with Type 2 diabetes. *Diabetic Medicine*, Vol. 21, No. 2, (Feb. 2004), pp. 103-113,doi:10.1046/j.1464-5491.2003.00985.x

Bergman, RN. (1989). Lilly lecture. Toward physiological understanding of glucose tolerance. Minimal-model approach. *Diabetes*, Vol. 38, No. 12, (Dec. 1989), pp. 1512-1527, doi:10.2337/diabetes.38.12.1512

Bianchi, C.; Miccoli, R., Bonadonna, RC., Giorgino, F., Frontoni, S., Faloia, E., Marchesini, G., et al. (2010). Metabolic syndrome in subjects at high risk for type 2 diabetes: The genetic, physiopathology and evolution of type 2 diabetes (GENFIEV) study. *Nutrition, Metabolism, and Cardiovascular Diseases*, Epub (Nov. 2010), in press, doi:10.1016/j.numecd.2010.03.006

Bo, S.; Menato, G., Gallo, M., Bardelli, C., Lezo, A., Signorile, A., Gambino, R., et al. (2004a). Mild gestational hyperglycemia, the metabolic syndrome and adverse neonatal outcomes. *Acta Obstetricia et Gynecologica Scandinavica*, Vol., 83, No. 4, (April 2004), pp. 335-340, doi:10.1111/j.0001-6349.2004.00314.x

Bo, S.; Monge, L., Macchetta, C., Menato, G., Pinach, S., Uberti, B. & Pagano, G. (2004b). Prior gestational hyperglycemia: a long-term predictor of the metabolic syndrome. *Journal of Endocrinological Investigation*, Vol. 27, No. 7, (July-Aug 2004), pp. 629-635.

Bo, S.; Menato, G., Botto, C., Cotrino, I., Bardelli, C., Gambino, R., Cassader, M., et al. (2006). Mild gestational hyperglycemia and the metabolic syndrome in later life. *Metabolic Syndrome and Related Disorders*, Vol. 4, No. 2, (Summer 2006), pp. 113-121, doi:10.1089/met.2006.4.113

Boney, CM.; Verma, A., Tucker, R., & Vohr, BR. (2005). Metabolic Syndrome in childhood: Association with birth weight, maternal obesity, and gestational diabetes mellitus. *Pediatrics*, Vol. 115, No. 3, (March 2005), pp. e290-6. Am Acad Pediatrics. doi:10.1542/peds.2004-1808

Borges, RL.; Ribeiro, AB., Zanella, MT. & Batista, MC. (2010). Uric acid as a factor in the metabolic syndrome. *Current Hypertension Reports*, Vol. 12, No. 2 (March 2010), pp. 113-119, doi:10.1007/s11906-010-0098-2

Brand, JS.; van der Tweel, I., Grobbee, DE., Emmelot-Vonk, MH. & van der Schouw, YT. (2011). Testosterone, sex-hormone-binding globulin and the metabolic syndrome: A systematic review and meta-analysis of observational studies. *International Journal of Epidemiology*, Vol. 40, No. 1, (April 2000), pp. 189-207, doi:10.2337/diacare.23.4.490

Bruce, KD. & Hanson, MA. (2010). The developmental origins, mechanisms, and implications of metabolic syndrome. *The Journal of Nutrition*, Vol. 140, No. 3, (March 2010), pp. 648-652, doi:10.3945/jn.109.111179

Buchanan, TA. (2001). Pancreatic B-cell defects in gestational diabetes: implications for the pathogenesis and prevention of type 2 diabetes. *JCEM*, Vol. 86, No. 3, (March 2001), pp. 989-993, doi:10.1210/jc.86.3.989

Buchanan, TA. & Xiang, AH. (2005). Gestational diabetes mellitus. *The Journal of Clinical Investigation*, Vol. 115, No. 3, (March 2005), pp. 485-491, doi:10.1172/JCI24531

Carr, DB.; Utzschneider, KM., Hull, RL., Tong, J., Wallace, TM., Kodama, K., Shofer, JB., et al. (2006). Gestational diabetes mellitus increases the risk of cardiovascular disease in women with a family history of type 2 diabetes. *Diabetes Care*, Vol. 29, No. 9, (Sept. 2006), pp. 2078-2083, doi:10.2337/dc05-2482

Cheung, NW. & Byth, K. (2003). Population health significance of gestational diabetes. *Diabetes Care*, Vol. 26, No. 7, (July 2003), pp. 2005-2009, doi:10.2337/diacare.26.7.2005

Christoffersson, M. & Rydhstroem, H. (2002). Shoulder dystocia and brachial plexus injury: a population-based study. *Gynecologic and ObstetricInvestigation*, Vol. 53, No. 1, (Jan. 2002), pp. 42-47, doi:10.1159/000049410

Clark, CM.; Qiu, C., Amerman, B., Porter, B., Fineberg, N., Aldasouqi, S. & Golichowski, A. (1997). Gestational diabetes: should it be added to the syndrome of insulin resistance? *Diabetes Care*, Vol. 20, No. 5, (May 1997), pp. 867-871, doi:10.2337/diacare.20.5.867

Clausen, TD.; Mathiesen, ER., Hansen, T., Pedersen, O., Jensen, DM., Lauenborg, J. & Damm, P. (2008). High prevalence of type 2 diabetes and pre-diabetes in adult offspring of women with gestational diabetes mellitus or type 1 diabetes: The role of intrauterine hyperglycemia. *Diabetes Care*, Vol. 31, No. 2, (Feb. 2008), pp. 340-346, doi:10.2337/dc07-1596

Cutchie, WA.; Cheung, NW. & Simmons, D. (2006). Comparison of international and New Zealand guidelines for the care of pregnant women with diabetes. *Diabetic Medicine*, Vol. 23, No. 5, (May 2006), pp. 460-468, doi:10.1111/j.1464-5491.2006.01850.x

Damm, P. (2009). Future risk of diabetes in mother and child after gestational diabetes mellitus. *International Journal of Gynaecology and Obstetrics*, Vol. 104, Suppl 1, (March 2009) pp. S25-6, doi:10.1016/j.ijgo.2008.11.025

DeFronzo, RA. & Ferrannini, E. (1991). Insulin resistance. A multifaceted syndrome responsible for NIDDM, obesity, hypertension, dyslipidemia, and atherosclerotic cardiovascular disease. *Diabetes Care*, Vol. 14, No. 3, (March 1991), pp. 173-194, doi:10.2337/diacare.14.3.173

Després, JP.; Lemieux, I., Bergeron, J., Pibarot, P., Mathieu, P., Larose, E., Rodés-Cabau, J., et al. (2008). Abdominal obesity and the metabolic syndrome: Contribution to global cardiometabolic risk. *Arteriosclerosis, Thrombosis, and Vascular Biology*, Vol. 28, No. 6, (March 2008), pp. 1039-1049, doi:10.1161/ATVBAHA.107.159228

Dornhorst, A.; Paterson, CM., Nicholls, JS., Wadsworth, J., Chiu, DC., Elkeles, RS., Johnston, DG., et al. (1992). High prevalence of gestational diabetes in women from ethnic minority groups. *Diabetic Medicine*, Vol. 9, No. 9, (Nov. 1992), pp. 820-825, doi:10.1111/j.1464-5491.1992.tb01900.x

Egeland, GM. & Meltzer, SJ. (2010). Following in mother's footsteps? Mother-daughter risks for insulin resistance and cardiovascular disease 15 years after gestational diabetes. *Diabetic Medicine*, Vol. 27, No. 3, (March 2010), pp. 257-265. doi:10.1111/j.1464-5491.2010.02944.x

Expert Panel on Detection, Evaluation, and Treatment of High Blood Cholesterol in Adults. (2001). Executive Summary of The Third Report of The National Cholesterol Education Program (NCEP). Expert Panel on Detection, Evaluation, And Treatment of High Blood Cholesterol In Adults (Adult Treatment Panel III) *JAMA*, Vol. 285, No. 19, (May 2001), pp. 2486-2497, doi:10.1001/jama.285.19.2486

Ferrara, A.; Weiss, NS., Hedderson, MM., Quesenberry, CP., Selby, JV., Ergas, IJ., Peng, T., et al. (2007). Pregnancy plasma glucose levels exceeding the American Diabetes Association thresholds, but below the National Diabetes Data Group thresholds for gestational diabetes mellitus, are related to the risk of neonatal macrosomia, hypoglycaemia and hyperbilirubinaemia. *Diabetologia*, Vol. 50, No. 2, (Nov. 2006), pp. 298-306, doi:10.1007/s00125-006-0517-8

Forbes, S.; Taylor-Robinson, D., Patel, N., Allan, P., Walker, BR. & Johnston, DG. (2011). Increased prevalence of non-alcoholic fatty liver disease in European women with a history of gestational diabetes. *Diabetologia*, Vol. 54, No. 3, pp. 641-647, doi:10.1007/S00125-010-2009-0

Ford, ES. (2004). The metabolic syndrome and mortality from cardiovascular disease and all-causes: findings from the National Health and Nutrition Examination Survey II Mortality Study. *Atherosclerosis*, Vol. 173, No. 2, (April 2004), pp. 309-314, doi:10.1016/j.atherosclerosis.2003.12.022

Ford, ES. (2005). Prevalence of the metabolic syndrome defined by the International Diabetes Federation among adults in the U.S. *Diabetes Care*, Vol. 28, No. 11, (Nov. 2005), pp. 2745-2749, doi:10.2337/diacare.28.11.2745

Ford, ES.; Li, C. & Sattar, N. (2008). Metabolic syndrome and incident diabetes: current state of the evidence. *Diabetes Care*, Vol. 31, No. 9, (Sept. 2008), pp. 1898-1904, doi:10.2337/dc08-0423

Giuffrida, FM.; Sallum, CF., Gabbay, MA., Gomes, MB., Pires, AC. & Dib, SA. (2010). Relationship between glycated hemoglobin and metabolic syndrome of type 1 and type 2 diabetes: A factor analysis study. *Diabetes Care*, Vol. 33, No. 6, (June 2010), pp. e80, doi:10.2337/dc09-2280

Gunderson, EP.; Jacobs, DR., Chiang, V., Lewis, CE., Tsai, A., Quesenberry, CP., & Sidney, S. (2009). Childbearing is associated with higher incidence of the metabolic syndrome among women of reproductive age controlling for measurements before pregnancy: The CARDIA study. *AJOG*, Vol. 201, No. 2, (Aug. 2009), pp. 177.e1-9, doi:10.1016/j.ajog.2009.03.031

Guzder, RN.; Gatling, W., Mullee, MA. & Byrne, CD. (2006). Impact of metabolic syndrome criteria on cardiovascular disease risk in people with newly diagnosed type 2 diabetes. *Diabetologia*, Vol. 49, No. 1, 49-55, doi:10.1007/s00125-005-0063-9

Haffner, S. & Taegtmeyer, H. (2003). Epidemic obesity and the metabolic syndrome. *Circulation*, Vol. 108, No. 13, pp. 1541-1545, doi:10.1161/01.CIR.0000088845.17586.EC

Hedderson, MM. & Ferrara, A. (2008). High blood pressure before and during early pregnancy is associated with an increased risk of gestational diabetes mellitus. *Diabetes Care*, Vol. 31, No. 12, (Sept. 2008), pp. 2362-2367, doi:10.2337/dc08-1193

Hillier, TA.; Pedula, KL., Vesco, KK., Schmidt, MM., Mullen, JA., LeBlanc, ES. & Pettitt, D. J. (2008). Excess gestational weight gain. Obstetrics and gynecology, Modifying Fetal Macrosomia Risk Associated With Maternal Glucose, Vol. 112, No. 5, (Nov. 2008), pp. 1007-1014, doi:10.1097/AOG.0b013e31818a9779

Hu, G.; Qiao, Q., Tuomilehto, J., Balkau, B., Borch-Johnsen, K., Pyorala, K. & DECODE Study Group. (2004). Prevalence of the metabolic syndrome and its relation to all-cause and cardiovascular mortality in nondiabetic European men and women. *Archives of Internal Medicine*, Vol. 164, No. 10, (May 2004), pp. 1066-1076, doi:10.1001/archinte.164.10.1066

Hunt, KJ.; Resendez, RG., Williams, K., Haffner, SM. & Stern, MP. (2004). National Cholesterol Education Program versus World Health Organization metabolic syndrome in relation to all-cause and cardiovascular mortality in the San Antonio Heart Study. *Circulation*, Vol. 110, No. 10, pp. 1251-1257, doi:10.1161/01.CIR.0000140762.04598.F9

International Association of Diabetes and Pregnancy Study Groups Consensus Panel, Metzger, BE., Gabbe, SG., Persson, B., Buchanan, TA., Catalano, PA., Damm, P., et al. (2010). International association of diabetes and pregnancy study groups recommendations on the diagnosis and classification of hyperglycemia in pregnancy. *Diabetes Care*, Vol. 33, No. 3, (Feb. 2010), pp 676-682, doi:10.2337/dc09-1848

Isomaa, B.; Almgren, P., Tuomi, T., Forsén, B., Lahti, K., Nissén, M., Taskinen, MR., et al. (2001). Cardiovascular morbidity and mortality associated with the metabolic syndrome. *Diabetes Care*, Vol. 24, No. 4, (April 2001), pp. 683-689, doi:10.2337/diacare.24.4.683

Ix, JH.; Wassel, CL., Kanaya, AM., Vittinghoff, E., Johnson, KC., Koster, A., Cauley, JA., et al. (2008). Fetuin-A and incident diabetes mellitus in older persons. *JAMA*, Vol. 300, No. 2, (July 2008), pp. 182-188, doi:10.1001/jama.300.2.182

Joffe, GM.; Esterlitz, JR., Levine, RJ., Clemens, JD., Ewell, MG., Sibai, BM. & Catalano, PM. (1998). The relationship between abnormal glucose tolerance and hypertensive disorders of pregnancy in healthy nulliparous women. Calcium for Preeclampsia Prevention (CPEP) Study Group. *AJOG*, Vol. 179, No. 4, (Oct. 1998), pp. 1032-1037.

Kahn, R.; Buse, J., Ferrannini, E. & Stern, M. (2005). The metabolic syndrome: Time for a critical appraisal. Joint statement from the American Diabetes Association and the

European Association for the Study of Diabetes. *Diabetes Care*, Vol. 28, No. 9, (Sept. 2005), pp. 2289-2304, doi:10.2337/diacare.28.9.2289

Kantartzis, K.; Machann, J., Schick, F., Fritsche, A., Häring, H. & Stefan, N. (2010). The impact of liver fat vs visceral fat in determining categories of prediabetes. *Diabetologia*, Vol. 53, No. 5, pp. 882-889, doi:10.1007/s00125-010-1663-6

Kim, CH. & Younossi, ZM. (2008). Nonalcoholic fatty liver disease: A manifestation of the metabolic syndrome. *Cleveland Clinic Journal of Medicine*, Vol. 75, No. 10, (Oct. 2008), pp. 721-728, doi:10.3949/ccjm.75.10.721

Kim, CH.; Newton, KM. & Knopp, R. H. (2002). Gestational diabetes and the incidence of type 2 diabetes: A systematic review. *Diabetes Care*, Vol. 25, No. 10, (Oct. 2002), pp. 1862-1868, doi:10.2337/diacare.25.10.1862

Lain KC.; Daftary, AR., Ness, RB. & Roberts, JM. (2008). First trimester adipocytokine concentrations and risk of developing gestational diabetes later in pregnancy. *Clinical Endocrinology*, Vol. 69, No. 3, (Sept. 2008), pp. 407-11, doi:10.1111/j.1365-2265.2008.03198.x

Lann, D. & LeRoith, D. (2007). Insulin resistance as the underlying cause for the metabolic syndrome. *The Medical clinics of North America*, Vol. 91, No. 6, (Nov. 2007), pp. 1063-77, doi:10.1016/j.mcna.2007.06.012

Lauenborg, J.; Hansen, T., Jensen, DM., Vestergaard, H., Mølsted-Pedersen, L., Hornnes, P., Locht, H., et al. (2004). Increasing incidence of diabetes after gestational diabetes: A long-term follow-up in a Danish population. *Diabetes Care*, Vol. 27, No. 5, (May 2004), 1194-1199, doi:10.2337/diacare.27.5.1194

Lauenborg, J.; Mathiesen, E., Hansen, T., Glümer, C., Jørgensen, T., Borch-Johnsen, K., Hornnes, P., et al. (2005). The prevalence of the metabolic syndrome in a Danish population of women with previous gestational diabetes mellitus is three-fold higher than in the general population. *JCEM*, Vol. 90, No. 7, (July 2005), pp. 4004-4010, doi:10.1210/jc.2004-1713

Laughon, SK.; Catov, J., Provins, T., Roberts, JM. & Gandley, RE. (2009). Elevated first-trimester uric acid concentrations are associated with the development of gestational diabetes. *AJOG*, Vol. 201, No. 4, (Oct. 2009), pp. 402.e1-5, doi:10.1016/j.ajog.2009.06.065

Lee, JM.; Kim, SR., Yoo, SJ., Hong, OK., Son, HS. & Chang, SA. (2009). The relationship between adipokines, metabolic parameters and insulin resistance in patients with metabolic syndrome and type 2 diabetes. *The Journal of International Medical Research*, Vol. 37, No. 6, pp. 1803-1812.

Leon, DA. (1998). Fetal growth and adult disease. *European Journal of Clinical Nutrition*, Vol. 52, Suppl 1, (Jan. 1998), S72-8, discussion S78-82.

Ley, SH.; Harris, S. B., Mamakeesick, M., Noon, T., Fiddler, E., Gittelsohn, J., Wolever, T. M. S., et al. (2009). Metabolic syndrome and its components as predictors of incident type 2 diabetes mellitus in an Aboriginal community *CMAJ*, Vol. 180, No. 6, (March 2009), pp. 617-624, doi:10.1503/cmaj.080972

Matsubara, M. (2004). Plasma adiponectin decrease in women with Nonalcoholic Fatty Liver. *Endocrine Journal*, Vol. 51, No. 6, (Jan. 2005), pp. 587-593.

Matsuura, F.; Yamashita, S., Nakamura, T., Nishida, M., Nozaki, S., Funahashi, T., Matsuzawa, Y. (1998). Effect of visceral fat accumulation on uric acid metabolism in male obese subjects: Visceral fat obesity is linked more closely to overproduction of uric acid than subcutaneous fat obesity. *Metabolism*, Vol. 47, No. 8, (Aug. 1998), pp. 929–933, doi:10.1016/S0026-0495(98)90346-8.

McNeill, AM.; Rosamond, WD., Girman, CJ., Golden, SH., Schmidt, MI., East, HE., Ballantyne, CM., et al. (2005). The metabolic syndrome and 11-year risk of incident cardiovascular disease in the atherosclerosis risk in communities study. *Diabetes Care*, Vol. 28, No. 2, (Feb. 2005), pp. 385-390, doi:10.2337/diacare.28.2.385

Mello, G.; Parretti, E., Mecacci, F., Lucchetti, R., Cianciulli, D., Lagazio, C., Pratesi, M., et al. (1997). Anthropometric characteristics of full-term infants: Effects of varying degrees of "normal" glucose metabolism. *Journal of perinatal medicine*, Vol. 25, No. 2, pp. 197-204.

Mestman, JH.; Anderson, GV. & Guadalupe, V. (1972). Follow-up study of 360 subjects with abnormal carbohydrate metabolism during pregnancy. *Obstetrics and Gynecology*, Vol. 39, No. 3, (March 1972), pp. 421-425.

Metzger, BE. (2007). Long-term outcomes in mothers diagnosed with gestational diabetes mellitus and their offspring. *Clinical Obstetrics and Gynecology*, Vol. 50, No. 4, (Dec. 2007), pp. 972-979, doi:10.1097/GRF.0b013e31815a61d6

Metzger, BE. & Coustan, DR. (1998). Summary and recommendations of the Fourth International Workshop-Conference on Gestational Diabetes Mellitus. *Diabetes Care*, Vol. 21, Suppl 2 (Aug. 1998), pp. B161-7.

Nakano, S.; Kuboki, K., Matsumoto, T., Nishimura, C. & Yoshino, G. (2010). Small, dense LDL and high-sensitivity C-reactive protein (hs-CRP) in metabolic syndrome with type 2 diabetes mellitus. *Journal of Atherosclerosis and Thrombosis*, Vol. 17, No. 4, (April 2010), pp. 410-415.

Nanda, S.; Savvidou, M., Syngelaki, A., Akolekar, R. & Nicolaides, KH. (2011). Prediction of gestational diabetes mellitus by maternal factors and biomarkers at 11 to 13 weeks. *Prenatal Diagnosis*, Vol. 31, No. 2, (Dec. 2010), pp. 135-141, doi:10.1002/pd.2636

Ninomiya, JK.; L'Italien, G., Criqui, MH., Whyte, JL., Gamst, A. & Chen, RS. (2004). Association of the metabolic syndrome with history of myocardial infarction and stroke in the Third National Health and Nutrition Examination Survey. *Circulation*, Vol. 109, No. 1, (Jan. 2004), pp. 42-46, doi:10.1161/01.CIR.0000108926.04022.0C

Nolan, CJ. (2011). Controversies in gestational diabetes. Best practice & research. *Clinical Obstetrics & Gynaecology*, Vol. 25, No. 1, (Feb. 2011), pp. 37-49, doi:10.1016/j.bpobgyn.2010.10.004

O'Sullivan, JB. (1991). Diabetes mellitus after GDM. *Diabetes*, Vol. 40, Suppl 2, (Dec. 1991), pp.131-135.

O'Sullivan, JB., & Mahan, CM. (1964). Criteria for the oral glucose tolerance test in pregnancy. *Diabetes*, Vol. 13, (May-June 1964), pp. 278-285.

Porepa, L.; Ray, JG., Sanchez-Romeu, P. & Booth, GL. (2010). Newly diagnosed diabetes mellitus as a risk factor for serious liver disease. *CMAJ*, Vol. 182, No. 11, (Aug. 2010), pp. E526-31, doi:10.1503/cmaj.092144

Qiu, C.; Sorensen, TK., Luthy, DA., et al. (2004). A prospective study of maternal serum C-reactive protein (CRP) concentrations and risk of gestational diabetes mellitus. *Paediatr Perinat Epidemiol.*, Vol. 18, No. 5, (Sept. 2004), pp. 377-384, doi:10.1111/j.1365-3016.2004.00578.x

Ray, JG.; Vermeulen, MJ., Shapiro, JL. & Kenshole, AB. (2001). Maternal and neonatal outcomes in pregestational and gestational diabetes mellitus, and the influence of maternal obesity and weight gain: The DEPOSIT study. Diabetes Endocrine Pregnancy Outcome Study in Toronto. *QJM*, Vol. 94, No. 7, (July 2001), pp. 347-356, doi:10.1093/qjmed/94.7.347

Ray, JG.; Berger, H., Lipscombe, LL. & Sermer, M. (2010). Gestational prediabetes: A new term for early prevention. *The Indian Journal of Medical Research*, Vol. 132, (Sept. 2010), pp. 251-255.

Reaven, GM. (1988). Banting lecture 1988. Role of insulin resistance in human disease. Diabetes, Vol. 37, No. 12, (Dec. 1988), pp. 1595-1607, doi:10.2337/diabetes.37.12.1595

Reaven, GM. (2009). Is diagnosing metabolic syndrome a uniquely simple way to predict incident type 2 diabetes mellitus. *CMAJ*, Vol. 180, No. 6, (March 2009), pp. 601-602, doi:10.1503/cmaj.090092

Reece, EA.; Leguizamón, G. & Wiznitzer, A. (2009). Gestational diabetes: The need for a common ground. *Lancet*, Vol. 373, No. 9677, (May 2009), pp. 1789-1797, doi:10.1016/S0140-6736(09)60515-8

Retnakaran, R.; Hanley, AJ., Raif, N., Connelly, PW., Sermer, M. & Zinman, B. (2003). C-reactive protein and gestational diabetes: The central role of maternal obesity. *JCEM*, Vol. 88, No. 8, pp. 3507-3512, doi:10.1210/jc.2003-030186

Retnakaran, R.; Hanley, AJ., Raif N., Connelly, PW., Sermer, M. & Zinman, B. (2004) Reduced adiponectin concentration in women with gestational diabetes: a potential factor in progression to type 2 diabetes. *Diabetes Care*, Vol. 27, No. 3, pp. 799-800, doi:10.2337/diacare.27.3.799

Retnakaran, R.; Hanley AJ., Raif, N., Hirning, CR., Connelly, PW., Sermer, M., Kahn, SE. & Zinman, B. (2005). Adiponectin and beta cell dysfunction in gestational diabetes: Pathophysiological implications. *Diabetologia*, Vol. 48, No. 5, (May 2005), pp. 993-1001, doi:10.1007/s00125-005-1710-x

Retnakaran, R.; Connelly, PW., Maguire G., Sermer, M., Zinman, B. & Hanley, AJ. (2007).Decreased high molecular weight adiponectin in gestational diabetes: implications for the pathophysiology of type 2 diabetes. *Diabetic Medicine*,.Vol. 24, No. 3, pp.245-252, doi:10.1111/j.1464-5491.2007.02077.x

Retnakaran, R.; Qi, Y., Sermer, M., Connelly, PW., Hanley, AJ. & Zinman, B. (2008a). Glucose intolerance in pregnancy and future risk of pre-diabetes or diabetes. *Diabetes Care*, Vol. 31, No. 10, (Oct. 2008), pp. 2026-2031, doi:10.2337/dc08-0972

Retnakaran, R.; Qi, Y., Sermer, M., Connelly, P. W., Zinman, B. & Hanley, A.J. (2008b). Isolated hyperglycemia at 1 hour on oral glucose tolerance test in pregnancy resembles gestational diabetes mellitus in predicting postpartum metabolic dysfunction. *Diabetes Care*, Vol. 31, No. 7, (July 2008), pp. 1275-1281, doi:10.2337/dc08-0126

Retnakaran, R. (2009a). Glucose tolerance status in pregnancy: A window to the future risk of diabetes and cardiovascular disease in young women. *Current Diabetes Reviews*, Vol. 5, No. 4, (Nov. 2009), pp. 239-244, doi:10.2174/157339909789804378

Retnakaran, R. & Shah, BR. (2009b). Mild glucose intolerance in pregnancy and risk of cardiovascular disease: A population-based cohort study. *CMAJ*, Vol. 181, No. 67, (Aug. 2009), pp. 371-376, doi:10.1503/cmaj.090569

Retnakaran, R.; Qi, Y., Sermer, M., Connelly, PW., Hanley, AJ. & Zinman, B. (2009c). The antepartum glucose values that predict neonatal macrosomia differ from those that predict postpartum prediabetes or diabetes: Implications for the diagnostic criteria for gestational diabetes. *JCEM*, Vol. 94, No. 3, (March 2009), pp. 840-845, doi:10.1210/jc.2008-2434

Retnakaran, R.; Qi, Y., Sermer, M., Connelly, PW., Hanley, AJ. & Zinman, B. (2009d). An abnormal screening glucose challenge test in pregnancy predicts postpartum metabolic dysfunction, even when the antepartum oral glucose tolerance test is normal. *Clinical Endocrinology*, Vol. 71, No. 2, (Aug. 2009), pp. 208-214, doi:10.1111/j.1365-2265.2008.03460.x

Retnakaran, R, & Shah, BR. (2009e). Abnormal screening glucose challenge test in pregnancy and future risk of diabetes in young women. *Diabetic Medicine*, Vol. 26, No. 5, pp. 474-477, doi:10.1111/j.1464-5491.2009.02712.x

Retnakaran, R.; Qi, Y., Sermer, M., Connelly, PW., Hanley, AJ. & Zinman, B. (2010a). Beta-cell function declines within the first year postpartum in women with recent glucose intolerance in pregnancy. *Diabetes Care*, Vol. 33, No. 8, (Aug. 2010), pp. 1798-1804, doi:10.2337/dc10-0351

Retnakaran, R.; Qi, Y., Connelly, PW., Sermer, M., Zinman, B. & Hanley, AJ. (2010b). Glucose intolerance in pregnancy and postpartum risk of metabolic syndrome in young women. *JCEM*, Vol. 95, No. 2, pp. 670-677, doi:10.1210/jc.2009-1990

Retnakaran, R.; Qi, Y., Connelly, PW., Sermer, M., Hanley, AJ., & Zinman, B. (2010c). Risk of early progression to prediabetes or diabetes in women with recent gestational dysglycaemia but normal glucose tolerance at 3-month postpartum. *Clinical Endocrinology*, Vol. 73, No. 4, (Oct. 2010), pp. 476-483, doi:10.1111/j.1365-2265.2010.03834.x

Retnakaran, R.; Qi, Y., Connelly, PW., Sermer, M., Hanley AJ., & Zinman, B. (2010d). Low adiponectin concentration during pregnancy predicts postpartum insulin resistance, beta-cell dysfunction and fasting glycaemia *Diabetologia*, Vol. 53, No. 2, pp. 268-276, doi:10.1007/s00125-009-1600-8

Ridker, PM. (1998). Inflammation, infection, and cardiovascular risk: How good is the clinical evidence. *Circulation*, Vol. 97, No. 17, pp. 1671-1674.

Ridker, PM.; Cushman, M., Stampfer, MJ., Tracy, RP. & Hennekens, CH. (1997). Inflammation, aspirin, and the risk of cardiovascular disease in apparently healthy men. *NEJM*, Vol. 336, No. 14, (July 1997), pp. 973-979, doi:10.1056/NEJM199704033361401

Ridker, PM.; Buring, JE., Cook, NR. & Rifai, N. (2003). C-Reactive Protein, the metabolic syndrome, and risk of incident cardiovascular events. *Circulation*, Vol. 107, No. 3, pp. 391-397, doi:10.1161/01.CIR.0000055014.62083.05

Ridker, PM.; Wilson, PW. & Grundy, SM. (2004). Should C-Reactive Protein be added to the metabolic syndrome and to assessment of global cardiovascular risk? *Circulation*, Vol. 109, No. 23, pp. 2818-2825, doi:10.1161/01.CIR.0000132467.45278.59

Rudge, MV.; Calderon, IM., Ramos, MD., Abbade, JF. & Rugolo, LM. (2000). Perinatal outcome of pregnancies complicated by diabetes and by maternal daily hyperglycemia not related to diabetes. A retrospective 10-year analysis. *Gynecologic and Obstetric Investigation*, Vol. 50, No. 2, pp. 108-112, doi:10.1159/000010293

Sattar, Nl; Gaw, A., Scherbakova, O., et al. (2003). Metabolic syndrome with and without C-reactive protein as a predictor of coronary heart disease and diabetes in the West of

Scotland Coronary Prevention Study. *Circulation,* Vol. 108, No. 4, pp. 414–419, doi:10.1161/01.CIR.0000080897.52664.94

Savitz, D.; Janevic, T., Engel, S., Kaufman, J. & Herring, A. (2008). Ethnicity and gestational diabetes in New York City, 1995-2003. *BJOG,* Vol. 115, No. 8, (July 2008), pp. 969-978, doi:10.1111/j.1471-0528.2008.01763.x

Savvidou, M.; Nelson, SM., Makgoba, M., Messow, CM., Sattar, N. & Nicolaides, K. (2010). First-trimester prediction of gestational diabetes mellitus: Examining the potential of combining maternal characteristics and laboratory measures. *Diabetes,* Vol. 59, No. 12, (Dec. 2010), pp. 3017-3022, doi:10.2337/db10-0688

Schmidt, MI.; Duncan, BB., Reichelt, AJ., Branchtein, L., Matos, MC., Costa e Forti, A., Spichler, ER., et al. (2001). Gestational diabetes mellitus diagnosed with a 2-h 75-g oral glucose tolerance test and adverse pregnancy outcomes. *Diabetes Care,* Vol. 24, No. 7, (July 2001), pp. 1151-1155, doi:10.2337/diacare.24.7.1151

Scholl, TO.; Sowers, M., Chen, X. & Lenders, C. (2001). Maternal glucose concentration influences fetal growth, gestation, and pregnancy complications. *American Journal of Epidemiology,* Vol. 154, No. 6, (Sept. 2001), pp. 514-520, doi:10.1093/aje/154.6.514

Seghieri, G.; Breschi, MC., Anichini, R., De Bellis, A., Alviggi, L., Maida, I. & Franconi, F. (2003). Serum homocysteine levels are increased in women with gestational diabetes mellitus. *Metabolism,* Vol. 52, No. 6, (June 2003), pp. 720-723, doi:10.1016/S0026-0495(03)00032-5

Sermer, M.; Naylor, CD., Gare, DJ., Kenshole, AB., Ritchie, JW., Farine, D., Cohen, HR., et al. (1995). Impact of increasing carbohydrate intolerance on maternal-fetal outcomes in 3637 women without gestational diabetes. The Toronto Tri-Hospital Gestational Diabetes Project. *AJOG,* Vol. 173, No. 1, (July 1995), pp. 146-156.

Shah, BR.; Retnakaran, R. & Booth, G. L. (2008). Increased risk of cardiovascular disease in young women following gestational diabetes mellitus. *Diabetes Care,* Vol. 31, No. 8, (Aug. 2008), pp. 1668-1669, doi:10.2337/dc08-0706

Smirnakis, KV.; Plati, A., Wolf, M., Thadhani, R. & Ecker, JL. (2007) Predicting gestational diabetes: Choosing the optimal early serum marker. *AJOG,* Vol. 196, No. 4, (April 2007), pp. 410.e1-6, doi:10.1016/j.ajog.2006.12.011

Stefan, N.; Fritsche, A., Weikert, C., Boeing, H., Joost, H., Häring, H. & Schulze, M. B. (2008). Plasma fetuin-A levels and the risk of type 2 diabetes. *Diabetes,* Vol. 57, No. 10, (Oct. 2008), 2762-2767, doi:10.2337/db08-0538

Stern, MP. (1995). Diabetes and cardiovascular disease. The "common soil" hypothesis. *Diabetes,* Vol. 44, No. 4, (April 1995), pp. 369-374, doi:10.2337/diabetes.44.4.369

Targher, G.; Bertolini, L., Poli, F., Rodella, S., Scala, L., Tessari, R., Zenari, L., et al. (2005). Nonalcoholic fatty liver disease and risk of future cardiovascular events among type 2 diabetic patients. *Diabetes,* Vol. 54, No. 12, (Dec. 2005), pp. 3541-3546, doi:10.2337/diabetes.54.12.354

Tarim, E.; Yigit, F., Kilicdag, E., Bagis, T., Demircan, S., Simsek, E., Haydardedeoglu, B. &Yanik, F. (2006). Early onset of subclinical atherosclerosis in women with gestational diabetes mellitus. *Ultrasound in Obstetrics and Gynecology,* Vol. 27, No. 2, (Feb. 2006), pp. 177-182, doi:10.1002/uog.2687

Thadhani, R.; Wolf, M., Hsu-Blatman, K., Sandler, L., Nathan, D. & Ecker, J. L. (2003). First-trimester sex hormone binding globulin and subsequent gestational diabetes mellitus. *AJOG,* Vol. 189, No. 1, (July 2003), pp. 171-176, doi:10.1067/mob.2003.343

Tiikkainen, M.; Tamminen, M., Häkkinen, A., Bergholm, R., Vehkavaara, S., Halavaara, J., Teramo, K., et al. (2002). Liver-fat accumulation and insulin resistance in obese women with previous gestational diabetes. *Obesity Research*, Vol. 10, No. 9, (Sept. 2002), pp. 859-867, doi:10.1038/oby.2002.118

Utzschneider, KM. & Kahn, SE. (2006). Review: The role of insulin resistance in nonalcoholic fatty liver disease. *JCEM*, Vol. 91, No. 12, pp. 4753-4761, doi:10.1210/jc.2006-0587

Utzschneider, KM.; van de Lagemaat, A., Faulenbach, MV., Goedecke, JH., Carr, DB., Boyko, EJ., Fujimoto, WY., et al. (2010). Insulin resistance is the best predictor of the metabolic syndrome in subjects with a first-degree relative with type 2 diabetes. *Obesity*, Vol. 18, No. 9, (Sept. 2010), pp. 1781-1787, doi:10.1038/oby.2010.77

Vambergue, A.; Nuttens, MC., Verier-Mine, O., Dognin, C., Cappoen, JP. & Fontaine, P. (2000). Is mild gestational hyperglycaemia associated with maternal and neonatal complications? The Digest Study. *Diabetic Medicine*, Vol. 17, No. 3, (March 2000), pp. 203-208, doi:10.1046/j.1464-5491.2000.00237.x

Verma, A.; Boney, CM., Tucker, R. & Vohr, B. R. (2002). Insulin resistance syndrome in women with prior history of gestational diabetes mellitus. *JCEM*, Vol. 87, No. 7, pp. 3227-3235.

Ward, WK.; Johnston, CL., Beard, JC., Benedetti, TJ., Halter, JB. & Porte, D. (1985). Insulin resistance and impaired insulin secretion in subjects with histories of gestational diabetes mellitus. *Diabetes*, Vol. 34, No. 9, (Sept. 1985), pp. 861-869, doi:10.2337/diabetes.34.9.861

Wen, SW.; Liu, S., Kramer, MS., Joseph, KS., Levitt, C., Marcoux, S. & Liston, R. M. (2000). Impact of prenatal glucose screening on the diagnosis of gestational diabetes and on pregnancy outcomes. *American Journal of Epidemiology*, Vol. 152, No. 11, pp. 1009-14, doi:10.1093/aje/152.11.1009

WHO Expert Consultation. (2004). Appropriate body-mass index for Asian populations and its implications for policy and intervention strategies. *Lancet*, Vol. 363, No. 9403, (Jan. 2004), pp. 157-163, doi:10.1016/S0140-6736(03)15268-3

Wild, S.; Roglic, G., Green, A., Sicree, R. & King, H. (2004). Global prevalence of diabetes: Estimates for the year 2000 and projections for 2030. *Diabetes Care*, Vol. 27, No. 5, (Oct. 2004), pp. 1047-1053, doi:10.2337/diacare.27.10.2569

Wildman, R.P.; Muntner, P., Reynolds, K., McGinn, AP., Rajpathak, S., Wylie-Rosett, J. & Sowers, M. R. (2008). The obese without cardiometabolic risk factor clustering and the normal weight with cardiometabolic risk factor clustering: Prevalence and correlates of 2 phenotypes among the US population (NHANES 1999-2004). *Archives of Internal Medicine*, Vol. 168, No. 15, (Aug. 2008), pp. 1617-1624, doi:10.1001/archinte.168.15.1617

Williams, MA.; Qiu, C., Muy-Rivera, M., et al. (2004). Plasma adiponectin concentrations in early pregnancy and subsequent risk of gestational diabetes mellitus. *JCEM*, Vol. 89, No. 5, pp. 2306-11, doi:10.1210/jc.2003-031201

Wilson, PW.; D'Agostino, RB., Parise, H., Sullivan, L. & Meigs, JB. (2005). Metabolic syndrome as a precursor of cardiovascular disease and type 2 diabetes mellitus. *Circulation*, Vol. 112, No. 20, pp. 3066-3072, doi:10.1161/CIRCULATIONAHA.105.539528

Winzer, C.; Wagner, O., Festa, A., Schneider, B., Roden, M., Bancher-Todesca, D., Pacini, G., et al. (2004). Plasma adiponectin, insulin sensitivity, and subclinical inflammation in women with prior gestational diabetes mellitus. *Diabetes Care*, Vol. 27, No. 7, (July 2004), pp. 1721-1727, doi:10.2337/diacare.27.7.1721

Wolf, M.; Sandler, L., Hsu, K., et al. (2003). First-trimester C-reactive protein and subsequent gestational diabetes. *Diabetes Care*, Vol. 26, No. 3, (July 2003), pp. 819-824, doi:10.2337/diacare.26.3.819

Youssef, W. & McCullough, AJ. (2002). Diabetes mellitus, obesity, and hepatic steatosis. *Seminars in Gastrointestinal Disease*, Vol. 13, No. 1, (Jan. 2002), pp. 17-30.

Zhang, Y.; Lu, X., Hong, J., Chao, M., Gu, W., Wang, W. & Ning, G. (2010). Positive correlations of liver enzymes with metabolic syndrome including insulin resistance in newly diagnosed type 2 diabetes mellitus. *Endocrine*, Vol. 38, No. 2, pp. 181-187, doi:10.1007/s12020-010-9369-6

9

Insulin Resistance in the Third Trimester of Pregnancy Suffering from Gestational Diabetes Mellitus or Impaired Glucose Tolerance

Mohammed Helmy Faris Shalayel[1], Mohammed Chyad Al-Noaemi[2] and Salah A.M. Ahmed[3]
[1]National College for Medical and Technical Studies,
[2]Al-Yarmouk College, Khartoum,
[3]Nile College - Khartoum,
Sudan

1. Introduction

Pregnancy results in a state of insulin resistance (Dahlgren, 2006) that appears to include a decrease in maximum insulin sensitivity or responsivity (Baban et al., 2010). This insulin resistance abates in the postpartum period (Kuhl, 1991). Insulin resistance is defined as the decrease of the biological action of insulin (Catalano, 2010; Robert, 1995), and it mainly presents as hyperinsulinemia (Baban et al., 2010; Robert, 1995) or decreased ability of insulin to regulate glucose utilization (Kim et al., 1996).

The resistance to insulin can be characterized as pre-receptor (insulin antibodies), receptor (decreased number of receptors on the cell surface), or post-receptor (defects in the intracellular insulin signaling pathway). In pregnancy, the decreased insulin sensitivity is best characterized as a post-receptor defect resulting in the decreased ability of insulin to bring about glucose transporter (GLUT4) mobilization from the interior of the cell to the cell surface (Catalano, 2010).

Most pregnant women are able to counteract the insulin resistance state by increasing their insulin secretion. However, when the capacity of insulin secretion is not sufficiently large to meet the insulin resistance, glucose intolerance develops and the women develop gestational diabetes (Kuhl et al., 1985).

Gestational diabetes mellitus (GDM) is defined as a carbohydrate intolerance of varying severity with onset or first recognition during the present pregnancy (Kaaja & Rönnemaa, 2008; Damm et al., 1994; Summary and recommendation of the second international workshop conference of gestational diabetes, 1985; Shalayel et al., 2010). GDM has onset or discovery of glucose intolerance during pregnancy (Reece et al., 2009), usually in the second or third trimester (Shalayel et al., 2007). GDM carries long-term implications for the subsequent development of type 2 diabetes in the mother and increased risk for obesity and glucose intolerance in the offspring (Barbour et al., 2007). The world health organization defines diabetes in pregnancy as a fasting glucose ≥ 7.9 mmol/L or a value >11 mmol/L 2-hour after a 75g glucose load (Shalayel et al., 2010; Campbell & Lees, 2000).

Impaired Glucose Tolerance (IGT) was previously known as *chemical diabetes* or *subclinical diabetes* (Shalayel et al., 2007). It may be defined as an intermediate group of individuals whose carbohydrate metabolism does not constitute diabetes but is not entirely normal (Brudenell, 1993). Thus, IGT designed glucose tolerance results intermediate between normal glucose homeostasis and overt diabetes (Kahn et al., 2005; Bilous & Donnelly, 2010; Burch, 1994). It is diagnosed if fasting glucose ≥ 6 but < 7.8 m mol/L or 2-hour glucose > 7.8 m mol/L and <11.1 mmol/L (Shalayel et al., 2010; Hope et al., 1993). About 25% of patients with IGT eventually become diabetic (Shalayel et al., 2007).
In fact there are significant alterations in glucose metabolism during pregnancy (Catalano, 1994). The carbohydrate tolerance is reduced, especially in the last trimester due to reduced sensitivity to insulin action (Hod &, Yogev, 2007).
Insulin resistance is defined where a normal or elevated insulin level produces an attenuated biological response classically this refers to impaired sensitivity to insulin mediated glucose disposal (Wilcox, 2005).
The objectives of this study were to stand on the state of insulin resistance that occurs in pregnancy and to assess the possible role of cortisol, human placental lactogen and prolactin in augmentation of such state. The study also showed the effect of some maternal risk factors such as age, parity, previous heavy babies and first-degree family history of diabetes in glucose tolerance impairment in pregnancy.

2. Subjects and methods

The study was carried on Sudanese pregnant women in the third trimester (34.2±0.63, 35.97±0.71 and 36.53 ±0.64 current week of gestation for the GDM, IGT and control groups respectively).

2.1 Subjects

Thirty pregnant women with the GDM,30 pregnant women with IGT and 30 pregnant women with a normal glucose tolerance (control group) chosen from Khartoum teaching hospital, Khartoum north hospital, Soba hospital, Ibrahim Malik hospital, Maternity hospital and Fath-Elrahman Elbasheer referral center. Oral consent was obtained from all the participants involved in the present study.
All subjects overnight fasted before the test. A fasting blood sample was drawn at 6:00 O'clock a.m. then 75 g oral glucose dissolved in 200 cc water was given for each, waiting for 2 hours and then another blood sample was drawn from each.

2.2 Parameters analysis

The concentration of fasting serum c-peptide, serum cortisol, human placental lactogen and prolactin (2-h after 75-g glucose load) were measured with the specific radio-immunoassay.
Insulin: the concentrations of serum insulin in the fasting sample (0 min) and in the 2-hour after 75 g glucose load sample were measured with the specific immunoradiometric assay (IRMA).
Anti insulin antibodies (AIA): the presence of circulating anti-insulin antibodies is semi-quantitatively estimated by determination of the binding of tracer to AIA in the serum fraction.
Plasma levels of glucose were assayed with a glucose oxidase kit while serum levels of cholesterol and triacylglycerols (TAGs) were estimated by the specific enzymatic colorimetric methods.

2.3 Statistical analysis

Data were expressed as mean, standard deviation (S.D.), standard error of mean (S.E.), and 95% confidence interval (CI) for mean. Comparisons were made using one-way analysis of variance (one-way ANOVA) and the significant differences among mean values were indicated by Scheffe test. Data of anti-insulin antibodies (AIA) of different groups of the study were compared by Kruskal–Wallis one-way ANOVA. The differences among the incidence percentages of family history of diabetes and previous heavy babies in the different groups of the study were assessed by calculation of z-values and their corresponding p-values. The correlation coefficient (r) is used to measure the closeness of the linear relationship between age and 2h-plasma glucose and between parity and 2h-plasma glucose. Calculations were performed using Statistical Packages for Social Sciences (SPSS) program.

3. Results

The GDM and the IGT pregnant women were found to be significantly older than the control women [32.8 ±0.93 year (mean ± S.E.) and 31.1±1.1 vs. 23.9 ±0.82 respectively, $p<0.0001$].
Incidence of previous heavy babies (≥ 4.5 kg at birth) of the IGT group was significantly higher than that of the control group (33.3% vs 6.7%, z=2.25 and $p<0.05$). Also, incidence of previous heavy babies of the GDM group was significantly higher than that of the control group (46.7% vs 6.7%, z=3.2 and $p<0.01$).
Percentage of first degree family history of diabetes was significantly higher in the IGT group when compared with that of the control group (36.7% vs 10%, z=2.1 and $p < 0.05$). Much higher significant difference was shown between the GDM group and the control group (53.3% vs 10%, z=3.3 and $p<0.001$).

3.1 Plasma levels of glucose

The GDM women were found to have higher mean levels of plasma glucose when compared with the IGT and the control pregnant women as shown in table 1 and table 2 ($p<0.0001$).

	Mean	S.D.	S.E.	95% CI
GDM	7.59**	1.85	0.34	6.9-8.28
IGT	5.9*	0.45	0.082	5.73-6.07
Control	2.91	0.43	0.079	2.75-3.07

* Significant ** Highly significant

Table 1. Fasting plasma glucose levels (0 min) in the three studied groups (mmol/L)

	Mean	**S.D.**	**S.E.**	**95% CI**
GDM	12.35**	3.11	0.57	11.19-13.51
IGT	7.98*	0.69	0.13	7.72-8.23
Control	4.35	0.65	0.12	4.11-4.6

* Significant ** Highly significant

Table 2. 2h-plasma glucose levels (120 min) in the three studied groups (mmol/l)

3.2 Serum cholesterol and triacylglycerols results

It was found that the mean levels of serum cholesterol of the IGT group and that of the GDM group were significantly higher than that of the control group [252.5±13.17 mg/dl (mean ±S.E.), 239.07±14.82 vs 195.73±8.47 respectively, F=6.22 and p<0.003].
Also, it was found that the mean levels of serum triacylglycerols of the GDM group and that of the IGT group were significant higher than that of the control group [278.47±15.90 mg/dl (mean ±S.E.), 259.37±11.6 vs 188.63 ±8.92 respectively, F=17.81 and p<0.0001].
But, there was no significant difference between the mean levels of TAGs of the GDM group and that of the IGT group although the serum TAGs levels were greater in the GDM group.

3.3 Serum c-peptide results

Fasting c-peptides mean of the IGT group was not significantly higher than that of the GDM and control groups [0.34±0.04 p mol/l (mean ± S.E.) vs 0.26±0.03 and 0.28±0.04 respectively, p>0.05].

3.4 Serum levels of cortisol

There was a highly significant difference (p<0.0003) between serum level of cortisol of the GDM group and the IGT group from one hand and between the GDM group and the control group from other hand (table 3).

	Mean	S.D.	S.E.	95% CI
GDM	937.2**	434.8	79.38	774.9-1099.6
IGT	794.2*	331.5	60.52	670.4-918
Control	597.3	169.4	30.93	534-660.5

* Significant ** Highly significant

Table 3. Serum cortisol (nmol/l) values of the three studied group

3.5 Serum levels of insulin

There was no significant difference among the mean fasting serum insulin levels of the studied groups [12.29±0.83 MIU/ml (mean ±S.E.), 14.93±2.17 and 2.39±2.25 for the GDM, IGT and control groups respectively, p>0.05].
The men level of 2h-serum insulin of the IGT group was significantly higher than that of the GDM group (68±6.71 vs 36.5±3.06, p<0.002) while, it was not significantly higher than that of the control group (68±6.71 vs 54.88±8.15).

3.6 Serum anti-insulin antibodies (AIA) results

The results of AIA binding percentage to the tracer (table 4) showed significant difference among the three studied groups [X^2 (df=2) = 7.34,p<0.025].

	Mean	S.D.	S.E.	95%CI for mean	Mean rank
GDM	25.11**	31.01	5.66	13.53-36.69	54.25
IGT	7.18*	2.47	0.45	6.25-8.10	46.23
Control	6.04	1.50	0.27	5.48-6.60	36.02

* Significant ** Highly significant

Table 4. Percent bound results of serum AIA

3.7 Serum hPL results

Although the mean HPL levels of the IGT group and that of the GDM group were higher than that of the control group, there were no significant differences among them [7.15±0.49Mg/ml (mean ± S.E.), 6.85+0.58 and 5.73±0.24, p> 0.05].

3.8 Serum prolactin results

Although the control group recorded the highest levels of serum prolactin and the GDM recorded the lowest results, there were no significant differences among the studied groups [123.6±9.61 ng/dl (mean ± S.E.), 145±15 and 150.2±9.7 for the GDM, IGT and control groups respectively, p>0.05].

4. Discussion

There is an increased frequency of gestational diabetes in oriental women and those from the Indian subcontinent and the Middle East (Stewart & Taylor, 1994). Pregnancy and diabetes mellitus aggravate each other (Potemkin, 1989). Hormonal changes occur in pregnancy, which profoundly affect carbohydrate metabolism. The levels of estrogen, progesterone, human placental lactogen, free cortisol and prolactin rise progressively as pregnancy advances. Of these a number, notably human placental lactogen and cortisol are insulin antagonists. So, insulin resistance develops in the mother as the pregnancy progresses, and it is most marked in the last trimester. This leads to deterioration in glucose tolerance (Brudenell, 1993). This explains why IGT and GDM were only discovered in the third trimester of gestation.

The results showed that many maternal risk factors affect the incidence of abnormal glucose tolerance (IGT & GDM) in Sudanese pregnant women.

Maternal age is an established risk factor for gestational diabetes mellitus (GDM), but there is no consensus on the age above which there is significantly increased risk of GDM (American Diabetes Association, 2004). The finding that the IGT and the GDM groups were significantly older than those with normal glucose tolerance (control) group, agrees with many previous studies that approved the direct relation between advanced maternal age (<35) and greater risk for incidence of GDM (Solomon et al., 1997; Cianni et al., 2003). Moreover, the presence of a linear relationship between the age and the 2h-plasma glucose ensure that there is an age related deterioration of glucose tolerance and makes the age a very important maternal risk factor to affect glucose intolerance incidence.

The association between parity and diabetes seems consistent in different studies. Women with highest parity are frequently older and heavier. Therefore, no study that evaluates parity could ignore a proper age adjustment (Dode & dos Santos, 2009). Multiparity has been associated with GDM in some studies but not in other ones (Seghieri et al., 2005; Ben-Haroush et al., 2004).

Kumari et al. (2002) found that grand multiparous women with parity $\geq$ 10 had greater gestational diabetes mellitus incidence.

Significant higher mean parity of the IGT and the GDM groups when compared with the mean parity of the control (normal glucose tolerance) group as well as the existence of a linear relationship between parity and the 2h-plasma glucose, make the parity a very important maternal risk factor in impairment of glucose tolerance. This may be explained in terms of the diabetogenicity of the pregnancy, which is related to a pronounced peripheral resistance to insulin (Kuhl, 1991). Parity reflects the duration of exposure to the insulin resistance (Peters et al., 1995). Thus, one can conclude that higher parity may lead to accumulation of the diabetogenic effect of pregnancy. Consequently, much more glucose impairment occurs.

Genetic factors play a part in the development of diabetes although the exact mode of inheritance is not established (Brudenell, 1993). Recent evidence suggests that the gestational diabetes has a strong genetic component and is usually NIDDM. Both GDM and NIDDM are characterized by insulin deficiency and by insulin resistance (Dornhorst et al., 1990). This evidence agrees with that of Csorba and Edwards (1995) who showed that the development of both type II and GDM is probably governed by a complex and variable interaction of genes and environments. Moreover, they suggest that both beta cell dysfunction and insulin resistance is operative in the manifestation of these disorders. This may explain why the incidence of first degree family history of diabetes was significantly higher in the GDM and in the IGT groups when compared with that of the control group. Therefore, family history of diabetes is a very important maternal risk factor from the obstetrician's point of view (Brudenell, 1993).

The result that the GDM and the IGT groups have incidence of previous heavy babies significantly higher than that of control group, make previous delivery of a large baby to be a very important maternal risk factor since a tendency to bear heavy babies may precede the development of clinical diabetes by many years (Brudenell, 1993).

Changes in lipid metabolism occur during pregnancy. Plasma levels of triglycerides, cholesterol and free fatty acids rise, and there is a greater tendency to ketosis (Campbell & Lees, 2000). Some studies showed that total triglycerides increase with gestational time in pre-gestational diabetic women, GDM women and healthy control women (Montelongo et al., 1992).

Every aspect of lipid metabolism is affected by pregnancy. The plasma level of free fatty acids falls from early to mid-pregnancy and thereafter shows a significant rise. The same is true for the plasma level of glycerol. This is in keeping with the accumulation of body fat that occurs during the anabolic phase of pregnancy (first two trimesters). In the catabolic phase of pregnancy (last trimester), raised free fatty acids and glycerol levels are available as fuel to the maternal tissues to offset the increasing diversion to the rapidly growing fetus of glucose and amino acids. As with free fatty, glycerol and triglycerides, plasma levels of cholesterol and phospholipids are increased in pregnancy (Brudenell, 1993) taking in account that plasma triglycerides may be a physiological contributor to infant birth weight (Knopp et al., 1992). Thus, one can expect more increase of these lipid substances when the glucose tolerance deteriorates in pregnancy. Therefore, the mean level of serum cholesterol and triglycerides were significantly higher in the GDM and in the IGT groups when compared with the control (normal glucose tolerance) group.

The changes in lipid metabolism are mediated by hormonal changes and fit into the general pattern of an increase in storage of glycogen and fat in most maternal tissues during the metabolic first two trimesters of pregnancy, followed by the mobilization of fuel for the benefit of both mother and fetus in catabolic third trimester (Brudenell, 1993).

Boden (1996) demonstrated that in early pregnancy, insulin secretion in response to glucose is increased, peripheral insulin sensitivity is normal or increased and glucose tolerance is normal or slightly enhanced. In addition, there is maternal fat accumulation. During late pregnancy, there is increased fetal growth and increased fetal demand for nutrients.

Maternal responses to these demands consist of an accelerated switch from carbohydrate to fat utilization that is facilitated by peripheral insulin resistance and by high blood levels of lipolytic hormones. In patients with GDM, insulin resistance is either comparable or greater than in non-diabetic pregnancy whereas insulin secretion appears to be compromised.

Changes in hepatic and adipose metabolism alter circulating concentrations of triacylglycerols, fatty acids, cholesterol, and phospholipids. After an initial decrease in the first 8 wk of pregnancy, there is a steady increase in triacylglycerols, fatty acids, cholesterol, lipoproteins, and phospholipids (Butte, 2000). There is a two- to threefold increase in basal triglyceride and cholesterol concentrations with advancing gestation. The increases are more pronounced in the GDM as compared with the normal glucose tolerant pregnant woman (Catalano, 2010). The higher concentration of estrogen and insulin resistance are thought to be responsible for the hypertriglyceridemia of pregnancy (Butte, 2000).

Thus, it is concluded that in the third trimester of pregnancy, there is a competition between mother and her fetus on glucose uptake. This competition will be directed towards the benefit of the fetus. For this reason, the pregnant women do switch to other energy source rather than glucose such as fat to overcome the state of insulin resistance.

The syndrome of insulin resistance is a group of clinically diverse disorders (Catalano, 2010; Flier, 1992). Pregnancy induces complex changes in energy metabolism, manifested clinically by insulin resistance (Bedalov & Balasubramanyam, 1997). Glucose tolerance deteriorates in all pregnant women, but only in 2-3% of all pregnancies is the deterioration sufficiently large to fulfill the diagnostic criteria for gestational diabetes1. Many previous studies demonstrated that pregnancy result in a state of insulin resistance and women with gestational-onset diabetes appear to have a greater degree of insulin resistance (Ryan et al., 1985).

Why pregnancy is capable of inducing the temporary diabetic state is still partly unknown, although many other studies tried to put general points to explain this state.

Bergstrom et al. (1990) revealed that an increased fasting c-peptide reflects insulin resistance. In fact, insulin and c-peptide are secreted in equimolar amount. However, because of its longer half-life, the plasma concentration of c-peptide is higher than that of insulin. Within limits, c-peptides levels can serve as valuable index to insulin secretion. Thus, low c-peptide levels are to be expected when insulin secretion is diminished whereas elevated c-peptides may result from increased beta-cells activity.

Regarding our results, the serum fasting c-peptide mean level was the highest in the IGT groups (0.337± 0.038 Pmol/L) when compared with the GDM group (0.262 ± 0.025) and the control group (0.284 ± 0.041) although the differences were not significant ($P > 0.05$). This gives prediction to the higher insulin resistance in the IGT group when compared with the control group.

Most pregnant women are able to counteract the insulin resistance in pregnancy by increasing their insulin secretion. This also explains the highest mean levels of insulin in the IGT group when compared with the control group.

Although the insulin levels, (fasting and 2h-insulin) were lower in the control group than that of the IGT group, the glucose tolerance kept normal. This may support the suggestion that during normal pregnancy, the Staub-Traugott effect i.e., improved glucose disposal after successive glucose load administrations occurs and appears to be caused by mechanisms other than enhanced insulin secretion with successive glucose loads (Lewis et al., 1993).

However, when the capacity of insulin secretion is not sufficiently large to meet the resistance, glucose intolerance develops and the women develop gestational diabetes

(Shalayel et al., 2010; Buchanan & Xiang, 2005). This may be due to the presence of high levels of insulin antagonistic hormones as hPL and cortisol (Carr & Gabbe, 1998) as well as high level of circulating anti-insulin antibodies which may make the pregnant women secrete more insulin to overcome the insulin resistance and eventually may lead to exhaustion of beta-cells of the pancreas. This explain the lowest mean levels of fasting c-peptide, fasting serum insulin and 2h-serum insulin in the GDM group when compared with the IGT and the control groups.

Damm et al. (1995) demonstrated that women who develop GDM have a relative insulin secretion deficiency, the severity of which is predictive for later development of diabetes. Furthermore, their relatively reduced beta-cells functions may be a significant pathogenic factor in relation to the high incidence of subsequent diabetes in women with GDM. This agrees with Paulus et al. (1995) who showed that the diagnoses of gestational diabetes mellitus are at a greater risk for developing diabetes in later life.

Homko et al (2001) reported that patients with GDM during late pregnancy not only had severe deficiencies in insulin secretion rate (ISR) and were more insulin resistant than controls. In addition, the women with GDM had a major ß-cell defect that made it impossible for them to compensate for their increased level of insulin resistance, which occurred during late pregnancy.

Our study also showed that the cortisol increases progressively as pregnancy advances and the mean cortisol level was significantly the highest in the GDM group when compared with the IGT and the control groups while its level was the lowest in the control group in the third trimester. This ensures the possibility role of cortisol as an insulin antagonist in the deterioration of the glucose tolerance in pregnancy.

Cortisol is bound in the circulation to alpha-globulin called *transcortin* or *corticosteroid-binding globulin* (CBG). The bound cortisol functions as circulating reservoir of hormone that keeps a supply of free cortisol available to the tissues. At normal levels of total plasma cortisol (13.5μg/dL), there is very little free cortisol in plasma, but the binding sites on CBG become saturated when the total plasma cortisol exceeds 20μg/dL. CBG is synthesized in the liver, and its production is increased by estrogen and its level is elevated during pregnancy. When the CBG level rises, more cortisol is bound, and initially there is a drop in the free cortisol level which stimulates adrenocorticotrophic hormone (ACTH) secretion. Therefore, more cortisol is secreted until a new equilibrium is reached at which the bound cortisol is elevated but the free cortisol is normal. Changes in the opposite direction occur when the CBG level falls. This explains why pregnant women have higher total plasma levels of cortisol without symptoms of glucocorticoids excess (Barrett et al., 2010). Cortisol is nearly totally (90%) bound to CBG up to concentrations of 25μg/dL. But, when cortisol concentrations rise above this level, as occurred in the IGT group (serum cortisol mean level = 28.57μg/dL) and in the GDM group (serum cortisol mean level = 33.71μg/dL), the binding capacity of CBG is exceeded and the proportion of unbound, free, cortisol rises greatly (Burch, 1994). This free cortisol increases glucose tolerance deterioration therefore confirms the dominating role of cortisol as a regulator of stress dependent insulin resistance (Lehrke et al., 2008).

Human placental lactogen (hPL) is a single protein of 191 amino acids, which is encoded by two genes hPL/CS-A and hPL/CS-B, which are identical except for one minor difference in the single sequence coding region. The hPL/CS genes are clustered together with the pituitary growth hormone gene (hGH-N) and a variant GH gene, hGH-V, on the long arm of chromosome (Davis, 1990). Human PL has only a limited homology with prolactin, but a very high homology with the growth hormone mRNA coding sequence, although in other species there is a more homology with prolactin than growth hormone. The hormone is synthesized in the syncytiotrophoblastic villous epithelium of the placenta and it is secreted into maternal blood (Davis, 1990; Strauss & Barbieri, 2009). Maternal serum hPL levels rise progressively from the first trimester through till term (Strauss & Barbieri, 2009) and this agrees with our results of serum hPL in the control group. Although, there were no significant differences among hPL mean level of the IGT and the GDM groups were higher than that of the control group. This non-significant slight increase in the IGT and the GDM groups may share in increasing insulin resistance in these groups when compared with control group.

Some authors reported that pronounced fetal macrosomia may occur even with adequate maternal blood glucose control. The severe fetal hyperinsulinemia in this case may be imputed to some factor other than excessive glucose load, possibly hPL, which induces proliferation and enhanced function of pancreatic ß-cells. In concert with this hypothesis, maternal serum hPL concentrations measured in the third trimester are higher in diabetic pregnancies complicated by fetal macrosomia (Persson et al., 1995; Reis et al., 2002).

The regulation of hPL secretion is not fully understood. Progesterone exerts stimulatory effects in early gestation, but not in late gestation. Finally the hPL/CS gene contains a binding site for the glucocorticoids receptor, suggesting a potential modulatory role for corticosteroids, and also has binding sites for a pituitary protein factor that is thought to regulate both prolactin and growth hormone gene expression (Davis, 1990). Furthermore, the very high levels of circulating estrogen that occur during pregnancy result in a parallel increase in the circulating levels of prolactin (Schlechte, 2007). This may explain the interconnection between hPL and prolactin since, it seems that prolactin, growth hormone and placental lactogen hormone are phylogenetically ancient hormones which in vertebrates have evolved from common ancestral molecules. These hormones share common effects in growth stimulation and lactation. Hypersomatotropism is associated with disturbance of glucose tolerance and insulin resistance. Hyperprolactinaemia, like hypersomatotropism, is associated with decreased insulin sensitivity (Foss et al., 1995).

The present study (on control group) demonstrated that prolactin increases progressively from the first trimester through till third trimester. Moreover, our study revealed that there were no significant differences among the levels of serum prolactin in GDM, IGT, and control groups. This agrees with what has been mentioned by Grigorakiz et al. (2000). Consequently, there is no evidence that prolactin may be directly incorporated with the pathogenesis of glucose intolerance in pregnancy. This may agree with the study of Milasinović et al. (1997) who reported that there is no evidence of the functional connection between prolactin and glucose metabolism.

Prolactin is found in large amounts in the amniotic fluid of humans and other primates, and it is now clearly established that the source of this prolactin is the placenta rather than the maternal or fetal pituitary. The endometrial lining of the uterus is greatly modified during pregnancy to form the decidua. This decidual tissue has been confirmed as the site of placental prolactin production by a number of different groups and the mature peptide hormone is immunologically indistinguishable from pituitary prolactin. Immunocytochemical studies have shown that the hormone is predominantly located in the parietal decidual cells and only very rarely in the chorionic cytotrophoblast. Amniotic fluid prolactin levels are very low in ectopic tubal pregnancy, confirming the role of the decidualized endometrium (Davis, 1990).

Amniotic fluid prolactin levels rise progressively after the 14th week human gestation and decline somewhat during the 3rd trimester. Prolactin secretion by the deciduas appears to be regulated quite differently from that in the pituitary gland. The first striking difference in regulation is that dopamine and dopamine agonists' drugs have no inhibitory effect on decidual prolactin secretion or amniotic fluid prolactin levels. Estrogen exerts a strong stimulation on pituitary lactotrophs but appears at most to have only small effects on decidual prolactin production (Davis, 1990).
The very high levels of circulating estrogen during pregnancy result in a parallel increase in the circulating levels of prolactin in pregnancy. The prolactin increase is to prepare the breasts for lactation. Prolactin levels begin to rise at 5-8 weeks of gestation and parallel the increase in the size and number of lactotrophs (Schlechte, 2007; Corenblum, 2008).
Progesterone appears to stimulate decidual prolactin secretion although it has little or no effect on decidual cells obtained in early pregnancy. Insulin stimulates both acute secretion and de novo synthesis of decidual prolactin (Davis, 1990). This may explain why prolactin mean level was the lowest in the GDM group as the level of insulin, which stimulates prolactin secretion, is the lowest when compared with the other groups (IGT and the control groups).

5. Conclusion

Now, it is clear that pregnancy is diabetogenic and characterized by increased insulin resistance which may be explained in term of reduced insulin secretion, reduced tissue sensitivity to insulin and increased secretion of hormones with an anti-insulin effect such as human placental lactogen, free cortisol and prolactin. All these characteristics with the incorporation of some maternal risk factors such as age, parity, previous heavy babies and family history of diabetes may lead to the impairment of glucose tolerance in some pregnant women. Most pregnant women are able to counteract the insulin resistance in pregnancy by increasing their insulin secretion or by switching to other energy source rather than glucose such as fat particularly in the third trimester to preserve glucose to the fetus. However, when the capacity of insulin secretion is not sufficiently large to meet the resistance, glucose intolerance develops and women develop gestational diabetes.

6. Abbreviation

GDM, gestational diabetes mellitus; IGT, impaired glucose tolerance; hPL, human placental lactogen; TAGs, triacylglycerol; NIDDM, non-insulin dependent diabetes mellitus; CBG, corticosteroid-binding globulin; ACTH, adrenocorticotrophic hormone.

7. References

American Diabetes Association. (2004). Gestational diabetes mellitus. *Diabetes Care*, 27 (Suppl. 1):S88–S90.

Baban RS, Kasar KAK, Al-Karawi IN. (2010). Fasting glucose to leptin ratio as a new diagnostic marker in patients with diabetes mellitus. OMJ, 25(4):269-275.

Barbour LA, Carrie E. McCurdy, Teri L. Hernandez, John P. Kirwanet et al. (2007). Cellular Mechanisms for Insulin Resistance in Normal Pregnancy and Gestational Diabetes. *Diabetes Care,* 30 (2): S112-S119.

Barrett K, Brooks H, Boitano S, Barman S. (2010). The adrenal medulla and adrenal cortex, In: *Ganong's Review of Medical Physiology* (23rd edition), pp. 346-347, The Mc Grow Hill Companies, ISBN: 978-0-07-160567-0, USA.

Bedalov A. and Balasubramanyam A. (1997). Glucocorticoid- induced ketoacidosis in gestational diabetes: Sequela of the acute treatment of preterm labor. A case report. *Diabetic Care,* 20(6): 922-924.

Ben-Haroush, A., Yogev, Y., Hod, M. (2004). Epidemiology of gestational diabetes mellitus and its association with type 2 diabetes. *Diabetic Medicine,* 21: 103-113.

Bergstrom R.W., Newell-Morris L.L., Leonetti D. L., et al. (1990). Association of elevated fasting C-peptide level and increased intra-abdominal fat distribution with development of NIDDM in Japanese- American men. *Diabetes,* 39 (1): 104-111.

Bilous R, Donnelly R. (2010). *Hand book of Diabetes* (4th edition), Wiley-Blackwell, ISBN: 9781405184090, UK.

Boden G. (1992). Fuel metabolism in pregnancy and in gestational diabetes mellitus. *Obstet-gynecol. Clin. North Am.,* 23 (1): 1-10.

Brudenell M. (1993) Diabetic pregnancy. In: *Obstetrics* (2nd edition), Turnbull S. A., Chamberlain G. (eds). pp. 585-602, Churchill Livingstone, Edinburgh, London, Melbourne and Newyork.

Buchanan TA, Xiang AH. (2005). Gestational diabetes mellitus. *J Clin Invest,* 115(3): 485–491.

Burch W. M. (1994). *Endocrinology* (3rd edition), Mass Publishing Co., ISBN: 977-269-018-7, Egypt.

Butte N.F. (2000). Carbohydrate and lipid metabolism in pregnancy: normal compared with gestational diabetes mellitus. *American Journal of Clinical Nutrition,* 71(5): 1256S-1261S.

Campbell S. and Lees C. (Eds). (2000). *Obstetrics by Ten Teachers,* 17th edition. Arnold, ISBN 0 340 74082 5, London.

Carr DB, Gabbe S. (1998). Gestational Diabetes: Detection, Management, and Implications. *Clin Diabetes,* 16(1): 4-11.

Catalano P. M. (1994). Carbohydrate metabolism and gestational diabetes. Clin. *Obstet. Gynecol,* 37(1): 25-38.

Catalano PM. Obesity, insulin resistance, and pregnancy outcome. *Reproduction* (2010) 140 365-371.

Cianni GD, Volpe L, Lencioni C, et al. (2003). Prevalence and risk factors for gestational diabetes assessed by universal screening. *Diabetes research and clinical practice,* 62(2): 131-137.

Corenblum B. (2008). Pituitary Disease and Pregnancy, In: *eMedicine from WebMD.* Article Last Updated: Jun 25, 2008. http://emedicine.medscape.com/article/127650-overview.

Csorba T. R. and Edwards A. L. (1995). The genetic and pathophysiology of type II and gestational diabetes. *Crit. Rev. Clin. Lab. Sci.,* 32 (5-6): 509-550.

Dahlgren J. (2006). Pregnancy and insulin resistance. *Metabolic Syndrome and Related Disorders*, 4(2): 149-152.

Damm P., Kuhl C., Buchard K., et al. (1994). Prevalence and predictive value of islet cell antibodies and insulin autoantibodies in women with gestational diabetes. *Diabetic Medicine*, 11: 558-563.

Damm P., Kuhl C., Hornnes P. and Molsted-Pedersen L. (1995). A longitudinal study of plasma insulin and glucagon in women with previous gestational diabetes. *Diabetes care*, 18 (5): 654-665.

Davis JRE. (1990). Prolactin and related peptides in pregnancy. *Baillière's Clinical Endocrinology and Metabolism*, 4(2): 273-290.

Dode MAS, dos Santos I S. (2009). Non classical risk factors for gestational diabetes mellitus: a systematic review of the literature. *Cad. Saúde Pública*, 25 (supl.3) Rio de Janeiro.

Dornhorst A., Nicholls J. S. D. and Johnston D.G. (1990). Diabetes and diet in pregnancy. *Bailliere's Clinical Endocrinology and Metabolism*, 4 (2): 291-311.

Flier J. S. (1992). Lilly lecture: Syndromes of insulin resistance- From patient to gene and back again. *Diabetes*, 41: 1207-1219.

Foss M. C., Paula F. J. A., Paccola G. M. G. F. and Piccinato C. E. (1995). Peripheral glucose metabolism in human prolactinaemia. *Clinical Endocrinology*, 43 (6): 721 -726.

Grigorakis SI, Alevizaki M, Beis C, et al. (2000). Hormonal parameters in gestational diabetes mellitus during the third trimester: High glucagon levels. *Gynecological and Obstetric investigation*, 49: 106 – 109.

Hod M., Yogev Y. (2007). Goals of Metabolic Management of Gestational Diabetes- Is it all about the sugar? *Diabetes Care*, 30(Supplement 2): S180-S187.

Homko C, Sivan E, Chen X, et al. (2001). Insulin Secretion during and after Pregnancy in Patients with Gestational Diabetes Mellitus. *The Journal of Clinical Endocrinology & Metabolism*, 86(2): 568-573.

Hope R. A., Longmore J. M., Hodgetts T. J. & Ramrakha P. S. (1993). *Oxford handbook of clinical medicine* (3rd edition), Oxford University Press, ISBN-13: 9780192621153, USA.

Kaaja R, Rönnemaa T. (2008). Gestational Diabetes: Pathogenesis and Consequences to Mother and Offspring. *Rev Diabet Stud*, 5(4):194-202.

Kahn CR. Weir GC. King GL. et al. (2005). *Joslin's Diabetes Mellitus* (14th edition), Lippincott Williams & Wilkins. ISBN: 0-7817-2796-0. USA. Pp 332-336.

Kim J. K., Wi J. K. and Young J. H. (1996) Plasma free fatty acids decrease insulin-stimulated skeletal muscle glucose uptake by suppressing glycolysis in conscious rats. *Diabetes*, 45: 446-453.

Knopp R. H., Magee M. S., Walden C. E., et al. (1992). Prediction of infant birth weight by GDM screening test-Immportance of plasma triglycerides. *Diabetes Care*, 15(11): 1605-1613.

Kuhl C. (1991). Aetiology of gestational diabetes. *Bailliere's Clinical Obstetrics and Gynaecology*, 5(2): 279-292.

Kuhl C., Hornnes P. J. and Andersen O. (1985). Etiology and pathophysiology of gestational diabetes mellitus. *Diabetes*, 34 (suppl.2): 66-70.

Kumari AS, Badrinath P. (2002). Extreme grandmultiparity: is it an obstetric risk factor? *Eur J Obstet Gynecol Reprod Biol.*, 101:22-5.

Lehrke M, BroedlUC, Biller-Friedmann IM, et al. (2008). Serum concentrations of cortisol, interleukin 6, leptin and adiponectin predict stress induced insulin resistance in acute inflammatory reactions. *Critical Care*, 12 (6): R157.

Lewis G. F., McNally C., Blackman J. D., et al. (1993). Prior feeding alters the response to the 50-g glucose challenge test in pregnancy- The Staub-Traugott effect revisited. *Diabetes Care*, 16 (12): 1551-1556.

Milasinović L, Djurdjević J, Dokmanović-Djordjević M, et al. (1997). Prolactin levels in pregnant women with glucose intolerance at full-term delivery. *Med Pregl*, 50:269-73.

Montelongo A. Lasunciaon M. A., Pallardo L. F. and Herrera E. (1992). Longitudinal study of plasma lipoproteins and hormones during pregnancy in normal and diabetic women. *Diabetes*, 41 (12): 1651-1659.

Paulus W. E., Stoz F., Bugan S. and Kreienberg R. (1995). Disorder of glucose metabolism and insulin resistance after gestational diabetes. *Zentralblatt fur Gynakologie*, 117 (8): 417-422.

Persson B, Hanson U, Marcus C. (1995). Gestational diabetes mellitus and paradoxical fetal macrosomia—a case report. *Early Hum Dev.*, 41:203–213.

Peters R., Kjos S., Xiang A. and Buchanan T. (1995). Effect of a second pregnancy on the risk of non-insulin-dependent diabetes in women with recent gestational diabetes. *Diabetes*, Abstracts book. 44(suppl.1): 14A (abstract no. 45).

Potemkin V. (1989). Diseases of the Ilet Apparatus of the Pancreas, In: *Endocrinology* (2nd edition), pp. (185-243), Mir Publishers, ISBN: 5-03-000754-7, Moscow.

Reece EA, Leguizamon G, Wiznitzer A. (2009). Gestational diabetes: the need for a common ground. *Lancet*, 373(9677): 1789-97. [abstract]

Reis FM, D'Antona D and Petraglia F. (2002). Predictive Value of Hormone Measurements in Maternal and Fetal Complications of Pregnancy. *Endocrine Reviews*, 23 (2): 230-257.

Robert J.J. (1995). Methods de mesure de la resistance a l'insulin-clamp hyperinsulinemique euglycemique. *La press Medicale*, 24 (15): 730-734.

Ryan E. A., O'sullivan M. J. and Skyler J. S. (1985). Insulin action during pregnancy- Studies with the euglycemic clamp technique. *Diabetes*, 34: 380-389.

Schlechte JA. (2007). Long-term management of prolactinomas. *J Clin Endocrinol Metab*, 92(8):2861-5.

Seghieri, G., De Bellis, A., Anichini, R., et al. (2005). Does parity increase insulin resistance during pregnancy? *Diabetic Medicine*, 22: 1574-1580.

Shalayel MH, Ahmed SA, Khattab AH, Satti GM. (2007). Prevalence of gestational diabetes mellitus and impaired glucose tolerance in pregnant Sudanese women in the third trimester. *Sudan Medical Monitor*, 2(2): 59-61. ISSN: 1858-5000.

Shalayel MH, Elrobh MS, Idris SA, Mohammed MS, Ahmed SA. (2010). Prolactin and insulin estimates in pregnancy with glucose intolerance. *Pak J Med Sci.*, 26(1):102-106.

Solomon GC, Willet WC, Carey VJ. et al. (1997). A Prospective Study of Pregravid Determinants of Gestational Diabetes Mellitus. *JAMA*, 278(13):1078-1083.

Stewart M. and Taylor R. (1994). Gestational diabetes mellitus. *Prof. Care-Mother-child*, 4(5): 136-138.

Strauss JF & Barbieri RL. (2009). The endocrinology of human pregnancy and fetoplacental neuroendocrine development, In: *Yen and Jaffe's Reproductive Endocrinology – Physiology, pathophysiology and clinical management* (6th edition), Strauss JF & Barbieri RL, pp. 256, Saunders Elsevier, ISBN: 978-1-4160-4907-4, Philadelphia.

Summary and recommendation of the second international workshop conference of gestational diabetes. (1985). *Diabetes*, 34 (suppl.2): 123-126.

Wilcox G. (2005). Insulin and Insulin Resistance. *Clin Biochem Rev*, 26(2): 19–39.

10

The Impact of Polycystic Ovarian Syndrome on Gestational Diabetes

Stefanie Aust and Johannes Ott
Medical University of Vienna, Department of Gynecologic Endocrinology and Reproductive Medicine, Austria

1. Introduction

When Stein and Leventhal, in 1935, observed a group of women who suffered from sterility, oligomenorrhoea, or amenorhhoea, hirsutism, and enlarged polycystic ovaries, the disorder that became known as the polycystic ovarian syndrome (PCOS) or the Stein-Leventhal syndrome, was diagnosed for the first time (Stein, 1958). The variability of individual presentation, as well as a varying collection of signs and characteristic features, with no single diagnostic test justify the categorization of the PCOS as a syndrome that affects not only reproductive health, but also the metabolic and cardiovascular systems. Although PCOS is one of the most common endocrinopathies in women, with an incidence of about 5-10% throughout the reproductive age span (Metalliotakis, 2006), there are divergent opinions about how to define and diagnose PCOS, as well as different types of treatment options throughout Europe and the US (Badawy & Elnashar, 2011). The high prevalence of women with this endocrine disorder highlights the importance of understanding the clinical presentation, pathophysiology, associated disorders, and treatment options. Up to 40% of women of reproductive age with PCOS have Type 2 diabetes or an impaired glucose tolerance (Legro et al., 2005), a form of insulin resistance that occurs equally in obese, normal weight, and thin women with PCOS (Matalliotakis et al., 2006). PCOS has been associated with an increased risk for gestational diabetes mellitus (GDM), but solid evidence confirming PCOS as a risk factor for GDM is still missing (Toulis et al., 2009). GDM, a well-known state of carbohydrate intolerance with a high, and rising, prevalence, causes not only maternal but also fetal pregnancy complications. GDM has a presentation similar to PCOS, and both are considered risk factors for Type 2 diabetes mellitus (Retnakaran et al., 2008).
The aim of this review is to summarize the available evidence about the risk of impaired glucose tolerance and GDM in PCOS women, as well as to review the pathophysiological aspects. In addition, the potential beneficial influence of several PCOS-specific treatment options on PCOS and GDM will be discussed.

2. Diagnostic criteria for polycystic ovary syndrome

The National Institutes of Health (NIH) has published criteria for diagnosing PCOS, based on an international conference on PCOS held in 1990. Accordingly, diagnostic criteria for the syndrome includes chronic anovulation, combined with clinical or biochemical hyperandrogenism, where other causes have been excluded (diagnosis of exclusion) (Huang et al. 2010). An expanded definition can be found in the revised Rotterdam criteria, a consensus on diagnostic criteria of the American Society for Reproductive Medicine and the European Society of Human Reproduction and Embryology. At least two of three criteria must be present: (i) oligoamenorrhoea or amenorrhoea; (ii) hyperandrogenism (clinical/biochemical); and (iii) polycystic ovaries on ultrasound, defined as more than 12 cysts of 2-9mm, or >10ml volume (Rotterdam ESHRE/ASRM-Sponsored PCOS Consensus Workshop Group, 2004). The revised Rotterdam criteria are considered the current standard diagnostic criteria.

In 2006, the Androgen Excess Society (AES) attempted to define evidence-based guidelines for diagnosis and future research in a review (Azziz et al., 2006). The AES task force suggested that androgen excess must be considered a central feature of the disease, and that PCOS should be defined by the presence of hyperandrogenism (clinical and/or biochemical) together with signs of ovarian dysfunction (oligoovulation or anovulation and/or polycystic ovaries), where similar disorders have been excluded (Azziz et al., 2006). Conditions for exclusion must be clarified in the diagnostic procedure. Premature ovarian failure with oligo-/amenorrhea that might be associated with other autoimmune endocrinopathies, hyperprolactinoma, or Cushing's syndrome are a few clinical possibilities that merit attention.

3. Pathophysiologic aspects of polycystic ovary syndrome

The heterogeneity of the syndrome and the unclear etiology favor the theory of multiple underlying pathophysiologic mechanisms that have yet to be fully elucidated. A heritable etiology for PCOS has been investigated intensively and several associated polymorphisms have been identified. However, to date, none of the possible candidate genes (e.g., regulators of the microbiological action of insulin) could be correlated with the onset of PCOS (Dumesic et al., 2007). In the research field of PCOS, studies on polymorphisms gained on importance within the last years. Moreover, environmental factors (e.g.: lifestyle, nutrition) together with certain genetic mutations might lead to the individual manifestation of PCOS but the diversity of clinical presentations aggravates the identification of genes involved in the origin of PCOS.

Although the definition of "polycystic ovary syndrome" might be ambiguous, it is important to emphasize that polycystic ovaries need not be present to diagnose this syndrome. Nevertheless, PCOS patients who demonstrate ovaries with multiple subcortical cysts on ultrasound and an increased proportion of primary follicles (Dumesic et al., 2007) have a greater rate of hyperandrogenism than women with PCOS without abnormal follicle development. The presence of polycystic ovaries might indicate a major clinical alteration of PCOS, and the presence of polycystic ovaries in childhood has been suggested as an indicator of a genetic predisposition (Battaglia et al., 2002). Moreover, an abnormal autoimmune history has been considered in PCOS, in which functional autoantibodies might favor the development of PCOS (Ott et al., 2010, Gleicher et al., 2007). Assuming a relation between insulin resistance, ovarian function, and thyroid function, elevated antiTPO levels have been found to influence treatment response in women with PCOS and infertility (Ott et al., 2010). Notably, PCOS has been called a marker for "reduced ovarian aging," since serum anti-Müller hormone (AMH) levels are higher in anovulatory women and have been found to be elevated in women with PCOS. AMH concentrations correspond

to the number of antral follicles and can be correlated to the level of ovarian dysfunction in infertility. Thus, it is possible that the process leading to ovarian aging is delayed in PCOS, which might also lead to a later onset of menopause in these women (Mulders et al., 2004).
Three hypotheses are frequently discussed in literature about how defects in primary cellular control mechanisms might result in PCOS: (i) an elevated luteinizing hormone (LH) pulse frequency and amplitude, and relatively low follicle stimulating hormone (FSH) serum levels (LH+/FSH-) lead to anovulation and ovarian hyperandrogenism; (ii) a defect in the sex steroid metabolism within the ovaries (theca cells) causes an exaggerated ovarian androgen secretion; and (iii) a regulatory dysfunction of the insulin pathway results in hyperinsulinemia and insulin resistance and contributes to the development of PCOS (Franks et al., 1998). These pathophysiologic mechanisms might be of special interest regarding the risk for GDM. Indeed, several possible insulin-mediated pathways have been identified that might contribute to hyperandrogenism in PCOS patients (see Figure 1).

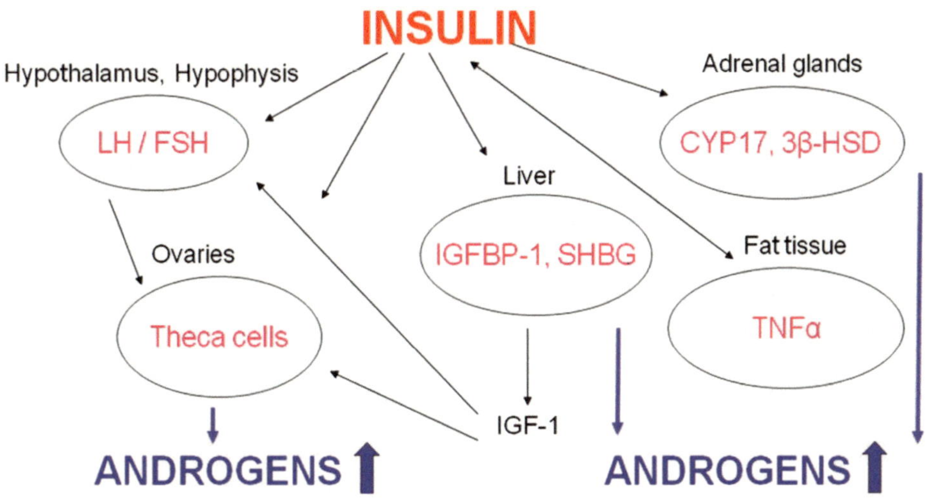

Fig. 1. How increased insulin levels might contribute to hyperandrogenism

These pathophysiologic hypotheses are related in a variety of ways. Elevated hypothalamic gonadotropin-releasing hormone (GnRH) pulsatility influences LH secretion; consequently, dysfunctional pulse frequency and amplitude lead to an increased 24-hour secretion of LH. High LH combined with high levels of insulin result in increased ovarian androgen production. Hypersecretion of LH also affects oocyte development. A defect in androgen synthesis that results in an increased enzymatic activity involved in the synthesis of dehydroepiandrosterone (DHEA), dehydroepiandrosterone sulfate (DHEA-S), and androstenedione leads, consequently, to an inadequate production of testosterone in ovarian theca cells. The synergistic interaction between LH and insulin on the ovarian theca cells leads to stimulation of androgen production. Several studies have provided useful information about a correlation between hyperandrogenism and a state of increased insulin resistance (Balen, 2004) (Baptiste et al., 2010). In women with PCOS, an another cause of high androgen levels can be explained by the influence of compensatory hyperinsulinemia on the hepatic synthesis and secretion of the sex hormone-binding globulin (SHBG). SHBG levels are reduced and the blood concentrations of biologically active androgens are thus increased. In addition, it has been suggested that adipose tissue dysfunction also plays a central role in the metabolic and endocrine abnormalities observed in PCOS (Villa J et al., 2011).

4. Clinical manifestation of polycystic ovary syndrome

A variety of signs and symptoms can be found in women who suffer from PCOS in which ovarian hyperandrogenism is considered the cardinal characteristic. The variable clinical presentation includes gynecological symptoms that include dysfunctional menstrual bleeding, such as oligo- or amenorrhea, or any kind of abnormal uterine bleeding combined with infrequent or absent ovulation, infertility resulting from elevated androgen levels, and polycystic ovaries (Dumesic et al., 2007). With regard to gynecologic malignancies, chronic anovulation over a long period of time is associated with a higher risk of developing endometrial adenocarcinoma and a higher incidence of endometrial hyperplasia, compared to age-matched controls (Badawy & Elnashar, 2011). Elevated serum androgen levels lead to androgenic disorders, such as acne, hirsutism, and alopecia androgenica, where hyperandrogenism is differently expressed in the PCOS phenotypes, resulting in cosmetic issues and psychological effects that can be burdensome and difficult to cope with.

Last not least, PCOS has been considered to be associated with a increased risks for type II diabetes mellitus and GDM. When considering the association with GDM, it is notable that both PCOS and GDM share some common characteristic features, including obesity, increased insulin resistance, dyslipidemia, and other metabolic abnormalities. The common presence of lipid abnormalities, such as elevated serum triglyceride- and low-density lipoprotein levels due to negative hormonal influences on the lipid homeostasis coexist with obesity and increased insulin resistance. PCOS shares components with the metabolic syndrome characterized by a combination of insulin resistance, dyslipidemia, and hypertension (Boomsma et al., 2006). Although a high BMI is associated with a higher risk of arterial disease, an increased cardiovascular risk (up to two-fold) in women with PCOS cannot be completely ascribed to a higher BMI (de Groot et al., 2011). Obesity and PCOS show, on the one hand, an independent influence, but, on the other hand, seem to have additive adverse effects on insulin action.

Up to 50% of women with PCOS suffer from an imbalance in carbohydrate homeostasis, central fat deposition, and increasing insulin resistance during pregnancy (Huang et al., 2010). It has been estimated that 25–70% of women with PCOS show a rise in insulin resistance and have an increased risk of developing complications during pregnancy, first and foremost of which is GDM (Godoy-Matos et al., 2009).

5. The risk of gestational diabetes in women with polycystic ovary syndrome

GDM is defined as the onset or first recognition and diagnosis of glucose intolerance during pregnancy. The diagnostic criterion for GDM is the 75g, two-hour oral glucose tolerance test (OGTT).

In fact, recent meta-analyses of pregnancy outcomes in women with PCOS demonstrated a significantly higher chance of developing GDM for PCOS women (odds ratios of about 2.90) (Boomsma et al., 2006) (Toulis et al., 2009). However, when analyzing the available evidence separately, there were largely conflicting results: while most of the studies demonstrated an increased risk for GDM in PCOS women (odds ratios ranging from 1.15 to 22.15) (Wortsman et al., 1991 as cited in Boomsma et al., 2006) (Radon et al., 1999, as cited in Boomsma et al., 2006), a few found odds ratios from 0.31 to 0.96 (Turhan et al., 2003, as cited in Boomsma et al., 2006) (Haakova et al., as cited in Boomsma et al., 2006). A comparison between the study designs revealed that the increased risks were predominantly found in cohort studies rather than in case-control studies. In addition, meta-analyses revealed a significant heterogeneity between the analyzed studies.

Conversely, some studies did not seem to support a higher prevalence and previous history of PCOS in women diagnosed with GDM, when compared to pregnancies in women with normal glucose homeostasis (Wijeyaratne et al., 2006) (Kousta et al., 2000). Obesity, PCOS, and diabetes in first-degree relatives have been described as risk factors for developing GDM and gestational impaired glucose tolerance, especially in young women and teenage pregnancies (<20 years) (Karcaaltincaba et al., 2011).

All in all, there is no solid evidence proving the increased risk for GDM in PCOS patients, but a trend assuming that the risk is, indeed, increased in women with PCOS, is recognizable. Confronted with the wide clinical and pathophysiological spectrum associated with the syndrome, further studies are warranted to validate the existing data.

5.1 Diagnostic aspects

The guidelines developed by the International Association of Diabetes and Pregnancy Study Groups (IADPSG) consider a screening for pre-gestational diabetes in high-risk women at the first prenatal visit and universal screening between the 24th and 28th week of gestation (Holt et al., 2011). In daily routine, an OGTT is performed in the third trimester. According to the diagnostic recommendations published in March 2010 by the IADPSG, fasting blood glucose concentrations that exceed 92 mg/dl, one-hour and two-hour glucose levels of more than 180 mg/dl, or 153 mg/dl measured during the OGTT, lead to the diagnosis of GDM (Metzger et al., 2010). Increased measurements in each of the three values raise the possibility of an adverse pregnancy outcome. A benefit of generalized testing to evaluate glycaemia levels in all pregnant women before the usual window is still a subject of controversy in the literature and must be decided individually (Karagiannis et al., 2010, Hadar et al., 2009). If increased levels of glucose are found in urine samples, or if GDM was present in a previous pregnancy, an OGTT in the second trimester should be performed. Since women who suffer from PCOS are considered to be at higher risk for developing GDM, it could be argued that they should undergo a more detailed and earlier screening for GDM.

5.2 Pathophysiological hypotheses about the risk of gestational diabetes in women with polycystic ovary syndrome

Several pathophysiologic mechanisms have been discussed that might contribute to the phenomenon of the increased GDM risk associated with PCOS.

5.2.1 Genetic predisposition

It has been hypothesized that a particular genetic background could contribute to the association between PCOS and GDM. In women with familial partial lipodystrophy due to LMNA (lamin A/C) mutations, a rare disorder characterized by a selective loss of adipose tissue and insulin resistance, the prevalence of PCOS and gestational diabetes was found to be higher than in the general population (Vantyghem et al., 2008). Moreover, mutations of the VNTR (variable number of tandem repeats) locus, upstream of the insulin gene (INS) where insulin expression is regulated, have been found in both women who suffer from PCOS and in women with GDM (Waterworth et al., 1997) (Lambrinoudaki et al., 2010).

5.2.2 Preexisting insulin resistance

In pregnancy, rising blood levels of lipolytic placental hormones lead to an elevation of free fatty acids that are commonly associated with the development of a dose-dependent insulin resistance. Affecting skeletal muscle glucose uptake, free fatty acids create a state of local insulin resistance and, as concentrations are elevated in late pregnancy, an increase in tissue insulin resistance can be observed during pregnancy (Sivan & Boden, 2003). In the presence of PCOS and a preexisting state of increased insulin resistance accompanying the syndrome, hyperglycemia seems to be induced more easily. The high pre-conception insulin resistance might have a deleterious additive effect on pancreatic beta cells, which are incapable of coping with the additive physiological insulin resistance of pregnancy (Khattab et al., 2011), thereby leading to an increased incidence of GDM (Toulis et al., 2009).

5.2.3 SHBG levels

Hyperinsulinemia stimulates in much the same way as LH-agonist ovarian testosterone production and decreases the serum sex hormone-binding globulin (SHBG) concentration. SHBG is known to have biologic functions beyond the regulation of free estrogen and testosterone serum levels. It has also been emphasized that low SHBG levels are associated with a minor glucose tolerance, thus, attributing a role to these low SHBG levels in the maintenance of glucose homeostasis. A possible explanation might be a modulation of the biologic effects of both estrogen and testosterone on liver, fat, and muscle tissue, as well as on other peripheral tissues (Ding et al., 2009). Furthermore, low plasma SHBG levels has been suggested as predictive for the risk of developing Type 2 diabetes mellitus (Ding et al., 2009). As an early indicator of GDM risk, low preconception levels of SHBG concentrations have been identified as strong predictors in PCOS women, independently of obesity and measures of insulin resistance. One study suggested that assessment of SHBG levels before conception might be a useful tool to by which to identify PCOS patients at risk for GDM during pregnancy (Veltman-Verhulst et al., 2010). However, the pathophysiologic pathways of this effect are unknown. It remains unclear whether the association between GDM and SHBG is direct or indirect. A lower SHBG results in higher free androgens that have already been demonstrated to be associated with an increased GDM risk (Bartha et al., 2000).

5.2.4 Insulin-like growth factor and insulin-like growth factor binding protein-1

The risk for GDM has been connected to maternal plasma concentrations of insulin-like growth factor-1 (IGF-1) and insulin-like growth factor binding protein-1 (IGFBP-1), suggesting that these determinants of glucose homeostasis play a potential role in the pathophysiologic process and contribute to the development of GDM (Qiu et al., 2005). Increased serum insulin concentrations lead to an inhibition of IGFBP-1 production, resulting in elevated serum levels of free IGF-1. A recent meta analysis on the interaction between IGFBP-1 and PCOS described lower levels of IGFBP-1 in affected patients (Kelly et al. 2011). Notably, a lower risk for developing GDM was correlated with increased levels of free IGF-1 and IGFBP-1, where higher C-peptide levels were positively associated with the development of GDM (Qiu et al., 2005). It should be emphasized that lower levels were found in obese women with/or without PCOS, compared to normal weight controls, suggesting that body weight has a certain influence on serum IGFBP-1 levels. The physiologic processes underlying the role of IGF-1 in glucose regulation are unclear. Infusions of IGF-1 are known to suppress glucose counter-regulatory hormones, such as glucagon and growth hormone (Jones & Clemmons, 1995). IGF-1 may also contribute to changes in insulin sensitivity and glucose uptake via direct IGF receptor-mediated effects on skeletal muscle (Sjogren et al., 2001). Alterations in IGFBP-1 concentrations may be due to variations in insulin secretion or hepatic insulin sensitivity, both known to be important factors in glucose regulation (Lee et al., 1997).

5.2.5 The influence of infertility treatments

PCOS is often accompanied by infertility that necessitates ovulation induction, using clomiphene citrate, gonadotropins, or even *in vitro* fertilization (IVF) (Boomsma et al., 2006). These treatment methods are known to increase the incidence of multiple pregnancies, as well as some negative consequences, including a rise in the risk for GDM (Schwartz et al., 1999). Furthermore, pregnancies established after IVF carry an increased risk for maternal complications (Pinborg et al., 2004) (Shevell et al., 2005). However, the increased risk of developing GDM has been suggested to occur independently of obesity, as well as in populations without assisted reproductive techniques (Boomsma et al., 2006) (Toulis et al., 2009).

6. Therapeutic considerations

The therapeutic challenges in the treatment of women with PCOS and GDM or impaired glucose tolerance arise from the diversity of recommendations and research conclusions. If adequately managed, the incidence of adverse perinatal outcomes in PCOS patients who develop GDM was found to be not significantly elevated (Li et al., 2010). Several treatment options exist for each of the symptoms of PCOS, and management of these patients depends on the individual symptoms. Clinical management of PCOS involves risk assessment for metabolic disorders, as diabetes and dyslipidemia, and for hypertension, cardiovascular complications, and liver diseases (Setji & Brown, 2007). Insulin-sensitizing drugs, such as metformin and/or oral contraceptives, are thought to improve the clinical features of PCOS, but limited data is available that assesses the true influence and safety of these drugs in this population (Setji & Brown, 2007). Targeting androgen symptoms, such as acne, hirsutism, and alopecia androgenica, estrogen-containing oral contraceptives, antiandrogens and topical agents are considered first-line therapy for women who do not want to conceive, as they effectively reduce serum androgen levels. In addition, treatment with oral contraceptives is associated with an improvement in the menstrual pattern. However, when trying to achieve pregnancy, other treatment options are offered to the patient. All of these might also independently influence the risk for GDM.

6.1 Lifestyle modifications

Addressing life-style factors before conception should be the first-line approach to reduce any further therapeutic strategies during pregnancy. The appearance of the varying phenotypes of PCOS depends, to a great extent, on lifestyle and environmental factors (Garruti et al., 2009). Reducing weight improves the endocrine profile and has the most significant impact on the likelihood of ovulation and pregnancy, the most relevant endpoints in infertile PCOS women. Dietary composition has been considered to improve the initial metabolic and reproductive situation in these patients. It has been suggested that low fat diets be recommended to these patients to produce a decrease in hyperinsulinemia (Reaven, 2005). Since it has been well-established that obesity is not only associated with anovulation, infertility, and early miscarriage, but also with late pregnancy complications in women with PCOS (Badawy & Elnashar, 2011), lifestyle modifications, including dietary recommendations and increased exercise in order to achieve weight reduction, should be recommended to these patients. Bariatric surgery has also been advocated as a possible strategy for weight loss in PCOS women, at least in the morbidly obese, and is effective in restoring ovulation and improving insulin resistance. Reducing weight, along with lifestyle modifications that affect the patients' behavior in a continuing way, is considered the most relevant therapeutic approach in women with PCOS (Hirschberg, 2009). Whether it affects the risk of developing GDM in subsequent pregnancies remains an open question (Escobar-Morreale et al., 2005).

6.2 Insulin-sensitizing drugs

Elevated insulin resistance plays an important part in the pathophysiology of PCOS and GDM. Insulin-sensitizing drugs, particularly metformin, are thought to reduce androgen symptoms, positively influence reproductive deregulations (oligo-amenorrhoe, anovulation), and increase pregnancy rates in PCOS patients (Dunaif, 2008). Large placebo-controlled trials are available only for metformin, as this is the only insulin-sensitizing drug with extensive clinical use in women with PCOS (De Leo et al., 2003).

6.2.1 Metformin as a PCOS-specific therapy

Metformin, a biguanide (see Figure 2), is a therapeutic option for restoration of ovulation in PCOS women. Moreover, several studies have suggested metformin as a promising medication in pregnancy in order to reduce the incidence of developing GDM and to minimize the risk for an adverse pregnancy outcome (Carlsen & Vanky, 2010). A variety of studies have been performed to determine the beneficial effects of metformin in PCOS, although the mechanisms of action–a broad spectrum of endocrine, metabolic, vascular, and even anti-inflammatory effects–of this drug have not been completely clarified, as yet (Khattab et al., 2011).

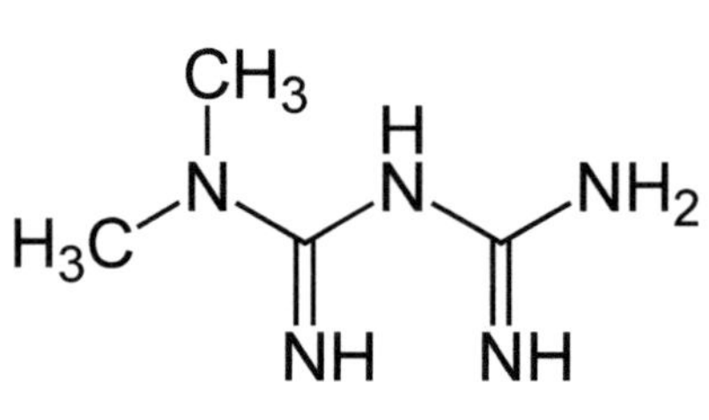

Fig. 2. Formula of metformin

Metformin affects the hepatic glucose output and the insulin-mediated glucose consumption in peripheral tissues, and suppresses the free fatty acid concentrations, which results in a lower substrate level for gluconeogenesis. Metformin improves insulin sensitivity and reduces insulin blood levels by increasing peripheral glucose utilization without negatively influencing normal blood glucose concentrations. With regard to pregnancy, a positive impact on uterine vascularity and blood flow and a reduction in plasma endothelin-1 levels, as well as androgen and LH concentrations, have been mentioned, suggesting that metformin is a possible positive therapeutic drug in the prevention of pregnancy complications in PCOS (Khattab et al., 2011). Thus, it has been assumed that metformin treatment combined with a special diet reduces pregnancy complications, and also prevents the fetus from elevated androgen concentrations (Glueck et al., 2004a).

Several studies have investigated a possible beneficial effect of metformin in the pregnancies of PCOS patients, particularly with regard to the risk of GDM. Some trials even report about a nine-fold (Begum et al., 2009) or ten-fold reduction (Glueck et al., 2002) of GDM after metformin treatment throughout pregnancy. However, the literature is controversial. The anticipated reduction in the prevalence of GDM after treatment with metformin during pregnancy could not be verified in randomized controlled trials, although metformin therapy had improved insulin sensitivity (Legro et al., 2007) (Fougner et al., 2008). In particular, recent large randomized controlled studies and meta analyses could not verify a relevant reduction of pregnancy complications due to metformin treatment (Vanky et al., 2010). Thus, the general use of metformin during pregnancy in non-diabetic women with PCOS cannot be recommended.

Metformin is associated with low gastrointestinal disturbances, but the available trials did not describe any serious adverse events. Classified as a category B drug in pregnancy, metformin appears to be non-teratogenic (Glueck et al., 2004b). However, results from placebo-controlled trials on maternal and fetal health risk have not yet been clarified. The pathogenesis of PCOS has been related to increased intrauterine androgen exposure; thus, the effect of therapeutic investigations on maternal and fetal hormone levels must be considered when treating pregnant women with PCOS. metformin seems to pass the placental barrier and was found to be present in the fetal circulation. However, androgen and estrogen levels did not seem to be influenced and remained within normal range (Carlsen & Vanky, 2010), whereas elevated SHBG levels have been reported in newborns after intrauterine metformin exposure (Vanky et al., 2005). The clinical relevance of these findings remains unclear.

6.3 Other methods of ovulation induction

With regard to pregnancy outcome, there are different possibilities of infertility treatment in women with PCOS and ovulatory dysfunction. Pregnancy induction by assisted reproductive techniques (ART) is offered if women fail to conceive spontaneously. Ovulation induction is based on two principles: (i) ovaries are exposed to a higher level of follicle stimulating hormone; and/or (ii) hormonal derangements are corrected. After exclusion of other causes of infertility, the fertility medication, clomiphen citrate (CC), is considered the first-line therapeutic approach to ovulation induction. In this approach, the development of a single ovulatory follicle is the main goal, since the risk for multiple pregnancies has to be kept as low as possible.

Literature on the risk for GDM as it relates to CC stimulation is scarce. To date, only one retrospective study has been published that compared the effects of CC stimulation and laparoscopic ovarian drilling in women pre-treated with metformin to those treated with metformin only. For all groups, there was a rate of GDM of about 30%, suggesting that neither CC stimulation nor laparoscopic ovarian drilling exert any effect on the risk for GDM (Ott et al., 2010).

For CC-resistant anovulatory PCOS patients, second-line therapeutic approaches include laparoscopic ovarian drilling and gonadotropin stimulation (Rotterdam ESHRE/ASRM-Sponsored PCOS Consensus Workshop Group, 2004). As mentioned above, only one trial has evaluated whether laparoscopic ovarian drilling would alter the risk for GDM and found no influence (Ott et al., 2010). Whether gonadotropin stimulation is associated with an increased rate of GDM remains controversial. While some studies found no difference in the prevalence of GDM between PCOS patients and controls (Vollenhoven et al., 2000), data from prospective studies suggest that medicamentous ovulation induction leads to an increased risk for GDM (Shevell et al., 2005).

When all of these treatment options fail, IVF remains the last option by which to achieve pregnancy (Badawy & Elnashar, 2011). It has been reported that the prevalence of GDM is substantially increased in women after pregnancy induction via ART than in PCOS patients who conceive spontaneously (Bals-Pratsch et al., 2011). Proceeding on the assumption of a - possibly genetically determined - highly deranged insulin metabolism that may lead to this state of infertility where women cannot conceive spontaneously or with the help of lower-dose stimulation protocols, the higher rate of GDM could be explained. One might raise the question whether the maternal endocrine status before placentation and/or after IVF stimulation possibly influences glucose tolerance in women with PCOS. Furthermore, elevated estrogen levels lead to an excessive stimulation of estrogen receptor alpha in the pancreatic beta cells, producing exaggerated insulin signaling that may cause an increased state of insulin resistance in peripheral tissues (Nadal et al., 2009).

Moreover, IVF is known to lead to an increased risk for maternal complications, including GDM independently of the presence of PCOS (Pinborg et al., 2004) (Shevell et al., 2005). When IVF stimulation is complicated by ovarian hyperstimulation syndrome (OHSS), the risk for GDM increases even more (Raziel et al., 2009). Notably, PCOS is a known risk factor for the development of OHSS. Higher rates of GDM, but also placental abruption prematurity and low birth weight have been reported for pregnancies complicated by severe OHSS. Therefore, these pregnancies should be considered high-risk pregnancies, and followed/treated as such. The best option to prevent OHSS is to use mild stimulation protocols (Raziel et al., (2009). However, metformin has also been mentioned as leading to a significant reduction in OHSS rates (Khattab et al., 2006).

7. Perinatal outcome of women with polycystic ovary syndrome and gestational diabetes

Hyperglycemia negatively influences not only maternal, but also fetal health. Obesity, fertility treatments, and other characteristics of patients with PCOS are associated with a higher incidence of pregnancy complications, such as hypertension and preeclampsia (Boomsma et al., 2008). Compared to normal pregnancies, PCOS patients demonstrate a higher incidence of early pregnancy loss (Li et al., 2010). Likewise, perinatal mortality seems to be increased among women with PCOS, and neonatal complications are observed more frequently (Boomsma et al., 2006). A potential additive effect of co-existent PCOS and GDM on obstetrical complications advocates for a closer antenatal and intrapartal monitoring of these patients (Alshammari et al., 2010). According to the Barker hypothesis, an altered maternal nutrition and metabolism is thought to lead both to an altered fetal nutrition and to changes in the endocrine and metabolic environment in which the fetus develops (de Boo & Harding 2006). This explains why PCOS complications might affect the fetus.

Maternal glucose levels correlate with fetal birth weight, development of fetal macrosomia, fetal hyperinsulinemia, and fetal body-fat percentage (Yang et al., 2002) (Metzger et al., 2010). Cesarean section is performed more frequently in women with GDM, as the diagnosis "large for gestational age" due to elevated maternal glucose levels is associated with a higher incidence of adverse pregnancy outcomes in spontaneous delivery (e.g., shoulder dystocia). PCOS also seems to correlate with a lower rate of vaginal delivery compared to healthy controls (Bjercke et al., 2002), although the higher incidence of Caesarean sections correlates with the occurrence of obesity, since women with a normal BMI and PCOS have an incidence of Caesarean section equal to that of age-matched controls (Boomsma et al., 2006).

Accordingly, the perinatal outcome of women with PCOS who develop GDM has been investigated intensively within the last several years. Both PCOS and associated factors, such as obesity or the treatment methods for fertility induction, can be considered responsible for the poorer pregnancy outcomes (Thatcher & Jackson, 2006, Boomsma et al., 2008). However, with regard to the risk of macrosomia, preeclampsia, neonatal complications, neonatal anomalies, and death of the fetus in women with GDM and PCOS, compared to women with GDM alone, no significant differences have been observed (Li et al., 2010). Manifest obesity before pregnancy and total weight gain during pregnancy must be closely monitored and addressed insistently, not only to minimize the risk for GDM, but also to achieve better global well-being in women with PCOS.

8. Conclusion and future research areas

The diverse observations regarding the elevated risk of GDM in women with PCOS have presented scientists and clinicians with a challenge. Caution is advised when interpreting clinical and statistical heterogeneous studies on PCOS and pregnancy complications, as a variety of contradictory results are present throughout the literature. The diagnosis of PCOS is inconsistent, as some investigators use only ultrasound criteria alone, and others rely on hormonal or clinical parameters, whereas the revised Rotterdam criteria are considered the current valid diagnostic criteria for the diagnosis of PCOS.

Women with PCOS who want to have children must be informed about the increased risk for developing GDM in their pregnancies. Metabolic findings in PCOS include increased insulin resistance, dyslipidemia, and elevated androgen levels - often accompanied by infertility and infertility treatments in order to achieve pregnancy. Confounding factors, such as obesity and the diverse ovulation induction treatments in infertile women with PCOS, can be considered potentially risk-increasing variables. Those coexisting factors, together with additional predisposing factors, such as a positive family history for diabetes mellitus, have been suggested to correlate with a generally increased risk for developing GDM and impaired glucose tolerance (Toulis et al., 2009).

Comparable pathophysiological mechanisms of insulin resistance and impaired glucose tolerance can be found in GDM and in women with PCOS who demonstrate an increased tissue resistance to insulin. However, the exact pathophysiologic link between PCOS and GDM has not yet been fully elucidated. Future scientific research could aim to clarify the association between PCOS and GDM and shed some new light on the possible underlying pathomechanisms. Moreover, further investigations to evaluate a potential benefit of early GDM screening are warranted, particularly as GDM is a well-known risk factor for fetal and maternal complications (Tieu et al., 2010).

The presence of increased glucose levels might lead to considerable pregnancy complications and stress on the mother and fetus. Accurate screening for GDM, together with regular consultations and monitoring, as well as addressing additional preventable stress factors, reduce the risk for developing GDM. Primary prevention can be further improved by lifestyle modification in women with PCOS. With regard to early diagnosis, screening in PCOS patients with a variety of risk factors might be justified. One might focus on the development of alternative markers to identify a woman at risk for developing GDM, in addition to the available parameters, such as fasting plasma glucose and OGTT, which enable clinicians to select patients at risk even before the manifestation of GDM. Thus, such markers as androgen levels, SHBG levels, fasting insulin levels, baseline proinsulin levels, and the hip-waist ratio might be of future interest.

Metformin has been highlighted as a promising substance for reducing the risk of GDM in PCOS patients. However, a relevant reduction of obstetrical complications due to metformin treatment could not be verified in a recent randomized and controlled multicenter study (Vanky et al., 2010). The general use of metformin during pregnancy in non-diabetic women with PCOS cannot be considered a valid recommendation.

Even with all the evidence and comparative studies, PCOS, still remains a challenging diagnostic and research issue, particularly with regard to its impact on GDM.

9. References

Azziz, R., Carmina, E., Dewailly, D., Diamanti-Kandarakis, E., Escobar-Morreale, H. F., Futterweit, W., Janssen, O. E., Legro, R. S., Norman, R. J., Taylor, A. E. & Witchel, S. F. (2006). Positions statement: criteria for defining polycystic ovary syndrome as a predominantly hyperandrogenic syndrome: an Androgen Excess Society guideline. J Clin Endocrinol Metab, Vol.91, No.11, pp. 4237-45, ISSN: 0021-972X

Badawy, A. & Elnashar, A. (2011). Treatment options for polycystic ovary syndrome. Int J Womens Health, Vol.3, pp. 25-35, ISSN: 1179-1411

Balen, A. (2004). The pathophysiology of polycystic ovary syndrome: trying to understand PCOS and its endocrinology. Best Pract Res Clin Obstet Gynaecol, Vol.18, No.5, (Octoberober 2004), pp. 685-706, ISSN: 1521-6934

Bals-Pratsch, M., Grosser, B., Seifert, B., Ortmann, O. & Seifarth, C. (2011). Early Onset and High Prevalence of Gestational Diabetes in PCOS and Insulin Resistant Women Before and After Assisted Reproduction. Exp Clin Endocrinol Diabetes, (March 3 2011), ISSN: 1439-3646

Baptiste, C. G., Battista, M. C., Trottier, A. & Baillargeon, J. P. (2010). Insulin and hyperandrogenism in women with polycystic ovary syndrome. J Steroid Biochem Mol Biol, Vol.122, No.1-2, (October 2010), pp. 42-52, ISSN: 1879-1220

Bartha, J. L., Comino-Delgado, R., Romero-Carmona, R. & Gomez-Jaen, M. C. (2000). Sex hormone-binding globulin in gestational diabetes. Acta Obstet Gynecol Scand, Vol.79, No.10, (October 2000), pp. 839-45, ISSN: 0001-6349

Battaglia, C., Regnani, G., Mancini, F., Iughetti, L., Flamigni, C. & Venturoli, S. (2002). Polycystic ovaries in childhood: a common finding in daughters of PCOS patients. A pilot study. Hum Reprod, Vol.17, No.3, (March 2002), 771-6, ISSN: 0268-1161

Begum, M. R., Khanam, N. N., Quadir, E., Ferdous, J., Begum, M. S., Khan, F. & Begum, A. (2009). Prevention of gestational diabetes mellitus by continuing metformin therapy throughout pregnancy in women with polycystic ovary syndrome. J Obstet Gynaecol Res, Vol.35, No.2, (April 2009), pp. 282-6, ISSN: 1341-8076

Boomsma, C. M., Eijkemans, M. J., Hughes, E. G., Visser, G. H., Fauser, B. C. & Macklon, N. S. (2006). A meta-analysis of pregnancy outcomes in women with polycystic ovary syndrome. Hum Reprod Update, Vol.12, No.6, (November-December 2006), pp. 673-83, ISSN: 1355-4786

Boomsma, C. M., Fauser, B. C. & Macklon, N. S. (2008). Pregnancy complications in women with polycystic ovary syndrome. Semin Reprod Med, Vol.26, No.1, (January 2008), 72-84, ISSN: 1526-8004

Carlsen, S. M. & Vanky, E. (2010). Metformin influence on hormone levels at birth, in PCOS mothers and their newborns. Hum Reprod, Vol.25, No.3, (March 2010), pp. 786-90, ISSN: 1460-2350

De Groot, P. C., Dekkers, O. M., Romijn, J. A., Dieben, S. W. & Helmerhorst, F. M. (2011). PCOS, coronary heart disease, stroke and the influence of obesity: a systematic review and meta-analysis. Hum Reprod Update, (February 2011), ISSN: 1460-2369

De Leo, V., la Marca, A. & Petraglia, F. (2003). Insulin-lowering agents in the management of polycystic ovary syndrome. Endocr Rev, Vol.24, No.5, (October, 2003), pp. 633-67, ISSN: 0163-769X

Ding, E. L., Song, Y., Manson, J. E., Hunter, D. J., Lee, C. C., Rifai, N., Buring, J. E., Gaziano, J. M. & Liu, S. (2009). Sex hormone-binding globulin and risk of type 2 diabetes in women and men. N Engl J Med, Vol.361, No.12, (September 2009), pp. 1152-63, ISSN: 1533-4406

Dumesic, D. A., Abbott, D. H. & Padmanabhan, V. (2007). Polycystic ovary syndrome and its developmental origins. Rev Endocr Metab Disord, Vol.8, No.2, (November 2006), pp.127-41, ISSN: 1389-9155

Dunaif, A. (2008). Drug insight: insulin-sensitizing drugs in the treatment of polycystic ovary syndrome--a reappraisal. Nat Clin Pract Endocrinol Metab, Vol.4, No.5, (May 2008), pp. 272-83, ISSN: 1745-8374

Escobar-Morreale, H. F., Botella-Carretero, J. I., Alvarez-Blasco, F., Sancho, J. & San Millan, J. L. (2005). The polycystic ovary syndrome associated with morbid obesity may resolve after weight loss induced by bariatric surgery. J Clin Endocrinol Metab, Vol.90, No.12, (December 2005), pp. 6364-9, ISSN: 0021-972X

Fougner, K. J., Vanky, E. & Carlsen, S. M. (2008). Metformin has no major effects on glucose homeostasis in pregnant women with PCOS: results of a randomized double-blind study. Scand J Clin Lab Invest, Vol.68, No.8, pp. 771-6, ISSN: 1502-7686

Franks, S., Gharani, N., Waterworth, D., Batty, S., White, D., Williamson, R. & McCarthy, M. (1998). Current developments in the molecular genetics of the polycystic ovary syndrome. Trends Endocrinol Metab, Vol.9, No.2, (February 1998), pp. 51-4, ISSN: 1043-2760

Garruti, G., Depalo, R., Vita, M. G., Lorusso, F., Giampetruzzi, F., Damato, A. B. & Giorgino, F. (2009). Adipose tissue, metabolic syndrome and polycystic ovary syndrome: from pathophysiology to treatment. Reprod Biomed Online, Vol.19, No.4, (October 2009), pp. 552-63, ISSN: 1472-6491

Gleicher, N., Barad, D. & Weghofer, A. (2007). Functional autoantibodies, a new paradigm in autoimmunity? Autoimmun Rev, Vol.7, No.1, (November 2007), 42-5, ISSN: 1568-9972

Glueck, C. J., Wang, P., Kobayashi, S., Phillips, H. & Sieve-Smith, L. (2002). Metformin therapy throughout pregnancy reduces the development of gestational diabetes in women with polycystic ovary syndrome. Fertil Steril, Vol.77, No.3, (March 2002), pp. 520-5, ISSN: 0015-0282

Glueck, C. J., Goldenberg, N., Wang, P., Loftspring, M. & Sherman, A. (2004a). Metformin during pregnancy reduces insulin, insulin resistance, insulin secretion, weight, testosterone and development of gestational diabetes: prospective longitudinal assessment of women with polycystic ovary syndrome from preconception throughout pregnancy. Hum Reprod, Vol.19, No.3, (March 2004), pp. 510-21, ISSN: 0268-1161

Glueck, C. J., Goldenberg, N., Pranikoff, J., Loftspring, M., Sieve, L. & Wang, P. (2004b). Height, weight, and motor-social development during the first 18 months of life in 126 infants born to 109 mothers with polycystic ovary syndrome who conceived on and continued metformin through pregnancy. Hum Reprod, Vol.19, No.6, (June 2004), pp. 1323-30, ISSN: 0268-1161

Godoy-Matos, A. F., Vaisman, F., Pedrosa, A. P., Farias, M. L., Mendonca, L. M. & Pinheiro, M. F. (2009). Central-to-peripheral fat ratio, but not peripheral body fat, is related to insulin resistance and androgen markers in polycystic ovary syndrome. Gynecol Endocrinol, Vol.25, No.12, (December 2009), pp. 793-8, ISSN: 1473-0766

Hadar, E., Oats, J. & Hod, M. (2009). Towards new diagnostic criteria for diagnosing GDM: the HAPO study. J Perinat Med, Vol.37, No.5, 447-9, ISSN: 1619-3997

Hirschberg, A. L. (2009). Polycystic ovary syndrome, obesity and reproductive implications. Womens Health (Lond Engl), Vol.5, No.5, (September 2009), pp. 529-40; quiz 541-2, ISSN: 1745-506

Holt, R. I., Coleman, M. A. & McCance, D. R. (2011). The implications of the new International Association of Diabetes and Pregnancy Study Groups (IADPSG) diagnostic criteria for gestational diabetes. Diabet Med, (January 2011), ISSN: 1464-5491

Huang, A., Brennan, K. & Azziz, R. (2010). Prevalence of hyperandrogenemia in the polycystic ovary syndrome diagnosed by the National Institutes of Health 1990 criteria. Fertil Steril, Vol.93, No.6, (April 2010), pp. 1938-41, ISSN: 1556-5653

Jones, J. I. & Clemmons, D. R. (1995). Insulin-like growth factors and their binding proteins: biological actions. Endocr Rev, Vol.16, No.1, (February 1995), 3-34, ISSN: 0163-769X

Karagiannis, T., Bekiari, E., Manolopoulos, K., Paletas, K. & Tsapas, A. (2010). Gestational diabetes mellitus: why screen and how to diagnose. Hippokratia, Vol.14, No. 3, (July 2010), pp. 151-4, ISSN: 1790-8019

Karcaaltincaba, D., Buyukkaragoz, B., Kandemir, O., Yalvac, S., Kiykac-Altinbas, S. & Haberal, A. (2011). Gestational diabetes and gestational impaired glucose tolerance in 1653 teenage pregnancies: prevalence, risk factors and pregnancy outcomes. J Pediatr Adolesc Gynecol, Vol.24, No.2, (April 2011), pp. 62-5, ISSN: 1873-4332

Kelly, C. J., Stenton, S. R. & Lashen, H. (2011). Insulin-like growth factor binding protein-1 in PCOS: a systematic review and meta-analysis. Hum Reprod Update, Vol.17, No.1, (January-February 2011), 4-16, ISSN: 1460-2369

Khattab, S., Mohsen, I. A., Aboulfoutouh, I., Mohsen, M. N., Van Wely, M., Van der Veen, F. & Youssef, M. (2011). Can metformin reduce the incidence of gestational diabetes mellitus in pregnant women with polycystic ovary syndrome? Prospective cohort study. Gynecol Endocrinol, (January 2011), ISSN: 1473-0766

Kousta, E., Cela, E., Lawrence, N., Penny, A., Millauer, B., White, D., Wilson, H., Robinson, S., Johnston, D., McCarthy, M. & Franks, S. (2000). The prevalence of polycystic ovaries in women with a history of gestational diabetes. Clin Endocrinol (Oxf) Vol. 53, No.4, (October 2000), pp. 501-7, ISSN: 0300-0664

Lambrinoudaki, I., Vlachou, S. A. & Creatsas, G. (2010). Genetics in gestational diabetes mellitus: association with incidence, severity, pregnancy outcome and response to treatment. Curr Diabetes Rev, Vol.6, No.6, (November 2010), pp. 393-9, ISSN: 1875-6417

Lee, P. D., Giudice, L. C., Conover, C. A. & Powell, D. R. (1997). Insulin-like growth factor binding protein-1: recent findings and new directions. Proc Soc Exp Biol Med, Vol.216, No.3, (December 1997), pp. 319-57, ISSN: 0037-9727

Legro, R. S., Gnatuk, C. L., Kunselman, A. R. & Dunaif, A. (2005). Changes in glucose tolerance over time in women with polycystic ovary syndrome: a controlled study. J Clin Endocrinol Metab, Vol.90, No.6, (June 2005), pp. 3236-42, ISSN: 0021-972X

Legro, R. S., Barnhart, H. X., Schlaff, W. D., Carr, B. R., Diamond, M. P., Carson, S. A., Steinkampf, M. P., Coutifaris, C., McGovern, P. G., Cataldo, N. A., Gosman, G. G., Nestler, J. E., Giudice, L. C., Leppert, P. C. & Myers, E. R. (2007). Clomiphene, metformin, or both for infertility in the polycystic ovary syndrome. N Engl J Med, Vol.356, No.6, (February 8 2007), 551-66, ISSN: 1533-4406

Li, G., Fan, L., Zhang, L., Zhang, W. & Huang, X. (2010). Metabolic parameters and perinatal outcomes of gestational diabetes mellitus in women with polycystic ovary syndrome. J Perinat Med, Vol.38, No.2, (November 2005), 141-6, ISSN: 1619-3997

Matalliotakis, I., Kourtis, A., Koukoura, O. & Panidis, D. (2006). Polycystic ovary syndrome: etiology and pathogenesis. Arch Gynecol Obstet, Vol.274, No.4, (July 2006), 187-97, ISSN: 0932-0067

Metzger, B. E., Gabbe, S. G., Persson, B., Buchanan, T. A., Catalano, P. A., Damm, P., Dyer, A. R., Leiva, A., Hod, M., Kitzmiler, J. L., Lowe, L. P., McIntyre, H. D., Oats, J. J., Omori, Y. & Schmidt, M. I. (2010). International association of diabetes and pregnancy study groups recommendations on the diagnosis and classification of hyperglycemia in pregnancy. Diabetes Care, Vol.33, No.3, (March 2010), pp.676-82, ISSN: 1935-5548

Mulders, A. G., Laven, J. S., Eijkemans, M. J., de Jong, F. H., Themmen, A. P. & Fauser, B. C. (2004). Changes in anti-Mullerian hormone serum concentrations over time suggest delayed ovarian ageing in normogonadotrophic anovulatory infertility. Hum Reprod, Vol.19, No.9, (September 2004), pp. 2036-42, ISSN: 0268-1161

Nadal, A., Alonso-Magdalena, P., Soriano, S., Quesada, I. & Ropero, A. B. (2009). The pancreatic beta-cell as a target of estrogens and xenoestrogens: Implications for blood glucose homeostasis and diabetes. Mol Cell Endocrinol, Vol.304, No.1-2, (May 25 2009), pp. 63-8, ISSN: 1872-8057

Ott, J., Kurz, C., Nouri, K., Wirth, S., Vytiska-Binstorfer, E., Huber, J. C. & Mayerhofer, K. (2010). Pregnancy outcome in women with polycystic ovary syndrome comparing the effects of laparoscopic ovarian drilling and clomiphene citrate stimulation in women pre-treated with metformin: a retrospective study. Reprod Biol Endocrinol, Vol.8, pp. 45, ISSN: 1477-7827

Ott, J., Aust, S., Kurz, C., Nouri, K., Wirth, S., Huber, J. C. & Mayerhofer, K. (2010). Elevated antithyroid peroxidase antibodies indicating Hashimoto's thyroiditis are associated with the treatment response in infertile women with polycystic ovary syndrome. Fertil Steril, Vol.94, No.7, (December 2010), pp. 2895-7, ISSN: 1556-5653

Pinborg, A., Loft, A., Schmidt, L., Langhoff-Roos, J. & Andersen, A. N. (2004). Maternal risks and perinatal outcome in a Danish national cohort of 1005 twin pregnancies: the role of in vitro fertilization. Acta Obstet Gynecol Scand, Vol.83, No.1, (January 2004), pp. 75-84, ISSN: 0001-6349

Qiu, C., Vadachkoria, S., Meryman, L., Frederick, I. O. & Williams, M. A. (2005). Maternal plasma concentrations of IGF-1, IGFBP-1, and C-peptide in early pregnancy and subsequent risk of gestational diabetes mellitus. Am J Obstet Gynecol, Vol.193, No.5, (November 2005), pp. 1691-7, ISSN: 1097-6868

Raziel, A., Schachter, M., Friedler, S. & Ron-El, R. (2009). Outcome of IVF pregnancies following severe OHSS. Reprod Biomed Online, Vol.19, No.1, (July 2009), 61-5, ISSN: 1472-6491

Reaven, G. M. (2005). Insulin resistance, the insulin resistance syndrome, and cardiovascular disease. Panminerva Med, Vol.47, No.4, (December, 2005), pp. 201-10, ISSN: 0031-0808

Retnakaran, R., Qi, Y., Sermer, M., Connelly, P. W., Hanley, A. J. & Zinman, B. (2008). Glucose intolerance in pregnancy and future risk of pre-diabetes or diabetes. Diabetes Care, Vol.31, No. 10, (Octoberober 2008), pp. 2026-31, ISSN: 1935-5548

Schwartz, D. B., Daoud, Y., Zazula, P., Goyert, G., Bronsteen, R., Wright, D. & Copes, J. (1999). Gestational diabetes mellitus: metabolic and blood glucose parameters in singleton versus twin pregnancies. Am J Obstet Gynecol, Vol.181, No.4, (October 1999), pp. 912-4, ISSN: 0002-9378

Setji, T. L. & Brown, A. J. (2007). Comprehensive clinical management of polycystic ovary syndrome. Minerva Med, Vol.98, No.3, (June 2007), pp. 175-89, ISSN: 0026-4806

Shevell, T., Malone, F. D., Vidaver, J., Porter, T. F., Luthy, D. A., Comstock, C. H., Hankins, G. D., Eddleman, K., Dolan,

S., Dugoff, L., Craigo, S., Timor, I. E., Carr, S. R., Wolfe, H. M., Bianchi, D. W. & D'Alton, M. E. (2005). Assisted reproductive technology and pregnancy outcome. Obstet Gynecol, Vol.106, No.5, pp. 1039-45, ISSN: 0029-7844

Sivan, E. & Boden, G. (2003). Free fatty acids, insulin resistance, and pregnancy. Curr Diab Rep, Vol.3, No.4, (August 2003), pp. 319-22, ISSN: 1534-4827

Sjogren, K., Wallenius, K., Liu, J. L., Bohlooly, Y. M., Pacini, G., Svensson, L., Tornell, J., Isaksson, O. G., Ahren, B., Jansson, J. O. & Ohlsson, C. (2001). Liver-derived IGF-I is of importance for normal carbohydrate and lipid metabolism. Diabetes, Vol.50, No.7, (July 2001), 1539-45, ISSN: 0012-1797

Stein, I. F., Sr. (1958). The Stein-Leventhal syndrome; a curable form of sterility. N Engl J Med, Vol.259, No.9, pp. 420-423, ISSN: 0028-4793

Thatcher, S. S. & Jackson, E. M. (2006). Pregnancy outcome in infertile patients with polycystic ovary syndrome who were treated with metformin. Fertil Steril, Vol.85, No.4, (April 2006), 1002-9, ISSN: 1556-5653

Thessaloniki ESHRE/ASRM-Sponsored PCOS Consensus Workshop Group. (2004). Revised 2003 consensus on diagnostic criteria and long-term health risks related to polycystic ovary syndrome. Fertil Steril, Vol.81, No.1, pp.19-25, ISSN: 0015-0282

Tieu, J., Middleton, P., McPhee, A. J. & Crowther, C. A. (2010). Screening and subsequent management for gestational diabetes for improving maternal and infant health. Cochrane Database Syst Rev, CD007222, ISSN: 1469-493X

Toulis, K. A., Goulis, D. G., Kolibianakis, E. M., Venetis, C. A., Tarlatzis, B. C. & Papadimas, I. (2009). Risk of gestational diabetes mellitus in women with polycystic ovary syndrome: a systematic review and a meta-analysis. Fertil Steril, Vol.92, No.2, (August 2009), 667-77, ISSN: 1556-5653

Vanky, E., Zahlsen, K., Spigset, O. & Carlsen, S. M. (2005). Placental passage of metformin in women with polycystic ovary syndrome. Fertil Steril, Vol. 83, No.5, (May 2005), pp. 1575-8, ISSN: 1556-5653

Vanky, E., Stridsklev, S., Heimstad, R., Romundstad, P., Skogoy, K., Kleggetveit, O., Hjelle, S., von Brandis, P., Eikeland, T., Flo, K., Berg, K. F., Bunford, G., Lund, A., Bjerke, C., Almas, I., Berg, A. H., Danielson, A., Lahmami, G. & Carlsen, S. M. (2010). Metformin versus placebo from first trimester to delivery in polycystic ovary syndrome: a randomized, controlled multicenter study. J Clin Endocrinol Metab, Vol.95, No.12, (December 2010), pp. 448-55, ISSN: 1945-7197

Vantyghem, M. C., Vincent-Desplanques, D., Defrance-Faivre, F., Capeau, J., Fermon, C., Valat, A. S., Lascols, O., Hecart, A. C., Pigny, P., Delemer, B., Vigouroux, C. & Wemeau, J. L. (2008). Fertility and obstetrical complications in women with LMNA-related familial partial lipodystrophy. J Clin Endocrinol Metab, Vol.93, No.6, (June 2008), pp. 2223-9, ISSN: 0021-972X

Veltman-Verhulst, S. M., van Haeften, T. W., Eijkemans, M. J., de Valk, H. W., Fauser, B. C. & Goverde, A. J. (2010). Sex hormone-binding globulin concentrations before conception as a predictor for gestational diabetes in women with polycystic ovary syndrome. Hum Reprod, Vol.25, No.12, (December 2010), pp. 3123-8, ISSN: 1460-2350

Vollenhoven, B., Clark, S., Kovacs, G., Burger, H. & Healy, D. (2000). Prevalence of gestational diabetes mellitus in polycystic ovarian syndrome (PCOS) patients pregnant after ovulation induction with gonadotrophins. Aust N Z J Obstet Gynaecol, Vol.40, No.1, (February 2000), pp. 54-8, ISSN: 0004-8666

Waterworth, D. M., Bennett, S. T., Gharani, N., McCarthy, M. I., Hague, S., Batty, S., Conway, G. S., White, D., Todd, J. A., Franks, S. & Williamson, R. (1997). Linkage and association of insulin gene VNTR regulatory polymorphism with polycystic ovary syndrome. Lancet, Vol.349, No.9057, (April 5 1997), pp. 986-90, ISSN: 0140-6736

Wijeyaratne, C. N., Waduge, R., Arandara, D., Arasalingam, A., Sivasuriam, A., Dodampahala, S. H. & Balen, A. H. (2006). Metabolic and polycystic ovary syndromes in indigenous South Asian women with previous gestational diabetes mellitus. BJOG, Vol.113, No.10, (October 2006), pp. 1182-7, ISSN: 1470-0328

11

Impact and Mechanisms of Pancreatic Beta-Cell Mass Programming by Maternal Diabetes - Insight from Animal Model Studies

Audrey Chavey, Jamileh Movassat and Bernard Portha
Laboratoire B2PE (Biologie et Pathologie du Pancréas Endocrine),
Unité BFA (Biologie Fonctionnelle et Adaptive),
Université Paris-Diderot, Paris,
France

1. Introduction

The incidence of type 2 diabetes mellitus (T2D) is growing worldwide. It is now established that interactions between the individual genetic makeup and environment contribute to the development of T2D. In this review, we first discuss the evidence for beta-cell dysfunction in IUED (*in utero* exposure to maternal diabetes), IUEO (*in utero* exposure to maternal overnutrition) and IUGR (*in utero* growth restriction) humans. We then evaluate relevant animal models of IUED, IUEO and IUGR focusing on the strengths and limits of each, in order to define critical periods and types of alterations that can lead to impaired beta-cell function. Finally, we discuss several potential mechanisms dissected in relevant animal models that begin to explain these outcomes.

2. Perinatal risk factors for diabetes in later life: Human studies

There are strong arguments showing that T2D is more prevalent among subjects that were exposed to maternal diabetes *in utero* (IUED). The role of maternal inheritance in T2D was first suggested by epidemiological studies. A higher susceptibility for diabetes is described in descendents from diabetic great grand mothers via the maternal line than via the paternal line (Dörner et al., 1984). A higher incidence of T2D and of gestational diabetes (GD) is seen in children of diabetic mothers as compared to those of diabetic fathers (Martin et al., 1985). A decreased prevalence of diabetes is seen in children from diabetic mothers, after starting a systematic treatment of diabetic pregnant women (Dörner et al., 1987). Especially interesting in this context are the studies on the Pima Indians, a population with an exceptionally high T2D incidence. The prevalence of impaired glucose tolerance, of T2D and of GD is much higher (7 fold increased) in children from mothers who had diabetes during pregnancy, than in children from mothers who developed diabetes only after their pregnancy. Moreover, paternal diabetes has a much smaller effect on the prevalence of diabetes in these offspring than maternal diabetes (Pettitt, 1996).
The maternal influence in the development of T2D was reported in a majority of studies (Alcolado et al., 2002). Although some studies did not find a maternal effect, none reported a

higher paternal transmission (Mitchell et al., 1993; Mc Carthy et al., 1996; Viswanathan et al., 1996; Frayling et al., 1999). The prospective Framingham Offspring Study in which all offspring and parents were formally tested for diabetes, demonstrated that the risk of impaired glucose tolerance or T2D was greater in offspring of mothers with early diabetes onset (before 50), suggesting the role of fetal environment (Meigs et al., 2000). However, the effects of fetal exposure to diabetes may be confounded by genetic factors. Mothers who had T2D before or during pregnancy have, by definition, early diabetes. Therefore, they may carry T2D susceptibility genes, which are transmitted to their offspring. To determine the role of the intrauterine diabetic environment per se, the prevalence of diabetes was compared in Pima nuclear families in which at least one sibling was born before and one after the mother was diagnosed with T2D. Offspring born after their mother displayed diabetes had a 4-fold higher risk of diabetes and a higher body mass index (BMI) than their full siblings born before their mother developed diabetes (Dabelea et al., 2000). These findings indicate that intrauterine exposure to a diabetic environment increases risk of obesity and T2D beyond that attributable to genetic factors, at least in Pima Indians. In Caucasians, offspring whose mothers had pregestational diabetes (type 1 or 2) or gestational diabetes had a higher frequency of impaired glucose tolerance (IGT). (Plagemann et al., 1997). Carriers of mutations in the MODY gene hepatocyte nuclear factor 1 alpha whose mothers had diabetes when they were *in utero*, were diagnosed with diabetes 8 years earlier than those who inherited the mutation from the father (Stride et al. 2002). To circumvent the confounding effect of genes linked to early onset T2D and transmitted by the pregnant T2D mother, the effect of fetal exposure to T1D was evaluated in adult offspring lacking T1D immunological markers. A 33% prevalence of IGT was reported in offspring of T1D mothers compared with none in offspring of T1D fathers (control group) (Sobngwi et al., 2003). Altogether, these findings suggest that fetal exposure to maternal diabetes is indeed associated with abnormal glucose homeostasis in offspring and may participate in the excess of maternal transmission in T2D.

There are some studies related to the metabolic defects associated with fetal exposure to maternal diabetes in human offspring. The typical feature of infants of diabetic mothers is fetal macrosomia and high birth weight. A correlation between high birth weight and later impairment of glucose tolerance therefore is expected. Among Pima Indians high birth weight increases the risk of developing diabetes in later life (Pettitt, 1996). In the population of Malta, with a high prevalence of type-2 diabetes, woman with high birth weight have an increased risk of developing gestational diabetes. Birth weight is significantly higher in mothers with a family history of diabetes from the maternal side than from the paternal side, and than in those with no family history of diabetes (Savona-Ventura & Chircop, 2002). The relation between large babies and later impaired glucose tolerance in these studies appears to be related to the macrosomia of babies from diabetic mothers.

Two studies reported that IGT in offspring exposed to intrauterine diabetic environment resulted from decreased insulin action based on finding of a high insulin-to-glucose ratio during oral glucose challenge (Plagemann et al., 1997; Silverman et al., 1995). However, fetal exposure to maternal T1D was not associated with reduced insulin sensitivity (minimal model) in young offspring (Hunter et al., 2004). Offspring of T2D mothers tended to have decreased insulin action, but were heavier compared with offspring of healthy mothers (Hunter et al., 2004). In adult Pima Indians with normal glucose tolerance and who had been exposed to an intrauterine diabetic environment, acute insulin response to iv glucose was found reduced in those offspring whose mother was diabetic before pregnancy while it remained normal in those whose mother developed diabetes after pregnancy (Gautier et al., 2001). Body fat and insulin sensitivity (euglycemic hyperinsulinemic clamp) were similar in the two groups of subjects (Gautier et al., 2001). In the same study, acute insulin response was found reduced in offspring of parents (mother or father) with early onset of T2D (Gautier et al., 2001), suggesting that gene(s) linked to early onset diabetes is(are) associated with reduced insulin secretory response to glucose (Hanson et al., 1995). Offspring of T1D mothers had reduced insulin secretion, more pronounced in IGT subjects, but similar fat mass and insulin action compared with offspring of T1D fathers (Sobngwi et al., 2003). Also in non-diabetic offspring of mothers with young-onset T2D (diagnosed under age 50), beta-cell function (early insulin release after oral glucose) was found decreased as compared to that of offspring of fathers with young-onset T2D (Singh et al., 2006).

Therefore human studies suggest that insulin secretion defect participates to the abnormal glucose tolerance observed in adult offspring exposed to maternal diabetes during fetal life. Importantly, they showed that insulin secretion may be reduced even in normal glucose-tolerant offspring. Nevertheless, in children and adolescent offspring, insulin resistance involvement was suggested and may be related, at least in part, to their higher body weight.

Besides IUED populations, evidence continues to mount showing that T2D is also more prevalent among subjects that were intrauterine growth restricted (IUGR). The first study to link low birth weight to increased T2D risk was conducted in a group of men born in Hertfordshire, UK, who were 64 years old at the time of the study. Those men who had the lowest birth weight were 6 times more likely to currently have either impaired glucose tolerance or T2D than those men who were heaviest at birth (Hales et al., 1991). These findings have been reproduced in over 40 populations worldwide, including many ethnic groups. In some cohorts where there is a high prevalence of maternal obesity, there is also increased risk of diabetes at the high-birth weight end of the spectrum (U-shaped curve for diabetes risk distribution). This is thought to reflect the increased risk of diabetes in the macrosomic offspring of women with gestational diabetes (Nathanielsz et al., 2007). Some of the strongest evidence in support of the role for environment in underlying the relationship between fetal growth and T2D had come from the study of twins. Studies of adult twins in Denmark revealed that, in both monozygotic (identical) and dizygotic (nonidentical) twin pairs who were discordant for T2D, the diabetic twin had a significantly lower birth weight than the normoglycemic cotwin (Poulsen et al., 1997). If it is assumed that the monozygotic twins are genetically identical, then, the difference in birth weight must be related to the fetal environment. These studies thus provide strong evidence for the importance of a nongenetic intrauterine factor in the development of type 2 diabetes in later life. Assessing the impact of maternal nutrition on the health of offspring in humans is difficult. Investigations involving individuals conceived during conditions of famine have provided direct evidence of the effects exerted by maternal nutrition during gestation and lactation on the overall health of the adult offspring. The Dutch famine, which occurred in the western part of The Netherlands at the end of World War II, was a short period of famine lasting from December 1944 to May 1945. Prior to the onset of the famine, the affected area of The Netherlands consisted of a reasonably well-nourished population. The occurrence of this abrupt famine therefore granted researchers a unique opportunity to retrospectively study the effect of maternal nutrition on offspring's glucose tolerance. Compared with individuals born the year before the famine, those who were in utero during the famine had higher plasma glucose levels, 2 h after a standard oral glucose tolerance test (Ravelli et al., 1998).

However this association was not observed in the Leningrad Siege Study (Stanner et al., 1997). The inconsistent results might be due to differences in postnatal environmental life exposures. Although the Dutch population rapidly developed into a wealthy and rich population after the famine, the Leningrad people remained relatively poor. In a more recent study of a large sample of Chinese adults, a significant association was found between severe famine exposure during the fetal period and an increased risk of hyperglycemia in adulthood (Li et al., 2010). The association was stronger in subjects with a Western dietary pattern or higher economic status in adulthood. No consistent association was observed between famine exposure during childhood and hyperglycemia. These studies therefore provided direct evidence that poor maternal nutrition leads to increased susceptibility to T2D in the offspring.

The mechanisms that underlie the association between poor maternal nutrition and T2D are unclear. Several studies in children and adults have shown that non-diabetic and pre-diabetic subjects with low birth weight are insulin resistant and, thus, predisposed to develop T2D (Barker, 2004; Valdez et al., 1994; Bhargawa et al., 2004; Li et al., 2001; Boney et al., 2005; Clausen et al., 1997; Flanagan et al., 2000). Adults born small for gestational age showed a significantly higher percentage of body fat (Jaquet et al., 2000) and their insulin sensitivity adjusted for either BMI or total fat mass, was markedly decreased. In fact in was first thought that the adverse effect of IUGR on glucose homeostasis is mediated through programming of the fetal endocrine pancreas (Hales et al., 1991), since IUGR infants have reduced plasma concentrations of insulin (Economides et al., 1989) and beta-cell numbers (Van Assche et al., 1977). However, several studies found no impact of low birth weight on insulin secretion in humans (Barker, 2004; Clausen et al., 1997; Flanagan et al., 2000). To address this discrepancy and since insulin sensitivity per se has a profound impact on insulin secretion, Jensen et al. (2002) measured both insulin secretion and insulin sensitivity in well-matched Caucasian glucose-tolerant men either IUGR or controls. To eliminate the major confounders, such as 'diabetes genes', none of the participants had a family history of diabetes, hypertension and ischemic heart disease. There was no difference between the groups with regard to current weight, body mass index (BMI), body composition and lipid profile. When adjusted for insulin sensitivity, insulin secretion was found reduced by 30%. However insulin sensitivity was found normal in the IUGR subjects. The authors hypothesized that defects in insulin secretion might precede defects in insulin action and that when IUGR individuals accumulate body fat, they develop insulin resistance (Jensen et al., 2002). This is entirely consistent with the concept that despite insulin resistance being a crucial component of T2D in humans, the failure of beta-cell function and growth determines progression to the diabetic phenotype (Weir et al., 2001). Thus, decreased substrate availability to the IUGR fetus caused by uteroplacental insufficiency might have permanently impaired pancreatic beta-cell growth by neogenesis and proliferation processes which take place mostly during the fetal-neonatal period. This is consistent with the observation that pancreatic tissue taken from human fetuses with severe IUGR is characterized by a reduction in endocrine cell mass (Van Assche & Aerts, 1979). However this has not been confirmed since no difference was also found between IUGR and control human fetuses in insulin-positive area or islet organization during the last two months of pregnancy (Beringue et al., 2002).

To summarize, what are the more common factors that confer coincident risk of T2D and low birth weight? Although alterations in both insulin secretion and insulin action are possible, a number of points support the hypothesis that early impairment in beta-cell development leads to fetal growth and predispose individuals to development of T2D later in life. Indeed, beta-cell mass deficit has been increasingly recognized as a central cause of T2D over the years (Meier, 2008). The importance of beta-cell mass for T2D risk has been further highlighted by the results of recent genome-wide scans that have linked the likelihood of developing T2D to genetic defects in insulin secretion (Saxena et al., 2007; Scott et al., 2007; Zeggini et al., 2007). Importantly, among these T2D loci, two of them (CDKAL1 and HHEX-IDE) which are associated with significant impairments in beta-cell function (Pascoe et al., 2008; Groenewoud et al., 2008), have been related to low birth weight (Freathy et al., 2009). In this case, the most likely explanation for the association between low birth weight and T2D risk seems to be a genetically determined defective development of beta-cells leading to insufficient insulin secretion. The intrauterine insulin deficiency may then impair fetal growth (Terauchi et al., 2000), while insufficient insulin secretion later in life may confer T2D risk.

3. Perinatal risk factors for diabetes in later life - Animal studies

Thank to abundant studies, mostly in rodents in which the foetal environment can be manipulated, a substantial body of data now addresses the mechanisms involved in the developmental programming of glucose intolerance and T2D.

3.1 IUED models

In rat, maternal diabetes may be induced experimentally by streptozotocin (STZ) injection that selectively destroys beta-cells. Mild or severe diabetes ensue depending on the dose used. At birth, the progeny of mild diabetic mothers had normal weight or slight macrosomia and an enhanced percentage of pancreatic endocrine tissue due to hyperplasia and hypertrophy of the islet cells (Aerts et al., 1990 ; Reusens-Billen et al., 1984), leading to a higher beta-cell mass that was hyper-vascularized (Reusens & Remacle, 2001). The pancreatic insulin content and insulin secretion were raised in these fetuses (Kervran, et al., 1978). On the other hand, fetuses from severe diabetic dams were small at birth and had decreased pancreatic weight (Aerts et al., 1997). Their beta-cells were almost degranulated, leading to low pancreatic insulin content and low plasma insulin (Kervran, et al., 1978). Similar endocrine pancreas/beta-cell alterations with low beta-cell mass have been reported in fetuses from spontaneous diabetic BB rats (Verhaeghe et al., 1989) or spontaneous diabetic GK rats (Serradas et al., 1998; Miralles & Portha, 2001). The long-term consequences have been evaluated in the progeny of these models. Impaired glucose tolerance was observed in the offspring of mild STZ diabetic rats due to lower insulin secretion in response to glucose, while insulin resistance was reported in the offspring of the severe STZ diabetic mothers (Aerts & Van Assche, 2006; Han et al., 2007; Grill et al., 1991). Glucose tolerance was also impaired in offspring of normal mothers receiving glucose infusion during late gestation, and it was associated to decreased glucose-induced insulin secretion (Ktorza et al., 1990; Aerts et al., 1990; Oh et al., 1988; Gauguier et al., 1991).
The greatest difficulty in most animal models of diabetic pregnancy has been the attainment of a stable degree of mild hyperglycemia during gestation. Though useful, most techniques used to achieve models of diabetes in pregnancy have some drawbacks. Maternal glucose infusions limited to the last trimester of pregnancy result in hyperglycemia and

hyperinsulinemia, and do not mimic the relative insulin deficiency of gestational diabetes (Bihoreau et al., 1986). The multiple lipid and protein abnormalities associated with diabetes may be as important in the induction of fetal abnormalities as hyperglycemia, but they are not replicated by the maternal glucose infusion model. A concern of studies using STZ during pregnancy is the possibility that the toxin might cross the placenta and be directly harmful to the fetal pancreas and other fetal tissues, and thus make any analysis of the long-term effects of hyperglycemia *in utero* difficult (Ryan et al., 1995). The problem may be circumvented by giving STZ to female neonates who will later become pregnant: this will result in moderate gestational hyperglycemia (Triadou et al., 1982). Finally it must be recognized that none of the previously mentioned models will serve directly as a model of human gestational diabetes.

An ideal animal model to test the isolated impact of diabetic pregnancy would enter the pregnancy in a euglycemic state, become exposed to hyperglycaemic during whole pregnancy and return postpartum to normoglycemic environment. Such a model also would allow study of the long-term effects of diabetes independent of any genetic influence. It was recently proposed that the pregnant GK rat being transferred normal Wistar (W) rat embryo represents a more relevant paradigm in such a perspective (Gill-Randall et al., 2004). Using the GK/Par rat we have transferred W rat oocytes to diabetic GK/Par females and at their birth the W neonates were suckled by non-diabetic W foster mothers. Under these unique conditions, we have found that maternal diabetes negatively imprints the growth of a genetically normal (Wistar) beta-cell mass in a way as the insult is still present later at adult age as a decreased beta-cell population (Chavey et al., 2008; Portha et al., 2009).

3.2 IUGR models

Not only maternal diabetes but also intrauterine undernutrition induced by several means such as protein or calorie restriction, or alteration in the availability of the nutrients by placental insufficiency alter early islet development and provoke lasting consequences in rodents.

Global restrictions (to 40-50% of normal intake) in the last week of rat pregnancy results in low birth weight offspring with decreased beta-cell mass. Although these animals can regain their body and pancreatic weights upon normal postnatal feeding, they still demonstrate a reduced beta-cell mass and insulin content in adulthood (Garofano et al., 1997; Bertin et al., 2002). Extending this level of nutrient restriction during suckling results in a permanent reduction of beta-cell mass (Martin et al., 1997; Garofano et al., 1998) and subsequent age-dependent loss of glucose tolerance in the offspring (Garofano et al., 1999). Underfeeding the rat mothers during the first two trimesters of gestation exerts no adverse effect upon insulin secretion and insulin action in the adult male offspring (Portha et al., 1995).

The maternal protein restriction (5-8% as compared to 20% in normal diet) model has been one of the most extensively studied models of IUGR. The low-protein-fed mothers give birth to growth-restricted offspring (Snoeck et al., 1990; Dahri et al., 1991; Langley-Evans et al., 1998; Desai et al., 1996; Fernandez-Twinn et al., 2005), and when suckled by their mothers maintained on the same low-protein diet, they remain permanently growth restricted, despite being weaned on a normal diet (Desai et al., 1996). Reduced placental weight and endocrine and metabolic abnormalities are also observed (Dahri et al., 1991; Fernandez-Twinn et al., 2003; Ozanne et al., 1998). Despite young offspring of low-protein-fed dams demonstrating improved glucose tolerance (Ozanne et al., 1998; Shepherd et al., 1997), the male offspring undergo an age-dependent loss in glucose tolerance, such that by 17 months of age they develop T2D and insulin resistance (Petry et al., 2001). Female offspring only develop hyperinsulinemia and impaired glucose tolerance at a much later age (21 months) (Fernandez-Twinn et al., 2005). Studies in this model have also demonstrated reductions in beta-cell mass (Snoeck et al., 1990;), skeletal muscle mass (Desai et al., 1996), central adipose deposit weights (Shepherd et al., 1997; Ozanne et al., 2000) and insulin signalling defects in muscle, adipocytes and liver (Ozanne et al., 1996; Ozanne et al., 2000; Ozanne et al., 2005). This IUGR model has also been associated with the development of hypertension with the kidney and the renin–angiotensin system as playing a role (Langley-Evans et al., 2003).

Administration of either dexamethasone or carbenoxolone (to inhibit 11 beta-hydroxysteroid dehydrogenase type 2) to normal pregnant rats also causes fetal growth retardation and the adult offspring are hypertensive and hyperglycemic, with hyperactive hypothalamic-pituitary-adrenal axis (Seckl, 2004). Fetal growth retardation may also result from experimental uteroplacental insufficiency (UPI). Fetal UPI rats have decreased levels of glucose, insulin, IGF1, amino acids and oxygen (Ogata et al., 1986; Simmons et al., 1992; Unterman et al., 1990). UPI offspring develop diabetes in later life (Simmons et al. 2001; Boloker et al., 2002) with a phenotype that is similar to that observed in T2D humans with alterations in insulin secretion and action and a failure of beta-cell function and growth (Holemans et al. 2003; Stoffers et al., 2003).

3.3 IUEO models

There are several reports on the consequences of a high fat diet (during gestation only or both gestation and lactation) on the adult progeny. High fat diet consumption by female rats malprograms the male offspring for glucose intolerance and increased body weight in adulthood (Srinivasan et al., 2006). Some of the observed consequences include reduced whole body insulin sensitivity, impaired insulin secretion and changes in the structure of pancreas (Guo & Jen, 1995; Taylor et al., 2005), defective mesenteric artery endothelial function (Khan et al., 2005), hypertension (Khan et al., 2003; Langley-Evans et al., 1996), alterations in renal functions (Armitage et al., 2005), increased body adiposity (Guo & Jen, 1995; Khan et al., 2005), deranged blood lipid profile (Guo & Jen, 1995; Karnik et al., 1989; Khan et al., 2003), hyperleptinemia (Taylor et al., 2005), and proatherogenic lesions (Palinski et al., 2001). There are not many reports on fetal islet adaptations due to a high fat dietary modification in the dam. Cerf et al. (2005) demonstrated that feeding female rats with a high fat diet throughout gestation resulted in significant decreases in beta-cell volume and number resulting in hyperglycemia in 1-day-old newborn rat pups without changes in serum insulin concentrations. However, the report of fetal hyperinsulinemia in the high fat term rat fetus (Srinivasan et al., 2006) is not consistent with this finding.

Also male mice whose mothers consumed a high fat diet were heavier, glucose intolerant and insulin resistant, and produced second-generation offspring who were insulin resistant, although not obese (Dunn & Bale, 2009). Whether this is a consequence of paternal *in utero* exposure or their adult sequelaes of obesity and diabetes, is unclear. It was recently reported that chronic high fat diet consumption in father rats induced increased body weight, adiposity, impaired glucose tolerance and insulin sensitivity in their offspring (Ng et al., 2010). Relative to controls, their female offspring had an early onset of impaired insulin secretion and glucose tolerance that worsened with time, and normal adiposity. Among the differentially expressed islet genes, hypomethylation of the Il13ra2 gene was demonstrated.

This is a proof of concept that paternal high-fat-diet exposure programs beta-cell dysfunction in rat F1 female offspring. This is the first report in mammals of non-genetic, intergenerational transmission of metabolic sequelae of a high fat diet from father to offspring (Ng et al., 2010).
Among the many types of maternal metabolic stress used to produce IUGR, hypercholesterolemia combined to high fat diet was recently added since feeding LDL receptor null (LDLR-/-) mice a high fat resulted in litters with significant growth retardation. The LDLR-/- high fat diet offspring developed significantly larger atherosclerotic lesions by 90 days compared with chow diet offspring (Bhasin et al., 2009). Importantly, maternal hypoaminoacidemia proved to be an important antecedent in this hypercholesterolemic IUGR mouse (Bhasin et al., 2009) as in a protein-deficient IUGR mouse model (Bhasin et al., 2009) and a IUED rat model (Aerts et al., 1989). An important between these mechanisms may contribute to adult glucose intolerance onset, obesity, and atherosclerosis. In this study beta-cell mass was not investigated.
To sum-up, it turns to be manifest that despite differences in the type, timing, and duration of intrauterine insult, most animal models of IUED, IUEO or IUGR have outcomes of impaired glucose tolerance or T2D, similar to IUED, IUEO or IUGR humans.

4. Various early life stressors, the same target: The developing beta-cell mass

As abundantly illustrated in animal models, many early life stressors such as maternal hyperglycaemia, undernutrition, overnutrition, hypercholesterolemia, corticosteroid therapy, uteroplacental insufficiency, or hypoxia, trigger a beta-cell mass adaptive response in the fetus.

4.1 Critical windows for beta-cell adaptive response to early life stressors

The development of the endocrine pancreas starts from a pool of common precursor cells that become progressively committed to the endocrine lineage under the control of a hierarchical network of transcription factors. During late fetal and early postnatal life , the beta cell mass is determined by the recruitment of undifferentiated precursors, as well as the replication and apoptosis rates of the beta cells. Obviously, any disturbance of the environment of the endocrine cells at a specific developmental time-point, as it occurs in a perturbed intra-uterine milieu, may modify the balance of controlling factors, thereby contributing to an adaptive beta-cell growth response which is metabolically appropriate on the short term. However this adaptive response may turn to be detrimental if maintained on the long term, as it may foster beta-cell failure and diabetes later in life. We are largely ignorant of when programming may be initiated during development.

4.1.1 Pre-implantation

An early onset for programming was indicated, as maternal low protein diet during only the preimplantation period of rat development (0-4 days after mating), before return to control diet for the remainder of the gestation, induced blastocyst abnormalities and programming of postnatal growth rate and hypertension (Kwong et al., 2000). More specifically it was shown that preimplantation embryos collected from dams after 0-4 days of maternal low protein diet displayed significantly reduced cell numbers, within the inner cell mass and trophectoderm lineages, apparently induced by a slower rate of cellular proliferation. The low protein diet significantly reduced insulin and essential amino acid levels, and increased glucose levels within maternal serum by day 4 of development. These data indicate that the mildly hyperglycemic and amino acid-depleted maternal environment generated by undernutrition may act as an early mechanism of programming and initiate conditions of 'metabolic stress', restricting early embryonic proliferation and the generation of appropriately sized stem-cell lineages. In chemically or genetically obtained rat diabetes models in which maternal serum insulin depletion and hyperglycemia are induced, proliferation of inner cell mass or total cell numbers within blastocysts is inhibited (Lea et al., 1996; Pampfer et al., 1997). Therefore the preimplantation embryo is particularly sensitive to metabolic modifications that may have programming consequences (Reik et al., 1993; Dean et al., 1998), and one possibility is that the preimplantation embryo itself is programmed.

4.1.2 Post-implantation

Embryo transfer experiments may also help to dissociate the impact of the maternal environment into early (pre-implantation) versus late gestation (postimplantation). We recently found that embryos (blastocysts) from a nondiabetic Wistar strain, placed into a diabetic GK/Par uterus, develop a reduced beta-cell mass which remains low on the long term (Chavey et al., 2008). Data with rat models of prenatal undernutrition (Dumortier et al., 2007) also illustrate that low-energy and low-protein diets that reduce the development of the beta-cell mass in both cases, act at different critical time-windows. The beta-cell mass is deficient in the low-energy pancreas because this diet reduces neogenesis, probably because of high glucocorticoid levels, rather than by impairing vascularisation and proliferation. Early gestation is thus a very sensitive period in this model. By contrast, pancreatic alterations take place at a later fetal stage in the low-protein model and the beta-cell mass is deficient in this case because this diet reduces beta-cell vascularisation and proliferation without altering beta-cell differentiation (Dumortier et al., 2007).

4.1.3 Postnatal versus prenatal

Further support for the crucial impact of prenatal nutritional environment is the recent report that prenatal nutrient restriction in both male and female rats led to an inappropriate postnatal beta-cell mass formation attributed to a decrease in the rate of beta-cell replication and beta-cell neogenesis (Matveyenko et al., 2010). In contrast, male and female rats exposed to postnatal nutrient restriction alone (with normal prenatal nutrient exposure) were characterized by decreased pancreatic and body weights, but a weight-adjusted beta-cell mass higher than control animals (Matveyenko et al., 2010). Another illustration is offered by observations in normal rat pups reared artificially on a high carbohydrate milk formula (Patel & Srinivasan, 2002): such alteration of nutrition during the suckling period only, induced persistent adaptation of energy metabolism in adulthood (obesity, glucose intolerance, impaired insulin secretion).

4.2 Molecular mechanisms mediating the perinatal beta-cell adaptive response

Molecular mechanisms responsible for impaired beta-cell mass formation after IUGR have come under investigation. First, it has been proposed that IUGR can result in a reduction of the embryonic beta-cell progenitor pool, leading to inappropriate postnatal beta-cell formation. Stanger et al. (2007) demonstrated that selective genetic reduction in the size of Pdx1+ pancreatic progenitors during the fetal period results in impaired beta-cell formation during the postnatal period with consequent development of glucose intolerance during adulthood. Consistent with this, maternal food restriction leads to significant reduction in Pdx1+ and Ngn3+ (Neurogenin 3) pancreatic precursors during embryonic development in rats, decreased postnatal beta-cell formation, and inability to expand beta-cell mass in response to pregnancy (Garofano et al., 1998; Blondeau et al., 2002). Another mechanism proposed to explain reduced beta-cell formation after IUGR is related to prenatal glucocorticoid exposure. Maternal undernutrition significantly increased both fetal and maternal corticosterone concentrations in rats (Blondeau et al., 2001). Subsequently, maternal and/or fetal overexposure to glucocorticoids (via administration of dexamethasone) impairs both fetal and postnatal beta-cell formation in rodents and nonhuman primates (Blondeau et al., 2002; Bréant et al, 2006; De Vries et al., 2007; Gesina et al., 2004). Blondeau et al. (2001) have shown that fetal corticosterone concentrations are inversely correlated with fetal insulin content and postnatal beta-cell formation in rats. Evidence suggests that glucocorticoids can exert a direct effect on the developing fetal pancreas via transcriptional modulation of transcription factors involved in beta-cell formation and differentiation (Bréant et al., 2006). Glucocorticoid receptors are present in the pancreas during embryonic development of rodents and humans (Bréant et al., 2006) and glucocorticoids can bind to the Pdx1 promoter and thus suppress fetal endocrine cell differentiation (Bréant et al., 2006). Glucocorticoid treatment has been shown to significantly reduce fetal expression of key endocrine transcription factors such as Pdx1 and Pax6 but simultaneously increase expression of transcription factors that regulate development of the exocrine pancreas (Gesina et al., 2006).

The UPI model of IUGR (due to bilateral uterine artery ligation) is also characterized by a permanent decrease in islet Pdx1 mRNA expression. This decrease has recently been shown to be due to progressive epigenetic silencing of the Pdx1 gene locus secondary to proximal promoter methylation (Stoffers et al., 2003; Park et al., 2008) and it may be responsible for the decreased rate of beta-cell replication and inappropriate postnatal beta-cell mass development (Stoffers et al., 2003; Kulkarni et al., 2004).

It has also been demonstrated that the UPI or the low protein IUGR offspring experience increased oxidative stress and impaired mitochondrial function (Simmons et al., 2005). The mitochondrial dysfunction was not limited to just the beta-cell, as mitochondria from both the liver and skeletal muscle exhibit decreased oxidation of pyruvate, subsequently leading to the development of features commonly found in T2D (Peterside et al., 2003; Selak et al., 2003). Also exposure to a Western-style diet before and during pregnancy (an IUEO model) alters the redox state as early as preimplantation development, leading to mild oxidative stress associated with inflammation. The finding that administration of antioxidants to the dam reverses oxidative stress and completely prevents the development of glucose intolerance and increased adiposity in the adult offspring suggests that oxidative stress plays an important role in the development of adiposity in this case (Sen & Simmons, 2010).

Some studies in the low protein IUGR model have demonstrated that oxidative stress is not limited to just mitochondrial DNA damage, but also genomic DNA, impacting on cell-cycle regulation and gene expression (Chen et al., 2007). While DNA is being targeted throughout by ROS, there are particular regions that are known to be more sensitive to ROS-mediated damage, for example telomeres. Telomeres comprise GC-rich repeats and are found at the ends of each chromosome. They are known to shorten with each cellular division and, hence, can act as a mitotic clock, registering the number of replicative divisions to have taken place within the cell. Investigations using a low protein IUGR model have indeed reported a decrease in longevity in the offspring (Jennings et al., 1999; Chen et al., 2009) accompanied by reduction in mitochondrial antioxidant defences (Tarry-Adkins et al., 2009) and telomere length in islets (Tarry-Adkins et al., 2009).

Pancreatic islet development has been shown to be influenced by a number of growth factors including the insulin-like growth factors, IGF-I and IGF-II whose expression *in utero* is regulated by nutrient and hormone concentrations. IUGR modify expression of both IGF genes in a variety of fetal tissues. In a low protein IUGR rat model with a decreased beta-cell mass and beta-cell replication and an increased rate of beta-cell apoptosis, gene expression for IGF-II but not IGF-I was found reduced in the fetal pancreas and this was (Petrik et al., 1999). In a different IUGR model with more severe global food restriction which induced hyperinsulinemia and an increase in beta-cell mass in their fetuses (Alvarez et al., 1997), the fetal phenotype was associated with an increase in pancreatic IGF-I expression, islet IGF-1R (Martın et al., 2005) and IRS-2 (Fernandez et al., 2007). In the fetal GK/Par rat exposed to mild hyperglycemia during gestation (a model of IUED), data from our group suggest that the beta-cell deficit (reduced by more than 50%) starts as early as fetal age 16 days E16 and reflects decreased beta-cell proliferation, a limitation of beta-cell neogenesis from precursors and increased apoptosis of both beta-cells and their precursors (Calderari et al., 2007). Notably, Pdx1 and Ngn3 expression were decreased on E18 but normally expressed on E13 (Calderari et al., 2007). Defective signalling through the IGF2/IGF1-R pathway may represents the primary instrumental anomaly since IGF2 and IGF1-R protein expressions are already decreased within the GK/Par pancreatic rudiment at E13, at a time when beta-cell mass (first wave of beta cell expansion) is in fact normal (Miralles & Portha, 2001). Low levels of pancreatic IGF2, associated with beta-cell mass deficiency, are maintained thereafter within the fetal pancreas (Serradas et al., 2002). Crossbreeding protocols between non-diabetic W and diabetic GK rats showed that in late gestation (E18), pancreatic IGF2 protein expression was as low in GKmother/GKfather and Wmother/GKfather crosses than in GKmother/GK father crosses (Serradas et al., 2002). These findings rather support the hypothesis that the pancreatic IGF2 anomaly in the GK diabetic model is linked to a genetic determinism. This view is also consistent with the results of genetic analyses that linked a locus containing the gene encoding IGF2 to diabetes in the GK rat (Gauguier et al., 1996). The Igf2 gene is subjected to paternal genomic imprinting. However, because the Igf2 expression is similarly affected in fetuses, regardless of whether the father is W or GK (Serradas et al., 2002), we cannot conclude to a simple change of Igf2 gene imprinting in the GK rat.

Finally, studies have demonstrated that the maintenance of methylated histone H3 Lys4 by Set7/9 a member of the SET methyltransferase family, is crucial to Pdx1 activity in beta-cell lines (Chakrabarti et al., 2003; Francis et al., 2005; Deering et al., 2009). This led to the hypothesis that Set7/9 may represent a novel chromatin-modifying protein that functions in part through its recruitment to target genes by cell-specific transcription factors such as Pdx1. Since, a role of histone methyl transferases, particularly set7, has also been demonstrated in the sustained deleterious effects of chronic hyperglycemia on human microvascular endothelial cells (Siebel et al., 2010), such an epigenetic change could potentially be involved in the deleterious effect of high glucose upon the fetal pancreas in the IUED models.

5. Various early life stressors, one ultimate programming agent: Perinatal hyperglycemia

As abundantly illustrated in animal models, early life stressors such as maternal undernutrition, overnutrition, hypercholesterolemia, corticosteroid therapy, uteroplacental insufficiency, or hypoxia, program metabolic adaptations that favor survival initially, but are ultimately detrimental to adult health. Interestingly, a crucial commonality exists between these models with quite different etiologies: in most of the cases, the altered maternal/fetal metabolism appears to be associated with a diabetogenic effect in the adult offspring either male or female, resulting in a permanent deficiency of the endocrine pancreatic function (F1). In females, the combination of a latent diabetogenic tendency (low insulin response) and the metabolic stress of pregnancy promotes gestational diabetes. F1 gestational diabetes per se is an inducing factor for impaired glucose tolerance and gestational diabetes again in the next female generation (F2).

Finally, the relevant message is that programming of the endocrine pancreas ultimately originates from hyperglycemia experienced during the fetal and/or early postnatal life, whatever the etiology of maternal hyperglycemia is primary (in F0 diabetic mothers) or secondary (in F1 diabetic mothers issued from F0 mothers exposed to undernutrition, UPI, or high glucocorticoid).

6. Transgenerational inheritance of beta-cell mass programming

While a large number of animal studies have shown the effects of undernutrition during foetal/perinatal development on the glucose metabolism of offspring (F1) in adulthood, several studies have shown that glucose metabolism is also altered in the offspring (F2) as well as grand offspring (F3) of fetally malnourished F1 females, even when the F1 and F2 females have been well nourished since weaning (Aerts & Van Assche, 2006; Benyshek et al., 2006). With a aim to dissect the relative parental contributions that lead to F2 offspring outcomes in these models of maternal (F0) undernutrition, it was recently reported that F1 males exhibit moderate hyperglycemia and IGT with aging and impaired glucose-stimulated insulin secretion and that all F2 offspring of F1 males or F1 females develop glucose intolerance (Jimenez-Chillaron et al., 2005). Therefore, intergenerational progression of glucose intolerance can derive from both the maternal and paternal lines. This is an experimental proof that transgenerational transmission of IGT may also occur through the paternal lineage, besides the more widely accepted maternal and grand maternal inheritance of diabetes (Zambrano et al., 2005; Drake et al., 2005; Blondeau et al., 2002; Benyshek et al., 2006).

Conceptually, transgenerational inheritance of disease risk may be mediated by nongenomic mechanisms, including either 1) epigenetic mechanisms (Ozanne & Constancia, 2007; Pinney & Simmons, 2009; Drake & Liu, 2009; Waterland & Michels, 2007) or 2) other broader indirect mechanisms associated with parental physiology (Gluckman et al., 2007). First, alterations in nutrition during development can alter epigenetic marks, thus regulating gene expression through DNA methylation and/or histone modifications. Interestingly, such epigenetic modifications may progress with aging during postnatal life, in association with metabolic phenotypes, as recently observed at the Pdx1 and GLUT4 loci in UPI rats (Park et al., 2008; Raychaudhuri et al., 2008). If these epigenetic changes occur in the germ line, they can be inherited through meiosis (Chong et al., 2007), thus providing a plausible explanation for intergenerational effects, transmitted via either maternal or paternal lines. In addition, other indirect biological processes may influence phenotypes in subsequent generations. For example, physical constraints may alter birth size through the maternal lineage: since uterine size is reduced in girls that are born small and remain short, this may influence fetal growth and reduce weight in their progeny (Gluckman et al., 2007).

Furthermore, maternal metabolism may also influence cross-generational phenotypes (Aerts & Van Assche, 2006). Maternal undernutrition during pregnancy (F0) increases risk for developing diabetes and obesity in her offspring (F1). When these high-risk adult F1 females become pregnant, the metabolic stress of pregnancy may result in hyperglycemia and/or overt gestational diabetes that may, in turn, contribute to defective beta-cell mass and increased diabetes risk in F2 offspring (Aerts & Van Assche, 2006). By this mechanism gestational diabetes may pass from one generation to the next one. In these last examples, intergenerational transmission of phenotypes would occur exclusively through the maternal lineage, as opposed to the epigenetic mechanisms mentioned above. Such a scenario is relevant to the GK/Par rat, since the GK/Par mothers are mildly hyperglycemic through their gestation and during the suckling period. It offers a rationale to elucidate several clues: 1/ the initiation of pancreas programming in the F1 offspring of the first founders (F0), since the GK line is issued from intercrosses between Wistar females and males with borderline IGT but otherwise normal basal blood glucose level (Goto et al., 1975); 2/ the progression of the IGT phenotype until a stable mild diabetic phenotype was reached among the generations (n=35) (Goto et al., 1975); 3/ the lack of attenuation of the diabetic GK phenotype overtime (along more than 20 years and 80 generations), since offspring of GK female/W male crosses were more hyperglycemic than those of W female/GK male crosses (Gauguier et al., 1994).

7. Epigenetic mechanisms mediating the diabetes risk associated with beta-cell mass programming

Several lines of evidence indicate that epigenetic modification may be a key unifying mechanism mediating risk associated with a perturbed intrauterine environment. First, disruption of physiologic responses and functional capacity as observed in multiple tissues in of IUED or IUGR animals and humans, including muscle, adipose, pancreas, liver, and CNS may be related to histone modification and DNA methylation thereby altering related gene expression (Waterland & Michels, 2007).

The preimplantation embryo is particularly sensitive to epigenetic modifications that might permanently alter the phenotype in the adult (Reik et al., 1993; Doherty et al., 2000). For example, in the agouti mouse model, folate supplementation of the maternal diet at conception increases DNA methylation of the agouti gene and increases longevity of the offspring (Cooney et al., 2002). Maternal protein restriction has been shown to alter the methylation status of the promoters of the glucocorticoid receptor (Lillycrop et al., 2005), PPARa (Lillycrop et al., 2008), and the angiotensin receptor (Bogdarina et al., 2007) with parallel changes in gene expression. More recent studies have shown that histone modifications can also be influenced by the early environment. Alterations in histone modifications have also been implicated in mediating the effect of caloric restriction during the second half of pregnancy on the programmed reduction of GLUT4 expression in the offspring (Raychaudhuri et al., 2008). In the case of the UPI rat model and the pancreatic tissue, Simmons and colleagues have reported a progressive reduction in expression of Pdx1, a key transcription factor regulating pancreatic development and function (Stoffers et al., 2003). Pdx1 expression is reduced by 50% in UPI fetuses and by 80% in adult UPI offspring. Notably, these changes precede the onset of beta-cell dysfunction, suggesting a primary pathogenic role. Since the Pdx1 promoter is a target for epigenetic modification, as it contains a conserved CpG islands and is associated with high levels of histone acetylation. Interestingly, binding of both acetylated histone H3/H4 and the transcription factor USF1 was found abolished in UPI fetuses (Park et al., 2008). While there was methylation at multiple CpGs in UPI adult offspring, no methylation was detected in UPI neonates, indicating that methylation was unlikely to explain Pdx1 repression early in life. Together, these data indicate that progressive silencing of gene expression is largely initiated by early epigenetic changes and is maintained thereafter even in the absence of further experimental insults during postnatal life. UPI also increases histone acetylation of the PPARalpha coactivator PGC-1 and carnitine–palmitoyltransferase I (CPT1) promoters in newborn and young rats, and these changes are associated with increased PGC-1 and CPT1 mRNAs (Fu et al., 2004). Finally, there is now little doubt that epigenetic regulation of gene expression also occurs in humans as a response to early nutritional insult: a recent study has revealed that individuals who were exposed to famine *in utero* during the Dutch Hunger Winter had altered methylation of the Igf2 gene in white blood cells in adulthood (Heijmans et al., 2008).

8. Implications for human health

Although the focus of most studies in the metabolic programming field has been on delineating the effects of reduced maternal nutrition, there is now a growing interest in the role of maternal overnutrition in the programming of diabetes risk. The worldwide prevalence of obesity continues to increase, in association with an increase in the risk of metabolic T2D. Indeed, a recent study estimated that the number of people worldwide with diabetes would increase from 171 million in 2000 to 366 million by 2030 if the prevalence of obesity remained constant (Wild et al., 2004), which has major implications for public health strategies worldwide (WHO, 2000). This global trend to increasing obesity is reflected in the increasing numbers of women who are obese during pregnancy (Kanagalingam et al., 2005). Given that the offspring of obese mothers have an increased risk of developing obesity and T2D themselves (Boney et al., 2005; Catalano, 2003; Catalano et al., 2009), the potential impact of the intergenerational consequences of maternal obesity is of great concern for public health policy makers.

Moreover, maternal hyperglycemia per se increases the probability of adolescent obesity and future T2D. To what extent maternal hyperglycemia is fuelling the global rise in obesity and T2D is unknown, but its contribution is highly significant. The exact degree of hyperglycemia that has this effect and the exact timing in pregnancy at which hyperglycemia is impressionable on fetal programming is unknown. The need to identify and treat all women with gestational diabetes is very much dependent on us knowing this. Meanwhile, achieving rigorous glycemic control in women with diabetic pregnancy has to remain a major therapeutic goal.

Several interventions (dietary or pharmacological) to reduce the long-term sequelae of early life programming effects have been used in animal models. For example, the administration of folic acid with a low protein diet during pregnancy prevents the altered phenotype and epigenotype in rat offspring (Lillycrop et al., 2005), and administration of a diet rich in methyl donors prevents the transgenerational increase in obesity in agouti yellow mice (Waterland et al., 2008). Importantly, the timing of such interventions can be crucial. Examples include neonatal leptin treatment which reverses the programming effects of prenatal undernutrition (Vickers et al., 2005). In the UPI rat model, epigenetic silencing of the Pdx1 gene can be reversed during a critical developmental window in the neonatal period, using trichostatin A which inhibit HDACs (Park et al., 2008). In the same model, exposure to Exendin-4 in the neonatal period reversed the detrimental fetal programming of the beta-cell mass and prevented the development of diabetes in adulthood: this was closely related to restoration of pdx1 expression and beta-cell proliferation rate (Stoffers Diabetes 2003). A GLP-1 or Exendin-4 treatment limited to the neonatal pre-diabetic period was also shown to delay the installation and limit the severity of T2D in the GK/Par model (Tourrel et al., 2002). In such context, it is important to note that GLP1-derived drugs that are currently used to treat patients with T2D may target chromatin remodelling. Treating beta-cells from the INS1 cell line or dispersed mouse islet cells with GLP-1 increased global acetylation of histone H3 and increased its phosphorylation in a concentration-dependent manner (Kim et al., 2009). Such histone modifications increased association with the transcription factor phospho- CREB and with cAMP-response CREB coactivator 2. Taken as a whole, these data may provoke optimism - that there may be a window for potential postnatal therapeutic interventions to prevent/modify the "programmed" diabetes risk.

9. Acknowledgments

The studies from our lab and referred to in this review have been funded by the French ANR (programme Physio 2006 - Prograbeta - ref ANR-06-PHYSIO-028), EGIDE (PHC franco-espagnol PICASSO 2008-2009) and NEB Association. A. Chavey received a CNRS postdoctoral fellowship and was granted by NESTLE-France and SFD/Lilly.

10. References

Aerts, A & Van Assche, FA (2006). Animal evidence for the transgenerational development of diabetes mellitus. *Int J Biochem Cell Biol* 38 : 894–903.

Aerts, L, Vercruysse, L & Van Assche, FA (1997). The endocrine pancreas in virgin and pregnant offspring of diabetic pregnant rats. *Diabetes Research and Clinical Practice*, 38, 1-19.

Aerts, L, Holemans, K & Van Assche, FA (1990). Maternal diabetes during pregnancy: Consequences for the offspring. *Diabetes Metabolic Review*, 16, 147–197.

Aerts, L et al. (1989). Plasma amino-acids in diabetic pregnant rats and in their fetal and adult offspring. *Biol. Neonate*, 56, 31–39.

Alcolado JC, Laji K & Gill-Randall R (2002). Maternal transmission of diabetes. *Diabet Med* 19:89–98.

Alvarez C, et al. (1997). Contrasted impact of maternal rat food restriction on the fetal endocrine pancreas. *Endocrinology* 138: 2267–2273.

Armitage JA, et al. (2005). Developmental programming of aortic and renal structure in offspring of rats fed fat-rich diets in pregnancy. J Physiol 565: 171–184,.

Barker, DJP (2004). The developmental origins of adult disease. *J. Am. Coll. Nutr.* 23, 588S–595S.

Benyshek, DC; Johnston, CS & Martin, JF (2006). Glucose metabolism is altered in the adequately-nourished grand-offspring (F3 generation) of rats malnourished during gestation and perinatal life. Diabetologia 49:1117–1119.

Beringue, F; et al. (2002). Endocrine pancreas development in growth-retarded human fetuses. *Diabetes* 51:385-391.

Bertin, E, et al. (2002). Development of β-cell mass in fetuses of rats deprived of protein and/or energy in last trimester of pregnancy. *Am. J. Physiol. Regul. Integr. Comp. Physiol.* 283, R623–R630.

Bhargava, SK, et al. (2004). Relation of serial changes in childhood body-mass index to impaired glucose tolerance in young Aadulthood. *N. Engl. J. Med.* 350, 865–875.

Bhasin, KKS, et al. (2009). Maternal low-protein diet or hypercholesterolemia reduces circulating essential amino acids and leads to intrauterine growth restriction. *Diabetes* 58:559–566.

Bihoreau, MT, Ktorza, A, Kinebanyan, MF & Picon, L (1986). Impaired glucose homeostasis in adult rats from hyperglycemic mothers. *Diabetes* 35:979–984.

Blondeau, B, Avril, I, Duchene, B & Bréant, B (2002). Endocrine pancreas development is altered in foetuses from rats previously showing intra-uterine growth retardation in response to malnutrition. *Diabetologia* 45:394–401.

Blondeau, B, et al. (2001). Glucocorticoids impair fetal_beta-cell development in rats. *AmJ Physiol Endocrinol Metab* 281:E592–E599.

Bogdarina, I, Welham, S, King, PJ, Burns, SP & Clark AJ (2007). Epigenetic modification of the reninangiotensin system in the fetal programming of hypertension. *Circ Res.*;100:520–6.

Boloker, J, Gertz, SJ, & Simmons, RA (2002). Offspring of Diabetic Rats Develop Obesity and Type II Diabetes in Adulthood. *Diabetes* 51, 1499–1506.

Boney, CM, Verma, A, Tucker, R & Vohr, BR (2005). Metabolic syndrome in childhood: association with birth weight, maternal obesity, and gestational diabetes mellitus. *Pediatrics* 115, e290–296.

Bréant, B, Gesina, E & Blondeau, B (2006). Nutrition, glucocorticoids and pancreas development. *Horm Res* 65(Suppl 3):98–104.

Calderari, S, et al. (2007). Defective IGF-2 and IGF-1R protein expressions in embryonic pancreas precede beta-cell mass anomaly in GK rat. *Diabetologia* 50, 1463–1471.

Catalano, PM (2003). Obesity and pregnancy - the propagation of a viscous cycle? *J. Clin. Endocrinol. Metab.* 88, 3505–3506.

Catalano, PM, et al. (2009). Perinatal risk factors for childhood obesity and metabolic dysregulation. *Am. J. Clin. Nutr.* 90, 1303–1313.

Cerf, ME, et al. (2005). Islet cell response in the neonatal rat after exposure to a high-fat diet during pregnancy. *Am J Physiol Regul Integr Comp Physiol* 288: R1122–R1128.

Chakrabarti, SK, Francis, J, Ziesmann, SM, Garmey, JC & Mirmira, RG (2003): Covalent histone modifications underlie the developmental regulation of insulin gene transcription in pancreatic beta cells. *J Biol Chem* 278:23617–23623.

Chavey, A, et al. (2008). Intrauterine programming of beta-cell development and function by maternal diabetes. What does embryo-transfer experiments in GK/Par rats tell us?.*Diabetologia* 51[Suppl1]:151A.

Chen, JH, Hales, CN & Ozanne, SE (2007). DNA damage, cellular senescence and organismal ageing: causal or correlative? *Nucleic Acids Res.* 35, 7417–7428.

Chen, JH, Martin-Gronert, MS, Tarry-Adkins, JL & Ozanne, SE (2009). Maternal protein restriction affects postnatal growth and the expression of key proteins involved in lifespan regulation in mice. *PLoS ONE* 4, e4590.

Chong, S, et al. (2007). Modifiers of epigenetic reprogramming show paternal effects in the mouse. *Nat Genet* 39:614–622.

Clausen, JO, Borch-Johnsen, K & Pedersen, O (1997). Relation between birth weight and the insulin sensitivity index in a population sample of 331 young, healthy Caucasians. *Am. J. Epidemiol.* 146, 23–31.

Cooney, CA, Dave, AA & Wolff, GL (2002). Maternal methyl supplements in mice affect epigenetic variation and DNA methylation in offspring. *J. Nutr.* 132, 2393S–2400S.

Dabelea, D, et al. (2000). Intrauterine exposure to diabetes conveys risks for type 2 diabetes and obesity: a study of discordant sibships. *Diabetes* 49:2208–2211

Dahri, S, Snoeck, A, Reusens-Billen, B, Remacle, C & Hoet, JJ (1991). Islet function in offspring of mothers on low-protein diet during gestation. *Diabetes* 40, 115–120.

De Vries, A, et al. (2007). Prenatal dexamethasone exposure induces changes in nonhuman primate offspring cardiometabolic and hypothalamic-pituitary-adrenal axis function. *J Clin Invest* 117:1058–1067.

Dean, W, et al. (1998). Altered imprinted gene methylation and expression in completely ES cell-derived mouse fetuses: association with aberrant phenotypes. *Development*; 125: 2273–2282.

Deering, TG, Ogihara, T, Trace, AP, Maier, B & Mirmira, RG (2009). Methyltransferase Set7/9 maintains transcription and euchromatin structure at islet-enriched genes. *Diabetes*;58:185–93.

Desai, M, Crowther, NJ, Lucas, A & Hales, CN (1996). Organ-selective growth in the offspring of protein-restricted mothers. *Br. J. Nutr.* 76, 591–603.

Doherty, AS, Mann, MR, Tremblay, KD, Bartolomei, MS & Schultz, RM (2000). Differential effects of culture on imprinted H19 expression in the preimplantation mouse embryo. *Biol. Reprod.* 62, 1526–1535.

Dörner, G, Plagemann, A, & Reinagel, H (1987). Familial diabetes aggregation in type I diabetics: Gestational diabetes an apparent risk factor for increased diabetes susceptibility in the offspring. *Exp. Clin. Endocrinol.*, 89, 84–90.

Dörner, G, Steindel, E & Thoelke, H (1984). Evidence for decreasing prevalence of diabetes mellitus in childhood apparently produced by prevention of hyperinsulinism in the foetus and newborn. *Exp. Clin. Endocrinol.*, 84, 134–142.

Drake, AJ, Walker, BR & Seckl, JR (2005). Intergenerational consequences of fetal programming by in utero exposure to glucocorticoids in rats. *Am J Physiol Regul Integr Comp Physiol* 288:R34-R38.

Drake, AJ & Liu, L (2009). Intergenerational transmission of programmed effects: public health consequences. *Trends Endocrinol Metab* 21:206-212.

Dumortier, O, et al. (2007). Different mechanisms operating during different critical time-windows reduce rat fetal beta-cell mass due to a maternal low-protein or low-energy diet. *Diabetologia* 50, 2495–2503.

Dunn, GA & Bale, TL (2009). Maternal high-fat diet promotes body length increases and insulin insensitivity in second-generation mice. *Endocrinology* 150, 4999–5009.

Economides, DL, Nicolaides, KH, Gahl, WA, Bernardini, I & Evans, MI. (1989). Plasma insulin in appropriate and small for gestational age fetuses. *Am. J. Obstet. Gynecol.* 160, 1091–1094.

Fernandez, E; Martin, MA, Fajardo, S, Escriva, F & Alvarez, C (2007). Increased IRS-2 content and activation of IGF-1 pathway contribute to enhance beta-cell mass in fetuses from undernourished pregnant rats. *Am j Physiol Endocrinol Metab* 292:E187-E195.

Fernandez-Twinn, DS, et al. (2003). The maternal endocrine environment in the low-protein model of intra-uterine growth restriction. *Br. J. Nutr.* 90, 815–822.

Fernandez-Twinn, DS, et al. (2005). Maternal protein restriction leads to hyperinsulinaemia and reduced insulin-signaling protein expression in 21-mo-old female rat offspring. *Am. J. Physiol. Regul. Integr. Comp. Physiol.* 288, R368–R373.

Flanagan, DE, et al. (2000). Fetal growth and the physiological control of glucose tolerance in adults: a minimal model analysis. *Am. J. Physiol. Endocrinol. Metab.* 278, E700–E706.

Francis, J, Chakrabarti, SK, Garmey, JC & Mirmira, RG (2005). Pdx-1 links histone H3-Lys-4 methylation to RNA polymerase II elongation during activation of insulin transcription. *J Biol Chem* 280:36244 -36253.

Frayling, TM, et al.(1999). Parent-offspring trios: a resource to facilitate the identification of type 2 diabetes genes. *Diabetes* 48:2475–2479.

Freathy, RM, Bennett, AJ, Ring, SM, et al. (2009). Type 2 diabetes risk alleles are associated with reduced size at birth. *Diabetes*;58:1428–1433.

Fu, Q, et al. (2004). Uteroplacental insufficiency induces site-specific changes in histone H3 covalent modifications and affects DNA-histone H3 positioning in day 0 IUGR rat liver. *Physiol. Genomics* 20, 108–116.

Garofano, A., Czernichow, P & Breant, B (1997). In utero undernutrition impairs rat β-cell development. *Diabetologia* 40, 1231–1234.

Garofano, A, Czernichow, P & Breant, B (1998). β-Cell mass and proliferation following late fetal and early postnatal malnutrition in the rat. *Diabetologia* 41, 1114–1120.

Garofano, A, Czernichow, P & Breant, B (1999). Effect of ageing on β-cell mass and function in rats malnourished during the perinatal period. *Diabetologia* 42, 711–718.

Gauguier, D, Bihoreau, MT, Picon, L, Ktorza, A (1991). Insulin secretion in adult rats after intrauterine exposure to mild hyperglycemia during late gestation. *Diabetes* 40(Suppl 2):109–114.

Gauguier, D, et al. (1994). Higher maternal than paternal inheritance of diabetes in GK rats. *Diabetes* 43:220–224.

Gauguier, D, et al. (1996). Chromosomal mapping of genetic loci associated with non-insulin dependent diabetes in the GK rat. *Nat. Genet.* 12, 38–43.

Gautier, JF, et al. (2001). Low acute insulin secretory responses in adult offspring of people with early onset type 2 diabetes. *Diabetes* 50:1828–1833.

Gesina, E, et al. (2004). Dissecting the role of glucocorticoids on pancreas development. *Diabetes* 53:2322–2329.

Gill-Randall, R, Adams, D, Ollerton, RL, Lewis, M & Alcolado, JC (2004). Type 2 diabetes mellitus-genes or intrauterine environment? An embryo transfer paradigm in rats. *Diabetologia* 47:1354–1359.

Gluckman, PD, Hanson, MA & Beedle, AS (2007). Non-genomic transgenerational inheritance of disease risk. *Bio Essays* 29:145–154.

Goto, Y, Kakizaki, M & Masaki, N (1975). Spontaneous diabetes produced by selective breeding of normal Wistar rats. *Proc Jpn Acad;* 51: 80–85.

Grill, V, Johansson, B, Jalkanen, P & Eriksson, UJ (1991). Influence of severe diabetes mellitus early in pregnancy in the rat: effects on insulin sensitivity and insulin secretion in the offspring. *Diabetologia* 34:373-378.

Groenewoud, MJ, Dekker, JM, Fritsche, A, et al. (2008). Variants of CDKAL1 and IGF2BP2 affect first-phase insulin secretion during hyperglycaemic clamps. *Diabetologia;*51:1659–1663.

Guo, F & Jen, KL (1995). High-fat feeding during pregnancy and lactation affects offspring metabolism in rats. *Physiol Behav* 57: 681–686.

Hales, CN, et al. (1991). Fetal and infant growth and impaired glucose tolerance at age 64. *BMJ.;*303:1019–22.

Han, J, Xu, J, Long, YS, Epstein, PN & Liu, YQ (2007). Rat maternal diabetes impairs pancreatic beta-cell function in the offspring. *Am J Physiol Endocrinol Metab* 293: E228-E236.

Hanson, RL, Elston, RC, Pettitt, DJ, Bennett, PH, Knowler, WC (1995). Segregation analysis of non-insulin-dependent diabetes mellitus in Pima Indians: evidence for a major-gene effect. *Am J Hum Genet* 57:160–170.

Heijmans, BT, et al. (2008). Persistent epigenetic differences associated with prenatal exposure to famine in humans. *Proc Natl Acad Sci USA.;*105:17046–9.

Holemans, K, Aerts, L & Van Assche, FA (2003). Lifetime consequences of abnormal fetal pancreatic development. *J. Physiol.* 547, 11–20.

Hunter, WA, et al. (2004). Insulin sensitivity in the offspring of women with type 1 and type 2 diabetes. *Diabetes Care* 27:1148–1152.

Jaquet, D, Gaboriau, A, Czernichow, P & Levy-Marchal, C (2000). Insulin resistance early in adulthood in subjects born with intrauterine growth retardation. *J. Clin. Endocrinol. Metab.* 85, 1401–1406.

Jennings, BJ, Ozanne, SE, Dorling, MW & Hales, CN (1999). Early growth determines longevity in male rats and may be related to telomere shortening in the kidney. *FEBS Lett.* 448, 4–8.

Jensen, CB, et al. (2002). Early differential defects of insulin secretion and action in 19-year old Caucasian men who had low birth weight. *Diabetes* 51, 1271–1280.

Jimenez-Chillaron, JC, et al. (2005). Beta-cell secretory dysfunction in the pathogenesis of low birth weight associated diabetes: a murine model. *Diabetes* 54:702–711.

Kanagalingam, MG, Forouhi, NG, Greer, IA & Sattar, N (2005). Changes in booking body mass index over a decade: retrospective analysis from a Glasgow maternity hospital. *Br. J. Obstet. Gynaecol.* 112, 1431–1433.

Karnik, HB, Sonawane, BR, Adkins, JS & Mohla, S (1989). High dietary fat feeding during perinatal development of rats alters hepatic drug metabolism of progeny. *Dev Pharmacol Ther* 14: 135–140.

Kervran, A, Guillaume, M & Jost, A (1978). The endocrine pancreas of the foetus from diabetic pregnant rat. *Diabetologia,* 15, 387– 393.

Khan, IY, et al. (2005). A high-fat diet during rat pregnancy or suckling induces cardiovascular dysfunction in adult offspring. *Am J Physiol Regul Integr Comp Physiol* 288: R127–R133.

Khan, IY, et al. (2003). Gender-linked hypertension in offspring of lard-fed pregnant rats. *Hypertension* 41: 168–175.

Kim, DJ, et al. (2004). Lack of excess maternal transmission of type 2 diabetes in a Korean population. *Diabetes Res Clin Pract* 65:117–124.

Kim, SJ, Nian C & McIntosh CH (2009). Glucose-dependent insulinotropic polypeptide and glucagon-like peptide-1 modulate b-cell chromatin structure. *J. Biol. Chem.* 284, 12896–12904.

Ktorza, A, Gauguier, D, Bihoreau, MT, Berthault, MF & Picon, L (1990). Adult offspring from mildly hyperglycemic rats show impairment of glucose regulation and insulin secretion which is transmissible to the next generation. *In Frontiers in Diabetic Research. Lessons from Animal Diabetes,* ed. Shafrir, E., pp. 555–560. Smith-Gordon and Company Ltd, London.

Kulkarni, RN, et al. (2004). PDX-1 haploinsufficiency limits the compensatory islet hyperplasia that occurs in response to insulin resistance. *J Clin Invest* 114:828–836.

Kwong, WY, et al (2000). Maternal undernutrition during the preimplantation period of rat development causes blastocyst abnormalities and programming of postnatal hypertension. *Development*; 27: 4195–4202.

Langley-Evans, SC (1996). Intrauterine programming of hypertension in the rat: nutrient interactions. *Comp Biochem Physiol A Physiol* 114: 327–333.

Langley-Evans, SC & Nwagwu, M (1998). Impaired growth and increased glucocorticoid-sensitive enzyme activities in tissues of rat fetuses exposed to maternal low protein diets. *Life Sci.* 63, 605–615.

Langley-Evans, SC, Langley-Evans, AJ & Marchand, MC (2003). Nutritional programming of blood pressure and renal morphology. *Arch. Physiol. Biochem.* 111, 8–16.

Lea, RG, et al. (1996). Disturbed development of the preimplantation embryo in the insulindependent diabetic BB/E rat. *Diabetes*; 45: 1463–1470.

Li, B, Xu, Y & Choi, J (1996). Applying Machine Learning Techniques, Proceedings of ASME 2010 *4th International Conference on Energy Sustainability*, pp. 14-17, ISBN 842-6508-23-3, Phoenix, Arizona, USA, May 17-22, 2010.

Li, C, Johnson, MS & Goran MI (2001). Effects of low birth weight on insulin resistance syndrome in Caucasion and African-American children. *Diabetes Care* 24, 2035-2042.

Li, Y, et al. (2010). Exposure to the chinese famine in early life and the risk of hyperglycemia and type 2 diabetes in adulthood. *Diabetes* 59: 2400-2406.

Lillycrop, KA, Phillips, ES, Jackson, AA, Hanson, MA & Burdge, GC (2005). Dietary protein restriction of pregnant rats induces and folic acid supplementation prevents epigenetic modification of hepatic gene expression in the offspring. *J Nutr.*;135:1382–6.

Lillycrop, KA, et al. (2008). Feeding pregnant rats a protein-restricted diet persistently alters the methylation of specific cytosines in the hepatic PPAR alpha promoter of the offspring. *Br J Nutr.*;100:278–82.

Martin, MA, Alvarez, C, Goya, L, Portha, B & Pascual-Leone, AM (1997). Insulin secretion in adult rats that had experienced different underfeeding patterns during their development. *Am J Physiol* 272:E634–E640.

Martin, AO, Simpson, JL, Ober, C, & Freinkel, N (1985). Frequency of diabetes mellitus in probands with gestational diabetes: Possible maternal influence on the predisposition to gestational diabetes. *Am. J. Obstet. Gynecol.*, 151, 471–475.

Martin, MA, et al. (2005). Protein-caloric food restriction affects insulin-like growth factor system in fetal Wistar rat. *Endocrinology* 146:1364–1371.

Matveyenko, AV; Singh, I, Shin, BC, Georgia, S, Devaskar, SU (2010). Differential effects of prenatal and postnatal nutritional environment on beta-cell mass development and turnover in male and female rats. *Endocrinology* 151: 5647–5656.

McCarthy, M, et al. (1996). Evaluation of the importance of maternal history of diabetes and of mitochondrial variation in the development of NIDDM. *Diabet Med* 13:420–428.

Meier, JJ (2008). Beta cell mass in diabetes: a realistic therapeutic target? *Diabetologia*;51:703–713.

Meigs, JB, Cupples, LA & Wilson, PW (2000). Parental transmission of type 2 diabetes: the Framingham Offspring Study. *Diabetes* 49:2201–2207.

Miralles, F & Portha, B (2001). Early development of beta-cells is impaired in the GK rat model of type 2 diabetes. *Diabetes* 50(suppl.1):S84-S88.

Mitchell, BD, et al. (1993). Differences in the prevalence of diabetes and impaired glucose tolerance according to maternal or paternal history of diabetes. *Diabetes Care* 16:1262–1267.

Nathanielsz, PW, Poston, L & Taylor, PD (2007). In utero exposure to maternal obesity and diabetes: animal models that identify and characterize implications for future health. *Clin Perinatol.*;34:515–26.

Ng, SF; Lin, R, Laybutt, DR, Barres, R, Owens, JA & Morris, MJ (2010). Chronic high-fat diet in fathers programs beta-cell dysfunction in female rat offspring. *Nature* 467:963-967.

Ogata, Es, Bussey, M & Finley, S (1986). Altered gas exchange,limited glucose, branched amino acids, and hypoinsulinism retard fetal growth in the rat. *Metabolism* 35, 950–977.

Oh, W, Gelardi, NL & Cha, CJ (1988). Maternal hyperglycemia in pregnant rats, its effect on growth and carbohydrate metabolism in the offspring. *Metabolism* 37, 1146–1151.

Ozanne, SE, Constancia, M (2007). Mechanisms of disease: the developmental origins of disease and the role of the epigenotype. *Nat Clin Pract Endocrinol Metab* 3:539 - 546.

Ozanne, SE, Dorling, MW, Wang, CL & Petry, CJ (2000). Depot-specific effects of early growth retardation on adipocyte insulin action. *Horm. Metab. Res.* 32, 71–75.

Ozanne, SE., Smith, GD, Tikerpae, J & Hales, CN (1996). Altered regulation of hepatic glucose output in the male offspring of protein-malnourished rat dams. *Am. J. Physiol.* 270, E559–E564.

Ozanne, SE, Wang, CL, Petry, CJ, Smith, JM & Hales, CN (1998). Ketosis resistance in the male offspring of protein-malnourished rat dams. *Metab. Clin. Exp.* 47, 1450–1454.

Ozanne, SE, et al. (2005). Low birthweight is associated with specific changes in muscle insulin-signalling protein expression. *Diabetologia* 48, 547–552.

Palinski, W, et al. (2001). Maternal hypercholesterolemia and treatment during pregnancy influence the long-term progression of atherosclerosis in offspring of rabbits. *Circ Res* 89: 991–996.

Pampfer, S, Vanderheyden, L, McCracken, JE, et al. (1997). Increased cell death in rat blastocysts exposed to maternal diabetes in utero and to high glucose or tumour necrosis factor-αin vitro. *Development*; 124: 4827–4836.

Park, JH, Stoffers, DA, Nicholls, RD & Simmons, RA (2008). Development of type 2 diabetes following intrauterine growth retardation in rats is associated with progressive epigenetic silencing of Pdx1. *J Clin Invest* 118:2316–2324.

Pascoe, L, et al. (2008). Beta cell glucose sensitivity is decreased by 39% in non-diabetic individuals carrying multiple diabetesrisk alleles compared with those with no risk alleles. *Diabetologia*; 51:1989–1992.

Patel MS, Srinivasan M. Metabolic programming: causes and consequences. *J Biol Chem* 2002; 277: 1629–1632.

Peterside, IE, Selak, MA & Simmons, RA (2003). Impaired oxidative phosphorylation in hepatic mitochondria in growth-retarded rats. *Am. J. Physiol. Endocrinol. Metab.* 285, E1258–E1266.

Petrik, J, et al. (1999). A low protein diet alters the balance of islet cell replication and apoptosis in the fetus and is associated with a reduced pancreatic expression of insulin-like growth factor-II. Endocrinology; 140: 4861–73.

Petry, CJ, Dorling, MW, Pawlak, DB, Ozanne, SE & Hales, CN (2001). Diabetes in old male offspring of rat dams fed a reduced protein diet. *Int. J. Diabetes Res.* 2, 139–143.

Pettitt, DJ (1996). Diabetes in subsequent generations. In A. Dornhorst & D. R. Hadden (Eds.), Diabetes and pregnancy. An international approach to diagnosis and management (pp. 367–376). *Chichester: John Wiley & Sons.*

Pinney, SE, & Simmons, RA (2009). Epigenetic mechanisms in the development of type 2 diabetes. *Trends Endocrinol Metab* 21:223-229.

Plagemann, A, Harder, T, Kohlhoff, R, Rohde, W & Dorner, G (1997). Glucose tolerance and insulin secretion in children of mothers with pregestational IDDM or gestational diabetes. *Diabetologia* 40:1094–1100.

Portha, B, et al. (2009). Des modèles animaux pour étudier l'origine développementale des maladies métaboliques de l'adulte : Application à l'étude du risque de diabète. *Cah. Nutr. Diétét.*, 44: 77-84.

Portha, B, Kergoat, M, Blondel, O & Bailbé, D (1995). Underfeeding rat mothers during the two first trimesters of gestation does not alter insulin action and insulin secretion in the progeny. *Eur.J.Endocrinol.* 133:475-482.

Poulsen, P, Vaag, AA, Kyvik, KO, Moller-Jensen, D & Beck-Nielsen, H (1997). Low birth weight is associated with NIDDM in discordant monozygotic and dizygotic twin pairs. *Diabetologia.*;40:439–46.

Ravelli, AC, et al. (1998). Glucose tolerance in adults after prenatal exposure to famine. *Lancet.*;351:173–7.

Raychaudhuri, N, Raychaudhuri, S, Thamotharan, M & Devaskar, SU (2008). Histone code modifications repress glucose transporter 4 expression in the intrauterine growth-restricted offspring. *J Biol Chem* 283:13611–13626.

Reik, W, et al. (1993). Adult phenotype in themouse can be affected by epigenetic events in the early embryo. *Development*; 119: 933–942.

Reusens, B, & Remacle, C (2001). Intergenerational effects of adverse intrauterine environment on perturbation of glucose metabolism. *Twin Research*, 4, 406–411.

Reusens-Billen, B, Remacle, C, Daniline, J & Hoet, JJ (1984). Cell proliferation in pancreatic islets of rat fetus and neonates from normal and diabetic mothers. An in vitro and in vivo study. *Hormone and Metabolic Research*, 16, 565–571.

Ryan, EA, Liu, D, Bell, RC, Finegood, DT & Crawford, J (1995). Long-term consequences in offspring of diabetes in pregnancy: studies with syngeneic islet-transplanted streptozotocin-diabetic rats. *Endocrinology* 136:5587-5592.

Savona-Ventura, C, & Chircop, M (2002). Birth-weight influence on the subsequent development of gestational diabetes mellitus.J. Mater. Fet. Neonate Med., 11, 56.

Saxena, R, et al. (2007). Genome-wide association analysis identifies loci for type 2 diabetes and triglyceride levels. *Science*;316: 1331–1336.

Scott, LJ, et al. (2007). A genome-wide association study of type 2 diabetes in Finns detects multiple susceptibility variants. *Science*; 316:1341–1345.

Seckl, JR (2004). Prenatal glucocorticoids and long-term programming. *Eur. J. Endocrinol.* 151 (Suppl 3), U49–U62.

Selak, MA, Storey, BT, Peterside, I & Simmons, RA (2003). Impaired oxidative phosphorylation in skeletal muscle of intrauterine growth-retarded rats. *Am. J. Physiol. Endocrinol. Metab.* 285:E130–E137.

Sen, S & Simmons, RA (2010). Maternal antioxidant supplementation prevents adiposity in the offspring of western diet-fed rats. *Diabetes* 59:3058-3065.

Serradas, P, Gangnerau, MN, Giroix, MH, Saulnier, C & Portha, B (1998). Impaired pancreatic beta-cell function in the fetal GK rat. Impact of diabetic inheritance. *J Clin Invest* 101:899–904.

Serradas, P, et al. (2002). Fetal insulin-like growth factor-2 production is impaired in the GK rat model of type 2 diabetes. *Diabetes* 51, 392–397.

Shepherd, PR, Crowther, NJ, Desai, M, Hales, CN & Ozanne, SE (1997). Altered adipocyte properties in the offspring of protein malnourished rats. *Br. J. Nutr.* 78, 121–129.

Siebel, AL, Fernandez, AZ & El-Osta, A (2010). Glycemic memory associated epigenetic changes. *Biochem Pharmacol.* 80:1853-1859.

Silverman, BL, Metzger, BE, Cho, NH & Loeb, CA (1995). Impaired glucose tolerance in adolescent offspring of diabetic mothers. Relationship to fetal hyperinsulinism. *Diabetes Care* 18:611–617.

Simmons, RA, Suponitsky-Kroyter, I & Selak, MA (2005). Progressive accumulation of mitochondrial DNA mutations and decline in mitochondrial function lead to β-cell failure. *J. Biol. Chem.* 280, 28785–28791.

Simmons, RA, Gounis, AS, Bangalore, SA & Ogata, ES (1992). Intrauterine growth retardation: Fetal glucose transport is diminished in lung but spared in brain. *Pediatr. Res.* 31, 59–63.

Simmons, RA, Templeton, LJ & Gertz, SJ (2001). Intrauterine Growth Retardation Leads to Type II Diabetes in Adulthood in the Rat. *Diabetes* 50, 2279–2286.

Singh, R, et al. (2006). Reduced beta cell function in offspring of mothers with young-onset type 2 diabetes. *Diabetologia* 49:1876-1880.

Snoeck, A, Remacle, C, Reusens, B & Hoet, JJ (1990). Effect of a low protein diet during pregnancy on the fetal rat endocrine pancreas. *Biol. Neonate* 57, 107–118.

Sobngwi, E, et al. (2003). Effect of a diabetic environment in utero on predisposition to type 2 diabetes. *Lancet* 361:1861–1865.

Srinivasan, M, Karewa, SD, Palaniyappan, A, Pandya, JD & Patel, MS (2006). Maternal high-fat diet consumption results in fetal programming predisposing to the onset of metabolic syndrome-like phenotype in adulthood. *Am J Physiol Endocrinol Metab* 291:E792-E799.

Stanger, BZ, Tanaka, AJ & Melton, DA (2007). Organ size is limited by the number of embryonic progenitor cells in the pancreas but not the liver. *Nature* 445:886–891.

Stanner, SA, et al. (1997). Does malnutrition in utero determine diabetes and coronary heart disease in adulthood? Results from the Leningrad Siege Study, a cross sectional study. *BMJ*;315:1342–1348.

Stoffers, DA, Desai, BM, DeLeon, DD & Simmons RA (2003). Neonatal exendin-4 prevents the development of diabetes in the intrauterine growth retarded rat. *Diabetes* 52:734–740.

Stride, A, et al. (2002). Intrauterine hyperglycemia is associated with an earlier diagnosis of diabetes in HNF-1_ gene mutation carriers. *Diabetes Care* 25:2287–2291.

Tarry-Adkins, J L, et al. (2009). Poor maternal nutrition followed by accelerated postnatal growth leads to telomere shortening and increased markers of cell senescence in rat islets. *FASEB J.* 23, 1521–1528.

Taylor, PD, et al. (2005). Impaired glucose homeostasis and mitochondrial abnormalities in offspring of rats fed a fat-rich diet in pregnancy. *Am J Physiol Regul Integr Comp Physiol* 288: R134–R139.

Terauchi, Y, et al. (2000). Insulin effect during embryogenesis determines fetal growth: a possible molecular link between birth weight and susceptibility to type 2 diabetes. *Diabetes*;49:82–86.

Theys, N, Bouckenooghe, T, Ahn, MT, Remacle, C & Reusens, B (2009). Maternal low-protein diet alters pancreatic islet mitochondrial function in a sex-specific manner in the adult rat. *Am J Physiol Regul Integr Comp Physiol* 297:R1516-1525.

Tourrel, C, et al. (2002). Persistent improvement of type 2 diabetes in the Goto-Kakizaki rat model by expansion of the beta-cell mass during the prediabetic period with Glucagon-like peptide-1 or Exendin-4. *Diabetes* 51: 1443-1452.

Triadou, N, Portha, B, Picon, L & Rosselin, G (1982). Experimental chemical diabetes and pregnancy in the rat. Evolution of glucose tolerance and insulin response. *Diabetes* 31:75-79.

Unterman, T, et al. (1990). Circulating levels of insulin-like growth factor binding protein-1 [IGFBP-1] and hepatic mRNA are increased in the small for gestational age fetal rat. *Endocrinology* 127, 2035–2037.

Valdez, R, et al. (1994) Birthweight and adult health outcomes in a biethnic population in the USA. *Diabetologia* 37, 624–631.

Van Assche FA & Aerts L (1979). The fetal endocrine pancreas. Contrib Gynecol Obstet 5:44–57.

Van Assche, FA, et al. (1977). The endocrine pancreas in small-for dates infants. *Br. J. Obstet. Gynaecol.* 84, 751–753.

Verhaeghe, J, et al. (1989). Maternal and fetal endocrine pancreas in the spontaneously diabetic BB rat. Biol Neonate 55, 298–308.

Vickers, MH, et al. (2005). Neonatal leptin treatment reverses developmental programming. *Endocrinology* 146, 4211–4216.

Viswanathan, M, McCarthy, MI, Snehalatha, C, Hitman, GA & Ramachandran, A (1996). Familial aggregation of type 2 (non-insulin-dependent) diabetes mellitus in south India; absence of excess maternal transmission. *Diabet Med* 13:232–237.

Waterland, RA, et al. (2008). Methyl donor supplementation prevents transgenerational amplification of obesity. *Int. J. Obes.* 32, 1373–1379.

Waterland, RA & Michels, KB (2007). Epigenetic epidemiology of the developmental origins hypothesis. *Annu. Rev. Nutr.* 27:363–88

Weir, GC, et al. (2001) Beta-cell adaptation and decompensation during the progression of diabetes. *Diabetes* 50 (Suppl. 1), S154–S159.

Wild, S, et al. (2004) Global prevalence of diabetes: estimates for the year 2000 and projections for 2030. *Diabetes Care* 27, 1047–1053.

World Health Organisation (2000). Obesity: preventing and managing the global epidemic. Report of a WHO consultation. In: WHO Technical Report Series. *World Health Organisation.* pp. 1–247.

Zambranon E, et al. (2005): Sex differences in transgenerational alterations of growth and metabolism in progeny (F2) of female offspring (F1) of rats fed a low protein diet during pregnancy and lactation. *J Physiol* 566:225–236.

Zeggini, E, et al. (2007). Replication of genome-wide association signals in UK samples reveals risk loci for type 2 diabetes. *Science*; 316:1336–1341.

Unravelling the Connection Between Gestational Diabetes Mellitus and Butyrylcholinesterase

Alexander E. Omu Frcog
Department of Obstetrics and Gynaecology,
Faculty of Medicine, Kuwait University,
Kuwait

1. Introduction

Gestational Diabetes Mellitus (GDM) is glucose intolerance first diagnosed during pregnancy (Metzger and Coustan 1998, World Health Organization 1999). Gestational diabetes is a condition that complicates 3-12.% of pregnancies (Gabbe and Graves 2003, Omu et al 2010) with wide variation in the incidence of gestational diabetes reported among ethnic groups.This could be newly diagnosed type 1 or type 2 Diabetes Mellitus or a new onset of hyperglycemia secondary to metabolic changes related to pregnancy (Yogev and Visser 2009). The rates of Gestational diabetes mellitus are increasing with the epidemic of obesity worldwide. Risk factors for GDM include advanced maternal age, multiparity, and racial or ethnic minority status (Table 1).

•	Body mass index more than 30 kg/m^2
•	Previous macrosomic baby weighing 4.5 kg or more
•	Previous gestational diabetes
•	Family history of diabetes (first-degree relative with diabetes)
•	Family origin with a high prevalence of diabetes:
	• South Asian (specifically women whose country of family origin is India, Pakistan or
	• Bangladesh)
	• Black Caribbean
	• Middle Eastern (specifically women whose country of family origin is Saudi Arabia, United Arab Emirates, Iraq, Jordan, Syria, Oman, Qatar, Kuwait, Lebanon or Egypt)

Reproduced from the National Institute for Health and Clinical Excellence guideline for diabetes in pregnancy (12) by RCOG Scientific Advisory Committee Opinion Paper 23: Diagnosis and Treatment of Gestational Diabetes (RCOG 2011).

Table 1. Risk factors for Gestational diabetes mellitus

There are health implications for both the mother and infant who remain at risk for complications such as embryopathies, spontaneous abortion and perinatal mortality and morbidity (Loeken 2006).
There has been considerable controversy surrounding the screening and diagnosis, natural history, management and outcome of women with gestational diabetes. The 2008 NICE guidelines (NICE 2008) on diabetes in pregnancy detailed a screening programme targeting biochemical screening to women with risk factors. Women with a history of gestational diabetes mellitus (GDM) have an increased risk for recurrence in subsequent pregnancies, according to the results of a population-based, retrospective cohort study (HAPO Study Cooperative Research Group 2008). Oxidative stress has been implicated in the pathogenesis and development of complications of diabetes in pregnancy (King and Loeken 2004, Loeken 2004, Marfella et al 2001, Morgan et al 2008, Rosen et al 2001, Wender-Ozegowska et al 2004). The role of Butyrylcholinesterase (BuChE) in the aetiology, screening and monitoring, complications and future drug development of Gestational Diabetes Mellitus has become an interesting area of speculative research (Mahmoud et al 2003, Mohmoud etal 2006, Mahmoud et al 2008, Rustemeijer et al 2001, Serlin et al 2009, Sternfield et al 1997).

2. The objective

The objective of this chapter is to elucidate the relationship between gestational diabetes mellitus (GDM) and BuChE in the pathogenesis, monitoring and future drug development.

3. Pathogenesis of GDM

The cornerstones of development of gestational diabetes mellitus are related to modern lifestyle, principally, a lack of exercise and an unhealthy diet, the environment and some degree of genetic profile (American Diabetic Association 2003, Hollander et al 2007, Serlin et al 2009). Elevated glucose in pregnancy may be caused by increased levels of diabetogenic factors of pregnancy such as glucocorticoids, human placental lactogen and oestrogens. Hyperglycaemia causes oxidative stress due to increased production of mitochondrial ROS, nonenzymatic glycation of proteins, and glucose autoxidation (Brownlee 2001). Elevated FFA can also cause oxidative stress due to increased mitochondrial uncoupling and ß-oxidation, leading to the increased production of ROS. In addition, hyperglycemia- and FFA-induced oxidative stress leads to the activation of stress-sensitive signaling pathways (Evans et al 2003). This, in turn, worsens both insulin secretion and action, leading to overt Gestational Diabetes Mellitus. Administration of glucocorticoids significantly decreases the catalytic activity of BuChE in plasma and liver regardless of sex (Vrdoljaki et al 2005).

3.1 Hyperglycemia and oxidative stress

The pathogenic effect of hyperglycaemia is mediated to a significant extent via increased production of reactive oxygen species (ROS) and reactive nitrogen species (RNS) and subsequent oxidative stress (King and Loeken 2004, Marfella2001, Rosen et al 2001, Wender-Ozegowska et al 2004). ROS and RNS directly oxidize and damage DNA, proteins, and lipids and thus adversely affect the pancreas especially the β Langerhan cells that produce insulin. Similarly, there is disruption of the alpha cells that produce glucagon. The paracrine relationship between the pancreatic beta and alpha cells is disrupted to cause β-cell dysfunction. There is also growing evidence that activation of stress-sensitive pathways, such as NF-kB, p38 MAPK, JNK/SAPK, and hexosamine, by elevations in glucose and possibly FFA levels leads to both insulin resistance and impaired insulin secretion through ß-cell dysfunction (Kyriakis et al 1992). Circulating serum levels of lipid peroxidation product malonedialdehyde (MDA) and protein oxidation markers are elevated in GDM compared to healthy normal pregnancy and give rise to a negatively strong correlation between MDA and BuChE in serum and placenta (Omu et al 2010). A third causal pathway may be through the induction of apoptosis of the beta cells by advanced glycation end-products. This would explain the varying severity of GDM among the patients. BuChE deficiency results in delayed metabolism of a number of compounds of clinical significance, including glucose, thus contributing to the pathogenesis of diabetes mellitus. Glucose metabolism is controlled by the hormone insulin produced in the pancreas. BuChE deficiency in pregnancy may be as a result of hereditary deficiency and haemodilution in second half of pregnancy.

3.2 Role of estrogen receptor alpha in glucose and lipid metabolism

The estrogen receptor ER-alpha is emerging as a key molecule involved in glucose and lipid metabolism. The activation of ER-alpha by physiological concentrations of E2 may play an important role in the adaptation of the endocrine pancreas to pregnancy. However, if ER-alpha is over stimulated by an excess of E2 or the action of an environmental estrogen such as Biphenol A (Nadal et al 2009, Paloma et al 2008, Ropero et al 2008), it can result in an excessive insulin signaling. This may provoke insulin resistance in the liver and muscle, as well as beta-cell exhaustion and therefore, contribute to the development of Gestational Diabetes. An association between oestrogen receptor alpha and BuChE has been reported (Combarros et al 2007).

3.3 Environmental factors

The increase of endocrine-disrupting chemicals (EDCs) in the environment has been implicated in the aetiology of GDM (Elobeid and Allison 2008, Newbold et al 2009, Rubin and Sato 2009). A connection at the epidemiologic level in humans has been recently proposed for dioxin, an environmental contaminant that acts through other than estrogen receptors (ERs) as an endocrine disruptor (Bertazzi et al 2001, Remillard et al 2002).

3.4 Autoimmunity and Treg in GDM

Autoimmune phenomena associated with type 1 diabetes mellitus (DM) can also be detected in a subgroup of women with GDM. Islet autoantibodies are present in sera from women with GDM with variable frequency. Distinct phenotypic and genotypic features may be recognised in this subset of women with GDM, which are representative of a distinct clinical entity. Women with previous autoimmune GDM may be candidates for potential immune intervention strategies (Mauricio et al 2001). Normal activity of Treg subpopulations are disrupted in GDM by mechanisms that threaten pregnancy and may contribute to other features of the disorder, with higher percentages of activated T cells than a matched population of healthy pregnant women. BuChE detoxifies anticholinesterases (AC) that are known to threaten pregnancy and one or more of these fetotoxins adversely impacts pregnancy outcome through a mechanism that may include Treg cells. In normal pregnancy, there is correlation between Treg activity and BuChE, whereas in women in whom adequate correlation between Treg cells and BuChE activity is not achieved (Mahmoud et al 2003, Mahmoud et al 2006, Mahmoud et al 2008, Saito et al 2005), there is failure of effective clearance of toxicants which adversely affect maternal immunomodulation in ways that can lead to GDM and other pregnancy-threatening conditions (Baccarelli et al 2002, Bertazzi et al 2001, Eskenazi et al 2004, Lappas et al 2010, Maussolie et al 1992, Remillard et al 2002).

3.5 Genetics of gestational diabetes mellitus

There is very little published data about the genetic basis for gestational diabetes mellitus (GDM) (Watanabe et al 2007). However, there is evidence for clustering of type 2 diabetes and impaired glucose tolerance in families with a GDM (McLellan et al 1995) and evidence for higher prevalence of type 2 diabetes in mothers of women with GDM (Martin et al 1985). HLA DR3 and DR4 antigens are in higher frequency in women with GDM than in women with normal pregnancies. Furthermore, an association between variation in the insulin receptor (*INSR*) in Caucasian and African-American women with GDM has been reported (Ober et al 1989). A β-cell defect is one of the primary characteristics of GDM and β-cell function is a highly heritable trait(Watanabe et al 2007).

4. Association between GDM and oxidative stress and diabetic complications

Pregnancy is susceptible to oxidative stress and antioxidant defenses that can be altered in response to elevated levels of oxidative stress (Chen and Scholl 2005. Marfella et al 2001, Maxwell et al 1997).

In GDM products of lipid peroxidation may be increased and antioxidant enzyme activities decreased and the oxygen free radicals may be involved in severe damage of cellular structure (Osawa andKato 2005, Twardowska-Saucha et al 1994) and pregnancy complicated by poor glycemic control is associated with a higher risk of embryopathies, spontaneous abortion and perinatal morbidity and mortality (Loeken 2006). Recently, Karacay et al (2010) demonstrated that plasma and serum maternal total antioxidant status (TAS) was decreased, while circulating levels of lipid peroxidation breakdown products (MDA) were increased between 24 and 36 weeks of gestation, thus showing that increased oxidative stress and reduction in antioxidant defense mechanisms may contribute to disease processes in GDM (Bertazzi et al 2001, Karacy et al 2010, Rustemeijer et al 2001). Carine et al (1993) and Zachara et al (1993) found no differences in glutathione peroxidase (GPX) levels between pregnant women at third trimester and non-pregnant women, but recent studies have demonstrated an association between GDM and impaired SOD activities and enhanced circulating lipid metabolite levels such as MDA (Grissa et al 2007). Catalase, the main regulator of hydrogen peroxide metabolism is involved in Glut 4 expression, insulin secretion, insulin signaling, protein tyrosine phosphatase regulation, and glucose transport stimulation (Goth et al 2005, Mueller et al 1997). Catalase is important in antioxidant defense against hydrogen peroxide and increased risk of diabetes has been reported in hereditary catalase deficiency (Goth and Eaton 2000, Sindhu et al 2004).

5. Biology of BuChE

The enzyme cholinesterase is present in all mammals and two classes have been identified :acetylcholinesterase (AChE, EC 3.1.1.7) and butyrylcholinesterase (BChE); AChE exists in the central nervous system, platelets and the erythrocyte membrane, while BChE is more abundant in the serum and is synthesized by the liver (Daresh et al 2003). BuChE was named "pseudocholinesterase" by Mendel and Rudney in 1943 (1943). Human plasma BuChE (EC 3.1.1.8) is a globular, tetrameric serine esterase with a molecular mass of ≈340 kDa that is stable in plasma with a half-life of 12 days (Lockridge et al 1987, Ostergaard et al 1988). BuChE acts on hydrophilic and hydrophobic choline esters, and that it hydrolyzes a variety of xenobiotics as shown in Table 2. Previous studies have reported a significant association between the serum BuChE activity and obesity, coronary artery disease, serum levels of triglycerides (TG), very low-density lipoprotein, low-density lipoprotein and Apo lipoprotein B, type 2 diabetes mellitus and the hepatic fat content (Alcantara et al 2005, Cucuianau et al 1999, Randell et 2005, Sridhar et al 2005). At variance with AChE-S, BuChE attenuates the fibril-formation process by the aromatic W8 residue. This residue can form heteroaromatic complexes with soluble monomeric or low-oligomeric Aβ conformers. That replacement of tryptophan to a polar residue abolishes the attenuation of Aβ fibril formation is fully compatible with this hypothesis. AChE mRNA is 20-fold more abundant than BuChE mRNA. In human blood, however, BuChE, at 50 nM, is 3-fold more abundant than AChE (Daresh et al 2003).

BuChE protein or mRNA has been found in almost every tissue of the body, showing that it has a function.	
1.	Acetylcholine and butyrylthiocholine hydrolysis.
2.	Protection from neurotoxins
-	OP nerve agents
-	OP pesticides
-	Carbamate pesticides
-	Alzheimer drugs-donepezil and rivastigmine
-	Physostigmine in the calabar beans
-	Cocaine from Erythroxylum coca plant
-	Solamidine from green potatoes
-	Luperzine A from the club moss
-	Anatoxina in the blue green algae.
3.	Hydrolysis of short-acting muscle relaxants
-	Succinylcholine
4.	Not clear yet
-	Glucose and lipid metabolism

Table 2. Functions of BuChE

5.1 Genetics of BuChE

The complete amino acid sequence of human serum BuChE have been described (Daresh et al 2003). The human butyrylcholinesterase (BuChE; EC 3.1.1.8) is encoded by a single gene which corresponds to the E1 locus *BuCHE* gene (3q26.1-q26.2) which presents four exons (Arpagaus et al 1993), with more than 70 already-described variants (Pantuck 1993, Souza et al 2005). Data from dizygotic twin pairs has shown linkage on chromosome 3 at the location of the BuChE gene and also on chromosome 5. BuChE is found in human plasma, either in homomeric viz. monomers (G1), dimers (G2), trimers (G3) and tetramers (G4), or heteromeric forms associated with other substances, such as albumin (G1-ALB) (Masson et al 1989, Pantuck 1993). The *BCHE-K* variant has been reported to show allelic association with Alzheimer disease (AD) in subjects who are also carriers of the e4 allele of apolipoprotein E (*APOE)*, especially in subjects over the age of 75 years. The K variant, is carried on one allele by one of four persons (Rao et al 2006). As BuChE is found common to both Alzheimer's disease and diabetes; it may play an etiological role via influencing insulin resistance and lipid metabolism (Arpagaus et al 1990, Lockridge et al 1987, Rao et al 2006). Similarly patients with Alzheimer's disease are more vulnerable to developing impaired fasting glucose and type 2 diabetes mellitus (Janson et al 2004, Johansen et al 1991)

5.2 BuChE and placental development

In utero exposure to poisons and drugs (e.g., anticholinesterases, cocaine) is frequently associated with spontaneous absorption and placental malfunction. The major protein interacting with these compounds is butyrylcholinesterase (BuChE), which attenuates the effects of such xenobiotics by their hydrolysis or sequestration. Sternfeld and Associates (1997) studied BuChE expression during placental development. RT-PCR revealed both BuChE mRNA and acetylcholinesterase (AChE) mRNA throughout gestation. Maximum butyrylcholinesterase activity has shown in week 12. In rat placenta, BuChE activity on gestational day 21 reached 150% of the level on gestational day 16. BuChE detoxifies anticholinesterases (AC) and other toxins including free radicals that are known to threaten pregnancy (Hollander et al 2007, Maxwell et al 1997, Osawa and Kato 2005, Twardowska-Saucha et al 1994). There is evidence that Kuwaiti women experiencing disorders of pregnancy like preeclampsia and diabetes mellitus in pregnancy exhibited lower serum activity of BuChE (Mahmoud et al 2003, Mahmoud et al 2006, Mahmoud et al 2008).

6. Clinical role of BuChE

BuChE (BuChE; EC 3.1.1.1.8) has well-defined pharmacologic functions:
BuChE and anaesthetic muscle relaxants: Mivacurium and succinylcholine are short-acting neuromuscular blocking drugs ideal for short surgical procedures as muscle relaxants used in anesthetic practice. The brief duration of action depends on rapid hydrolysis by plasma cholinesterase (Jensen et al 1991Pantuck 1993). An inherited or acquired deficiency of plasma BuChE can prolong the effect of mivacurium. When there is a deficiency of this enzyme due to the presence of one or more atypical alleles, mivacurium and succinylcholine are not properly metabolized and thus muscle paralysis can last for several hours (Davis et al 1997, Goudsouzian et al 1993, Petersen et al 1993, Savarese et al 1997).

6.1 Factors affecting BuChE activity

Different disease states and/or drug administrations may decrease BuChE activity.; such as extremes of age, pregnancy, renal and liver disease, malignancy, burns, chronic debility/malnutrition, myocardial infarction/cardiac failure, collagen diseases, myxedema, poisoning and protein energy malnutrition. Drugs that inhibit the enzyme's activity include acetylcholinesterase inhibitors (neostigmine, pyridostigmine, physostigmine, and edrophonium), anticholinesterases (especially echothlophate), cytotoxic agents (such as cyclophosphamide), steroids, ester-type local anesthetics, hexafluorenium, pancuronium, oral contraceptives and sertraline (Klein-Schwatz and Anderson 1996, MacQueen et al 2001, Muller et al 2002).

6.2 BuChE and Organophosphatase (OP) and cocaine hydrolysis

Another reason for continued interest in serum cholinesterase is its extraordinary sensitivity to organophosphate ester. Systemic administration of BuChE, at a dose sufficient to increase plasma BuChE levels 400-fold (5000 I.U.; i.v.), has been shown to significantly decrease cocaine-induced locomotor activity in rats over a 120-min session (Carmona et al 1997). The identification of BuChE variants that exhibit increased cocaine hydrolysis activity provides treatment options for cocaine-induced conditions such as cocaine overdose and addiction (Arkhypova et al 2004, Lockridge et al 2005), Lynch et al 1997).

6.3 BuChE activity and dyslipidemia and metabolic syndrome

Serum levels of BuChE are affected by dietary fat, obesity, hyperlipidemia and diabetes mellitus, alcohol and many drugs are known to increase BuChE activity (Alcantara et al 2005, Stefanello et al 2005, Vrdoljaki et al 2005). Therefore, BuChE may have a role in the altered lipoprotein metabolism in hypertriglyceridaemia associated with diabetes mellitus and insulin resistance. BuChE is synthesized in the liver, and is present in plasma and to a lesser extent in adipose tissue, small intestine and smooth muscle. Sridhar et al (2005) measured the serum level of BuChE levels in persons with type 2 diabetes mellitus and demonstrated a negative correlation between BuChE and serum total cholesterol and LDL cholesterol, thus further confirming that BuChE may be involved in lipid metabolism.

6.4 Serum determination of BuChE

The application of the techniques of molecular genetics has permitted precise identification of plasma cholinesterase variants and has resulted in the discovery of previously unrecognized variants. Serum BuChE activity has been determined by the method of Ellman et al (1961). In addition to colorimetric methods, HPLC, Electrophoresis, Immunoassay methods (ELIZA) and Biosensor methods have been used.

6.5 Production of human BuChE

Human BuChE has been obtained from human plasma by a large scale purification technique (Lockridge et al 2005). This procedure is severely limited by the volume of human plasma needed and may not be cost effective and it may not yield a sufficient amount of enzyme purified commercially. Large quantities of BuChE are needed for effective prophylaxis and treatment of exposure. BuChE has a broad spectrum of activity, a relatively long half-life, and few physiological side effects. Producing recombinant BuChE (rBuChE) is an alternative to purification of the enzyme from human plasma. A number of studies have shown the feasibility of producing large quantities of BuChE in transgenic animals (goats) and transgenic edible plants for prophylaxis or treatment of humans exposed to OP agents (Lockridge et al 2005, Podoly et al 2008, Protexia 2011) and cocaine overdose or addiction (Om et al 1993).

7. Association between BuChE and oxidative stress

Stefanello et al. (2005) investigated the effect of homocysteine administration on BuChE activity in the serum of rats. Acute and chronic administration of homocysteine significantly decreased BuChE activity but administration of vitamins A and C prevented the reduction of the activity. Delwing et al (2005) observed that acute proline administration provoked a 22% increase in BuChE activity in the serum of rats. In a similar study, Wyse et al (2004) demonstrated that vitamins E and C reversed the inhibition of BuChE activities provoked by arginine in the serum of rats, thus indicating that the reduction of BuChE activities caused by arginine was probably mediated by oxidative stress. In a similar fashion, Cederberg et al. (2001) have shown that combined treatment with vitamins E and C decreased oxidative stress and improved fetal outcome in experimental pregnancy. From the foregoing, BuChE may yet be another mechanism in the fight against oxidative stress.

7.1 Mechanisms of the association between BuChE and oxidative stress in GDM

In a recent report, we (Omu et al 2010) showed that BuChE activity was elevated in the serum and placenta in normal pregnancy as compared to diabetic cohorts ($p < 0.01$) and there was a higher activity level in gestational and type 2 diabetes on insulin ($p<0.05$) compared with diet controlled. Conversely, there was higher MDA and lower antioxidant activity in diet versus insulin controlled diabetes ($p < 0.01$). Both serum and placental BuChE activity showed a strong inverse correlation with MDA ($r = -0.876$, $p < 0.001$) and ($r = - 0.542$, $p < 0.01$), but strong positive correlation with total antioxidant activity in serum ($r = 0.764$, $p < 0.001$) and placenta ($r = 0.642$, $p < 0.01$). These results are therefore consistent with a mechanism in which BuChE acts to scavenge free radicals in the presence of oxidative stress. An interesting finding in the study was the higher BuChE activity in the two groups of insulin-treated diabetics compared with their counterparts on diet. This led to the speculation that the diabetic patients on diet only might not have had satisfactory glycogenic control. However, BuChE did not show any correlation with enzymatic antioxidants SOD and GPX (Omu et al 2010); indirectly showing that BuChE was not inhibiting MDA through the antioxidants pathway. While this is mere speculation, it has important clinical implication if the association between BuChE and glycemic control is confirmed by future research. HbA1c has been used for monitoring diabetic control of the last 3 months, maybe BuChE could be used for short term or immediate monitoring of glycemic control. BuChE is already a known marker of metabolic syndrome (Sridhar et al 2005), and its activity is high in human term placenta (Hahn et al 1993, Lappas et al 2010, Omu et al 2010, Simone et al 1994, Sternfield et al 1997). The lower level of placental BuChE activity compared with serum, shown in the study may be as a result of a high level of fetotoxic agents, including free radicals (oxidative stress), in the placenta that BuChE metabolises by hydrolysis.

7.2 Advanced glycation end-products (AGE), reactive oxygen species (ROS) and BuChE

Glycation reactions lead to the production of reactive oxygen species (ROS), which are harmful to cellular metabolism and cause cell damage. There are no research data of any relationship between AGE and BuChE activity. While it is highly speculative, BuChE may protect pregnancy from the effect of oxidative stress by preventing the (formation) of reactive oxygen species formation by hydrolyzing and inactivating advanced glycation end products upstream. This hypothesis is consistent with the finding of lack of correlation between BuChE and SOD and GPX (Omu et al 2010).

8. Gestational diabetes mellitus and BuChE

Another contributor to toxicant-induced immune dysregulation as a contributor to GDM might be that reactive products of inflammation expressed by the maternal immune system in response to paternal antigens adversely affect maternal health in ways that increase susceptibility to diabetes, thereby leaving women with naturally lower BuChE levels at greater risk for gestational and possibly Type 2 diabetes. The relationship between size of activated lymphocyte cohorts and BuChE activity in the RPL versus healthy cohorts provides additional support for the hypothesis that both immune activation and BuChE activity may be tied to some as-yet-unidentified systemic effector. For example, our observation of positive correlation between the frequency of CD3+CD16+CD56+ cells and BuChE activity in healthy individuals but not RPL-afflicted subjects would be expected if these cells which are often pathogenic, were expanded in response to environmental toxins. In the type 2 diabetes mellitus population serum BuChE activity has been correlated with insulin sensitivity ($r = -0.51$, $P < 0.001$). BuChE activity was elevated in the serum and placenta in normal pregnancy versus diabetic cohorts ($p < 0.01$) and there was a higher activity level in gestational and type 2 diabetes on insulin ($p < 0.05$) compared with diet controlled (Omu et al 2010, Mahmoud et al 2003, Mahmoud et al 2006, Mahmoud et al 2008, Rustemeijer et al 2001)

8.1 BuChE and congenital anomalies

BuChE may also play a significant role in congenital anomalies. Dupont et al. (1995) have reported that fetuses with anencephaly and open spinal bifida and gastroschisis revealed clearly dense band of BuChE in the amniotic fluid. A causative role for elevated free fatty acid (FFA) levels in the development of microvascular complications remains to be established, however. Increased levels of FFAs are positively correlated with both insulin resistance and the deterioration of ß-cell function in the context of concomitant hyperglycemia. These latter effects may result from oxidative stress (Evans et al 2003).

9. Future directions and hypotheses of connection between BuChE and GDM

There is need to explore a number of hypotheses to fully unravel the connection between GDM and BuChE through aggressive research efforts.

9.1 Role of estrogen alpha receptor and BuChE in pathogenesis of gestational diabetes

High levels of estrogens in the second half of pregnancy with high estrogen receptor alpha (ER α) lead to deterioration of glucose metabolism. Estrogens may reduce the risk of AD through enhancing or preserving cholinergic neurotransmission, and aromatase, the product of the CYP19 gene, is a critical enzyme in the peripheral synthesis of estrogens. There is evidence to suggest that the CYP19 and BuChE polymorphisms may interact in determining the risk of AD. Carriers of both the ER-a P/P genotype and the BuChE K variant would have decreased risk of developing AD (Conbarros et al 2007). ER alpha signaling activity and glucose metabolism may therefore be affected by CYP19 and BuChE polymorphisms.

9.2 Advanced glycation end products hydrolysis by BuChE

Advanced glycation end products may inhibit BuChE activities, probably as a result of the hydrolyzing effect of the latter, upstream before they cause oxidative stress.

10. Concluding remarks

Unraveling the connection between GDM and BuChE has become a veritable area of research in the pathogenesis, screening, prevention and management. With the large scale purification of BuChE from human plasma, milk of transgenic goats and edible transgenic plants and its suitability for prophylactic and therapeutic protection against cocaine and nerve agent toxicity, the way for therapeutic use in humans, especially during complicated pregnancy needs urgent scientific exploration as BuChE may have an important protective role in normal and diabetic pregnancy by reducing oxidative stress and therefore reduce diabetes induced complications. Mechanisms for attenuation of the effects of oxidative stress by BuChE should be investigated. Heritable factors may be an underlying biological thread in the connection between GDM and BuChE. In addition, genetic variants of BuChE exist, which may play a role in biological manifestation of individuals. Identification of such sequences would provide leads for further understanding of aetiological, therapeutic or prognostic aspects of Gestational diabetes mellitus. If future studies reveal that immune dysregulation is a contributor to the pathogenesis of GD or DM, characterization of the mechanisms will open additional avenues to development of therapeutic approaches to both disorders.

11. References

Alcantara VM, Oliveira LC, Rea RR, Suplicy HL, Chautard-Freire-Maia EA. Butyrylcholinesterase activity and metabolic syndrome in obese patients. *Clin Chem Lab Med.* 2005;43:285–8.

American Diabetes Association. Gestational diabetes mellitus. *Diabetes Care.* 2003; 26: S103–S105.

Arkhypova VN.,. Dzyadevychlexey S V, Soldatkin P, Korpan Y I. El'skaya A V, Gravoueille J-M, Martelet C and Jaffrezic-Renault N. Application of enzyme field effect transistors for fast detection of total glycoalkaloids content in potatoes. *Sensors and Actuators B: Chemical* 2004; 103: 416-422

Arpagaus M, Kott M, Vatsis KP, Bartels CF, La Du BN and Lockridge O Structure of the gene for human butyrylcholinesterase. Evidence for a single copy. *Biochemistry* 1990; 29:24-131.

Baccarelli A, Mocarelli P, Patterson DG, Bonzini M, Pesatori AC, Landi MT: Immunologic effects of dioxin: new results from Seveso and comparison with other studies. *Environ Health Persp* 2002; 110:1169–1173.

Bertazzi PA, Consonni PA, Bachetti S et al. Health effedts of dioxin exposure: a 20 years mortality study. *Am J Epidemiol* 2001; 153: 1031-1044

Brownlee M: Biochemistry and molecular cell biology of diabetic complications. *Nature* 2001; 414 :813 -820.

Carine D, Loverco G, Greko P, Capuno F, Scivaggi L. Lipid peroxidation products and antioxidant enzymes in red blood cells during normal and diabetic pregnancy. *Eur J Obstet Gynaecol Reprod Biol* 1993; 51: 103-109.2.

Carmona GN, Schindler CW, Shoaib M, Jufer R, Cone EJ, Goldberg SR, Greig NH, Yu QS and Gorelick DA. Attenuation of cocaine-induced locomotor activity by butyrylcholinesterase. *Exp Clin Psychopharmacol* 1998; 6:274-279.

Cederberg J, Siman CM, Eriksson UJ.. Combined treatment with vitamins E and C decrease oxidative stress and improves fetal outcome in experimental diabetic pregnancy. *Pediatric Research* 2001; 49: 755–762.

Chen X, Scholl TO. Oxidative stress: changes in pregnancy and with gestational diabetes mellitus. *Curr Diab Rep.* 2005; 5: 282-288.

Combarros O, Riancho JA, Arozamena J, Mateo I, Llorca J, Infante J et al. Interaction between estrogen receptor-alpha and butyrylcholinesterase genes modulates Alzheimer's disease risk. *J Neurol.* 2007; 254: 1290-1292.

Cucuianu M. Serum gamma glutamyltransferase and/or serum cholinesterase as markers of the metabolic syndrome. *Diabetes Care.* 1999;22:1381-1382.

Darvesh S, Hopkins D A. & Geula C. Neurobiology of butyrylcholinesterase *Nature Reviews Neuroscience* 2003; 4: 131–138.

Davis L, Britten JJ, Morgan M. Cholinesterase. Its significance in anaesthetic practice. *Anaesthesia.* 1997;52:714

Delwing D, Chiarani F, Wannmacher CMD, Wajner M, Wyse ATS. Effect of hyperprolinemia on acetylcholinesterase and butyrylcholinesterase activities in rat. *Amino Acids* 2005; .28:305–308.

Dupont M, Vallet B, Brun A, Boulot P, Demaille J. Scanning gel densitometry of amniotic fluid acetylcholinesterase and butyrylcholinesterase: quantification of 'faint-positive' bands in fetal malformations. *Biol Neonate.* 1995; 67: 244-247

Ellman GL, Courtney KD, Andres V, Featherstone RM, A new and rapid colorimetric determination of Acetycholinesterase activity. *Bioch Pharmacol* 1961; 7: 88-95

Elobeid, M.; Allison, D. "Putative environmental-endocrine disruptors and obesity: a review" *Current opinion in endocrinology, diabetes, and obesity* 2008; 15: 403–408.

Eskenazi B, Harley K, Bradman A, Weltzien E, Jewell NP, Barr DB, Furlong CE, Holland NT: Association of in utero organophosphate pesticide exposure and fetal growth and length of gestation in an agricultural population. *Environ Health Perspect* 2004; 112:1116–1124.

Evans J L, Goldfine I D, Maddux B A, and Grodsky G M.Are Oxidative Stress-Activated Signaling Pathways Mediators of Insulin Resistance and ß-Cell Dysfunction? *Diabetes* 2003; 52 :1-8.

Gabbe SG, Graves CR. Management of diabetes mellitus complicating pregnancy. *Obstet Gynecol* 2003; 102: 857–68.

Góth L, Eaton JW. Hereditary catalase deficiencies and increased risk of diabetes. *Lancet* 2000;356:1820-1821

Góth L, Tóth Z, Tarnai I, Bérces M, Török P and Bigler W N. Blood Catalase Activity in Gestational Diabetes Is Decreased but Not Associated with Pregnancy Complications *Clinical Chemistry.* 2005;51:2401-2404.

Goudsouzian NG, d'Hollander AA, Viby-Mogensen J. Prolonged neuromuscular block from mivacurium in two patients with cholinesterase deficiency. *Anesth Analg.* 1993;77:183–185.

Grissa O, Atègbo JM, Yessoufou A, Tabka Z, Miled A, Jerbi M, Dramane KL et al. Antioxidant status and circulating lipids are altered in human gestational diabetes and macrosomia. *Transl Res* 2007; 150:164-71.

Hahn T, Desoye G, Lang I, Skofitsch G. Location and activities of acetylcholinesterase and butyrylcholinesterase in the rat and human placenta. *Anat Embryol.* 1993;188: 435-40.

Hollander MH, Paarlberg KM, Huisjes AJ. Gestational diabetes: a review of the current literature and guidelines. *Obstet Gynecol Surv.* 2007;62:125–136.

HAPO Study Cooperative Research Group, Metzger BE, Lowe LP, Dyer AR, Trimble ER, Chaovarindr U, Coustan DR, et al. Hyperglycemia and adverse pregnancy outcomes. *N Engl J Med* 2008;358:1991–2002.

Janson J, Laedtke T, Parisi JE, Brien PO, Petersen RC, Butler PC: Increased risk of type 2 diabetes in Alzheimer disease. *Diabetes* 2004, 53:474-81].

Jensen FS, Viby-Morgensen J, Ostergaard D. Significance of plasma cholinesterase for the anaesthetist. *Curr Anaesth Crit Care.* 1991;2:232–237.

Johansen AE-M, Nielsen D, Andersen G, Hamid YH, Jensen DP, Glümer C, Drivsholm T, Borch-Johnsen K, Jørgensen T, Hansen T, Pedersen O: Large-scale studies of the functional K variant of the butyrylcholinesterase gene in relation to Type 2 diabetes and insulin secretion. *Diabetologia* 2004, 47:1437-41.

Karacay O, Sepici-Dincel A, Karcaaltincaba D, Sahin D, Yalvaç S, Akyol M, Kandemir O, Altan N. A quantitative evaluation of total antioxidant status and oxidative stress markers in preeclampsia and gestational diabetic patients in 24-36 weeks of gestation. *Diabetes Res Clin Pract.* 2010; 89: 231-8.

King GL, Loeken MR.Hyperglycemia-induced oxidative stress in diabetic complications. *Histochem Cell Biol.* 2004; 122: 333-8

Klein-Schwartz W, Anderson B. Analysis of sertraline-only overdoses. *Am J Emerg Med.* 1996;14:456–458.

Kyriakis, J.M., Banerjee, P. Nikolakaki, E., Dai, T., Rubie, E.A., Ahmad, M.F., Avruch, J. and Woodgett, J.R. The stress-activated protein kinase subfamily of c-Jun kinases. *Nature* 1994, 369: 156-60.

Lappas M, Mitton A, Permezel M. Release of Proinflammatory Cytokines and 8-Isoprostane from Placenta, Adipose Tissue, and Skeletal Muscle from Normal Pregnant Women and Women with Gestational Diabetes Mellitus. *J Endocrinol. 2010; 204; 75-84.*

Lockridge O, Bartels CF, Vaughan TA, Wong CK, Norton SE, Johnson LL. Complete amino acid sequence of human serum cholinesterase. *J Biol Chem.* 1987;262:549–557.

Lockridge O, Schopfer LM, Winger G, Woods JH Large scale purification of butyrylcholinesterase from human plasma suitable for injection into monkeys; a potential new therapeutic for protection against cocaine and nerve toxicity. *Journal of Medical Chemical, Biological and Radiological Defense.* 2005; 3:1–20.

Loeken MR. Advances in understanding the molecular causes of diabetes-induced birth defects. *J Soc Gynecol Investig*. 2006;13: 2-10.

Lynch TJ, Mattes CE, Singh A, Bradley RM, Brady RO, Dretchen KL. Cocaine detoxification by human plasma butyrylcholinesterase. Toxicol Appl Pharmacol 1997;145:363–371

MacQueen G, Born L, Steiner M. The selective serotonin reuptake inhibitor sertraline: its profile and use in psychiatric disorders. *CNS Drug Rev.* 2001;7:1–24.

Mahmoud F, Haines D, Abul H, Omu A. Butyrylcholinesterase activity and pregnancy-associated differences in immunologically relevant peripheral blood leukocyte populations. . *Am J Reprod Immunol.* 2003;50:77-82.

Mahmoud FF, Haines DD, Abul HT, Omu AE, Abu-Donia MB. Butyrylcholinesterase activity in gestational diabetes: correlation with lymphocyte subpopulations in peripheral blood. *Am J Reprod Immunol.* 2006; 56:185-92.

Mahmoud FF, Abul HT, Haines DD, Omu AE, Diejomaoh M, Wise JA, Abu Donia MB. Butyrylcholinesterase activity and lymphocyte subpopulations in peripheral blood of Kuwaiti women experiencing recurrent spontaneous abortion. *Reprod Immunol.* 2008;77:186-94.

Marfella R, Quagliaro L, Nappo F, Ceriello A and Giugliano D. Acute hyperglycemia induces an oxidative stress in healthy subjects. J Clin Invest 2001; 108 : 635-636.

Martin AO, Simpson JL, Ober C, Freinkel N: Frequency of diabetes mellitus in mothers of probands with gestational diabetes: possible maternal influence on the predisposition to gestational diabetes. *Am J Obstet Gynecol* 1985; 151:471–475.

Masson P A naturally occurring molecular form of human plasma cholinesterase is an albumin conjugate. *Biochim Biophys Acta* 1989; 988:258-266.

Massoulie´ J, Bon S, Anselmet A, Chatel J-M, Coussen F, Duval N, Krejici E, Legay C, Vallette F.Biosynthesis of the molecular forms of acetylcholinesterase. In Multidisciplinary Approaches to Cholinesterase Functions, A Shafferman, B Velan (eds). New York, Plenum Press, 1992, pp 17–24.

Mauricio D, de Leiva A. Autoimmune gestational diabetes mellitus: a distinct clinical entity? *Diabetes Metab Res Rev* 2001;17 : 422-2

Maxwell SRJ, Thomason H, Sandler D, Leguen C, Baxter MA, Thorpe GHG, Jones AF, Barnett AH Antioxidant status in patients with uncomplicated insulin-dependent and non-insulin-dependent diabetes mellitus. *Eur J Clin Invest* 1997; 27:484–490

McLellan JA, Barrow BA, Levy JC, Hammersley MS, Hattersley AT, Gillmer MD, Turner RC: Prevalence of diabetes mellitus and impaired glucose tolerance in parents of women with gestational diabetes. *Diabetologia* 1995;38: 693–698

Mendel B. and Rudney H. Cholinesterase and pseudo-cholinesterase. *Biochem. J.* 1943; 37: 59-63.

Metzger BE, Coustan DR, the Organizing Committee. Summary and recommendations of the Fourth International Workshop-Conference on Gestational Diabetes Mellitus. *Diabetes Care* 1998; 21: B161–167

Morgan SC, Relaix F, Sandell LL, Loeken MR. Oxidative stress during diabetic pregnancy disrupts cardiac neural crest migration and causes outflow tract defects. *Birth Defects Res A Clin Mol Teratol.* 2008; 82: 453-63.

Mueller S, Riedel HD, Stremmer W. Direct evidence for catalase as the predominant H_2O_2 removing enzyme in human erythrocytes. *Blood* 1997; 90: 4973-4978.

Müller TC, Rocha JB, Morsch VM, Neis RT, Schetinger MR. Antidepressants inhibit human acetylcholinesterase and butyrylcholinesterase activity. *Biochim Biophys Acta.* 2002;1587:92–98

Nadal A, Alonso-Magdalena P, Soriano S, Quesada I, Ropero AB. The pancreatic beta-cell as a target of estrogens and xenoestrogens: Implications for blood glucose homeostasis and diabetes. *Mol Cell Endocrinol.* 2009; 304: 63-8

National Institute for Health and Clinical Excellence. NICE clinical guideline 63: *Diabetes in pregnancy.Management of diabetes and its complications from pre-conception to the postnatal period.* London: NICE; 2008

Newbold R.; Padilla-Banks E.; Jefferson W. "Environmental estrogens and obesity". *Molecular and cellular endocrinology* 2009; 304: 84–89.

Ober C, Xiang KS, Thisted RA, Indovina KA, Wason CJ, Dooley S: Increased risk for gestational diabetes mellitus associated with insulin receptor and insulin-like growth factor II restriction fragment length polymorphisms. *Genet Epidemiol* 1989; 6:559–56.

Om A, Ellahham S, Ornato JP, Picone C, Theogaraj J, Corretjer GP, Vetrovec GW. Medical complications of cocaine: Possible relationship to low plasma cholinesterase enzyme. Am Heart J 1993; 125:1114–1117

Omu AE, Al-Azemi MK, Omu FE, Fatinikun T, Abraham S, George S, Mahnazhath N. Butyrylcholinesterase activity in women with diabetes mellitus in pregnancy: correlation with antioxidant activity. *J Obstet Gynaecol.* 2010; 30:122-6.

Osawa T, Kato Y. Protective role of antioxidative food factors in oxidative stress caused by hyperglycemia. *Ann N Y Acad Sci.* 2005; 1043:440-51.

Ostergaard D, Viby-Mogensen J, Hanel HK, Skovgaard LT. . Halflife of plasma cholinesterase. *Acta Anaesthesiol Scand.* 1988; 32:266–2696.

Paloma A M, Ropero A B, Carrera M. P,. Cederroth C R, Baquié M, Gauthier B R., Nef S, Stefani E and Nadal A. Pancreatic Insulin Content Regulation by the Estrogen Receptor ERα. PLoS ONE. 2008; 3: e2069.

Pantuck EJ. Plasma cholinesterase: gene and variations. Anesth Analg. 1993 ;77:380-86.

Petersen RS, Bailey PL, Kalameghan R, Ashwood ER. Prolonged neuromuscular block after mivacurium. *Anesth Analg.* 1993;76:194–196.

Podoly E, Bruck T, Diamant S, Melamed-Book N, Weiss A, Huang Y, Livnah O, Langermann S, Wilgus H, Soreq. Human recombinant butyrylcholinesterase purified from the milk of transgenic goats interacts with beta-amyloid fibrils and suppresses their formation in vitro. *Neurodegener Dis.* 2008;5: 232-6.

Protexia -Gene-Delivered Butyrylcholinesterase Is Prophylactic against the Toxicity of Chemical Warfare Nerve Agents and Organophosphorus Compounds *J. Pharmacol. Exp. Ther.* 2011: 337; 92-101

Randell EW, Mathews MS, Zhang H, Seraj JS, Sun G. Relationship between serum butyrylcholinesterase and the metabolic syndrome. *Clin Biochem.* 2005;38:799–805.

Rao A A, Sridhar G R, Thota H, Babu C S, Prasad A S, Divakar C. Alzheimer's disease and Type 2 diabetes mellitus: the cholinesterase connection? *Lipids in Health and Disease* 2006, 5:28-34.

RCOG Scientific Advisory Committee Opinion Paper 23: Diagnosis and Treatment of Gestational Diabetes. January 2011.

Remillard RBJ, Bunce NJ. Linking Dioxins to Diabetes: Epidemiology and Biologic Plausibility. *Environ Health Perspect* 2002; 110:853-858.

Ropero AB, Alonso-Magdalena P, Quesada I, Nadal A. The role of estrogen receptors in the control of energy and glucose homeostasis. *Steroids*.2008.; 73; 874-79.

Rosen P, Nawroth PP, King G, Moller W, Tritschler HJ, Packer L: The role of oxidative stress in the onset and progression of diabetes and its complications: a summary of a Congress Series sponsored by UNESCO-MCBN, the American Diabetes Association, and the German Diabetes Society. *Diabetes Metab Res Rev* 2001;17 :189 – 212,

Rubin B, Soto A. "Bisphenol A: Perinatal exposure and body weight". *Molecular and cellular endocrinology* 2009; 304: 55–62.

Rustemeijer C, Schouten JA, Voerman HJ, Beynen AC, Donker AJM, Heines, RJ. Is pseudocholinesterase activity related to markers of triacylglycerol synthesis in type II diabetes mellitus? *Clin Sci* 2001;101:29-35

Saito S, Sasaki Y, Sakai M. CD4(+)CD25 high regulatory T cells in human pregnancy. *J Reprod Immunol.* 2005; 65:111–120.

Savarese JJ, Lien CA, Belmont MR, Wastila WB. The clinical pharmacology of new benzylisoquinoline-diester compounds. with special consideration of cisatracurium and mivacurium. *Anesthetist.* 1997;46:840–849

Serlin DC and. Lash, R W. Diagnosis and Management of Gestational Diabetes Mellitus. *Am Fam Physician.* 2009 ; 80: 57-62.

Simone C, Derewlany LO, OskampM, Johnson D, Knie B, Koren GAcetylcholinesterase and butyrylcholinesterase activity in the human term placenta: implications for fetal cocaine exposure. *Journal of Laboratory and Clinical Medicine.* 1994. 123: 400–406

Sindhu RK, Koo JR, Roberts CK, Vazioori ND. Dysregulation of hepatic superoxide dismutase, catalase, and glutathione peroxidase in diabetes: responses to insulin and antioxidant therapies. *Clin Exp Hypertens* 2004;26:43-53

Souza RLR, Mikami LR, Maegawa ROB and Chautard-Freire-Maia EA Four new mutations in the *BCHE* gene of butyrylcholinesterase in a Brazilian blood donor sample. *Mol Genet Metab* 2005; 84:349-353.

Sridhar GR, Nirmala G, Apparao A, Madhavi AS, Sreelatha S, Rani J S and Vijayalakshmi P Serum butyrylcholinesterase in type 2 diabetes mellitus: a biochemical and bioinformatics approach. *Lipids Health Dis.* 2005; 4: 18-.

Stefanello FM, Franzon R, Tagliari B, Wannmacher C, Wajner M, Wyse AT. Reduction of butyrylcholinesterase activity in rat serum subjected to Hyperhomocysteinemia. Metabolic Brain Disease 2005; 20:97–103.

Sternfeld M, Ben-Ari S, Rachmilewitz J, Glick C, Loewenstein-Lichtenstein Y, Soreq H, Andres C, Zakut H, Timberg R: Normal and atypical butyrylcholinesterases in placental development, function, and malfunction. *Cell & Mol Neurobiol* 1997; 17:315–332.

Twardowska-Saucha K, Grzeszczak W, Lacka B, Frehlich J, Krywult D. Lipid peroxidation, antioxidant enzyme activity and trace element concentration in II and III trimesters of pregnancy in pregnant women with diabetes. *Poskie Archiwum Medycyny Wewnetrzne j.* 1994; .92: 313-21.

Vrdoljaki A L, Bradamante V, Radi B, Peraica M, Fuchs R, Reine E. Butyrylcholinesterase activity and plasma lipids in dexamethasone treated rats *Acta Pharm* 2005; 55: 177–185.

Watanabe R M, Black M H, Xiang A H., Allayee H, Lawrence J M., Buchanan T A. Genetics of Gestational Diabetes Mellitus and Type 2 Diabetes. *Diabetes Care* 2007; 30: S134-S140

Wender-Ozegowska E, Kozlik J, Biczysko R, Ozegowski S. Changes of Oxidative Stress Parameters in Diabetic Pregnancy. *Free Radical Research,* 2004; 38 : 795-803.

World Health Organization. *Definition, diagnosis and classification of diabetes mellitus and its complications. Report of a WHO consultation. Part 1. Diagnosis and classification of diabetes mellitus.* Geneva: WHO, 1999; WHP/NCD/NCS/99.26p.

Wyse ATS, Stefanello FM, Chiarani F, Delwing D, Wannmacher CMD, Wajner M. Arginine administration decreases cerebral cortex acetylcholinesterase and serum butyrylcholinesterase by oxidative stress induction. *Neurochemical Research 2004; .29:385–389.*

Yogev, Y. & Visser, G. Obesity, gestational diabetes and pregnancy outcome. Seminars in Fetal & Neonatal Medicine 2009, 14, 77-84

Zachara BA, Wardak C, Didkowski W, Maciage A, Marchaluk E. Changes in blood selenium and glutathione peroxidase concentrations and glutathione peroxidase activity in human pregnancy. *Gynecol Obstet Invest* 1993; 35: 12-17.

13

Gestational Hyperglycemia, Excessive Pregnancy Weight Gain and Risk of Fetal Overgrowth

Xinhua Chen, Theresa O. Scholl,
Robert A. Steer and T. Peter Stein
University of Medicine and Dentistry of New Jersey – School of Osteopathic Medicine
USA

1. Introduction

Between 1989 and 2004 the prevalence of gestational diabetes mellitus (GDM) in the US increased from 1.9% to 4.2% in parallel with the well documented obesity epidemic (Getahun et al., 2008; Mokdad et al., 2001). However, an additional 9-20% of pregnant women, with a milder form of glucose intolerance which does not meet the diagnostic criteria for GDM, may also be at risk of type 2 diabetes, cardiovascular disease and problems while pregnant (Stamilio et al., 2004; Mello et al., 1997; Bo et al., 2004; Nordin et al., 2006).

Fetal overgrowth, defined as macrosomia (birth weight >4000g) or large-for-gestational-age birth (LGA, birth weight >90th percentile for a given gestational age) increases maternal morbidity from operative delivery and also causes serious consequences to the offspring including birth trauma, obesity during childhood and type 2 diabetes and metabolic syndrome in adult life (Boney et al., 2005; Zhang & Bowes, 1995; Langer, 2000).

GDM and excessive pregnancy weight gain, especially in obese women are known risk factors for fetal overgrowth (Ray et al., 2001; Hillier et al., 2008). Although previous research has suggested that metabolic abnormalities are also present in pregnant women with less severe hyperglycemia, the clinical implications of milder maternal hyperglycemia are poorly described (Chen et al., 2010; Cheng et al., 2006; Nordin et al., 2006).

The primary objective of this chapter is to use prospective data from a population of low income and minority women to examine (i) the influence of maternal hyperglycemia including GDM and less severe maternal hyperglycemia on risk of fetal overgrowth; (ii) the association of longitudinally measured excessive pregnancy weight gain with risk of fetal overgrowth (IOM, 2009); (iii) the independent contribution of gestational hyperglycemia and excessive pregnancy weight gain to fetal overgrowth.

Because gestational hyperglycemia and excess weight gain during pregnancy are preventable risk factors, early detection and treatment of mild hyperglycemia and monitoring pregnancy weight gain may be important for reducing the risk of LGA, for reducing childhood and later obesity and for improving the long term risk for metabolic disease.

2. Maternal hyperglycemia and fetal overgrowth

2.1 Fetal overgrowth

Fetal growth is dependent on the capacity of mother to supply nutrients and also on the capacity of the placenta to transfer these nutrients to the fetus (Oken & Gillman., 2003; Ehrenberg et al., 2004). Maternal factors including parity, length of gestation, mother's adult size, and mother's own birth weight are strongly related to fetal growth and development (Langer, 2000). The prevalence of fetal overgrowth was reported as 8-16% from women without GDM and 15-40% from women with gestational hyperglycemia (Mello et al., 1997; Ostlund et al., 2003; Bo et al., 2004; Gruendhammer et al., 2003).

2.2 GDM and fetal overgrowth

Despite different diagnostic criteria, many studies confirmed that GDM increases the risk of macrosomia or LGA birth (Ricart et al., 2005; Ray et al., 2001; Ehrenberg et al., 2004). Maternal hyperglycemia increases fetal growth via delivery of excess maternal plasma glucose to the fetus, which results in fetal hyperinsulinemia and promotes fetal overgrowth (HAPO, 2008; Oken & Gillman., 2003). GDM women undergoing intensive diabetic care had similar neonatal birth weights and macrosomia rates compared to non-GDM women (Ogonowski et al., 2008) and a clinical trial of continuous glucose monitoring in GDM resulted in a significant improvement in infant birth weight with a reduced risk of macrosomia (Murphy et al., 2008).

2.3 Significance of mild gestational hyperglycemia and LGA birth

2.3.1 Prevalence of mild gestational hyperglycemia

Recent studies have paid more attention to pregnancy outcomes of women with gestational hyperglycemia less severe than overt GDM. The prevalence of mild hyperglycemia (defined as abnormal plasma glucose concentration during glucose challenge test with a diagnostic oral glucose tolerance test (OGTT) that did not meet the criteria of GDM) in women screened for GDM was 32% in Caucasian women (Mello et al, 1997), 25% in Mexican-Americans (Yogev et al, 2004) and 9% in multiethnic US population where 70% were African American (Stamilio et al., 2004). The relatively high prevalence of less severe maternal hyperglycemia raises important questions about effects on the fetus since these women are not provided the usual diabetic care for GDM.

2.3.2 The impact of mild gestational hyperglycemia on fetal overgrowth is inconsistent

Studies suggest that an impaired maternal OGTT is associated with adverse maternal-fetal outcomes especially risk of macrosomia and LGA birth (Vambergue et al., 2000; Ostlund et al., 2003). The degree of maternal glucose intolerance was associated with a graded increase in the incidence of fetal macrosomia (Sermer et al., 1995). Moreover, the recent hyperglycemia and adverse pregnancy outcome study (HAPO) found a strong association of maternal glucose concentrations below levels diagnostic of diabetes with increased infant birth weight (HAPO, 2008), but others found no significant increase in the risk of LGA in mildly hyperglycemic women (Nordin et al., 2006; Gruendhammer et al., 2003). Bo et al suggested that metabolic syndrome in mid-pregnancy might be an independent predictor of macrosomia in women with some degree of gestational hyperglycemia, including GDM and mild hyperglycemia without GDM (Bo et al., 2004).

Conflicting data on mild hyperglycemia and fetal overgrowth can be, at least in part, due to the different population studied and the criteria used for mild hyperglycemia. Although the HAPO study included multiple countries and populations and had a large sample size, it was focused on developing an international consensus for the diagnosis and treatment of carbohydrate intolerance during pregnancy, and was not designed to compare the difference in LGA between GDM and less severe hyperglycemic pregnancies (HAPO, 2008). Thus, to establish the risk of adverse fetal outcomes in relation to milder degrees of maternal hyperglycemia is clinically important, particularly in high risk US populations.

2.4 The Camden study

Camden Study is a prospective cohort study of pregnancy outcome and complications in young, generally healthy women residing in one of the poorest cities in the continental United States (Webster & Bishaw, 2006). Women with serious non-obstetric problems (e.g., Lupus, type 1 or 2 diabetes, seizure disorders, malignancies, acute or chronic liver disease, drug or alcohol abuse and psychiatric problems) were excluded from participation. The sample for this analysis totaled 2,373 pregnant women with live births who enrolled between 1996-2006.

2.4.1 Definition of GDM and mild hyperglycemia non-GDM in Camden study

The diagnosis of GDM was made using a two-step approach. All participants were initially screened by measuring the plasma glucose concentration 1h after a 50-g oral glucose challenge test (GCT) at 28±0.1 (mean±SE) weeks' gestation. A diagnostic OGTT was performed on that subset of women exceeding the glucose threshold value (>140 mg/dl). The diagnostic criteria for GDM was the Carpenter/Coustan conversion as recommended by the American Diabetes Association (ADA) which defines GDM by two or more glucose values over the cut points of 95,180,155,140 mg/dl at fasting, 1, 2, and 3 hours during a 100g OGTT (American Diabetes Association, 2000). Women with a positive GCT and fewer than two abnormal glucose values were identified as having an impaired GCT without GDM (impaired GCT non-GDM). All of patients diagnosed with GDM obtained dietary counseling and/or insulin treatment for their glycemic control; patients with impaired CGT non-GDM were untreated.

We identified 2,092 women (88.1%) with normal GCT, 182 women (7.7%) with impaired GCT non-GDM and 99 women (4.2%) with GDM (table 1). Ethnic composition of the cohort was 46% Hispanic, 37.6% African American and 16.6% Caucasian plus others. When the maternal characteristics were rank ordered with respect to glucose tolerance status, older maternal age, higher pre-pregnant body mass index (BMI), obesity and prior history of GDM, all were found to be positively associated with maternal glycemic status (normal GCT, impaired GCT non-GDM or GDM) and represented a linear increasing trend in terms of severity (p for trend <0.001 for each).

2.4.2 Maternal hyperglycemia and LGA birth

LGA is defined as a neonatal birth weight greater than the 90th percentile for gestational age that has been adjusted for ethnicity, parity and infant sex (Zhang & Bowes, 1995). Women with GDM or impaired GCT without GDM had a ~2-fold increased risk for bearing an LGA infant as compared to women with normal GCT (table 2, model 1) after controlling for maternal confounding variables and using a standard which adjusted LGA for maternal ethnicity, parity and fetal gender. This increased risk persisted after additional adjustments

Characteristics	All patients	Normal GCT	Impaired GCT non-GDM	GDM
N (%)	2373 (100)	2092 (88.1)	182 (7.7)	99 (4.2)
Age (yr)[1]	22.1±0.1	21.7±0.1	24.4±0.4	26.3±0.6
Pre-pregnant BMI (kg/m^2)[1]	25.7±0.1	25.4±0.1	26.6±0.5	29.8±0.8
BMI categories[1]				
<18.5	146 (6.2)	141 (6.7)	5 (2.8)	0
18.5-24.9	1157 (48.8)	1050 (50.2)	82 (45.1)	25 (25.3)
25-29.9	587 (24.7)	503 (24.0)	50 (27.5)	34 (34.3)
≥30	483 (20.4)	398 (19.0)	45 (24.7)	40 (40.0)
Cigarette smoking	440 (18.5)	381(18.2)	39 (21.4)	20 (20.2)
Ethnicity[2]				
Hispanic	1089 (45.9)	949 (45.4)	82 (45.0)	58 (58.6)
African American	891(37.6)	803 (38.4)	67 (36.8)	21 (21.2)
Caucasian & other	393 (16.6)	340 (16.3)	33 (18.1)	20 (20.2)
Medicaid	2323 (97.9)	2047 (97.9)	178 (97.8)	98 (99.0)
Prior GDM in multiparas[1]	33 (1.4)	15 (0.7)	8 (4.4)	10 (10.0)
Primiparas[2]	923 (38.9)	833 (39.8)	60 (33.0)	30 (30.3)

Data are mean ± SE or n (%).
Normal GCT, during a glucose challenge test, glucose ≤140mg/dl; Impaired GCT non-GDM, glucose >140mg/dl during a glucose challenge test and non-GDM; GDM, gestational diabetes mellitus (same in tables 2,4,5).
1. p for linear contrasts among groups <0.001 from ANOVA, or Mantel-Haenszel chi-square test;
2. p for linear contrasts among groups <0.05 from Mantel-Haenszel chi-square test.

Table 1. Characteristics of Study Participants

for pre-pregnant BMI and net maternal weight gain (net weight gain=total weight gain-infant birth weight) in women with impaired GCT non-GDM (Table 2, model 2), but it was non-significant in women with GDM.

		LGA	AOR (95% CI)[1]	
	N	Unadjusted %	Model 1[2]	Model 2[3]
GDM	99	10.1	2.05 (1.03, 4.10)	1.52 (0.74, 3.13)
Impaired GCT non-GDM	182	12.1	2.48 (1.50, 4.09)	2.50 (1.50, 4.14)
Normal GCT	2092	5.3	Reference	Reference

LGA, large-for-gestational age infant; AOR, adjusted odds ratio; 95% CI, 95% confidence interval (same as in tables 4-5).
1 p for linear trend <0.01.
2 Model 1 was adjusted for age and cigarette smoking in addition to using a standard which adjusted LGA for maternal ethnicity, parity and fetal gender.
3 Model 2 was adjusted for all variables in model 1 with additional adjustment for pre-pregnant BMI and net of weight gain (kg) during pregnancy.

Table 2. Maternal Hyperglycemia and LGA birth

2.4.3 What do we learn from the Camden study?

Complicating the interpretation of previous studies has been the inability to adjust the observations for important factors related to fetal growth such as pre-pregnant obesity or gestational weight gain, often because the data were not available (Hillier et al., 2008; Rosenberg et al., 2005; Aberg et al., 2001). Our study in Camden also differs because of the inclusion of several ethnic groups (Vambergue et al., 2000; Bo et al., 2004; Mello et al., 1997). With our large cohort, we had the power to control for known potential confounders that influence the fetal overgrowth, including pre-pregnant BMI and net gestational weight gain. We confirmed that untreated maternal mild hyperglycemia (impaired GCT with one abnormal or no abnormal glucose value at OGTT) in otherwise young and healthy women in the US was associated with a 2-3 fold increased risk of delivering an LGA infant (table 2). These observations are consistent with previous findings from populations studied worldwide by the HAPO group and other studies (HAPO, 2008; Stamilio et al 2004). In addition, increased risk of LGA birth in GDM women (all of whom were treated by diet or with insulin) was associated with high maternal pre-pregnant BMI.

3. Pregnancy weight gain and LGA birth

3.1 Significance of optimal pregnancy weight gain and fetal growth

To optimize gestational weight gain for both mother and fetus is critical and remains controversial. A large number of studies have found that excess gestational weight gain is associated with decreased risk of small-for-gestational age birth and with increased risk for LGA birth (Oken et al., 2009; Jensen et al., 2005; Hinkle et a., 2010), regardless the definition or the scales used for excess pregnancy weight gain (Kiel et al., 2007; Jain et al., 2007).

3.2 Weight gain and maternal obesity

The independent contribution of excess gestational weight gain and maternal obesity on the risk of LGA or macrosomia has been extensively investigated (Jensen et al., 2005; Jain et al., 2007), because obesity is a common problem during pregnancy (Chu et al., 2007; Sebire et al., 2001; Rosenberg et al., 2005). Even in women with a normal pre-pregnant BMI, a higher pregnancy weight gain was associated with an increased risk of LGA, while a normal weight gain by the 1990 The Institute of Medicine (IOM) guidelines was associated with a decreased risk of LGA (DeVader et al., 2007). The definition of an optimal gestational weight gain in obese pregnancy remains controversial (Nohr et al., 2008). Jain et al observed that overweight/obese women who gain weight within the IOM recommendation achieve better fetal outcomes (Jain et al., 2007), while others found weight gain within IOM ranges did not reduce the risk of LGA among the obese (Dietz et al., 2009). It was suggested that limited or no weight gain in more severely obese pregnant women may increase favorable neonatal outcomes (Kiel et al., 2007; Jensen et al., 2005). Thus, an optimal gestational weight gain may need to be further defined by obesity severity (Hinkle et al., 2010; Oken et al., 2009).

3.3 What are problems in the research of weight gain during pregnancy?

There are limited data that link excess pregnancy weight gain measured prior to screening for GDM and /or longitudinal gestational weight gain measures through out the pregnancy to adverse pregnancy outcomes. In 2009, the IOM published revised gestational weight gain guidelines for how much weight a woman should gain during pregnancy to optimize both maternal and child outcomes. The report highlighted the importance of intervention in pregnancy to prevent obesity in the post-partum for mother and child (IOM, 2009).

3.4 The US Institute of medicine new guidelines for gestational weight gain

The new 2009 IOM guidelines are based on the WHO BMI (kg/m^2) categories (WHO, 1998) and include the recommended total pregnancy weight gain (kg) or rates of weight gain during the 2nd and 3rd trimester (kg/week). Weight gain below or above the recommended range is defined as inadequate or excessive gain, respectively.

Prepregnancy BMI	BMI (kg/m^2) (WHO)	Total weight gain range		Rate of weight gain 2nd and 3rd trimester (mean, range)[2]	
		(lbs)	(kg)	(lbs/wk)	(kg/wk)
Under weight	<18.5	28-40	12.5-18.0	1.0 (1.0-1.3)	0.51 (0.44-0.58)
Normal weight	18.5-24.9	25-35	11.5-16.0	1.0 (0.8-1.0)	0.42 (0.35-0.50)
Overweight	25.0-29.9	15-25	7.0-11.5	0.6 (0.5-0.7)	0.28 (0.23-0.33)
Obese (includes all classes)	≥30.0	11-20	5.0-9.0	0.5 (0.4-0.6)	0.22 (0.17-0.27)

[1] IOM, Institute of Medicine in US.
[2] Calculations assume a 0.5-2kg (1.1-4.4 lbs) weight gain in the first trimester (based on Siega-Riz et. al., 1994; Abrams et al 1995, Carmichael et al 1997).

Table 3. New recommendations for total and rate of weight gain during pregnancy, by prepregnancy BMI (IOM, 2009)[1]

3.5 Assessment of pregnancy weight gain

We explored the associations between gestational weight gain assessed throughout pregnancy with LGA using the 2009 IOM guidelines for weight gain during pregnancy. Inadequate, adequate and excessive pregnancy weight gain at weeks 24, 28, 32 and at delivery was categorized according to IOM recommendations (table 3). Maternal obesity was defined as BMI ≥30 (WHO, 1998); height was measured with a stadiometer at entry. Gestational duration was based upon gestation from participants' last normal menstrual period confirmed or modified by ultrasound. Pregnancy weight was measured at week 12, 24, 28, 32 and at delivery. Total gestational weight gain was computed as the difference between weight at delivery and recalled pre-pregnant weight. Gestational weight gain during the 2nd and 3rd trimester was computed as the difference between weights measured at each visit minuses the weight measured at week 12. The rate of weight gain was the weight gain (kg) divided by gestational age (weeks).

3.6 Excess pregnancy weight gain measured mid to late gestations and LGA birth

The proportion of women with excess pregnancy weight gain at weeks 24, 28, and 32 was similar to delivery (48.5%, 52%, 54% and 50% respectively). Depending on the gestation, 21-27% had an adequate weight gain and 22-30% had an inadequate gain throughout the four time points.

Compared to women with adequate weight gain, excessive weight gain was associated with a 1.58-2.66 fold increased risk of LGA birth (table 4) after controlling for all the confounding variables with the exception of pre-pregnant BMI (p for trend <0.0001 for each model). Similar results were obtained when additional adjustment for pre-pregnant BMI. In addition, women with inadequate weight gain had a reduced risk of LGA birth at week 28 and 32 (p<0.05).

3.7 Contribution of Camden data

These data confirmed that excess pregnancy weight gain throughout the 2nd and 3rd trimesters and at delivery significantly increased risk of LGA, whereas inadequate pregnancy weight gain reduced LGA risk. The current study has several important strengths. Firstly, we used the most recent IOM recommendations (2009) for the estimation of excess weight gain by BMI categories and the analysis models were fully adjusted for potential confounding, including pre-pregnant BMI. In contrast, more arbitrary criteria were used to define excess weight gain in previous studies (Herring et al., 2009; Rosenberg et al., 2005), and pre-pregnant BMI either was not available or was not adjusted for in the analysis (Hillier et al., 2008; Rosenberg et al., 2005). Secondly, there are limited data on longitudinal measures of pregnancy weight gain (Herring et al., 2009; Saldana et al., 2006). We used multiple measures of pregnancy weight gain starting prior to the screen for GDM. The relationship between excess pregnancy weight gain assessed relatively early in pregnancy and risk of LGA could be important for preventive strategies. Total weight gain is not an ideal measure to evaluate in relation to fetal growth in GDM patients, because most of patients are treated and their weight gain is monitored after the diagnosis.

	Week 24		Week 28		Week 32		At delivery	
Weight gain	LGA (%)	AOR (95% CI)	LGA (%)	AOR (95% CI)	LGA (%)	AOR (95% CI)	LGA (%)	AOR (95% CI)
Adequate	3.5	Reference	5.1	Reference	6.1	Reference	3.6	Reference
Inadequate	3.2	0.90 (0.47,1.71)	2.6	0.50 (0.27, 0.95)	2.3	0.49 (0.24, 0.98)	2.3	0.62 (0.31, 1.25)
Excessive	8.7	2.62 (1.55, 4.43)	8.0	1.65 (1.05, 2.61)	7.6	1.58 (1.00, 2.50)	9.1	2.66 (1.69, 4.19)

[1] Models were adjusted for age and cigarette smoking in addition to using a standard which adjusted LGA for parity, ethnicity and infant gender.
[2] p for trend <0.0001 for week 24, 28, 32 and delivery respectively.

Table 4. Excess pregnancy weight gain and LGA birth[1,2]

4. Association of various degree of gestational hyperglycemia, excess pregnancy weight gain with LGA birth

4.1 Does excess gestational weight gain prior to screening GDM predict risk of GDM?

High gestational weight gain between early and mid pregnancy was positively associated with risk of GDM or impaired glucose tolerance (Hedderson et al., 2010; Herring et al., 2009). In the Camden study, we found a positive association between excess weight gain prior to or at the time of screening for GDM (weeks 24 and 28) with increased risk for GDM (AOR 1.57, 95% CI 1.01, 2.44 for week 24, AOR 1.94, 95% CI 1.28, 2.95 for week 28). This association was not significant at week 32 or at delivery which may suggest an effect of treatment and weight monitoring after the diagnosis of GDM. We did not observe a significant association between excess weight gain and impaired GCT non-GDM (p>0.05 for all time points).

4.2 The association of gestational hyperglycemia and excess weight gain with LGA

Combined association of gestational hyperglycemia and excess weight gain on the risk of LGA has not been examined extensively. Hillier et al observed at GDM screening that macrosomia risk was increased across the spectrum of maternal glucose levels and that this relationship was further modified by excessive maternal weight gain (Hillier et al., 2008). A weight gain of 40lbs or more nearly doubled the risk of fetal macrosomia among glucose intolerant women including those with GDM. However, results were not adjusted for pre-pregnancy BMI which can complicate the relationship between maternal hyperglycemia and pregnancy weight gain. Thus, our next goal was to examine the independent and combined contributions of hyperglycemia and excess weight gain on risk of LGA. An analysis stratified by excessive weight gain was used to index the influence of various degrees of maternal glycemic status on LGA risk, using women with non-excess pregnancy weight gain (adequate and inadequate gain combined) and a normal GCT as the reference group. Our results showed that excess weight gain (at week 24, 28, 32 or at delivery) was positively associated with a 2-6 fold increased risks for delivering an LGA infant (table 5) regardless of whether the women were diagnosed with GDM, impaired GCT non-GDM or normal GCT. Furthermore, women with non-excess weight gain and an impaired GCT non-GDM also had a 2-3 fold increased risk of LGA birth during all of four time points, whereas risk of LGA was not increased in the GDM group with non-excess weight gain.

	Weight gain at week 24		Weight gain at week 28		Weight gain at week 32		Weight gain at delivery	
	LGA (%)	AOR (95% CI)[3]	LGA (%)	AOR (95% CI)[3]	LGA (%)	AOR (95% CI)[3]	LGA (%)	AOR (95% CI)[3]
Excess weight gain								
GDM	11.5	4.03 (1.67, 9.73)	10.5	3.31 (1.39, 7.90)	11.3	3.20 (1.34, 7.63)	14.3	6.07 (2.58, 14.70)
Impaired GCT non-GDM	16.0	6.14 (3.16, 11.90)	14.6	4.97 (2.53, 9.71)	14.1	4.62 (2.18, 8.31)	14.9	6.42 (3.20, 12.88)
Normal GCT	7.8	2.91 (1.88, 4.48)	7.2	2.43 (1.58, 3.73)	6.8	2.02 (1.33, 3.10)	8.2	3.58 (2.29, 5.60)
Non-excess weight gain[2]								
GDM	5.6	1.64 (0.37, 7.21)	6.7	1.69 (0.38, 7.50)	5.9	1.31 (0.30, 5.71)	4.7	1.62 (0.37, 7.11)
Impaired GCT non-GDM	8.1	2.78 (1.17, 6.59)	9.5	2.98 (1.31, 6.77)	9.9	2.69 (1.19, 6.08)	9.1	3.79 (1.65, 8.68)
Normal GCT	2.8	Reference	3.1	Reference	3.6	Reference	2.5	Reference

[1] Model was adjusted for age, pre-pregnant BMI and cigarette smoking in addition to using a standard which adjusted LGA for maternal ethnicity, parity and fetal gender.
[2] Adequate and inadequate weight gain is combined.
[3] p for trend <0.0001.

Table 5. Maternal hyperglycemia and LGA infant: Stratified by excess weight gain[1]

4.3 What do we learn?

These data confirmed that hyperglycemia and excess weight gain are independently associated with risk of fetal overgrowth. Women with excess weight gain at any of four times in gestation and hyperglycemia, even a mild hyperglycemia, had a substantially increased risk of LGA. Risk of LGA was not increased among gestational diabetics without an excessive weight gain but only among the group with impaired GCT non-GDM. Thus, excess pregnancy weight gain and hyperglycemia are independent risk factors for LGA.

5. Conclusion

By using the most updated IOM guidelines (2009) on pregnancy weight gain, we found that healthy, young women with mild but untreated hyperglycemia were at increased risk for fetal overgrowth (LGA). The risk of LGA birth in women with GDM, who are treated by diet or with insulin after diagnosis, was dependent on maternal pre-pregnant weight. Excess pregnancy weight gain assessed longitudinally through out mid to late gestation consistently showed strong associations with LGA risk. In addition, excess pregnancy weight gain and hyperglycemia appeared to be independent risk factors for LGA. The risk for LGA was increased still further in women with excess weight gain, even in those with mild hyperglycemia. Because prepregnancy obesity, mild gestational hyperglycemia, and excess weight gain during pregnancy are preventable risk factors, these findings suggest that early detection and treatment of mild hyperglycemia and monitoring pregnancy weight gain during early gestation are both important for reducing the risk of LGA, for reducing childhood and later obesity and for improving the long term risk for metabolic disease in the offspring.

6. Acknowledgements

This work was supported by grants from the National Institute of Child Health and Human Development (HD18269 and HD38329 to T.O.S.) and National Institute of Diabetes and Digestive and Kidney Diseases (1R21DK078865-01 and 5R21DK078865-02 to X.C.).

7. References

Aberg, A., Rydhstroem H., & Frid, A. (2001). Impaired glucose tolerance associated with adverse pregnancy outcome: A population-based study in southern Sweden. *Amer J Obstet Gynecol* Vol.184, No.2, (January 2001), pp.77-83, ISSN 1097-6868.

Abrams, B., Carmichael, S., & Selvin, S. (1995). Factors associated with the pattern of maternal weight gain during pregnancy. *Obstet Gynecol* Vol.86, No.2, (August 1995), pp.170-6, ISSN 0029-7844.

American Diabetes Association. (2000). Gestational diabetes mellitus. *Diabetes Care* Vol.23, No. 1, (January 2000), pp. S77-9, ISSN 0149-5992.

Bo, S., Menato, G., Gallo, M., Bardelli, C., Lezo, A., Signorile, A. Gambino, R., Cassader, M., Massobrio, M., & Pagano, G. (2004). Mild gestational hyperglycemia, the metabolic syndrome and adverse neonatal outcomes. *Acta Obstet Gynecol Scand* Vol.83, No.4, (March 2004), pp.335-40, ISSN 0001-6349.

Boney, C., Verma, A., Tucker, R., & Vohr, B. (2005). Metabolic syndrome in childhood: association with birth weight, maternal obesity, and gestational diabetes mellitus. *Pediatrics* Vol.115, No.3, (March 2005), pp.e290-6, ISSN 1098-4275.

Carmichael, S., Abrams, B. & Selvin S. (1997). The pattern of maternal weight gain in women with good pregnancy outcomes. *Am J Public Health* Vol. 87, No.12, (December 1997), pp.1984-88, ISSN 1938-3207.

Chen X, Scholl TO, Leskiw M, Savaille J, Stein TP. (2010). Differences in maternal circulating fatty acids composition and dietary fat intake in women with gestational diabetes or mild gestational hyperglycemia. *Diabetes Care* Vol.33, No.9, (September), pp.2049-54, ISSN 0149-5992.

Cheng, Y., Esakoff, T., Block-Kurbisch, I., Ustinov, A., Shafer, S., & Caughey, A. (2006). Screening or diagnostic: markedly elevated glucose loading test and perinatal outcomes. *J Matern Fetal Neonatal Med* Vol. 19, No. 11, (November 2006), pp.729-34, ISSN 1476-7058.

Chu, S., Callaghan W., Kim S., Schmid C., Lau, J., England, L., & Dietz, P. (2007). Maternal obesity and risk of gestational diabetes mellitus. *Diabetes Care* Vol. 30, No.8, (August 2007), pp.2070-76, ISSN 0149-5992.

DeVader, S., Neeley, H., Myles, T., & Leet, T. (2007). Evaluation of gestational weight gain guidelines for women with normal prepregnancy body mass index. *Obstet Gynecol* Vol.110, No.4, (October 2007), pp.745-51, ISSN 0029-7844.

Dietz, P., Callaghan, W., & Sharma, A. (2009). High pregnancy weight gain and risk of excessive fetal growth. *Amer J Obstet Gynecol V*ol.201, No.1, (July 2009), pp.51.e1-6, ISSN 0002-9378.

Ehrenberg, H., Mercer, B., & Catalano, P. (2004). The influence of obesity and diabetes on the prevalence of macrosomia. *Amer J Obstet Gynecol V*ol.191, No.3, (September 2004), pp.964-8, ISSN 0002-9378.

Getahun, D., Nath, C., Ananth, C., Chavez, M., & Smulian, J. (2008). Gestational diabetes in the United States: temporal trends 1989 through 2004. *Amer J Obstet Gynecol V*ol.198, No.5, (May 2008), pp.525.e1-5, ISSN 0002-9378.

Gruendhammer, M., Brezinka, C., & Lechleitner, M. (2003). The number of abnormal plasma glucose values in the oral glucose tolerance test and the feto-maternal outcome of pregnancy. *Eur J Obstet Gynecol Reprod Biol* Vol.108, No.2, (June 2003), pp.131-6, ISSN 0301-2115.

Hedderson, M., Gunderson, E., & Ferrara, A. (2010). Gestational weight gain and risk of gestational diabetes mellitus. *Obstet Gynecol* Vol.115, No.3, (March 2010), pp.597-604, ISSN 0029-7844.

Herring, S., Oken, E., Rifas-Shiman, S., Rich-Edwards, J., Stuebe, A., Kleinman, K., & Gillman, M. (2009). Weight gain in pregnancy and risk of maternal hyperglycemia. *Amer J Obstet Gynecol V*ol.201, No.1, (July 2009), pp.61.e1-7, ISSN 0002-9378.

Hillier, T., Pedula, K., Vesco, K., Schmidt, M., Mullen, J., LeBlanc, E., & Pettitt, D. (2008). Excess gestational weight gain: modifying fetal macrosomia risk associated with maternal glucose. *Obstet Gynecol* Vol.112, No.5, (November 2008), pp.1007-14, ISSN 0029-7844.

Hinkle, S., Sharma, A., & Dietz, P. (2010). Gestational weight gain in obese mothers and associations with fetal growth. *Am J Clin Nutr* Vol.92, No.3, (September 2010), pp.644-51, ISSN 0002-9165.

IOM (Institute of Medicine). Weight gain during pregnancy: reexamining the guidelines. (April 2009). The National Academies Press, Washington DC. Available from: <http://www.nap.edu/catalog/12584.html>

Jain, N., Denk, C., Kruse, L., & Dandolu, V. (2007). Maternal obesity: can pregnancy weight gain modify risk of selected adverse pregnancy outcomes? *Am J Perinatol* Vol.24, No.5, pp. 291-8, ISSN 0735-1631.

Jensen, D., Ovesen, P., Beck-Nielsen, H., Mølsted-Pedersen, L., Sørensen, B., Vinter, C., & Damm, P. (2005). Gestational weight gain and pregnancy outcomes in 481 obese glucose-tolerant women. *Diabetes Care* Vol. 28, No.9, (September 2005), pp.2118-22, ISSN 0149-5992.

Kiel, D., Dodson, E., Artal, R., Boehmer, T., & Leet, T. (2007). Gestational weight gain and pregnancy outcomes in obese women. *Obstet Gynecol* Vol.110, No.4, (October 2007), pp.752-8, ISSN 0029-7844.

Langer, O. (2000). Fetal macrosomia: Etiologic factors. *Clinical Obstetrics Gynecology* Vol.43, No.2, (June 2000), pp.283-97, ISSN 0100-7203.

Mello, G., Parretti, E., Mecacci, F., Lucchetti, R., Lagazio, C., Pratesi, M., & Scarselli, G. (1997). Risk factors for fetal macrosomia: the importance of a positive oral glucose challenge test. *Eur J Endocrinol* Vol.137, No.1, (July1997), pp.27-33, ISSN 0804-4643.

Mokdad, A., Bowman B., Ford E., Vinicor, F., Marks, J., & Koplan, J. (2001). The Continuing Epidemics of Obesity and Diabetes in the United States. *JAMA* Vol.286, No.10, (September 2001), pp.1195-1200, ISSN 0098-7484.

Murphy, H., Rayman, G., Lewis, K., Kelly, S., Johal, B., Duffield, K., Fowler, D., Campbell, P., & Temple R. (2008). Effectiveness of continuous glucose monitoring in pregnant women with diabetes: randomised clinical trial. *BMJ* Vol.337, a1680. Published online 2008 September. doi: 10.1136/bmj.a1680, ISSN 0959-8146.

Nohr, E., Vaeth, M., Baker, J., Sørensen, T., Olsen, J., & Rasmussen K. (2008). Combined associations of prepregnancy body mass index and gestational weight gain with the outcome of pregnancy. *Am J Clin Nutr* Vol. 87, No.6, (June 2008), pp.1750-9, ISSN 0002-9165.

Nordin, N., Wei, J., Naing, N., & Symonds, E. (2006). Comparison of maternal-fetal outcomes in gestational diabetes and lesser degrees of glucose intolerance. *J Obstet Gynaecol Res* Vol.32, No.1, (February 2006), pp.107-14, ISSN 1341-8076.

Ogonowski, J., Miazgowski, T., Czeszyńska, M., Jaskot, B., Kuczyńska, M., & Celewicz, Z. (2008). Factors influencing risk of macrosomia in women with gestational diabetes mellitus undergoing intensive diabetic care. *Diabetes Res Clin Pract* Vol.80, No.3, (June 2008), pp. 405-10, ISSN 0168-8227.

Oken, E., & Gillman, M. (2003). Fetal origins of obesity. *Obesity Research* Vol.11, No.4, (April 2003), pp.496-506, ISSN 1930-7381.

Oken, E., Kleinman, K., Belfort, M., Hammitt J., & Gillman, M. (2009). Associations of Gestational Weight Gain With Short- and Longer-term Maternal and Child Health Outcomes. *Am J Epidemiol* Vol.170, No.2, (July 2009), pp.173-80, ISSN 0002-9262.

Östlund, I., Hanson, U., Björklund, A., Hjertberg, R., Eva, N., Nordlander E., Marja-Liisa, S., & Wager J. (2003). Maternal and fetal outcomes if gestational impaired glucose tolerance is not treated. *Diabetes Care* Vol.26, No.7, (July 2003), pp.2107-11, ISSN 0149-5992.

Ray, J., Vermeulen, M., Shapiro, J., & Kenshole, A. (2001). Maternal and neonatal outcomes in pregestational and gestational diabetes mellitus, and the influence of maternal obesity and weight gain: the Deposit study. *QJM* Vol.94, No.7, (July 2001), pp.347-56, ISSN 1460-2725.

Ricart, W., López, J., Mozas, J., Pericot, A., Sancho, M., González, N., Balsells, M., Luna, R., Cortázar, A., Navarro, P., Ramírez, O., Flández, B., Pallardo, L., Hernández, A.,

Ampudia, J., Fernández-Real, J., & Corcoy, R. (2005). Potential impact of American Diabetes Association (2000) criteria for diagnosis of gestational diabetes mellitus in Spain. *Diabetologia* Vol.48, No.6, (June 2005), pp.1135-41, ISSN 0012-186X.

Rosenberg, T., Garbers, S., Lipkind, H., & Chiasson, M. (2005). Maternal obesity and diabetes as risk factors for adverse pregnancy outcomes: differences among 4 racial/ethnic groups. *Am J Publ Hlth* Vol.95, No.9, (September 2005), pp.1544-51, ISSN 0090-0036.

Saldana, T., Siega-Riz, A., Adair, L., & Suchindran, C. (2006). The relationship between pregnancy weight gain and glucose tolerance status among black and white women in central North Carolina. *Am J Obstet Gynecol* Vol.195, No.6, (December 2006), pp. 1629-35, ISSN 0002-9378.

Sebire, N., Jolly, M., Harris, J., Wadsworth, J., Joffe, M., & Beard, R., Regan, L. & Robinson, S. (2001). Maternal obesity and pregnancy outcome: a study of 287 213 pregnancies in London. *International Journal of Obesity* Vol.25, No.8, (August 2001), pp.1175-82, ISSN 0307-0565.

Sermer, M., Naylor, D., Gare, D., Kenshole, A., Ritchie, J., Farine, D., Cohen, H., McArthur, K., Holzapfel, S., Biringer, A., & Chen, E. (1995). Impact of increasing carbohydrate intolerance on maternal-fetal outcomes in 3637 women without gestational diabetes: the Toronto tri-hospital gestational diabetes project. *Am J Obstet Gynecol* Vol.173, No.1, (July 1995), pp. 146-56, ISSN 0002-9378.

Siega-Riz, A., Adair, L., & Hobel, C. (1994). Institute of Medicine maternal weight gain recommendations and pregnancy outcome in a predominantly Hispanic population. *Obstetrics Gynecology* Vol.84, No.4, (October 1994), pp.565-73, ISSN 0029-7844.

Stamilio, D., Olsen, T., Ratcliffe, S., Sehdev, H., & Macones, G. (2004). False-positive 1-hour glucose challenge test and adverse perinatal outcomes. *Obstet Gynecol* Vol.103, No.1, (January 2004), pp. 148-56, ISSN 0029-7844.

The HAPO Study Cooperative Research Group. (2008). Hyperglycemia and adverse pregnancy outcomes. *N Engl J Med* Vol.358, No.19, (May 2008), pp. 1991-2002, ISSN 1533-4406.

Vambergue, A., Nuttens, M., Verier-Mine, O., Dognin, C., & Cappoen, J., & Fontaine P. (2000). Is mild gestational hyperglycaemia associated with maternal and neonatal complications? The Diagest Study. *Diabet Med* Vol.17, No. 3, (March 2000), pp. 203-8, ISSN 1464-5491.

Webster, B., & Bishaw, A. (2006). Income, earnings, and poverty data from the 2005 American community survey. (August 2006). US Government Printing Office, Washington, DC. Available from: <https://www.census.gov/prod/2007pubs/acs-08.pdf>

World Health Organization (WHO). (1998). Obesity: preventing and managing the global epidemic. WHO Consultation on Obesity Report, Geneva. Geneva, June, 1997.

Yogev, Y., Langer, O., Xenakis, E., & Rosenn, B. (2004). Glucose screening in Mexican-American women. *Obstet Gynecol* Vol 103, No.6, (June 2004), pp. 1241-5, ISSN 0029-7844.

Zhang, J. & Bowes, W. (1995). Birth-weight-for-gestational-age patterns by race, sex, and parity in the United States population. *Obstet Gynecol* Vol.86, No.2, (August 1995), pp. 200-8, ISSN 0029-7844.

14

Congenital Cardiopathies Screening Associated with Diabetes Mellitus Using Maternal Fructosamine Plasma Concentration

Zilma Silveira Nogueira Reis and Gabriel Costa Osanan
Obstetrics and Gynecology Department,
Universidade Federal de Minas Gerais
Brazil

1. Introduction

The consequences of uncontrolled diabetes mellitus during pregnancy are severe for both mother and fetus. The risk of congenital malformations among infants of diabetic mothers is related to the quality of the diabetic control (Allen et al., 2007; American Diabetes Association [ADA], 2004). In diabetic pregnancy, unsatisfactory glycemic control at the moment of diagnosis or delivery of care was associated with an increased risk of anomalies (Allen et al., 2007; Schaefer-Graf at al., 2000). The most common anomalies involve the cardiac, musculoskeletal, and central nervous systems (Sheffield at al., 2002). Despite this knowledge, it has been disappointing that so few diabetic women receive preconception counseling, plan their pregnancies or are early referred to tertiary centers (American Diabetes Association [ADA], 2004; Reis at al., 2010a). Considering this reality, it is important to study second trimester markers of congenital cardiopathies, in order to decrease fetal morbidity and mortality, at birth.

2. Congenital cardiopathies and diabetes mellitus

If maternal hyperglycemia is present during organogenesis there is an increased risk of congenital anomalies and miscarriage (American Diabetes Association [ADA], 2004). Experimental studies suggest that hyperglycemia is the major teratogen in diabetic pregnancies, but other diabetes-related factors may also affect fetal outcomes (Aberg at al., 2001; Buchanan & Kjos, 1999; Leonard et al., 1989; Ren et al., 2011). It is a fact that an uncontrolled diabetes mellitus in early gestation is associated with a teratogenic effect, causing primary cardiogenesis defects. Most types of cardiac structural lesions have been associated with diabetes mellitus, ranging from small septal defects to major heart disease (Sekhavat et al., 2010; Abu-Sulaiman & Subaih, 2004).
The exact teratogenic mechanism of maternal diabetes is not fully defined and is likely multifactorial (Hornberger, 2006; Kumar et al., 2007). Diabetes mellitus affects the fetal heart both structurally and functionally. In late gestation, it causes a unique form of hypertrophic cardiomyopathy (Ren et al., 2011; Hornberger, 2006; Chaudhari et al., 2008; Russell et al., 2008), illustrated at Fig. 1. Cardiomegaly is a common finding in stillborn infants of mothers

with diabetes mellitus and may contribute to the risk of fetal death in these pregnancies (Russell et al., 2008). Hypertrophic cardiomyopathy observed in the infant of the diabetic mother is characterized by thickening of the interventricular septum, and to a lesser extent the ventricular free walls (Hornberger, 2006). The presence of this pathology whether is associated with fetal hyperinsulinaemia and general somatic growth in maternal diabetes (Buchanan & Kjos, 1999; Ren et al., 2011). But, the wide variety of cardiac abnormalities suggests a complex pathogenesis. Experimental study proposed that the down-regulation of genes involved in development of cardiac neural crest could contribute to the pathogenesis of maternal diabetes-induced congenital heart defects (Kumar et al., 2007).

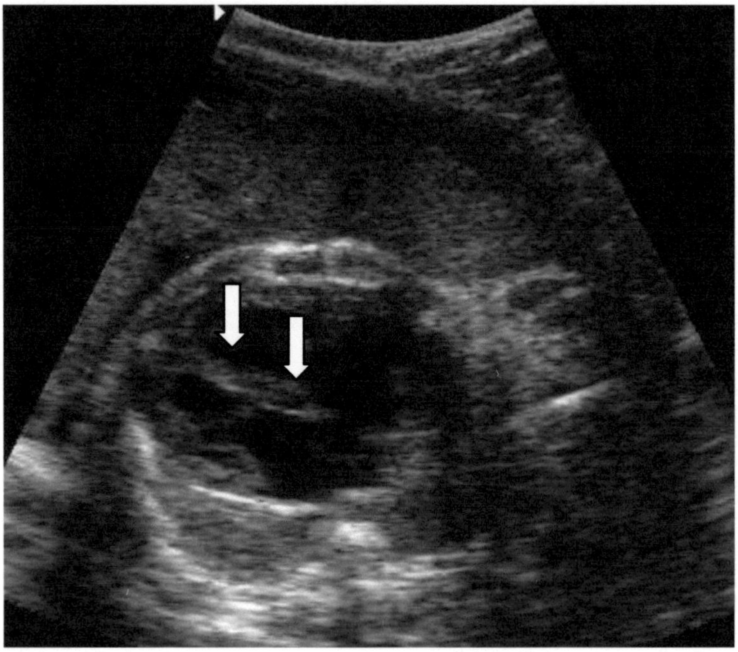

Fig. 1. Image of fetal ultrasonography: hypertrophic cardiomyopathy associated with Diabetes Mellitus

3. The strategies for prevention and management of the cardiac teratogenic effects in diabetes mellitus

The prevalence of pregestational diabetes among women early in their reproductive years is increasing. Thus, identifying women with diabetes is important because the diagnosis and appropriate therapy can decrease fetal and maternal morbidity (Crowtherl et al., 2005). Preconceptional evaluation and counseling of women with diabetes mellitus (type 1 or type 2) is fundamental point to minimize the risk to the fetus and mother. It is known that pregnancies in diabetes mellitus women should be planned, but that condition was not so frequent (American Diabetes Association [ADA], 2004; Reis at al., 2010a; Chaudhari et al., 2008). Unplanned pregnancy occurs in about two-thirds of women with diabetes leading to a persistent excess of malformations in their infants (American Diabetes Association [ADA], 2004).

Given the increased risk of congenital abnormalities among infants of diabetic mothers, an appropriate biochemical, ultrasonographic screening process and a detailed evaluation of fetal cardiac structure should be offered to all pregnant women with diabetes (Allen et al., 2007). A prenatal cardiac screening is purposed to identify defects that may require further evaluation and treatment, and to provide appropriate counselling to the family in a timely manner (American Diabetes Association [ADA], 2004; Sekhavat et al., 2010). Detailed fetal anatomic surveys in the early second trimester are common practice and typically include examination of both four-chamber and outflow tract views of the fetal heart.
The occurrence of congenital cardiopathies at echocardiography in fetuses whose mothers had preexisting diabetes mellitus was investigated in our tertiary university medical center (Reis at al., 2010a, 2010b). The most frequent conditions were hypertrophic cardiomyopathy (70%), pericardial effusion (15%), followed by intermittent or persistent bradycardia (15%). The most frequent structural congenital cardiopathies at echocardiography was interventricular communication (85.7%) associated or not to another heart malformations (Fig. 2). Functional findings at echocardiography were significantly more frequent among the poorly-controlled diabetic pregnancies.

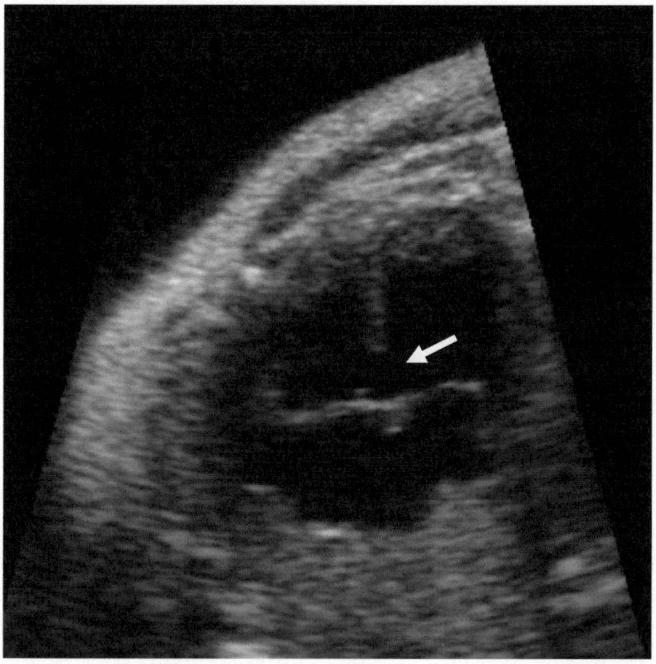

Fig. 2. Image of fetal ultrasonography: interventricular comunication associated with Diabetes Mellitus

In other reports, the malformations found in neonates, born of insulin-dependent diabetes mellitus gestations, included endocardial cushion defects, persistent truncus arteriosus and ventricular septal defects which appear to result from aberrant cardiac neural crest development (Sekhavat et al., 2010; Abu-Sulaiman & Subaih, 2004; Hornberger, 2006; Kumar et al., 2007; Russell et al., 2008). Hypertrophic cardiomyopathy was observed in 38% of neonates from insulin-dependent diabetes mellitus pregnant women, mainly hypertrophy of the interventricular septum (Abu-Sulaiman & Subaih, 2004).

4. The fructosamine level as a late marker (beyond the first trimester) for congenital cardiopathies

The measurement of glycated hemoglobin (HbAlc) and serum fructosamine in order to assess the recent glycemic control of diabetic patients has become well established. Maternal HbAlc at the beginning of pregnancy and maternal age at the onset of diabetes were associated with congenital malformations (Aberg at al., 2001).

Fructosamines are keto-amines formed by a non-enzymatic reaction between glucose and a protein (60-70% of which is glycosylated with albumin in serum), depending upon the severity and the duration of the hyperglycemia. Therefore, serum fructosamine directly reflects the dynamics of blood glucose concentration and correlates significantly with the mean plasma glucose levels from the preceding 1 to 3 weeks (Roberts et al., 1988; Weerasekera, 2000; Jenkins et al., 2007). Fructosamine testing has been available since the 1980s. Both fructosamine and HbA1c are used primarily as monitoring tools to help diabetics control their blood sugar, but the A1C test is much more popular and more widely accepted. However, the American Diabetes Association recognizes both tests and says that fructosamine may be useful in situations where the A1C cannot be reliably measured (Goldstein et al., 2004). In addition, the measurement of fructosamine can be a helpful adjunct to HbA1c glycaemic control monitoring during pregnancy (Chaudry et al., 2007). The role of fructosamine levels as a teratogenic marker is less studied.

Fetuses presenting a normal and abnormal echocardiography were compared using plasma fructosamine level means (Reis at al., 2010a). An association between congenital cardiopathies at echocardiography (functional and structural including isolated hypertrophic cardiomiopathy) and types of diabete mellitus (insulin-depending or not), was evaluated. An abnormal plasma fructosamine level at 20.4±8.0 weeks of gestation was associated with congenital cardiopathies at echocardiography, whether or not the cardiac embryogenesis happened in the first trimester. The congenital cardiopathies at echocardiography odds ratio was 9.6 (95% CI: 2.8 - 33.7) for abnormal plasma fructosamine (≥2.68mmol/L) and 10.9 (95% CI: 2.7 - 45.2) when adjusted for maternal age and insulin usage. There was also an increased chance (3.1, 95% CI: 1.1 - 8.8) of fetal heart anomaly with insulin usage, but only when evaluated individually by crude odds ratio.

In many underdeveloped countries, women do not have access or do not attend medical care early in pregnancy (Reis at al., 2010a, 2010b). Therefore, they are especially subject to the teratogenic effects of hyperglycemia. Analyzing results of our universitary referral center, it was disappointing that so few diabetic women receive preconception counseling and plan their pregnancies (Reis at al., 2010a). Therefore, considering this reality, without HbA1c early values, it was important to determine the correlation between fructosamine maternal levels and fetal malformations.

Based on our previous study, abnormal maternal fructosamine levels, even at the second trimester of pregnancy, predicts a high risk of fetal cardiac anomalies (Reis at al., 2010a). In this way, a fetal echocardiographic exam should be, routinely, performed in all diabetic mothers whose fructosamine levels are above 2.23 mmol/L (Reis et al., 2010b).

This recommendation was based on the significant capacity of maternal fructosamine levels to predict fetal heart anomaly in diabetic patients (Area Under Curve: 0.78 p-valor <0.0001), as shown in Fig. 3. However, different cut-off values from which fructosamine could indicate these malformations and they should be cautiously defined and discussed as shown in Table 1.

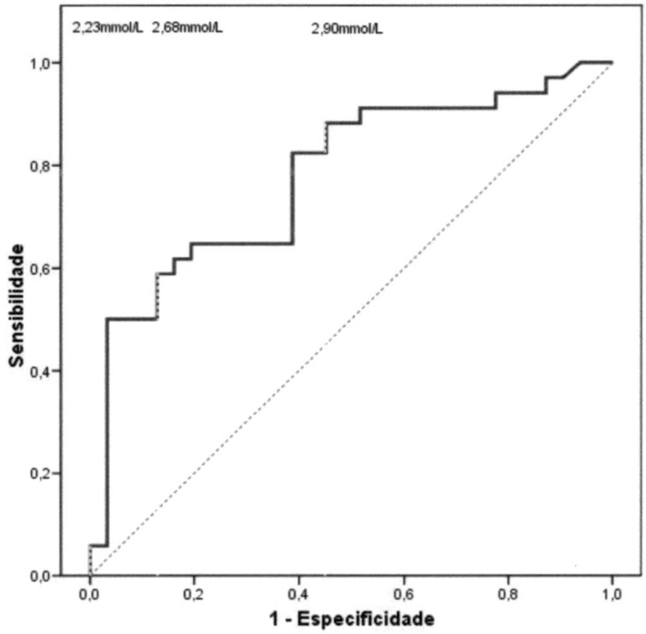

Fig. 3. Receiver-operating characteristics (ROC) curve for prediction of congenital cardiopathies at echocardiography for fetuses whose mothers had preexisting diabetes mellitus (n=65). AUC 0.78 (95% CI, 0.66–0.89), from: Reis et al., 2010

Cut-off points (maternal plasmatic levels of fructosamine)	Sensitivity	Specificity	False negative	Positive Likelihood ratio
2.23 mmol/L	88.2%	54.8%	11.8%	2.0
2.68 mmol/L	58.8%	87.1%	41.2%	4.6
2.90 mmol/L	44.1%	96.8%	55.9%	13.7

Table 1. Accuracy of the maternal fructosamine levels for the prediction of fetal cardiac anomalies in gestations complicated by diabetes mellitus. Reference: Reis et al., 2010b

If it is considered the cut-off value of fructosamine recommended for our local population (2.68mmol\L), this test will have a good specificity (87.1%) but a low sensitivity (58.8%), with a false negative rate of 41.2%. Even though, for an abnormal exam, the risk of fetal cardiac anomaly is increased 4.6-fold. If it is considered the cut-off value recommended by the manufacturer of the test (2.90mmol/L), the exam will have a high specificity (96.8%) but a low sensitivity (44.1%) with a false negative rate of 55.9%. In this case, for an abnormal test, the risk of fetal cardiac defects would be increased 13.7-fold. Finally considering the use of a cut-off point of 2.23mmol\L, the test will show a low specificity (54.8%) but a high sensitivity (88.2%), with a false negative rate of 11.8%. Thus, the cut-off point of 2.23 mmol/L is better than the other values tested, since it has the greatest sensitivity and lowest false negative rate among them.

5. Conclusions

Abnormal echocardiographic findings were associated with the first maternal plasma fructosamine levels in referral pregnancies complicated by diabetes mellitus. Hyperglycemia seems to be the most important determinant of these risks. Many pregnant diabetic women are referred at a late stage to a tertiary level of care. At this context, an abnormal plasma fructosamine level increases the chances of abnormalities at fetal echocardiography. It is possible to use a second trimester plasma fructosamine level to refer women with pregestational diabetes mellitus to a center of maternal-fetal medicine in order to offer them an appropriated assistance at birth. These findings are important for the management of women with diabetes mellitus and late prenatal care.

6. Acknowledgment

CAPES Foundation, Ministry of Education of Brazil, BEX 3105/10-5 process

7. References

Aberg, A.: Westbom, L. & Kallen, B. (2001). Congenital malformations among infants whose mothers had gestational diabetes or preexisting diabetes. *Early Human Development,* Vol.61, No.2, (Mar 2001), pp.85–95, ISSN 0378-3782.

Abu-Sulaiman, R.M. & Subaih, B: (2004). Congenital heart disease in infants of diabetic mothers: echocardiographic study. *Pediatr Cardiol,* Vol.25, No.2, (Mar-Apr 2004), pp.137-140, ISSN 1551-4439.

Allen, V.M.; Armson, B.A.; Wilson, R.D.; Allen, V.M.; Blight, C.; Gagnon, A.; Johnson, J.A.; Langlois, S.; Summers, A.; Wyatt, P.; Farine, D.; Armson, B.A.: Crane, J.; Delisle, M.F.; Keenan-Lindsay, L.; Morin, V.; Schneider, C.E.; Van Aerde, J. (2007) Teratogenicity associated with pre-existing and gestational diabetes. *J Obstet Gynaecol Can,* Vol.29, No.11, (Nov 2007), pp.927-944, ISSN 1701-2163.

American Diabetes Association [ADA]. (2004). Preconception care of women with diabetes. *Diabetes Care,* Vol.27, Suppl 1, pp. 76, (Jan 2004). ISSN 1935-5548.

Buchanan, T.A. & Kjos, S.L. (1999). Gestational Diabetes: Risk or Myth?. *The Journal of Clinical Endocrinology & Metabolism,* Vol.84, No.6, (1999), pp.1854-1857, ISSN 1945-7197.

Chaudhari, M.; Brodlie, M. & Hasan, A. (2008). Hypertrophic cardiomyopathy and transposition of great arteries associated with maternal diabetes and presumed gestational diabetes. *Acta Paediatr,* Vol.97, No.12, pp.1755-1757, (2008), ISSN 1651-2227.

Chaudry, R.; Gilby, P. & Carroll, V. (2007). Pre-existing (type 1 and type 2) diabetes in pregnancy. *Obstetrics, Gynaecology and Reproductive Medicine,* Vol.17, No.12, (Dec 2007), pp.339-334. ISSN 1751-7214.

Crowther, C.A.; Hiller, J.E.; Moss, J.R., et al. (2005). Effect of treatment of gestational diabetes mellitus on pregnancy outcomes. *N Engl J Med,* Vol.352, No.24, pp.2477, (Jun 2005), ISSN 1533-4406.

Goldstein, D.E.; Little, R.R.; Lorenz, R.A.; Malone, J.I.; Nathan, D.M.; Peterson, C.M. (2004) Tests of glycemia in diabetes. *Diabetes Care*, Vol.27, No.7, pp.1761-1763, (Jul 2004), ISSN 1935-5548.

Hornberger, L.K. (2006). Maternal diabetes and the fetal heart. *Heart*, Vol.92, No.8, pp.1125-1130, (May 2006), ISSN 1355-6037.

Jenkins, K.J.: Correa, A.: Feinstein, J.A.; Botto, L.: Britt, A.E.; Daniels, S.R.; Elixson, M.; Warnes, C.A.; Webb, C.L. (2007). Noninherited risk factors and congenital cardiovascular defects: current knowledge: a scientific statement from the American Heart Association Council on Cardiovascular Disease in the Young: endorsed by the American Academy of Pediatrics. *Circulation*, Vol.115, No.23, pp.2995-3014, (May 2007), ISSN 0009-7322.

Kumar, S.D.; Dheen, S.T. & Tay, S.S.W. (2007). Maternal diabetes induces congenital heart defects in mice by altering the expression of genes involved in cardiovascular development. *Cardiovascular Diabetology*, Vol. 6, No. 34, (Oct 2007), ISSN 1475-2840.

Leonard, C.L.; Bergman, M.; Frenz, D.A.; Macreery, L.A.; Newman, S.A. (1989). Abnormal ambient glucose levels inhibit proteoglycan core protein gene expression and reduce proteoglycan accumulation during chondrogenesis: Possible mechanism for teratogenic effects of maternal diabetes (extracellular matrix/skeletal birth defects). *Proc. Nati. Acad. Sci*, Vol.86, No.24, pp.10113-10117, (Dec 1989), ISSN 0027-8424.

Reis, Z.S.; Miranda, A.P.; Lage, E.M.; Bragança, R.D.; Costa, C.R.; Cabral, A.C.V. (2010a). Echocardiographic findings of congenital cardiopathies among fetuses of diabetic pregnant women and their relationship with plasma fructosamine levels. *J Matern Fetal Neonatal Med.* (Early on line, Dec 2010), ISSN 1476-7058.

Reis, Z.S.N.; Miranda, A.P.B.; Rezende, C.A.; Bragança, R.D.; Ribeiro, C.C.; Cabral, A.C.V. (2010b). [Congenital cardiopathies screening associated with diabetes mellitus using maternal fructosamine plasma concentration]. *Rev. Bras. Ginecol. Obstet*, Vol.32, No.2, pp. 66-71, (Feb 2010), ISSN 0100-7203.

Ren, Y.; Zhou1, Q.; Yan, Y.; Chu, C.; Gui, Y. Li, X. (2011). Characterization of fetal cardiac structure and function detected by echocardiography in women with normal pregnancy and gestational diabetes mellitus. *Prenat Diagn.* (Early on line, Mar 2011). ISSN 1097-0223.

Roberts, A.B.; Baker, J.R.; James, A.G.; Henley, P. (1988). Fructosamine in the management of gestational diabetes. *Am J Obstet Gynecol*, Vol.159, No.1, pp.66-71, (Jul 1988), ISSN 0002-9378.

Russell, N.E.; Holloway, P.; Quinn, S.; Foley, M.: Kelehan, P.; McAuliffe, F.M. (2008). Cardiomyopathy and cardiomegaly in stillborn infants of diabetic mothers. *Pediatr Dev Pathol*, Vol.11, No.1, pp.10-14, (Jan-Fev 2008), ISSN 1615-5742.

Schaefer-Graf, U.M.; Buchanan, T.A.; Xiang, A.N.; Songster, G. Montoro, M.; Kjos, S.L. (2000). Patterns of congenital anomalies and relationship to initial maternal fasting glucose levels in pregnancies complicated by type 2 and gestational diabetes. *Am J Obst Gynecol*, Vol.182, No.2, pp.313–320, (Feb 2000), ISSN 0002-9378.

Sekhavat, S.; Kishore, N.; Levine J.C. (2010). Screening fetal echocardiography in diabetic mothers with normal findings on detailed anatomic survey. *Ultrasound Obstet Gynecol*, Vol.35, No.2, pp.178–182, (Feb 2010), ISSN 1471-0528.

Sheffield, J.S.; Butler-Koster, E.L.; Casey, B.M.; McIntire, D.D.; Leveno, K.J. (2002). Maternal Diabetes Mellitus and Infant Malformations. *Obstet Gynecol*, Vol.100, No.5,pt1, pp.925–930, (Dec 2002), ISSN 1873-233X.

Weerasekera, D.S. & Peiris H. (2000). The value of serum fructosamine in comparison with oral glucose tolerance test (OGTT) as a screening test for detection of gestational diabetes mellitus. *Journal of Obstetrics and Gynaecology*, Vol.20, No.2, pp.136-138, (Mar 2000), ISSN 0144-3615.

15

Applications of Doppler Studies for Fetal Surveillance in Diabetic Pregnancies

William WK To
Department of Obstetrics & Gynaecology
United Christian Hospital, Hong Kong
China

1. Introduction

Diabetes mellitus complicating pregnancy is one of the most common antenatal complications that are associated with significant perinatal mortality and morbidity (Magee et al., 1993; Platt et al., 2002; Schmidt et al., 2001). Diabetic pregnancies can be divided into two categories: those with pre-gestational or pre-existing diabetes mellitus in which the diagnosis is made in the pre-pregnancy state, and those with gestational diabetes mellitus (GDM). Pre-existing diabetes consists of type I (insulin-dependent) diabetes mellitus (IDDM)with an incidence of around 0.5%, and type 2 (non-insulin-dependent) diabetes with an incidence of 2-3% (Kapoor et al., 2007). The incidence of gestational diabetes mellitus differs in different populations (Gunton et al., 2001) and ethnic groups, and was shown to be as high as 13% in Chinese populations (Ko et al., 2002). Effective treatment of pre-existing as well as gestational diabetes mellitus was shown to improve outcome and reduce perinatal mortality, as compared to untreated patients (Lao et al., 2001; Langer et al., 2005).

The pathological conditions encountered in fetuses of diabetic pregnancies differ in those with pre-existing diabetes mellitus and those with gestational diabetes. Pre-existing diabetics with persistent hyperglycaemia in the perinatal period are at higher risks of congenital malformations (Reece et al., 2007). In addition, those women with long-standing pre-existing diabetes before the index pregnancy run a higher risk of having diabetic vasculopathy that may affect various organ-systems in the body. Involvement of the uterine arteries will affect the development of an effective utero-placenta blood flow, which would be vital in maintaining normal growth and development in the fetus. The clinical manifestation of fetal growth restriction (also called intrauterine growth restriction) is thus more common in these pregnancies. The presence of significant congenital abnormalities and severe fetal growth restriction resulting from such conditions are logically directly related to increase in perinatal mortality and morbidity. On the other hand, gestational diabetes is usually only diagnosable either in a screening protocol or from clinical risk factors, by oral glucose tolerance test from mid trimester onwards, due to the effects of diabetogenic hormones from the placenta. The carbohydrate intolerance is thus short-lived and should last only from mid trimester to term. The hyperglycaemic states of the diabetes should revert to normal shortly after delivery with the removal of the placenta. Thus, chronic complications such as vasculopathy in the pregnant women will not have time to evolve during the course of pregnancy. On the contrary, the diabetic hyperglycaemic states in gestational diabetes would stimulate fetal hyperinsulinemia, which would in turn lead to over-secretion of insulin-like growth factors (IGF), leading to overgrowth of the fetus (Kapoor et al., 2007). Thus, in contrast to pre-gestational diabetes mellitus, where vasculopathy is rife and the incidences of pre-eclampsia and fetal growth restriction are commonly encountered, GDM pregnancies pose a different category of pathophysiology and clinical risks. The most common fetal problems for gestational diabetes will be macrosomia with associated polyhydramnios, as well as increased risks of near term stillbirths and neonatal metabolic complications in livebirths (Sacks, 2007). Indeed, recent data borne out by the HAPO study has demonstrated that in maternal hyperglycaemic states less severe than in diabetes mellitus is also associated with increased risks of adverse pregnancy outcomes (HAPO Study Cooperative Research Group, 2008)

A lot of emphasis has been put on fetal surveillance in these high-risk pregnancies in the attempt to optimise pregnancy outcome. There is, however, no consensus as to the best methods of antepartum surveillance (American College of Obstetricians & Gynecologists, 2001). The use of Doppler studies of the umbilical artery has been demonstrated to reduce perinatal adverse outcome in non-diabetic pregnancies (Alfirevic et al., 1995), but its use in diabetic pregnancies have shown conflicting results. While umbilical artery Doppler studies have been shown to be more predictive of adverse outcome than cardiotocography and biophysical profile in diabetic pregnancies (Bracero et al., 1996), fetal compromise would occasionally still be observed despite normal Doppler studies (Johnstone et al., 1992). Thus, the precise value of Doppler studies in the monitoring of GDM pregnancies remains controversial.

2. Serial growth scans for diabetic pregnancies

The recommendations for diagnosis and treatment of GDM of the Fifth International Workshop-Conference on Gestational Diabetes Mellitus (Metzger et al., 2007) suggest consideration of fetal growth patterns to guide metabolic management of pregnant women with GDM. However, estimation of fetal weight, particularly at term and in fetuses with high neonatal weight, is not as precise as desirable (Sacks et al, 2000). Fetal overgrowth and accelerated growth velocity of the abdominal circumference in the third trimester is known to predict large for gestational age babies (Kehl et al., 1996). Fetal overgrowth with macrosomia and associated polyhydramnios is associated with higher risks of near term stillbirth, as well as various neonatal metabolic derangements, including neonatal hypoglycaemia, electrolyte disturbances and neonatal jaundice. Previous randomized studies have demonstrated that measurement of fetal abdominal circumference throughout pregnancy in women with GDM is useful to identify pregnancies at high risk for fetal overgrowth and thus in need of more vigilant treatment including insulin therapy (Bonomo et al., 2004).

Serial measurements of the fetal abdominal circumference have been used to guide metabolic management of pregnancies complicated by gestational diabetes mellitus. There is at present no consensus as to the optimal protocol for such growth scans. A recent study evaluated the number of sonograms needed to reliably predict the absence of fetal overgrowth in GDM pregnancies. A total of 4478 ultrasound examinations were performed on 1914 subjects. Of 518 women with fetal abdominal circumference > 90th percentile, the diagnosis was detected in 73.9% with the first ultrasound examination at entry and in 13.1% with the second ultrasound examination. Of the fetuses, 85.9 and 86.9% of the fetuses were born non-large- for- gestational- age when abdominal circumference was < 90th percentile at 24-27 weeks and 28-32 weeks respectively; and 88% were born non-large-for-gestational-age when both scans showed normal growth. For those women who had no risk factors for fetal overgrowth, such as body mass index > 30 kg/m^2, history of macrosomia, and fasting glucose > 100 mg/dl, the accuracy of prediction of a non-large-for-gestational-age neonate was 90.0, 89.5 and 95.2%. The predictive ability did not increase with more than two normal scans. It was concluded that the yield of sonographic diagnosis of a large fetus dropped markedly after the finding if a large fetal abdominal circumference < 90th percentile on tow sonograms, which excludes with a high reliability the risk of a large for gestational age newborn. The ability was enhanced in women who had no risk factors for neonatal macrosomia (Schaefer-Graf et al., 2011). Thus, sonographic evaluation of fetal growth parameters is a crucial part of ultrasound assessment of diabetic pregnancies. The application of Doppler examination should take into account the data from such growth assessment parameters.

3. Use of Doppler studies for fetal surveillance

Various Doppler parameters have conventionally been utilized for fetal surveillance. The use maternal uterine artery Doppler as a screening tool to predict subsequent development of pre-eclampsia and fetal growth restriction in later gestation have gained acceptance in recent years. Umbilical artery Doppler, middle cerebral artery Doppler, or the combination of the two to produce a cerebral-placental ratio, have been widely used for the assessment of growth restricted fetuses. Less commonly used arterial Doppler parameters include fetal thoracic aorta or renal arteries. Venous Doppler assessment has been extensively investigated in recent years, including umbilical venous waveforms, intrahepatic venous Doppler and ductus venosus Doppler. The following sections attempt to review the application of the more commonly used Doppler parameters in diabetic pregnancies.

3.1 Maternal uterine artery

Maternal uterine artery remodelling is the hallmark sign of successful placentation, which can be demonstrated by progressive alterations in Doppler waveforms derived from the immediate extrauterine portion of the uterine artery. Pre-pregnancy uterine arteries show high resistance and elastic recoil in the form of early diastolic notches and low diastolic flow (Schulman et al., 1986). Successful placental invasion removes intimal muscle and reduces vascular resistance and elastic properties, giving more rigorous diastolic flow. In pregnancies with normal placentation, Doppler studies show that this remodelling is rapid, with loss of notching by 12 weeks and low resistance indices by 20 weeks or sooner. When placentation is deficient, notching of waveforms remains with high resistance (Papageorhiou et al., 2001). Such a picture of deficient placentation strongly predicts maternal hypertension, including proteinuric pre-eclampsia, fetal growth restriction and fetal demise (Coleman et al., 2000). Uterine artery Doppler screening using high resistance, persistent notching, or both, identifies such risks with a sensitivity up to 85% for severe proteinuric pre-eclampsia and for severe fetal growth restriction (Papageorghiou et al., 2002). However, there is so far no well established evidence of using such screening for adverse outcomes for either pre-existing or gestational diabetes mellitus alone.

When uterine artery Doppler were examined in a cohort of 43 pregnancies complicated by insulin-dependent diabetes, it was found that the uterine artery resistance indices were slightly higher in the presence of evident morphological vasculopathy, but could not predict diabetic specific fetal morbidity. It was concluded that in patients with diabetic vasculopathy, the uterine artery was also affected, but there was no relationship with long or short term parameters of glycaemic control. Based on the data, it was concluded that Doppler flow velocimetry of the uterine artery was a poor predictor of diabetes-specific fetal morbidity (Zimmermann et al., 1994).

In another prospective survey, 24 well controlled insulin dependent pregestational diabetic pregnancies were compared with 25 healthy pregnant women and Doppler ultrasound was performed on two occasions in the third trimester separated by a one-month interval. At the first examination, the median pulsatility index in the fetal thoracic aorta and in the uterine artery was significantly lower in the diabetic group as compared to healthy controls, whereas umbilical and uterine pulsatility indices were similar. At the second examination at a more advanced gestation, a significant physiological decrease in the median pulsatility index of the fetal aorta and uterine artery was observed in the controls, but not in the diabetic group. There was no correlation between the glycosylated haemoglobin or random blood glucose levels and the Doppler indices. An increased incidence of neonatal morbidity was noted in the diabetic group. Thus, the normal physiological third trimester fall in resistance indices in the uteroplacental and fetal placental indices was apparently absent in the diabetic group, and this was associated with increased neonatal morbidity. The pulsatility indices were not influenced by blood glucose regulation (Grunewald et al., 1996).

A similar retrospective study of 155 pre-gestational diabetic women between 22 weeks gestation and term also found that abnormal uterine artery Doppler with increased pulsatility index was related to pre-existing diabetic states with vasculopathy and adverse pregnancy outcome. There was an increased incidence of abnormal umbilical artery Doppler in those with abnormal uterine artery Doppler, indicating that the vasculopathy might influence placental perfusion and fetal well-being (Pietryga et al., 2006). Therefore, it is logical to expect that such screening by uterine artery Doppler will likely be effective only if the diabetic pregnancy is also complicated by gestational hypertension or fetal growth restriction. Given the higher incidence of such obstetric complications in pre-existing diabetes mellitus as compared to GDM, screening of diabetic pregnancies using uterine artery Doppler in mid trimester would probably produce a higher yield in the former group.

3.2 Fetal umbilical artery Doppler

The use of Doppler studies of the umbilical artery has been demonstrated to reduce perinatal adverse outcome in non-diabetic pregnancies (Alfirevic et al.,1995), but its use in diabetic pregnancies have shown conflicting results. Umbilical artery angle independent indices (systolic/diastolic ratio or pulsatility index) decrease with advancing gestation because of decreases in placenta vascular resistance, which physiologically occurs with advancing gestation. In pathologic conditions, such as intrauterine/ fetal growth restriction, the umbilical artery waveform change and the angle-independent indices become abnormal, giving values above their reference ranges. End-diastolic velocity may thus change from normal to reduced, absent or reversed. These changes represent an increased placental vascular resistance, and could pathologically be associated with a decrease in the number of placental arteries per high power field (Giles et al., 1985). The most common scenario for fetal growth restriction include placental insufficiency in singleton or multiple pregnancies from various aetiologies, which may or may not be associated with pre-eclampsia or other maternal conditions, or in fetuses with congenital malformations. Such a picture commonly occurs in women with pre-existing diabetes mellitus with vasculopathy. In pregnancies with suspected fetal growth restriction, the use of umbilical artery Doppler has been demonstrated to reduce the number of perinatal deaths and unnecessary obstetric interventions. In the context of diabetic pregnancies, however, the applications of umbilical artery Doppler remain controversial.

To investigate the vascular resistance by Doppler ultrasound in the umbilical artery of 53 IDDM pregnancies longitudinally over the course of pregnancy, the resistance index of the Doppler waveform was correlated with the mean value of a 24 hour blood glucose profile and the concentrations of glycosylated haemoglobin (HbA1C), which represented parameters of metabolic control. Regression analysis, however, showed no significant correlation between vascular resistance and mean blood glucose levels or HbA1C concentrations (Zimmermann et al., 1992).

In another study that included 67 normotensive women with pregnancies complicated by IDDM, the umbilical artery pulsatility index was compared with both pregnancy complications and perinatal outcome. The last umbilical pulsatility index value before delivery was used for analysis, and Doppler results were not used for patient management. Out of this cohort, 44 (66%) had pulsatility index values within the normal range between the 5th to 95th percentile, while 23 (34%) had abnormally high pulsatility index values. Among the group with pathologically abnormal umbilical pulsatility indices, analysis of the data revealed a significantly higher incidence of both caesarean section for acute fetal distress and perinatal complications. These complications include respiratory distress syndrome, hyperbilirubinemia, neonatal hypoglycaemia, and the need for neonatal intensive care unit admission. The authors concluded that in at least one third of IDDM patients, increased vascular resistance in the umbilical arteries were found, and these also suffered from higher incidences of perinatal complications (Fadda et al., 2001).

A retrospective study of 146 patients with gestational diabetes noted that Doppler examination of the umbilical arteries seemed to be of little clinical value unless pregnancy was complicated by pre-eclampsia or intrauterine growth restriction. The study included 227 patients with diabetes, and umbilical artery Doppler velocimetry and glycaemic control were examined in the third trimester. An elevated systolic/diastolic ratio and an abnormal glycosylated haemoglobin level were associated with adverse pregnancy outcome, but there was no stratification for vascular disease or fetal growth restriction in the data (Bracero et al., 1996).

In a prospective study of 65 well controlled diabetic pregnancies, Doppler measurements of uterine arteries, umbilical artery, the fetal descending thoracic aorta, and the middle cerebral artery (MCA) were performed together with cordocentesis for measurement of umbilical venous blood pH, pO_2 and haematocrit. It was found that the mean umbilical venous blood pH was significantly lower and the haematocrit significantly higher than the appropriate normal mean for gestation for these diabetic pregnancies. However, the Doppler indices of the placental and fetal circulations were essentially normal, except in some of the cases complicated by pre-eclampsia or intrauterine growth restriction (Salvesen et al., 1993). It was thus concluded that maternal diabetes mellitus was not associated with abnormalities in Doppler indices of the placental or fetal circulations.

To evaluate a random single Doppler study of the systolic/diastolic ratio of the umbilical artery as a predictor of perinatal outcome in diabetic pregnancies, a prospective double-blind study was performed in 92 diabetic pregnancies between 28 and 40 weeks gestation, and the results were associated with perinatal outcome parameters. The sensitivity and specificity of the Doppler studies as a predictor of poor perinatal outcome were 39% and

92% respectively. The positive and negative predictive values were 54% and 86% respectively. The authors suggested that the systolic/diastolic ratio of the umbilical artery offer no advantage over other well established tests in management of diabetic pregnancies (Ben-Ami et al., 1995).

In a cohort of 104 women with both type I and type II pre-existing diabetes mellitus, umbilical artery Doppler was performed at 28, 32, 36 and 38 weeks gestation. Overall, 22% had an elevated pulsatility index. If the Doppler examination was carried out within 2 weeks of delivery, 71% with abnormal umbilical artery Doppler had adverse perinatal outcome (likelihood ratio 4.2). However, the sensitivity of umbilical artery Doppler to predict such adverse outcome was only 35%, while specificity was 94%. The positive Predictive value was 80% and negative predictive value was 68%. Only 30% of women with adverse perinatal outcome had abnormal umbilical artery Doppler measurements. The authors thus concluded that the performance of umbilical artery Doppler was not satisfactory even in this group of high risk women with pre-existing diabetes, and that it was not a good predictor of adverse perinatal outcome (Wong et al., 2003).

To investigate whether complications were higher in diabetic pregnancies with cardiac maladaptation, fetal, uteroplacental and echocardiographic examinations were compared in the second and third trimester between diabetic and healthy pregnant women. Physiological cardiac hypertrophy was found in healthy women but was less prominent in patients with diabetes. While the majority of patients studied have normal Doppler results, the abnormal uteroplacental flow group consisted entirely of women with pregestational diabetes, especially IDDM patients. Neonatal complications were also more common in this subgroup. No relationship was found between echocardiographic findings, Doppler waveforms and perinatal outcome. Similar to previous studies, the findings confirmed that umbilical and uteroplacental Doppler were useful only in pre-existing diabetes, but not in GDM patients (Parlakgumus et al., 2010).

From the above studies, it can be seen that both observational data and randomized control data have failed to show any consistent association between maternal diabetes and abnormal umbilical artery Doppler indices. It is apparent that the current evidence supports the use of umbilical artery Doppler only in those patients with diabetes who have pregnancies complicated by hypertensive diseases, fetal growth restriction, or vasculopathy. Umbilical Doppler studies cannot be recommended as a routine screening for fetal surveillance especially in patients without pre-existing diabetes mellitus (Pietryga et al., 2006).

3.3 Middle cerebral artery Doppler

The middle cerebral artery (MCA) is the most studied cerebral artery because it is simple to sample, consistent and reproducible, and provides information on the cerebral blood flow in normal and growth restricted fetuses (Mari et al., 2008). In addition, the MCA can be sampled at an angle of near zero degrees between the ultrasound beam and the direction of the blood flow, so that the genuine velocity of the blood flow can be measured. In growth restricted foetuses, there is a redistribution of the blood flow from the fetal periphery to the brain, commonly known as the brain-sparing effect. In severe fetal growth restriction with abnormal umbilical artery, MCA Doppler is a valuable adjunct, with abnormal findings signifying the onset of compromise that should soon require delivery (Dubiel et al, 2002).Overt MCA changes appear as increased diastolic velocity, and an altered cerebral-placental ratio will thus be observed. Changes in cerebral-placental ratio may be at least partly pressure-dependent, reflecting structural placental deficiencies, whereas brain-sparing is attributed to hypoxia induced cerebrovascular dilatation (Baschat, 2003). In those pregnancies over 34 weeks gestation, placental functional decline may be more dominant that structural decline. Thus MCA changes in brain-sparing may appear in small fetuses with near-normal umbilical artery Doppler (Severi et al., 2002; To et al., 2005). Such findings are again more likely to occur in women with pre-existing diabetes mellitus with vasculopathy than in those with gestational diabetes mellitus.

Another use for examining the MCA is to detect fetal anaemia. The MCA can be insonated at an angle between zero and 15 degrees to measure the actual flow velocity in the vessel. The lowest intra- and inter-observer variability is obtained when the MCA proximal to the transducer is sampled near its origin from the internal carotid artery without the use of angle correction using a 1-2 mm sample volume (Mari et al., 2005). A peak systolic velocity (PSV) of 1.50 MoM in fetuses at risk of anaemia has a sensitivity for detecting anaemia of up to 100% (confidence interval 86-100%) in red cell alloimmunization as well as other cases of anaemia (Mari et al., 2000). In the context of diabetic pregnancies, maternal hyperglycemia is thought to cause an increase in fetal haematocrit, as cordocentesis has demonstrated a positive relationship between maternal hyperglycaemia and fetal polycythemia (Salvesen et al., 1992). Theoretically, the increase in blood viscosity due to polycythemia might be reflected by a corresponding decrease in blood flow velocity in the fetal circulation, which is opposite to the fetal anaemia model. This would be particularly prominent in affected macrosomic fetuses in gestational diabetes, who often suffer prolonged neonatal jaundice resulting from the polycythemia. However, such findings have not been consistently demonstrated in published reports.

In a prospective study of 138 singleton pregnancies with GDM, umbilical artery pulsatility index and middle cerebral artery pulsatility index were measured serially every 4 weeks from the diagnosis of GDM until delivery. A total of 305 Doppler examinations were performed with one to four examinations for each woman. About 27% (38) had one or more abnormal pregnancy outcomes: placental abruption, pre-eclampsia, preterm delivery, small-for-gestational-age, low Apgar scores, neonatal jaundice requiring treatment, sepsis, birth trauma, meconium aspiration syndrome, respiratory and neurological complications, However, there was extensive overlapping of the umbilical artery and MCA pulsatility indices, as well as MCA PSV values between those with normal and abnormal pregnancy outcomes. It was thus concluded that that Doppler studies of the umbilical and cerebral vessels were not useful for predicting outcome in these GDM pregnancies (Leung et al., 2004). In another cohort of 84 GDM pregnancies, it was found that stratifying the fetuses into appropriate, small- and large-for-gestational-age did not give any better correlation between the umbilical or middle cerebral impedance indices, but did apparently show that the bigger fetuses had lower MCA PSV and higher mean umbilical venous flow velocity than the smaller fetuses (To et al, 2009). It has been proposed that the pathophysiological basis of altered placental vascular flow patterns in diabetic pregnancies was functional, related to hyperglycemia induced thromboxane/ prostacyclin ratio imbalance (Saldeen et al., 2002), rather than to structural abnormalities related to trophoblastic invasion during development of the placental vascular bed. Thus, the abnormal umbilical waveforms and abnormal placental-cerebral Doppler ratios that were observable in non-diabetic pregnancies with fetal growth restriction would not be applicable to gestational diabetic pregnancies without significant growth restriction. The observation of lower MCA PSV in the larger or macrosomic fetuses might be compatible with this hypothesis. In short, in the absence of pre-eclampsia or significant fetal growth abnormalities, the use MCA Doppler in diabetic pregnancies appears to have limited value.

3.4 Umbilical Vein waveform and umbilical venous flow volume

Arterial waveforms describe downstream resistance in critical vascular beds, in which disease or response to pathological conditions causes blood flow alterations. Venous Doppler, however, provides important cardiac data about stressed fetal circulations. Potential targets include the umbilical vein, inferior vena cava and the ductus venosus, while regional networks such as the hepatic, superior vena cava, intracranial and pulmonary veins have not provided clinically relevant cardiac indicators (Harman et al., 2003). By mid second trimester, the fetal umbilical vein normally has a continuous blood flow pattern, but this pattern can become pulsatile in pathological conditions, such as in significant fetal growth restriction and in hydropic fetuses. Thus, for umbilical venous waveforms, it has been advocated that a qualitative assessment of continuous versus pulsatile blood flow is used (Mari et al., 2008). Such venous pulsations most likely represent severe and critical fetal myocardial dysfunction and usually only appear at very late stages of fetal compromise. Umbilical venous waveforms are therefore not useful as an early sign for assessment of fetal well being for timing delivery.

The use of umbilical venous volume flow based on calculations of the cross-sectional area of the umbilical vein has been used and reported in previous studies to have a high degree of reproducibility (Boito et al., 2003). There have been suggestions for using the intra-abdominal portion of the umbilical vein (Haugen et al., 2004), as the latter would be less mobile than a free cord loop. Empirical experience showed that the demand on technical expertise between the two sites were largely similar, though the variations in the diameter of the intra-hepatic umbilical vein along its length could be somewhat higher than that of the free cord loop, and calculations of its cross-sectional diameter more complicated. In addition, since routine umbilical arterial Doppler would be performed on a free cord loop, it would be practical and convenient to extend the measurements to the adjacent vein within the cord segment (To & Mok, 2009).

To evaluate whether umbilical and middle cerebral arterial Doppler indices and umbilical venous volume flow are reflective of maternal gestational diabetic states, and whether such indices would be associated with the size of the fetus, a prospective observational study was performed in a cohort of 84 GDM pregnancies and compared with 62 non-diabetic controls. It was found that the mean pulsatility index values for the umbilical artery and the mean total umbilical venous flow (TUVF) and TUVF per unit birth weight did not differ significantly between diabetic and non-diabetic pregnancies. Large-for-gestational-age fetuses showed higher TUVF than normal size fetuses, but the TUVF per unit birth weight was higher for small-gestational-age fetuses. These differences were independent of their diabetic status. The only significant differences between non-diabetic and diabetic pregnancies in the data appeared to be the difference in the diameter and the mean flow volume of the umbilical vein, which were again probably more likely to be related to the size of the fetus. It was thus concluded that umbilical venous Doppler measurements near term were unable to distinguish between diabetic and non-diabetic pregnancies, and that umbilical venous flow volume was apparently more sensitive to the size of the fetus than to the maternal diabetic state (To & Mok, 2009). As fetal size variations could be secondary to poor maternal glycemic control, and macrosomic fetuses would demonstrate such measurements, it might be argued that the total umbilical venous flow would still indirectly reflect fetal conditions, or the presence or absence of macrosomia. However, it is obvious that direct measurement of fetal growth parameters would be more precise in defining fetal overgrowth.

The mean total umbilical venous flow has been shown in previous studies to be related to the total cardiac output of the fetus, so that the larger fetus with a higher cardiac output would have higher flow volumes (Boito et al., 2003). It was not surprising that when controlled for birthweight, the mean total umbilical venous flow differences between large- and small-for-gestational-age fetuses were greatly attenuated. Recent data have shown that in growth restricted fetuses, there would be a preferential distribution of umbilical venous flow to the ductus venosus rather than via the fetal liver (Bellotti et al, 2004). However, whether such venous shunting mechanisms would be responsible for the observed higher mean umbilical venous flow per unit weight in small-for -gestational-age fetuses as compared to larger ones would require further evaluation. In diabetic pregnancies, on the other hand, it has been found that fetal liver volume could be associated with accelerated growth in these fetuses, though only marginal differences could be shown in the umbilical venous volume flow. Further studies to compare growth and TUVF volumes in fetuses within a large non-diabetic population would be of value to study the differences in circulatory volumes in relation to size of the fetus.

3.5 Artioventricular valves

The atrioventricular values (mitral and tricuspid) are characterized by two peaks - the "E" wave corresponding to the rapid filling of the ventricles and the "A" wave that corresponds to the atrial contraction. The "A" wave is taller than the "E" wave, and may reflect the stiffness of the fetal cardiac chambers. With advancing gestation, the E/A wave ratio increases. By contrast, after birth, the "E" wave will be taller than the "A" wave. In growth restricted fetuses, the two waves become abnormal (the E/A ratio increases) and in severe cases, there will be tricuspid and mitral regurgitation (Rizzo et al., 1988). Thus, in the study of diabetic pregnancies, such studies would be of value only if the pregnancy is complicated by severe fetal growth restriction.

3.6 Ductus venosus Doppler waveforms

The ductus venosus provides a unique combination of data, as it is the primary regulator of venous return in both normal and abnormal fetuses and is also a direct conduit of right atrial retrograde pulse waves (Harman et al., 2003). The ductus waveform is responsive to changes in oxygenation independent of cardiac function, and it is readily imaged because of its very high focal velocity on colour Doppler from early second trimester onwards. Ductus venosus waveforms are characterized by two peaks, the S and D, followed by a nadir, the atrial wave. Haemodynamically, these phases reflect the rapid chronologic change in pressure gradients between the umbilical vein and the right atrium. In normally grown fetuses, there is forward flow at the ductus venosus, and the pulsatility index for veins (S-D/a) decreases with advancing gestation. In growth restricted fetuses, the pulsatility index increases, and in the most severe cases, there will be reverse flow in the atrial wave.

Ductus venosus waveform deterioration precedes and predicts changes in biophysical profile score that indicate need for delivery (Baschat et al., 2003). This deterioration is

hypothesised to be the result of a volume/pressure effect, in which excess afterload is transmitted through the heart, and myocardial dysfunction appears as an end-stage compromise. A second indication of ductus venosus Doppler occurs at 12-14 weeks in conjunction with nuchal translucency screening and uterine artery screening. Abnormal retrograde atrial waves are a strong predictor of fetal cardiac abnormality, and also a good predictor of Down syndrome (Bilardo et al., 2001). Given the higher risks of congenital cardiac abnormalities in pregnancies complicated by pre-existing diabetes mellitus, ductus venosus screening at this gestation may have a role. There is as yet, scanty data in the literature that describe the use of ductus Doppler specific to diabetic pregnancies, and the application of ductus Doppler largely refers to that of growth restricted fetuses in general.
To evaluate the ability of the ductus venosus Doppler to predict adverse perinatal outcome in pregnancies complicated by pre-existing diabetes mellitus, a prospective study that included 82 women with pre-existing diabetes mellitus was performed. The ductus venosus Doppler index was defined as abnormal if the ductus venosus peak velocity index for veins was equal to or greater than the 95th percentile for gestation. Abnormal ductus venosus index was identified in 30.5% (n=25). Adverse perinatal outcome was identified in around one-third of these with abnormal indices (8/25) compared to 12.3% (5/57) with a normal ductus index. The sensitivity of the ductus venosus index in predicting adverse perinatal outcome in pre-existing diabetic pregnancies was thus 53.3% and specificity was 74.5%, with a positive predictive value of 32% and negative predictive value of 87.7%. The authors concluded that it should be useful to include ductus venosus Doppler indices as part of antenatal screening of pregnancies complicated by pre-existing diabetes mellitus (Wong et al., 2010).

4. Practical application of Doppler studies to diabetic pregnancies

It has thus been postulated that the degree of glycemic control would have more impact on the Doppler study results rather than directly related to the diabetic state (Bracero et al., 1991). The lack of association of Doppler parameters to maternal diabetic state was particularly true when the pregnancy was not complicated by fetal growth restriction or pre-eclampsia. While higher incidences of adverse outcome in diabetic pregnancies were related to the occurrence of such complications or to poor glycemic control with macrosomia, Doppler studies have apparently only limited effectiveness in predicting adverse perinatal outcome in these fetuses. Summing up the available data from the literature, a basic protocol for the sequential use of Doppler studies in both pre-existing and gestational diabetic pregnancies can be proposed (Table 1). Nevertheless, the clinical effectiveness of such a protocol still remains to be evaluated.

5. Summary

Available randomized control data and observational data have failed to demonstrate any consistent association between maternal diabetes and abnormal umbilical arterial Doppler indices. Doppler measurements of other fetal vessels apart from the umbilical arteries, such as the fetal descending aorta and the middle cerebral artery resistance indexes, or the peak systolic velocity of the middle cerebral arteries have also been studied in GDM pregnancies, and a similar lack of predictability for adverse outcome was generally found. The lack of

Gestation (weeks)	Vessel	Doppler parameters	Primary endpoint	PDM or GDM
12	DV	Retrograde atrial waves	aneuploidy; congenital cardiac abnormalities	P/GDM
	Uterine	Notching, PI	FGR	PGD
22-24	Uterine	Notching, PI	FGR	PGD
	UA, MCA	PI, CPR	FGR	PGD
3rd trimester	UA, MCA UV AV valves DV	PI, CRP, PSV PI, TUVF AV flow, TR, MR Retrograde atrial valves	FGR	PGD/ GDM

PDM: pre-existing diabetes mellitus, GDM: gestational diabetes mellitus, DV: ductus venosus
PI: pulsatility index, CRP: cerebral placental ratio, FGR: fetal growth restriction,
PSV: peak systolic velocity, AV: atrioventricular, TR: tricuspid regurgitation, MR: mitral regurgitation

Table 1. Sequential Doppler applications foe diabetic pregnancies

association of Doppler parameters to maternal diabetic state was particularly true when the pregnancy was not complicated by fetal growth restriction or pre-eclampsia. While higher incidences of adverse outcome in diabetic pregnancies were related to the occurrence of poor glycemic control with macrosomia and polyhydramnios, conventional arterial Doppler indexes and cerebral /placental Doppler ratios have not been shown to be effective in picking up these high risk fetuses. The use of umbilical venous Doppler and venous volume flow based on calculations of the cross-sectional area of the umbilical vein has been reported in various studies to have a high degree of reproducibility. Venous volume flow measurements have not been found to be consistently reflective of maternal gestational diabetic states. Such volume flow measurements apparently reflected well the fetal growth and size and thus indirectly the glycemic control and the risks of perinatal complications. Doppler studies of other venous sites, including the intraabdominal/ intrahepatic portion of the umbilical vein, or the ductus venosus have also been studied with variable results. Whether such measurements could be used directly for monitoring fetal well being requires further evaluation.

6. References

American College of Obstetricians & Gynecologists Practice Bulletin (2001). Clinical management guidelines for obstetrician-gynecologists. Number 30, September 2001. Gestational Diabetes. *Obstet Gynecol*, 98: 525-528.

Alfirevic Z, Neilson JP (1995). Doppler ultrasonography in high-risk pregnancies: systematic review with meta-analysis. *Am J Obstet Gynecol* , 172: 1379-1387.

Baschat AA (2003). Integrated fetal testing in growth restriction: combining multi-vessel Doppler and biophysical parameters. *Ultrasound Obstet Gynecol* , 21: 1-8

Bellotti M, Pennati G, De Gasperi C, Bozzo M, Battaglia FC, Ferrazzi E (2004). Simultaneous measurements of umbilical venous, fetal hepatic, and ductus venosus blood flow in growth-restricted human fetuses. *Am J Obstet Gynecol*, 190: 1347-1358.

Ben-Ami M, Battino S, Geslevich Y, Shalev E (1995). A random single Doppler study of the umbilical artery in the evaluation of pregnancies complicated by diabetes. Am J Perinatal, 12: 437-438.

Bilardo CM, Muller MA, Zikulnig L, Schipper M, Hecher K (2001). Ductus venosus studies in fetuses at high risk for chromosomal or heart abnormalities: relationship with nuchal translucency measurement and fetal outcome. *Ultrasound Obstet Gynecol*, 17: 288-294

Boito S, Struijk PC, Ursem NTC, Stijnen T, Wladimiroff JW. (2003) Assessment of fetal liver volume and umbilical venous volume flow in pregnancies complicated by insulin-dependent diabetes mellitus. *Br J Obstet Gynaecol*, 110: 1007-1013.

Bonomo M, Cetin I, Pisoni MP, Faden D, Mion E, Taricco E, Nobile de Santis M, Radaelli T, Motta G, Costa M, Solerte L, Morabito A (2004). Flexible treatment of gestaional diabetes modulated on ultrasound evaluation of intrauterine growth: a controlled randomized clinical trial. *Diabetes Metab*, 30: 237-244

Bracero LA, Schulman H (1991). Doppler studies of the uteroplacental circulation in pregnancies complicated by diabetes. *Ultrasound Obstet Gynecol*, 1: 391-394.

Bracero LA, Figueroa R, Byrne DW, Han HJ (1996). Comparison of umbilical Doppler velocimetry, nonstress testing and biophysical profile in pregnancies complicated by diabetes. *J Ultrasound Med* , 15: 301-308.

Coleman MA, McCowan LM, North RA (2000). Midtrimester uterine artery Doppler screening as a predictor of adverse pregnancy outcome in high-risk women. *Ultrasound Obstet Gynecol*, 15: 7-12.

Dubiel M, Gunnarsson GO, Gudmundsson S (2002). Blood redistribution in the fetal brain during chronic hypoxia. *Ultrasound Obstet Gynecol* , 20: 117-121

Fadda GM, Cherchi PL, D'Antona D, Ambrosini G, Marchesoni D, Capobianco G, Dessole S (2001). Umbilical artery pulsatility index in pregnancies complicated by insulin-dependent diabetes mellitus without hypertension. *Gynecol Obstet Invest*, 51: 173-177

Giles WB, Trudinger BJ, Baird PJ (1985). Fetal umbilical artery flow velocity waveforms and placental resistance: pathological correlation. *Br J Obstet Gynaecol*, 92: 31-38

Grunewald C, Divon M, Lunell NO (1996). Doppler velocimetry in last trimester pregnancy complicated by insulin-dependent diabetes mellitus. *Acta Obstet Gynecol Scand*, 75: 804-808.

Gunton JE, Hitchman R, McElduff A (2001). Effects of ethnicity on glucose tolerance, insulin resistance and beta cell function in 223 women with an abnormal glucose challenge test during pregnancy. *Aust NZ J Obstet Gynecol*, 41: 182-186.

HAPO Study Cooperative Research Group (2008). Hyperglycaemia and adverse pregnancy outcomes. New Engl J Med, 358: 1991-2002.

Harman CR, Baschat AA(2003). Comprehensive assessment of fetal wellbeing: which Doppler tests should be performed? *Curr Opin Obstet Gynecol*, 25: 147-157

Johnstone FD, Steel JM, Haddad NG, Hoskins PR, Greer IA, Chambers S (1992). Doppler umbilical artery flow velocity waveform in diabetic pregnancy. *Br J Obstet Gynaecol*, 99: 135-140

Kapoor N, Sankaran S, Hyer S, Shehata H (2007). Diabetes in pregnancy: a review of current evidence. *Curr Opin Obstet Gynecol*, 19: 586-590

Kehl RJ, Krew MA, Thomas A, Catalano PM (1996). Fetal growth and body composition in infants of women with diabetes mellitus during pregnancy. *J Matern Fetal Med*, 5: 273-280

Ko GTC, Tam WH, Chan JCN, Rogers M (2002). Prevalence of gestational diabetes mellitus in Hong Kong based on the 1998 WHO criteria. *Diabet Med,* 19: 80

Leung WC, Lam H, Lee CP, Lao TT (2004). Doppler study of the umbilical and fetal middle cerebral arteries in women with gestational diabetes mellitus. *Ultrasound Obstet Gynecol,* 24: 534-537

Langer O, Yogev Y, Most O, Xenakis EM (2005). Gestational diabetes: the consequence of not treating. *Am J Obstet Gynecol,* 192: 989-997

Lao TT, Tam KF (2001). Gestational diabetes diagnosed in third trimester pregnancy and pregnancy outcome. *Acta Obstet Gynecol Scand,* 80: 1003-1108

Magee MS, Walden CE, Benedetti TJ, Knopp RH (1993). Influence of diagnostic criteria on the incidence of gestational diabetes and perinatal morbidity. *JAMA,* 269: 609-615

Mari G, Deter RL, Carpenter RL, Rahman F, Zimmerman R, Moise KJ (2000). Non-invasive diagnosis by Doppler ultrasonography of fetal anaemia due to maternal red-cell alloimmunization. *N Engl J Med,* 342: 9-14

Mari G, Abuhammad A, Cosmi E, Segata M, Altaye M, Akiyama M (2005). Middle cerebral artery peak systolic velocity - technique and variability. *J Ultrasound Med,* 24: 425-430

Mari G, Hanif F (2008). Fetal Doppler: Umbilical artery, middle cerebral artery and venous system. *Semin Perinatol* , 32: 253-257

Metzger B, Buchanan T, Coustan D, De Leiva A, Dunger D, Hod M, Kitzmiller J, Kjos S, Oats J, Petitt D, Sacks D, Zoupas C (2007). Summary and recommendations of the Fifth International Workshop-Conference on Gestational Diabetes Mellitus. *Diabet Care,* 30 (Suppl): S251-S260

Papageorhiou AT, Yu CK, Bindra R, Pandis G, Nicolaides KH, Fetal medicine Foundation Second Trimetser Screening Group (2001). Multicenter screening for preeclampsia and fetal growth restriction by transvaginal uterine artery Doppler at 23 weeks of gestation. *Ultrasound Obstet Gynecol* , 18: 441 -449

Papageorghiou AT, Yu CK, Cicero S, Bower S, Nicolaides KH (2002). Second trimester uterine artery Doppler screening in unselected population: a review. *J Matern Fetal Neonatal Med,* 12: 78-88

Parlakgumus HA, Durukan T (2010). The relationship between cardiac adaptation to uteroplacental Doppler flow and perinatal outcome in pregnant women with diabetes. *Clin Exp Obstet Gynecol* , 37: 39-42

Pietryga M, Brazer J, Wender-Ozegowska E, Dubiel M, Gudmundsson S (2006). Placental Doppler velocimetry in gestational diabetes mellitus. *J Perinatol Med,* 34: 108-110

Platt MJ, Stanisstreet M, Casson IF, Howard V, Walkinshaw S, PennycookS, McKendrick O (2002). St Vincent's Declaration 10 years on: outcomes of diabetic pregnancies. *Diabet Med* , 19: 216-220

Reece EA, Homko CJ (2007). Prepregnancy care and the prevention of fetal malformations in the pregnancy complicated by diabetes. *Clin Obstet Gynecol,* 50: 990-997

Rizzo G, Arduini D, Romanini C, Mancuso S (1988). Doppler echocardiographic assessment of atrioventricular velocity waveforms in normal and small-for-gestational-age fetuses. *Br J Obstet Gynaecol,* 95: 65-69

Sacks DA, Chen W (2000). Estimating fetal weight in the management of macrosomia. *Obstet Gynecol Surv,* 55: 229-239

Sacks DA (2007). Etiology, detection and management of fetal macrosomia in pregnancies complicated by diabetes mellitus. *Clin Obstet Gynecol,* 50: 980-989

Saldeen P, Olofsson P, Laurini RN (2002). Structural, functional and circulatory placental changes associated with impaired glucose metabolism. *Eur J Obstet Gynecol Reprod Biol*, 105: 136-142

Salvesen DR, Brudenell MJ, Nicolaides KH (1992). Fetal polycythemia and thrombocytopenia in pregnancies complicated by maternal diabetes mellitus. *Am J Obstet Gynecol*, 166: 1287-1293

Salvesen DR, Higueras MT, Mansur CA, Freeman J, Brudenell JM, Nicolaides KH (1993). Placental and fetal Doppler velocimetry in pregnancies complicated by maternal diabetes mellitus. *Am J Obstet Gynecol*, 168: 645-652

Schaefer-Graf UM, Gaber B, Wendt L, Metzner S, Sacks DA, Vetter K, Kilavuz O, Abou-Dakn M (2011). How many sonograms are needed to reliably predict the absence of fetal overgrowth in gestational diabetes mellitus pregnancies? *Diabet Care*, 34: 39-43

Schmidt MT, Duncan BB, Reichelt AJ, Branchtein L, Matos MC, Forti AC, Spichler ER, Pousada JMD, Teixeira MM, YamashitaT (2001). Gestational diabetes mellitus diagnosed with a 2-h 75 g oral glucose tolerance test and adverse pregnancy outcomes. *Diabetes Care*, 24: 1151-1155

Schulam H, Fleischer A, Farmakides G, Bracero L, Rochelson B, Grunfeld L (1986). Development of uterine artery compliance in pregnancy as detected by Doppler ultrasound. *Am J Obstet Gynecol*, 155: 1031-1036

Severi FM, Bocchi C, Visentin A, Severi FM, Bocchi C, Visentin A, Falco P, Cobellis L, Florio P, Zagonari S, Pilu G (2002). Uterine and fetal cerebral Doppler predict the outcome of third trimester small-for gestational age fetuses with normal umbilical artery Doppler. *Ultrasound Obstet Gynecol*, 19: 225-228

To WWK, Chan AMY, Mok KM (2005). Use of umbilical-cerebral Doppler ratios in predicting fetal growth restriction in near term fetuses. *Aust NZ J Obstet Gynaecol* , 45: 130-136

To WWK, Mok KM (2009). Fetal umbilical arterial and venous Doppler measurements in gestational diabetic and non-diabetic pregnancies near term. *J Maternal Fetal Neonatal Med*, 22: 1176-1182

Wong SF, Chan FY, Cincotta RB, McIntyre DH, Stone M (2003). Use of umbilical artery Doppler velocimetry in the monitoring of pregnancy in women with pre-existing diabetes. *Aust NZ J Obstet Gynaecol*, 43: 302-306

Wong SF, Petersen SG, Idris N, Thomae M, McIntyre HD (2010). Ductus venosus velocimetry in monitoring pregnancy in women with pre-gestational diabetes mellitus. *Ultrasound Obstet Gynecol*, 36: 350-354

Zimmermann P, Kujansuu E, Tuimala R (1992). Doppler velocimetry of umbilical artery in pregnancies complicated by insulin-dependent diabetes mellitus. *Eur J Obstet Gynecol Reprod Biol*, 19: 47: 85-93

Zimmermann P, Kujansuu E, Tuimala R (1994). Doppler flow velocimetry of the uterine and uteroplacental circulation in pregnancies complicated by insulin-dependent diabetes mellitus. *J Perinatal Med*, 22: 137-147

16

The Influence of Diet to Control the Metabolism in Gestational Diabetes Mellitus

Rebeca Monroy-Torres[1] and Jaime Naves-Sanchez[2]
[1]*University of Guanajuato, Department Medicine and Nutrition;*
[2]*IMSS-48, HMI-SSG*
Mexico

1. Introduction

Gestational diabetes mellitus (GDM) is the intolerance to carbohydrates, first recognized during pregnancy. The prevalence of GDM has been increasing in the world and it affects more than 200,000 women every year.

This chapter emphasizes and discusses the role of the dietary and nutritional aspects of the GDM. First, we will do a general review about the transitional changes in food that are experienced worldwide, their phases-dietary habits, industrialization, globalization, culture, the media as television, video games which have led to changes in the eating patterns and how this diet style promotes a metabolic disease, wich will be supported with Mexican evidence. Second, we will do a general literature review of the most important nutritional and dietetic recommendations, findings, calculation and prescription of a correct diet (Distribution of: proteins, lipids and carbohydrates), in combination with counseling nutritional importance. Next, we will compare two recommended diets for GDM with the evidence we got from our research. Moreover, we will discuss the advantages and disadvantages of the glucemyc index and how a low and moderate one allows the control of blood glucose. The glycemic index is defined as the area under the curve of glucose response after eating a recomended amount of carbohydrates from a test food after a control food (white bread or glucose), and these had been considered part of the control of blood glucose. Besides, we present the methods for collecting diet information as a complement to improve the follow up and the adherence to GDM. Other important aspects to discuss are the importance of the preventive and promotional strategies in the medical nutrition therapy, physical activity, benefits, risk and the type of exercise for GDM, education, psychological support, insuline and drugs . The prevention and promotion should consider economical and social aspects because pregnant women use to change their food consumption because of economical influence. The health costs and long management of GDM mothers have a wide range of possible complications. These recommendations should result in adequate weight gain for the fetus and the woman. A deficit in the weight gain is associated with intrauterine growth restriction for the fetus. Dietary control is defined as a part of the comprehensive treatment of GDM and the diets low in carbohydrates, lipids, and proteins have demonstrated to reduce hyperglycemia and to prevent macrosomia compared with diets high in carbohydrates carbon.

The main goal of the dietary treatment is to maintain the maternal and fetal health and the diet with low carbohydrates help to the management of GDM, where the main goal is to achieve and to maintain blood glucose and glycated hemoglobin according to the practice guidelines for GDM and to avoid ketonuria. The adhesion to dietary treatment is difficult in most patients when they intake lower amount of carbohydrates. The findings reported in the control of the GDM such as changes in weight gain, energy intake, and macronutrients are part of a basic treatment to prevent complications for the fetus and the pregnant mother. We will review of promotion and prevention activities as part of the dietary treatment. Finally, we hope that this information let discuss new alternatives for GDM.

2. Diet: Transitional changes

Since the last century, many countries have experienced changes in health and food patterns that are characterized by an increasing prevalence of chronic diseases. These chronic diseases are the principal cause of death and commonly happen particularly particularly in pregnant women and children. There are many factors that may explain these changes and one of the most important one to consider is the dietary habits because they explain the metabolic diseases (Avila A, et al., 1995; ENSANUT, 2006). As mentioned above, there are other factors that might explain these changes and the principal ones are the alterations in dietary habits that are considered important to explain the metabolic diseases (Avila A, et al., 1995; ENSANUT, 2006). For example, México is living an epidemiological transition that has occurred in recent decades. For instance, the most common causes of death in this transition are cardiovascular diseases, cancer, accidents and diabetes. Fifty years ago, most of the causes of death in the Mexican population were related to diarrhea and respiratory diseases. The research done at the Mexican National Institute of Nutrition supports the idea that the proportion of animal products in the diet of Mexicans has increased sharply. In addition, fast food, ,in most countries, is considered as a frequent choice for many people who live in the city. The epidemiological changes that have occurred in many countries are not homogeneous throughout the world; for instance, they vary according to geographical, regional and socioeconomical factors. Based on the studies carried by Romieu, et al., it is possible to observe the coexistence of over nutrition and under nutrition in the same population. In underdeveloped countries, it is possible to observe that about one-third of children under 5 years are stunted, and 20% of women are obese. (Romieu I, et al., 1997).

The dynamic of the epidemiological aspects in many countries provides challenges and opportunities for studying dietary habits. These dietary habits can serve as the base for conducting studies about how the diet can modify the occurrence of chronic diseases, and the impact on the nutritional health can be investigated as well (Romieu I, et al., 1997; Ávila A, et al., 1995). Other then dietary habits, there are more factors to be considered at risk for developing obesity such as: excessive consumption, physical activity, sedentary and hereditary factors. Many countries have had an apparent economical development during the last decade and has contributed to the lifestyle, eating habits, customs, behaviors, etc. The diet of developed countries consist of cereals, legumes, fruits and vegetables. These changes are similar to those of the industrialized countries (high-energy diet, protein, animal fat and low fiber). This is the price we have had to pay for the globalization that our world is facing because this is the result of the free trade agreement in developed countries. Moreover, the powerful influence of the North American culture has affected the entire world. One example of this is the payment-saving culture „pay less, get more" so it is cheaper to be obese. The same phenomenon operates in fast food restaurants and convenience stores, among others.

The industrialization of a city has as a consequence that some products contain raw poor materials disguised with flavors that result in products of low nutritional value but tasty. They are also well supported with good marketing strategies and are aimed especially to children. Another important finding is that some Latin American countries spend from 20 to 30% of their income in food and they have the higest consumption of soft drinks in the world; hence, soft drinks have replaced water consumption. In additin to this, the presence of obesity in the family is an important factor to be considered because if both parents are obese then, the risk of obesity in children is 80%. Television and video games are other factors of great influence. In countries where the habit of reading is replaced by television and video games, it has been observed that there is an adjustement in children's behavior and habit consumptions of some products. For example, 85% of the commercials on TV promote soft drinks, desserts and fried food (Ramirez JA, et al., 2003).

Sciences such as demography and epidemiology help to understand the phenomenology behind food and nutrition in a sistematic way. Where the diet habits are related with the culture, traditional habits, climate, available foods, etc. These habits do not change inmediately. Transitional nutrition has five phases or periods that the majority of societies experienced and these are (Nielsen, S & Popkin, B, 2003):

a. Stage of "*food gathering*". The diet is high in carbohydrates and fiber but low in fat. This stage is characterized by the hunting and gathering of food.
b. Stage of "*starvation*". It occurred with the early development of agriculture when food was less varied and linked to periods of extreme food shortages.
c. Stage of "*increased consumption of fruits, vegetables and animal products*". Starches begin to be less important in the basic diet. This stage is related to the industrial and the second agricultural revolution.
d. Stage of "*Presence of chronic degenerative diseases*". It increases with the prevalence of obesity as a result of the consumption of diets high in fat, cholesterol, refined carbohydrates, small amounts of polyunsaturated fatty acids and fiber and physical inactivity. In this stage there is an increase in the population that migrate to big cities where home and work are located far away from traditional markets.
e. Stage of "*behavioral change*". This stage is characterized by the adoption of healthy diets, physical activity and the abandonment of traditional diets. Here, the consumption of cereals and tubers is very important. In this stage, there is a tendency to a global homogenization of the type of food that is consumed. Then, an intake of high energy, total fat, saturated fat and simple sugars is required. Moreover, physical activity decreases due to changes in occupational activities, transportation facilities, these contributed to increase the chronic diseases (diabetes mellitus, hypertension and atherosclerosis) related to overweight and other nutrition aspects.

Finally, it is necessary to say that each country goes through these periods of transition at different times and with a different speed.

The main characteristic of transactional nutrition is that these changes occur more rapidly in middle or low income countries than in the high-income ones. In low income countries, there is a negative impact in their economical growth due to that the fact that they spend more money in getting food of low nutritional value such as oils and fat of poor nutritional quality.

This is done with the purpose of getting cheaper food that can be obtained faster by people. However, the use of this kind of food promotes the appearance of cardiovascular diseases.
Changing of food consumption has altered in many countries because, they prefer to buy prepared food than to cooked it at home. As a result, the consumption of oilseeds, vegetable oils, fish and seafood has been decreasing but there is an increment in the consumption of animal fat, alcoholic beverages, meat and eggs consumption. These habits increase the costs and the quality of ingredients in food (Ortiz-Hernández, L, et al., 2006; Monroy-Torres R, et al., 2010). The changes mentioned above are part of the evidence that has been gathered from the population that lives in urban areas, people employ in the tertiary sectors and the actual role of woman (Ortiz-Hernández L, et al., 2006).
The determinants of the are located mainly in both, the social organization and the technological progress of the society (Ortiz-Hernández, et al., 2006). Another determinant that is also important to consider is the educational level. During the periods of 1988–1994 and, 2007-2008, the prevalence of childhood obesity in United State increased at all income and educational levels (CDC, 2010).
According to diet and disease, 20 years ago, it was discovered that low birthweight was associated with an increased risk of adult diabetes and cardiovascular disease (CVD). A hypothesis was formulated with this information,wich states that that the exposure to undernutrition in early life increased the risk to develop these disorders in the metabolic programation. In order to solve the problem caused in the metabolic programation, it has been proposed another hypothesis that claims that it would be important to improve the nutritional state from the pre gestational stage to the gestational stage and finally the nutritional attention to the new born to prevent common chronic diseases in the future. The research done with low birth weight children in many countries shows that they have increased CVD risk factors. The scientific findings gotten from maternal nutrition have contribute to understand the role of specific nutrients in the maternal diet, like low maternal vitamin B12 status,wich predicted the increased of adiposity and insulin resistance in children, especially if the mother had a folate deficiency. Both maternal undernutrition and gestational diabetes cause problems (glucose excess) They have also been associated with increased adiposity and insulin resistance in children. In underdeveloped countries, it has been noticed that undernutrition and overnutrition coexist. Recent intervention studies in developed countries have shown that CVD risk factors in the offspring can be improved by supplementing undernourished mothers during pregnancy. Of course, results differ according to the population, the intervention and the post-natal environment (Fall C., 2009).

3. Evidence in the diet management of gestational diabetes mellitus

Dietary therapy is the most important factor to be consider in the treatment of GDM. Therefore all women with GDM must receive counseling from a dietitian. Recommendations have to be individualized after a dietary evaluation of each patient. The two main objectives for the treatment of GDM are to achieve normoglycemia and to provide the required nutriments for normal fetal growth and maternal health. A third objective that is also considered to be important, is to prevent excessive maternal weight gain, particularly in women who are overweight or have gained excess weight in pregnancy.
Few trials have analyzed the efficacy of dietary therapy for GDM. A cluster randomized controlled study supports that Medical Nutrition Therapy (MNT) for GDM is recommended by the American Diabetes Association (ADA, 2010). The MNT is a lifestyle intervention that

consists of an integral component of diabetes prevention, management, and self-management education (Goldhaber-Fiebert JD, et al., 2003).

A recommended diet for the glucemia control in GDM must be low in carbohydrates,with a percentage between 35% and 50%; lipids from 30% to 40% and 20% of protein, of the total calories. This distribution has proved to reduce hyperglycemia and prevent macrosomia, when compared with diets high in carbohydrates (Franz M, et al., 2002).

These recommendations must include a nutritional counseling because the excessive restriction of carbohydrates (< 120g) increases the risk of ketonuria, low birth weight and defective supply of glucose to the fetus impact on the neurological development (Pastor JG , et al, 2002; ADA, 2007;ADA, 2003, 2010; Major CA, et al, 1998). Besides the aforementioned , it is necessary to say that low carbohydrates diets make it difficult for patients to adher to the treatment.

According to the American Diabetes Association (ADA 2010), a good diet control must, appart from getting glycated hemoglobin values (HbA1c) less than 6% and avoiding ketonuria (Standards of Medical Care in Diabetes-2008) maintain the capillary blood glucose concentrations in ≤95 mg/dl (Preprandial); ≤140 mg/dl (1-h postmeal); ≤120 mg/dl 2-h (postmeal). Regarding to plasma-referenced capillary blood glucose, the values suggested are ≤105 mg/dl (Preprandial), ≤155 mg/dl (1-h postmeal), ≤130 mg/dl (2-h postmeal)(Standards of Medical Care in Diabetes-2008). With these recommendations, patients with GDM should have an adequate weight gain for them and the fetus as well. The weight gain recomendation is calculated based on prepregnancy weight or with the body mass index (BMI). A deficit in weight gain is associated with intrauterine growth restriction (Pastor, et al, 2002).

Monroy-Torres R. et al. studied the influence of an individualized diet of low glycemic index to control GDM in woman between 24 and 26 gestational weeks. The diet was structured with 52% of complex carbohydrates and food of low and moderate glycemic index with 30% fat and 18% protein (plus 10 grams). The findings from the study were that the pregnant women with GDM did not have adverse effects related to blood glucose, glycosylated hemoglobin and weight gain. The newborns did not development macrosomia. The adherence observed was higher for calorie and macronutrient intake.

3.1 Glycemic index and glycemic load

According to Jenkins,the glycemic index (GI) is defined as the changes in blood glucose concentration after consuming food wich then has to be compared with standard amount of carbohydrate of a control food (white bread or glucose) (Jenkins DJA, 1984). The food with low and moderate GI has been considered as a part of a glycemic control; where the increased in the percentage of carbohydrates up to 60% of total calories is allowd when and if food of low and moderate glicemic control is given (Fraser RB, et al, 1988). The consumption of processed food or food with low fiber conten increases the glycemic index while the GI decreases with food high in fiber, fats, proteins and it depends on the cooking process. Moses R et al., 2006, compared the effects of a diet of low glycemic index with a diet of high GI. Both diets had 55% of carbohydrates. Women with GDM who had a diet with high glycemic index gave as a result that they had a newborn with high weight (large for gestational age) and higher ponderal index. Another important concept to discuss is the load Glycemic (LG) - that is the amount of carbohydrates in a specific food. The GI of food is not always easy to predict; for example, we could think that an ice cream has a high GI but it has low GI according to published charts. The reason is that an ice cream has fat and proteins, this combination decreases the digestion of glucose.

While the World Health Organization, the American Diabetes Association, Diabetes UK, and the Canadian Diabetes Association support both concepts (IG and LG),and many other health professionals consider that to use GI and GL is complex because both have many variables that change their values and responses in the blood glucose. This is why their use in the clinical practice is debatable (Franz M, 2003). Other explanation is that different tables; with GI and LG values for different food, show different values for GI among the existing tables which gives as a result that their use is consider controversial specially with new data has become available since the first tables were published in 2002 (Atkinson F, 2008; Foster-Powell K, 2002). However, the most important recommendation is to follow up the advice of the Standards of Medical Care in Diabetes 2008: choose a variety of grains, fruits, and vegetables, with an emphasis on whole grains and other high-fiber foods, to work with dietary and behavioral changes

3.2 Calculation and prescription of the diet

The American Diabetes Association consensus to manage GDM recommends to take into account the dietary calculation (ADA 2010) to consider the value of BMI. According to the clinical experience the diet prescription must be individualized (Jovanovic L, 2000). The diet may be calculated in a range between 1700 and 2000 kcal/day. It is important to avoid diets with caloric content lower than 1500 Kcal because the risk of ketonuria can be increased. The calculation and distribution of macronutrients can be as follows:

- Protein: 18% (range of 10 to 20%; add 10 g, of the gestational period)
- Fat: 30% (of these 7% saturated), range of 25 to 40% and reducing the intake of trans fat lowers LDL cholesterol
- Complex carbohydrates: 52% (range of 40 to 60%)

The American Diabetes Association (ADA, 2004) recommends to add 25 kcal per kilogram during pregnancy. A strategy to evaluate the adherence to energy consumption is to monitor weight gain which should not exceed 400 grams per week from the second trimester of pregnancy.

According to the table 1, ,we can see how the range of carbohydrates varies between 40% and 55% or more of the total calories. The American Diabetes Association of the United States recommends that all pregnant women with overweight and / or GDM should receive a diet with 35-40 grams of carbohydrates (simple carbohydrates), from food with low glycemic index. However, a consumption of carbohydrates less than 40% is risky because it results in ketonuria (ADA, 2010).

Variables	ADA 2010	**Euglycemic diets**
*BMI: 80 -120 %	35 Kcal / Kg (ideal weight)	30 Kcal / Kg (ideal weight)
*BMI: 121 -150%	35 Kcal / Kg (ideal weight)	24 Kcal / Kg (ideal weight)
*BMI: >= 151 %	35 Kcal / Kg (ideal weight)	12 Kcal / Kg (ideal weight)
Protein requirement	20 % of total calories	20 % of total calories
Fat intake	< 25 % of total calories	>= 40 % of total calories
Saturated fat intake	<7% of total calories	
Carbohydrates requirements	> 55 % of total calories	< 40 % of total calories
Cholesterol Requirements	300 mg/d	< 800 mg / d

* Relationship of BMI based on the percentage of body fat

Table 1. Comparison of diets recommended in GDM

We can observe in table 1 that the range of carbohydrates varies from less than 40% to over 55%. The American Diabetes Association of the United States recommends that all pregnant women with overweight and/or GDM must receive a diet with 35-40% of carbohydrates and food with low GI. The percentage of calories, that depends on carbohydrates , is reduced, a 20% of proteins and 30% of fat is recommended. This is done to keep the balance of macronutrients. In fact, it is advisable that the distribution to be similar to a normal diet but it is importan to have considered the quality of food and macronutrients (ADA 2004; 2010). It is important to control the intake of carbohydrates because they are the first nutrient that affects the postprandial glucose levels in addition to breakfast carbohydrate load.

During pregnancy, hormone levels of placental lactogen, cortisol, progesterone and prolactine increase and this affects the insuline to lower blood glucose levels. Therefore, breakfast carbohydrate load of 15 to 30 g is recommended. The total daily carbohydrates and calorie intake should be individualized according to glucose control. When a dietitian designs a meal plan, carbohydrates intake should be distributed during the day in a three time meal and two or three small meals (snacks) (Sheard, N.F., et al., 2004). For example, a diet of 2000 calories where the carbohydrates can represent a 40% of total calories; that in grams is equivalent to 200 grams, the total calories should be distributed during day as follow:

- Breakfast 7.5- 10%(15- 20g)
- Snack 10% (between breakfast and lunch)
- Lunch 35%
- Snack 15% (between lunch and dinner)
- Dinner 20%
- Evening Snack 10%

The minimum amount of carbohydrates required to prevent the starvation activation systems (ketosis) of fasting is between 100 and 150 grams per day. According to the Food and Nutrition Board in 2002, 130 grams per day of carbohydrate is enough to satisfy the glucose requirement of the brain (FNB, 2005). Moreover, this recommendation should provide a list of food of low and moderate glycemic index (≤ 55 and from 59 to 69, respectively). Each country has different patterns of food exchange that are based on the consumer habits and customs of each population. For example, Mexico has the Mexican Food System Equivalents (Marvan L, et al., 2008), it is a educational system that is provided to patients with GDM to explain the amount of food intake from different food groups. To understand better the amounts and real food portions, the dietitians often used food replicas. Based on what it was meal times explained above, food should be distributed depending on the glucose control in six or seven meals (three main meals and three or four snacks) (Jovanovic L, 2000, Monroy-Torres R, et al., 2008). Dietary and nutritional advice, lifestyle counseling and restriced food should be provided to patients in a written list. Adding proteins and fat to the meal plan for woman with GDM will not raise the postmeal glucose levels and to satisfy the woman´s hunger during the day (Monroy-Torres R, et al., 2008).

The methods to collect dietary information vary in their accurancy and ease use. The 24-hour recall is one of the easiest methods to collect information from the patient´s intake. It consists of obtaining information from food and fluid intake from a previous day (24 hours) and it is based on the assumption that the intake described is typical of a daily intake. However, the method has important problems; for example, the patient may not be able to recall the eaten food or not to estimate the amount of food eaten. On the other hand, the method offers the advantage of analizing the average consumption of energy, carbohydrates, fats and proteins from the diet. This allows to analyze to the amount of food and the adhesion to the diet from the beginning and to follow it up. Another method is the Food-frequency-questionnaire that is often used in combination with the 24-hour recall. The food-frequency-questionnaire provides a list of food or food group where the patient can have different options to answer like: rarely, never, frecuently, occasionally, daily, weekly and monthly. The Food-frequency- questionnaire is only recommended to use only at the beginning and the end of GDM treatment and this method is useful to evaluate changes in the eating habits and to analize the diet of patients within the next parameters: *adequate, complete, balanced, enough and varied* - these define a recommended diet. A diet is recommended for GDM when it has all these parameters: a) Enough: means to cover the energy requirements according to the individual characteristics like age, weight, physical activity and physiological conditions, b) *balanced*: means to intake nutrients based on references amounts (52% of complex carbohydrates, protein in 18%, fat in 30%); c) Complete: means to include at least three food groups at every meal and, d) varied: means to include different types of food within the same group, in a day (Marvan L, et al., 2008). Food records and postmeal monitoring of blood glucose can help to identify food that is less tolerated and to let individual nutrition and food recommendations changes (Sheard, N.F., et al., 2004).

If the modification of the food plan alone does not prove to achieve and mantain normoglicemya, then insuline therapy is needed. To achieve the goals with the use of insulin, women must eat the corrcect amounts of carbohydrates and they must eat at regular meal times (ADA, 2010), all above information is important to avoid unnecessary hypoglycemia risk. Exchange lists or counting carbohydrates are the methods that help patients with GDM select and decide themselves what to eat according their glucose levels and their insulin therapy. Since insulin is the therapy of choice for most diabetic women, several authors suggest to apply the method of carbohydrate counting or exchange lists during the first nutrition interview. In table 2, you can see the recommendations of a dietary treatment in combination with insulin that depend on the response to the glycemic control (Standards of Medical Care in Diabetes-2008).

Preconception stage	First strategy	Second strategy
Normal	Diet	Diet + Insulin
GDM controlled with insulin	Diet + Insulin	
GDM controlled hypoglycemic drugs	Diet +Insulin	Diet+ Insulin
GDM controlled with diet	Strict Diet	Diet+ Insulin

Adapted: Monroy-Torres-Sanchez Naves R & J, 2011

Table 2. Recommendations of dietary treatment in combination with insulin in GDM

The ADA (2010) mentions that all women should receive individualized counseling to provide adequate calories and nutrients during pregnancy. This counseling must help achieve the goal and maintain the blood glucose (fasting 105 mg/dl , 1 hr 155 mg/dl , and 2 hrs 130 mg/dl) and glycated hemoglobin (HbA1c)in 6%. For obese women, the treatment must be a 30%-33% of caloric restriction, it means near to 25 cal/kg per day is recommended, wich should be calculated with the current weight. Carbohydrate should be restricted to 35%-40% of calories. There are also data that support the use of low carbohydrate diets in pregnancy, and for carbohydrates to be low, the glycemic index. In a nonrandomized study, there was evidence that women with GDM on a diet comprising less than 42% carbohydrate, had lower post-prandial glucose levels, were less likely to require insulin, and had a lower incidence of large for gestational age. A small study with randomized pregnant women with low GI or high GI diets found that the former resulted in lower glucose levels, a blunting of the pregnancy associated rise in insulin resistance, and lower birthweight. In another study of GI, women assigned to a low GI diet during pregnancy gave birth to infants who were lighter and had a lower incidence of large for gestational age, compared to women given a high GI diet. Additional dietary measures are usually based upon the general recommendations for diabetes mellitus. A reduction in simple carbohydrates and fat intake is advisable. Emphasis is given to spreading the dietary intake over six meals daily, with three main meals and three snacks in order to avoid large carbohydrate loads at any time. Except for saccharin, which can cross the placenta and is therefore not recommended, other noncaloric sweeteners may be used in moderation (Moses, R., et al, 2006).

4. Preventive and promotional strategies

Medical nutrition therapy (MNT), including:

- Education
- Diet
- Physical activity
- Where justified, Insulin
- Psychological support to improve acceptance and adherence to disease treatment

We must consider that if GDM is not diagnosed at the early stage, mother' dietary habits and overall health in this period will have consequences in the short, medium and long term effecting the child as well. Regarding to the educational intervention, patients with GDM should know:

- What is GDM?
- The importance of metabolic control and risk of ketonuria
- Characteristics of recommended diet plan
- Self-monitoring techniques
- Goals of the blood glucose control
- Types of insulin, application techniques (where insulin is required)
- Importance of early intervention, monitoring and control postpartum
- Prevention of future type 2 diabetes mellitus

Weight loss is not recommended during pregnancy, even though the woman is obese. For during the GDM is necessary that weight gain should be in the lower ranks recommended, according to the start value of BMI except in the adolescent woman , where the weight increment must be higher.

The objectives of a diet plan are:

- Get optimal metabolic control and to prevent hypoglycemia
- Adequate weight gain during pregnancy

Some studies recommend energy consumption between 1800 and 2200 kcal, bearing in mind that weight gain should be among the lower ranks. In adolescents, low weight or great complexion is recommended to increase energy requirements.

The exercise is useful to help control metabolism. The type of exercise for pregnant women is with the work that can be done with the upper extremities. However it is contraindicated in the following cases:

- Increased uterine contractions
- Multiple pregnancy
- During hyperglycemia and hypoglycemia
- history of stroke or arrhythmia
- Hypertension

4.1 Physical activity

Currently more pregnant women want to have their pregnancy in natural and healthy conditions. Exercising in pregnant women is controversial as to the changes presented in their body and the hormonal levels. A long time ago, pregnancy was experienced as an illness, and had several myths related to it, including the exercise. The scientific arguments to restrict physical activity during pregnancy suggest that exercise causes an increment in maternal body temperature and therefore in the fetus too, with increased release of catecholamines, decreased circulating glucose and decreased blood flow to the placenta. However, there are other scientific studies that show the benefits of a regular physical activity during pregnancy to maintain health. When it is a normal pregnancy is recommended that pregnant women continue to perform normal physical effort.

For athletes, it is recommended to decrease the intensity, especially during the second trimester of pregnancy and especially during the last month. Pregnancy increases the elasticity of the ligaments by the effect of hormones released during pregnancy. For this reason, it is advisable to practice sports that do not require jumping, excessive stretching and to use appropriate footwear. Some reported benefits of regular moderate physical activity during pregnancy are (Artal, R. & Toole, M.O ., 2003):

- Helps improve fitness and body image of pregnant women, contributing to increased weight.
- Maintains cardiovascular function.
- Improved glycemic control.
- Promotes the welfare state joins mother and a better mood by providing psychological benefits.
- Decreases stress and anxiety.
- Provides better labor
- Promotes weight recovery after childbirth.

In people with type 2 diabetes, there is a lot of evidence that suggests that regular physical activity improves insulin sensitivity, weight loss, thereby improves glucose control. Several studies have examined whether regular exercise is also beneficial in the management of GDM, for example, Jovanovic L, (Jovanovic L, 2000) randomized 19 women with GDM to a regime of diet alone, or diet with 20 minutes of supervised aerobic training three days per week for six weeks. This modest amount of physical activity resulted in lower fasting glucose levels, lower glucose responses to a glucose challenge, and a lower HbA1c . Another study randomized 29 women with GDM to 30 minutes of exercise (70% of maximal heart rate) of three to four times per week. In this case the glucose levels did not improve in those who exercised. The action might be through the activation of AMPK, a kinase that is activated during exercise, it is possible that exercise may act through the same molecular cellular pathway and therefore there are not additive effects of these two treatment regimens (Hardie DG, 2004).

Another study found that women with a prepregnancy value BMI of 25 and who were in the exercise program were less likely to require insulin. Therefore, it seems reasonable to recommend that when there is not medical or obstetric contraindication, women with GDM should maintain a sensible level of light and moderate intensity if there is physical activity during the pregnancy. The above studies provide enough evidence that moderate physical activity such as walking between 20 and 30 minutes each day, or three to four times per week, through this they can achieve the glycemic control. The diet should provide with adequate nutrition for pregnancy. Carbohydrates should be distributed throughout the day over main meals and snacks. Limiting carbohydrates at 40% of the total caloric intake and having a higher proportion of carbohydrates of lower glycaemic index decreases postprandial glucose levels and reduces the need for insulin therapy (Smith, C.S. & Van Andel, R., 2001; Artal, R. & Toole, M.O ., 2003).

There is not enough evidence to support dietary or drug treatment in patients with gestational diabetes. Gestational diabetes and impaired glucose tolerance are associated with macrosomia and may be associated with an increased risk for cesarean delivery, shoulder dystocia, and birth trauma. Although preexisting diabetes has been shown to increase the risk of poor perinatal outcomes, it is not clear that data relating to preexisting diabetes can be extrapolated to patients with gestational diabetes.

Tuffnell and colleagues (Olwan N, 2009)researched the Cochrane Pregnancy and Childbirth Group trials register, the Cochrane Central Register of Controlled Trials, and bibliographies of relevant articles. They identified three studies of 223 women with impaired glucose tolerance; none of these studies was a randomized controlled trial comparing management strategies. Intensive management of gestational diabetes is time-consuming and resource-intensive. Overall, the evidence is insufficient to support the therapy for gestational diabetes. However, universal screening is the standard of care in most communities. When faced with abnormal results, most family physicians will opt to follow the consensus opinion of our specialist colleagues. For example, a study that analyzed the higher egg and cholesterol intakes found that they are associated with increased risk of type 2 diabetes mellitus. It was also observed that the higher egg and cholesterol intakes before and during pregnancy are associated with an increased risk of GDM. (Qiu C, et al., 2011).

Several lines of evidence indicate that realistic modifications of diet and lifestyle can prevent diabetes type 2. Some of the main determinants include lack of physical activity, hours of TV watching, low quality and energy dense diets, and high caloric sweetener intake. Caloric beverages have been recognized as an important source of energy and have been associated with an increased risk of overweight. (Schulze MB, 2005; Ludwig DS, 2001).

Lifestyle modification, to increase exercise and to modify diet habits are an effective way of to prevent and to delay the onset of type 2 diabetes in the future in women with GDM. One important aspect of combating the epidemics of obesity and type 2 diabetes has been through dietary strategies. Recently, very-low-carbohydrate diets have gained much popularity. Recently the effects of a diet lower in carbohydrates and higher in protein has been evaluated in obese and over-weight patients with type 2 diabetes for analyze the changes in blood glucose levels and in the insulin resistance. Because glucose is the major insulin secretagogue carbohydrate, its reduction would be expected to be beneficial in type 2 diabetes and the use of such diets. Although, as noted above, official recommendations generally continue to suggest low fat and high carbohydrate intake (Arora & McFarlane , 2005; Fioster GD, 2003) .

Efforts to change diets, physical activity patterns, and other aspects of lifestyle have traditionally attempted to educate individuals through schools, health care providers, worksites, and general media. These efforts will continue to play an important role, but they can be strongly reinforced by policy and environmental changes.

5. Conclusion

The control and prevention of GDM must be the principal goal. The dietary treatment must be based on the design and prescription of diets according to cultural habits, economical aspects and the diet must be accessible. The family, the health team and the society should be into the treatment of the GDM, mainly the prevention of diabetes mellitus type 2. To achieve this goal the authors suggest:

- To evaluate the best evidence in the dietary management of patients with GDM and to design programs that involve motivation.
- To monitor weight gain in pregnant women according to prepegnancy BMI and considering the biochemical markers, including glucose and glycated hemoglobin in order to adapt and correctly identify the nutritional treatment.
- To monitor not only fasting glucose, but the postprandial
- To increase surveillance and to monitor at intervals of 3 to 4 weeks in each appointment, for increasing the adherence to the diet.
- To perform several scientific studies to identify other factors that support control of the GDM.

Finally, it is important to consider the economical and social influence (Wilson C, 2003). Pregnant women usually modify their food intake according to the influence of their nutritional orientation . The full costs to achieve a behavioral change and the policies are complex and difficult to estimate. The efforts to reduce the increment of diabetes mellitus type 2, is screening pregnant women. In sum, the benefits will be for the fetus growth and health for both

6. Acknowledgment

Teacher Gabriela Ramirez-Tavares and Joseph Gerald Phillips for their contributions to this English version. Medical and Nutrition Department, Health and Science Division , Campus Leon, University of Guanajuato.

7. References

Alwan, N; Tuffnell, DJ; West J. (2009). Tratamiento para la diabetes gestacional: (Revision Cochrane traducida). En: *Biblioteca Cochrane Plus*; Num 3. Oxford: Update Software Ltd. Available in: http://www.update-software.com; http://www.bibliotecacochrane.com/BCPGetDocument.asp?SessionID=%2016594 02&DocumentID=CD003395#CD003395-fig-00120

American diabetes association. (2003). Position statement: Gestational diabetes mellitus. *Diabetes Care*; 26(suppl 1): S103-S5. ISSN: 0149-5992

American Diabetes Association. (2004). Gestational diabetes mellitus (Position Statement). *Diabetes Care*; 27(Suppl. 1): S88- S90. ISSN: 0149-5992

American Diabetes Association. (2007). Standards of medical care in diabetes 2007. *Diabetes care*; 30: suppl 1: S4-S41. ISSN: 0149-5992

American Diabetes Association. (2010). Standards of Medical Care in Diabetes—2010. *Diabetes care*;33 (suppl 1): 11s-61s. ISSN: 0149-5992

Arora, SK & Mcfarlane, SI (2005). The case for low carbohydrate diets in diabetes managerment. *Nutr Metab*; 2:16. ISSN: 1743-7075

Artal, R. & Toole, M.O . (2003). Guidelines of the American College of Obstetricians and Gynecologists for exercise during pregnancy and the postpartum period. *Br J Sports Med* ;37:6-12. ISNN: 1473-0480

Atkinson, F; Foster-Powell, K; Brand-Miller, JC. (2008). International Tables of Glycemic Index and Glycemic Load Values: 2008. *Diabetes Care*; 31:2281–2283. ISSN: 0149-5992

Avila, A; Shamah, T; Chávez, A. (1995). Encuesta urbana de alimentación y nutrición en la zona metropolitana de la cuidad de México. (Urban food and nutrition survey in the metropolitan area of Mexico City.) México City. *Instituto Nacional de la Nutrición.*

Briefel, RR; Wilson, A; Gleason PM. (2009). Consumption of Low-Nutrient, Energy-Dense Foods and Beverages at School, Home, and Other Locations among School Lunch Participants and Nonparticipants. *J Am Diet Assoc*; 109:S79-S90. ISSN: 0002-8223

Centers for Disease Control and Prevention. National Center for Health Statistics. National. Health and Nutrition Examination Survey. Available from: http://www.cdc.gov/nchs/nhanes/nhanes_questionnaires.htm. Accessed November, 2010.

Goldhaber-Fiebert, JD; Goldhaber-Fiebert, SN; Tristán, ML; Nathan DM.(2003). Randomized controlled community-based nutrition and exercise intervention improves glycemia and cardiovascular risk factors in type 2 diabetic patients in rural Costa Rica. *Diabetes Care*; 26: 24– 29. ISSN: 0149-5992

Fall C. (2009). Maternal nutrition: effects on health in the next generation. *Indian J Med Res*;130(5):593-9. ISSN: 0971-5916

Food and Nutrition Board (FNB). 2005. Dietary Reference Intakes for Energy, Carbohydrate, Fiber, Fat, Fatty Acids, Cholesterol, Protein, and Amino Acids (Macronutrients). This report may be accessed via www.nap.edu and is available in: http://books.nap.edu/openbook.php?record_id=10490&page=275

Foster, GD; Wyatt, HR; Hill, JO; McGuckin, BG; Brill, C; Mohammed, BS; Szapary, PO; Rader DJ; et al. (2003). A randomized trial of a low-carbohydrate diet for obesity. *N Engl J Med*; 348(21):2082-2090. ISSN 1533-4406.

Franz, M; Bantle, JP; Beebe, CA; Brunzell, JD; Chiasson, JL; Garg, A; Holzmeister, LA; Hoogwerf, B; Mayer-Davis, E; Mooradian, AD; Purnell, JQ; Wheeler, M. (2002). Evidence based nutrition principles and recommendations for the treatment and prevention of diabetes and related complications. *Diabetes Care*; 25:148-98. ISSN: 0149-5992

Franz M.(2003). The glycemic index: not the most effective nutrition therapy intervention. *Diabetes Care* 26:2466–2468. ISSN: 0149-5992

Foster-Powell, K; Holt, SH; Brand-Miller, JC. (2002). International table of glycemic index and glycemic load values: 2002. *Am J Clin Nutr*; 76:5–56. ISSN: 1938-3207

Fraser, RB; Ford, FA; Lawrence, GF. (1998).Insulin sensitivity in third trimester of pregnancy. A randomized study of dietary effects. *Br J Obstet Gynaecol*; 95: 223-9. ISSN 0306-5456

Hardie DG. (2004). AMP-activated protein kinase: a key system mediating metabolic responses to exercise. *Med Sci Sports Exerc*; 36:28-34. ISSN 1530-0315

Institución Nacional de Salud Pública, Secretaría de Salud, Instituto Nacional de Estadística, Geografía e Informática. (2006). Encuesta Nacional de Salud y Nutrición.

International Association of Diabetes and Pregnancy Study Groups Consensus Panel.(2010). International Association of Diabetes and Pregnancy Study Groups Recommendations on the Diagnosis and Classification of Hyperglycemia in Pregnancy. *Diabetes Care*;33:676-82. ISSN: 0149-5992

Jenkins, DJA; Wolever, TMS; Jenkins, AL; Josse, RG; Wong, GS. (1984).The glycaemic response to carbohydrate foods. *Lancet*; 2:388-91. ISSN 0140-6736

Jovanovic, L. (2000).Medical nutritional therapy in pregnant women with pregestational diabetes mellitus. *J Matern Fetal Neonatal Med*; 9: 21-8 . ISSN: 1476-7058

Kant, AK. (2000). Consumption of energy-dense, nutrient-poor foods by adult Americans: nutritional and health implications. The third National Health and Nutrition Examination survey, 1988-1994. *Am J Clin Nutr*; 72:929-936. ISSN: 1938-3207

Kim, C; Newton, KM; Knopp, RH. (2002). Gestational diabetes and the incidence of type 2 diabetes: a systematic review. *Diabetes Care*; 25: 1862– 1868. ISSN: 0149-5992

Ludwig, DS; Peterson, KE; Gortmaker, SL. (2001). Relation between consumption of sugar-sweetened drinks and childhood obesity: a prospective, observational analysis. *Lancet* ; 357(9255):505-508. ISSN 0140-6736

Nielsen, S & Popkin, B. (2003). Patterns and Trends in Food Portion Sizes, 1977-1998. *JAMA* ;289(4):450-453. ISSN: 00987484

Marvan, L; Pérez, AB; Palacios, B. (2008). Mexican Food System Equivalents. Third edition. Fomento de Nutrición y Salud; México D.F. ISBN: 978-970-94523-1-0

Major, CA; Henry, JM; De Veciana, M; Morgan, MA. (1998). The effects of carbohydrate restriction in patients with diet-controlled gestacional diabetes. *Obstet and Gynecol;* 91: 600-3. ISSN: 0029-7844

McLeroy, KR; Bibeau, D; Steckler, A; Glanz, K. (1998). An Ecological Perspective for Health Promotion Programs. *Health Educ Q* ; 15(4):351-378. ISSN: 0195-8402

Medical nutrition therapy: nutrition practice guidelines for gestational diabetes.(2001). *Am Dietetic assoc.* ISSN, 0002-8223

Monroy-Torres, R; Reeves-Aguirre, CC; Naves-Sánchez, J; Macias, AE. (2008). Influencia de una dieta individualizada de bajo en índice glucémico en el control de la diabetes mellitus gestacional. *Rev Ginecol obstetr Mex;* (76)12:722-729. ISSN 1561-3062

Monroy-Torres, R; Velásquez, A; Ortíz, A. (2010). Programa oportunidades sobre la seguridad alimentaria y nutricional en Atarjea: desde la percepción de sus participantes. *Avances en seguridad alimentaria y nutricional;* 1(1): 63-73 ISSN: 1659-326X.

Moses, R; Luebcke, M; Davis, W; Coleman, K; Tapsell,L; Petocz, P; Brand-Miller. (2006), "Effect of a low glycemic index diet during pregnancy on obstetric outcome". Am J Clin Nutr; 84, 807-812. ISSN: 1938-3207

Pastor, JG; Warshaw, H; Daly, A; Franz, M; Kulkarni, K. (2002). The evidence for the effectiveness of medical nutrition therapy in diabetes management. *Diabetes care;* 25: 608-13 . ISSN: 0149-5992

Qiu, C; Frederick, IO; Zhang, C; Sorensen, TK; Enquobahrie, DA; Williams, MA. (2011). Risk of gestational diabetes mellitus in relation to maternal egg and cholesterol intake. *Am J Epidemiol* ;173(6):649-58 ISSN 1476-6256

Ramírez, JA; García, M; Cervantes, R; Mata, N; Zárate, F; Mason, T; Villarreal, A. (2005).Transición alimentaria en México. *An Pediatr* ;58(6):568-73. ISSN: 1695-4033

Romieu, I; Hernandez-Avila, M; Rivera, JA; Ruel, MT; Parra, S. (1997).Dietary studies in countries experiencing a health transition:Mexico and Central America. *Am J Clin Nutr;* 65(suppl): 1159s-65s. ISSN: 1938-3207

Sheard, N.F.; Clark, N.G.; Brand-Miller, J.C.; Franz, M.J.; Pi-Sunyer, F.X.; Mayer-Davis, E.; Kulkarni, K.; Geil, P. (2004). Dietary carbohydrate (amount and type) in the prevention and management of diabetes: a statement by the american diabetes association. *Diabetes Care* ;27(9):2266-71. ISSN: 0149-5992

Schulze, MB & Hu, FB. (2005). Primary prevention of diabetes: what can be done and how much can be prevented? *Annu Rev Public Health;* 26:445-467. ISSN: 0163-7525

Smith, C.S. & Van Andel, R. (2001). Pregnancy and North American lifestyles: exercise, work, and diet in pregnancy. *Clin Fam Pract* ;3:167-181. ISNN: 00943509

Standards of Medical Care in Diabetes—2008. (2008). *Diabetes Care* ; 31: (Suppl 1): S12- S54. ISSN: 0149-5992

Wilson, C; Brown, T; Acton, K; Gilliland, S. (2003). Effects of clinical nutrition education and educator discipline on glycemic control outcomes in the Indian Health Service. *Diabetes Care*; 26:S23-S30. ISSN: 0149-5992

17

Insulin Use in Gestational Diabetes – Pragmatic Protocols for Self-Management and for Labour and Delivery

Sara J Meltzer and Rima Alsayari
McGill University Health Centre, Montreal, QC
Canada

1. Introduction

The expectation of treatment goals in the management of gestational diabetes are the most stringent and precise for control of diabetes in adults (American Diabetes Association, 2011; Canadian Diabetes Association Clinical Practice Guidelines Expert Committee, 2008). It is well accepted that the achievement of these goals requires an effective collaboration between a well-trained physician, a nurse educator and a qualified dietician experienced in working with pregnancy and, most importantly the woman with gestational diabetes (Canadian Diabetes Association Clinical Practice Guidelines Expert Committee, 2008; Murphy, et al., 2010; Jacqueminet S, 2010; Kim, 2010; Kjos S, 1999). The more involved the woman becomes in her own treatment plan, the more likely that she will succeed (Meltzer S. J., 2010).

2. Never underestimate the value of a well-planned, balanced diet

Once a diagnosis of gestational diabetes has been made, the initial step is always an assessment of the woman's present diet and the introduction of changes which would optimize her glucose control. Without an understanding and application of the concepts of medical nutrition therapy, further attempts at controlling glucose will always be limited. Individual dietary counselling with a trained dietician is preferable, whenever possible (Canadian Diabetes Association Clinical Practice Guidelines Expert Committee, 2008; International Diabetes Federation Writing Group, 2009).

The major concepts of the diet consist of identifying fast and more slowly absorbed carbohydrate sources: fruits and vegetables, starchy foods such as bread, pastas, rice, noodles, grains, and milk and milk products as the major carbohydrate in the diet. In any one meal, optimally there is a small portion of fruits and/or vegetables which will be absorbed quickly, a portion of starches/grains which will be absorbed more slowly, accompanied by a portion of protein and a small portion of fat. The mix of two forms of carbohydrate absorbed over different time periods, as well as the presence of fat and protein which, apart from being essential nutrients, slow further the absorption of glucose from the gut permits a more gradual and slower rise of glucose post-meal. This makes glucose much easier to control with either endogenous insulin or injected forms - presented conceptually in Figure 1. Additionally, use of foods with low glycemic index (higher in fibre and producing a lower post-ingestion glucose elevation) has been shown to be of help in minimizing effects of excess glucose in the pregnancy (Grant, Wolever, O'Connor, Nissenbaum, & Josse, 2011; Tzanetakou, Mikhailidis, & Perrea, 2011; Thomas D, 2009). Foetal growth, particularly asymmetric growth with increased central fat patterning relates to the effectiveness of glucose control of post-meal elevations and in general terms, excess post-prandial hyperglycaemia has negative effects on maternal and foetal well-being (Standl, Schnell, & Ceriello, 2011; Parretti, et al., 2001; DeVeciana, et al., 1995).

In gestational diabetes, as with early type 2 diabetes, the first phase of insulin release is impaired (Ornoy, 2011; Catalano, Kirwan, Haugel-de Mouzon, & King, 2003), thus more concentrated forms of carbohydrate (sugar added to coffee, juices, candies, cakes etc.) will be absorbed too quickly for the slow insulin response, allowing the glucose to go up quickly to above normal levels which may then affect the baby. The stimulation of insulin release can occur in response to certain amino acids. There may still be an intact protein-stimulated insulin release response even if the glucose-stimulated insulin release is compromised which can help avoid elevated glucose values (Catalano, Kirwan, Haugel-de Mouzon, & King, 2003). These concepts are relatively simple to understand and when explained to the woman with GDM helps her to understand the basis of her dietary efforts and concerns. Providing an explanation to the woman with visual tools suggesting the relative absorption times and how different foods work will make it easier for her to understand what she is trying to do when she goes home and plans her meals. (Figures 1 and 2 developed for this purpose).

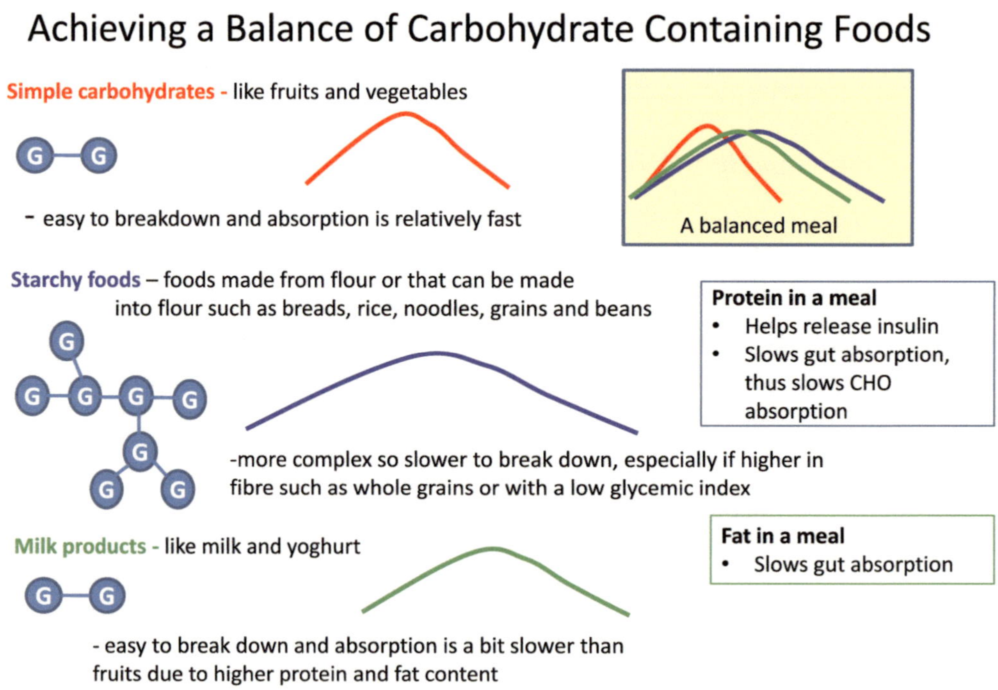

Fig. 1.

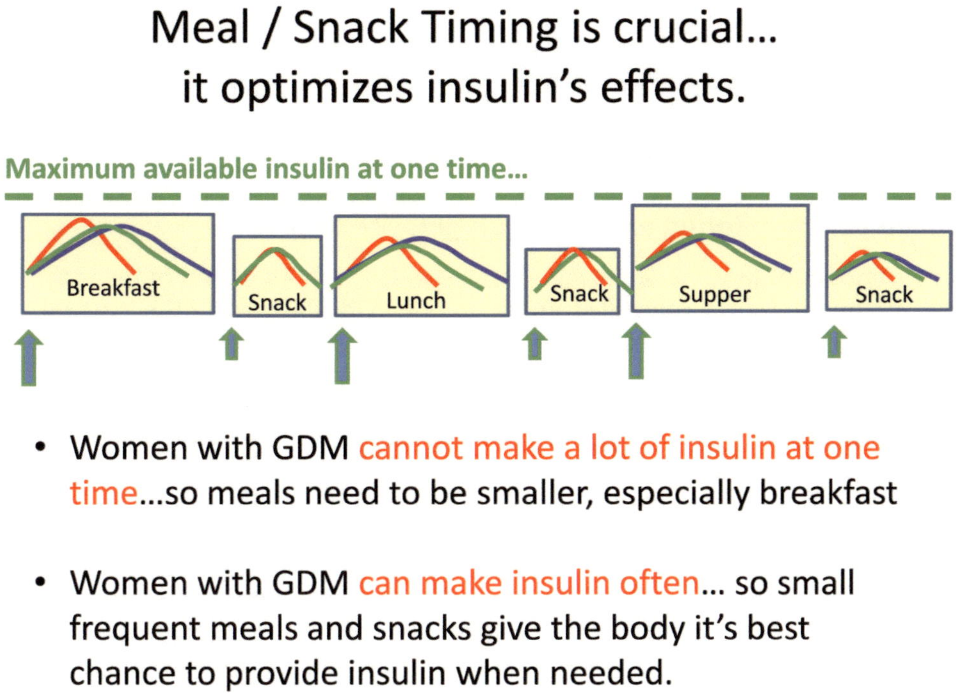

Fig. 2.

Author's statement: Sara J. Meltzer, MD, FRCPC, FACP
Figure 1 and 2 were developed by the author for use in clinical work teaching women with gestational diabetes the basic concepts of diet and are included here for those who may find them helpful.

To be sure that the diet has been effectively instituted - using food diaries and encouraging measuring and weighing can be very helpful to help the women understand successes and problems with her choices of foods in her normal environment (Burke, Wang, & Sevick, 2011). Unfortunately, some women will limit their food choices dramatically leaving out foods typical of their normal diet in an effort to reach glucose targets. Since it is important for the woman to understand how to incorporate the foods normally present in her diet including ethnically diverse foods while she has the help and time of a dietician's advice and can see the effects on her glycemic control with frequent testing, excessive limitation of her food choices should be discouraged. The effectiveness of long-term dietary adjustments to decrease insulin need is more likely if she understands the effects of her preferred foods on her glucose control. Since the mother is often in charge of family meal-planning and cooking, her application of learned knowledge should help her avoid future diabetes and reduce the risks to her offspring whose eating habits develop at home (Ratner, et al., 2008; Tuomilehto, et al., 2001; Verier-Mine, 2010; Diabetes Prevention Program Research Group, 2009; Egeland & Meltzer, 2010).

Pre-pregnancy BMI and actual weight gain are potentially modifiable risk factors so attention to both weight control pre-pregnancy and rate and total amount of weight gain in the pregnancy are important (Hutcheon, Platt, Meltzer, & Egeland, 2006; Radesky, Oken, Rifas-Shirman, Kleinman, Rich-Edwards, & Gillman, 2008). Recommended weight gain is often based on the Institute of Medicine recommendations, relate to pre-pregnancy BMI and intake will often be 25-30 kcal/kg (Institute of Medicine and National Research Council Committee to Re-examine IOM Pregnancy Weight Guidelines, 2009).

3. Teach self-monitoring and establish glucose targets

Another important facet of achieving glucose control will be to determine if the glucose values are appropriately controlled at various times of the day. In this situation, use of self-blood glucose monitoring (SBGM) is very effective. Avoiding starvation is also important so many centres will routinely test at some point for urine ketonuria to determine if the women are receiving adequate calories for their needs. The basic concepts of testing are easy to convey and ideally a qualified diabetes educator or pharmacist would review techniques in the use of the meter and lancet device chosen. In situations where this is not available, peer-to peer teaching may be equally effective. It is valuable to verify the accuracy of the woman's technique and device by asking her to do a comparative test against the laboratory value, ideally in a fasting state which provides a better comparator than in post-meal values which are in a state of flux and may differ in the capillary and venous system physiologically. This is important to clarify since the glucose targets required are within the normal range and many meters may have a small degree of consistent error which, if known, can be considered in defining her at-home meter glucose targets.

The usefulness of the testing is markedly enhanced if the woman is instructed on how to use this information to adjust her therapy (Hawkins J. S., Casey, Lo, Moss, McIntyre, & Leveno, 2009). The more pragmatic and useful the testing, the more likely compliance with management will be. Thus self-blood glucose monitoring is often done before breakfast and at 60-90 minutes after meals, since studies suggest that this is the highest level of glucose seen in the post-meal phase for the majority of women (Jovanovic L. G., 2008). The peak post-prandial glucose level in obese women tends to be higher and later - more around 90 minutes after the meal (Ben-Haroush, Yogev, Chen, Rosenn, Hod, & Langer, 2004). In many parts of the world, the post-meal test timing recommended may be closer to 120 minutes or 2 hours. Health providers must be aware that only testing before or after main meals may miss other parts of the day with significant increases in glucose so random testing at other times may also need to be suggested (Montaner, Ripolles, Pamies, & Corcoy, 2011)(29).

In most national guidelines, the goal of therapy is to achieve values which fall into the normal range, thus under 5.1 or 5.3 mmol/L (92-95mg/dl) fasting, under 7.8mmol/L (140mg/dl) at 1h post load, and under 6.7mmol/L (120mg/dl) at 2h post-load (American Diabetes Association, 2011; Canadian Diabetes Association Clinical Practice Guidelines Expert Committee, 2008). It must be realized that these numbers indicate the mean plus two standard deviations above the mean… the actual mean is lower…usually between 3.8 – 4.4 mmol/L in the fasting state and rarely above 6.5mmol/L at any point after the meal (Gillmer, Beard, Brooke, & Oakley, 1975; Parretti, et al., 2001; Rowan, Gao, Hague, & McIntyre, 2010; Yogev, Ben-Haroush, Chen, Rosenn, Hod, & Langer, 2004). Depending on the reliability of the individual, her meter accuracy and the evaluation of the pregnancy in terms of weight gain, macrosomia and relative risks for the offspring, lower achieved values are often possible and near-normal values can often be reached using the right insulin protocol and self-adjustment of insulin by the patient. There is no proven value of running blood glucose values at the top end of normal (or near the abnormal range) rather than the middle, so going for truly normal would appear to make sense if hypoglycemia does not occur. In a study of a Pima Indian cohort, diabetes conveyed excess offspring risk of obesity and glucose intolerance independent of genetic factors and other studies have explored the role of diet type and intake quantity in future offspring risks (Dabalea, et al., 2000; Reusens & Remacle, 2001). In fact, results of glucose targets achieved by any means in the MiG's study (metformin in gestational diabetes) suggest that outcomes are optimal in terms of appropriate fetal weight for dates with values closer to the mean of normal (Rowan, Gao, Hague, & McIntyre, 2010) and a long-term follow-up study (15 years) attaining similar lower mean values led to a very low incidence (1%) of teenage offspring glucose intolerance (Egeland & Meltzer, 2010). In the HAPO study, there was an association with maternal post-load glucose and clinical neonatal hypoglycemia; for the one hour glucose value (adjusted OR, 1.13; 95%CI; 1.03-1.26) and a weak association for the two hour glucose value (adjusted OR, 1.13; 95% CI 1.00-1.12) (HAPO Study Cooperative Research Group., 2009). Even within normal ranges, maternal glucose values have been linked to offspring insulin sensitivity and beta cell function (Reusens & Remacle, 2001; Bush, Chandler-Laney, Rouse, Granger, Oster, & Gower, 2011). In obese women particularly, achievement of the optimal glucose targets improves fetal outcomes (Langer, Yogev, Xenakis, & Brustman, 2005).

4. Physical activity should be encouraged unless precluded for obstetric reasons…

The effectiveness of a physically active lifestyle has been shown to help prevent the development of type 2 diabetes in those at risk such as women diagnosed with gestational diabetes (Ratner, et al., 2008; Sanz, Gautier, & Hanaire, 2010). Most guidelines recommend some form of regular exercise in pregnancy although only a few studies address this issue in detail (American Diabetes Association, 2011; Canadian Diabetes Association Clinical Practice Guidelines Expert Committee, 2008; Division of Nutrition PA, and Obesity, Centers for Disease Control; ACOG Committee Opinion, 2002; Bung, Artal, Khodiguian, & Kjos, 1991; Artal, Lockwood, & Brown, 2010). At the very least, encouraging women to walk after meals often for a total of 30 minutes per day is the recommendation and this can improve glucose results and will help the women understand during pregnancy how effective small amounts of exercise can be on glucose control. Care must be used in women with evidence of pre-term labour or any previous suggestions of cervical incompetence; however this is the minority of women with gestational diabetes.

5. Insulin adjustment algorithms with the patient self-adjusting are easy to teach and effective…

Initiation of insulin, if needed, is no longer a reason to hospitalize a patient. Insulin is often needed in about 10-50% of women, depending on the population and the criteria used for diagnosis (Langer, Berkus, Brustman, Anyaegbunum, & Mazze, 1991). Once the effect of diet on initial testing has been evaluated and if the woman's glucose values exceed the upper limits of glucose targets, it is a simple matter to initiate insulin in a logical and pragmatic way.

Consideration of the degree of macrosomia seen on ultrasound, particularly if increased abdominal girth is seen in the foetus may be used as a moderating factor in the need for initiation of insulin and potentially in the target glucose values aimed for (Buchanan, et al., 1998)(44). The HAPO study showed a clear correlation with macrosomia and the glucose values attained on the oral glucose tolerance test result at 28-32 weeks [fasting glucose adjusted OR, 1.38; 95% CI:1.32-1.44, one-hour adjusted OR, 1.46 ; 95% CI 1.39-1.53, two-hour adjusted OR, 1. 38 ; 95% CI: 1.32-1.44] (HAPO Study Cooperative Research Group, Metger BE; Lowe LR; Dyer AR et al, 2008). If there is no evidence of macrosomia on ultrasound and the initial A1c is below a pregnancy normal mean of 5.3%, it may be possible to accept slightly higher glucose values and still obtain a good foetal outcome.

The use of insulin pens has greatly simplified the teaching of insulin injection; however it is also relatively easy to teach injections using insulin syringes in a short teaching session, possibly in small groups. It is important that any woman being initiated on insulin (or any oral agent which is a secretogogue for that matter) be taught how to recognize and treat a hypoglycemic episode. The use of written and picture educational material often available from insulin producing companies will facilitate the educational essentials that must be explained. The concept of site use and rotation is another issue which should be addressed by the teaching nurse.

There have been studies using both metformin and glyburide as oral agents for the management of gestational diabetes showing reasonably comparative composite outcomes. There were 46% of the women in the metformin study who still required insulin and there was inadequate power in the glyburide randomized trial to determine macrosomia and neonatal hypoglycemia outcomes (Rowan, Hague, Gao, Battin, Moore, & and MiG Trial Investigators, 2008; Langer, Conway, Berkis, Xenakis, & Gonzales, 2000). At present in most countries, it remains "off-label" and most guidelines do not suggest its routine use or only if for some reason insulin cannot be used (American Diabetes Association, 2011; Canadian Diabetes Association Clinical Practice Guidelines Expert Committee, 2008; Jacqueminet S, 2010). For these reasons, it will not be addressed in detail in this chapter.

In terms of the actual insulin prescription, the concept of using a famous train robber's recommendation - Sutton's law "Go where the money is!" can be very helpful. In other words, pick the part of the day which is most abnormal from the point of view of glucose control. In general, improvement to absolutely normal of the fasting glucose value will facilitate the release of insulin by the woman and improve glucose much of the day (Pennartz, Schenker, Menge, Schmidt, Nauck, & Meier, 2011). In the majority of cases, bedtime insulin is the most effective first step although the women from South East Asia and Asia may have post-meal glucose which tends to be higher and may have normal fasting glucose values.

If the fasting glucose is the value which is above range, initiation of intermediate insulin at bedtime (neutral protamine Hagedorn or NPH in human or pork form) at a low dose should be done (can be as low as 2 units in a very nervous woman who is not too obese, but the usual starting dose would be 8 - 10 units minimum or 0.1 units/kg). In many clinics, the women return on a regular basis for adjustment of their insulin doses. As insulin needs increase progressively in response to placental growth and production of anti-insulin hormones, this often means that the initial period after adjustment is well controlled but over the two weeks the glucose control may deteriorate. It is very easy to have the women do the progressive adjustment of her own insulin based on her morning blood glucose (and thus her body's response to the insulin given); she can then increase the dose by specified increments until she achieves the desired range. The increments are largest for high glucose values (as much as 6 units at once) and gradually reduce to as little as 1 unit more insulin for the evening dose as the target range is reached (See Figure 3a). In someone who is markedly obese or may have evidence of acanthosis nigricans, often an initial dose may be 0.1-0.2 units/kg administered at bedtime again with an increase in dose the following day if the fasting glucose has not achieved the desired range. An important part of the algorithm is a glucose value below which she MUST REDUCE her evening dose of NPH. This avoids hypoglycaemia before it happens and discourages overzealous increases in insulin dosages. Our experience has been very effective and safe using the value of 4.2mmol/L below which a woman will reduce that night's dose as this glucose value is far away from the values of 3.2 or 2.8mmol/L which would be felt as a hypoglycemic reaction and require treatment (Snyder, Gray-Donald, & Koski, 1994; Meltzer, Snyder, Penrod, Nudi, & Morin, 2010).

In situations where women have markedly elevated fasting and post-meal glucose levels, an overall dose of 0.5 – 0.7u/kg can be used in the proportion of about 40% as bedtime NPH insulin and the remainder split over the day with a bit more at breakfast and less at lunch ie. 25% - 15% - 20% of the total calculated dose given as regular or rapid-acting insulin prior to breakfast, lunch and dinner respectively.

On very rare occasions likely explaining the lack of literature related to it, women develop a local allergy to NPH at the injection site with swelling and redness developing up to 12 hours after the last injection of NPH at that site and lasting for about one to two days. In virtually every situation where this has been seen and is deemed intolerable by the woman, switching to regular human insulin as a 10pm injection and retesting glucose at 0400 to adjust the 10 pm dose as well as adding a 0400h injection of human (preferably) or pork regular insulin which will be adjusted based on the pre-breakfast result will often correct the allergy problem and continue to effectively control the glucose. Usually the dose can be reduced from the previous insulin dose and given as one third at 2200h and about one third or a bit less at 0400h. Subsequent self-adjustment protocols can still be used with an added time of 0400h and will allow for safe correction of insulin to optimal doses. Unfortunately, this approach does interfere with the woman's sleep. The use of detemir or glargine insulin may be alternatives; however it has yet to be reported in this situation.

If the fasting glucose is normal and the post-meal is the glucose which is elevated (often related to ethnic differences), the insulin administered will be regular insulin or a rapid-acting analogue administered prior to the meal (See Figure 3b). If Regular insulin is used, the time it should be taken before the meal is often 20-30 minutes, which is why the rapid-acting analogues are often preferred, as they can be take much closer to the meal (0-15 minutes) and still effectively control the post-prandial 60-90 minute peak (Pettitt, Ospina, Kolaczynski, & Jovanovic, 2003). The effectiveness of the dose is evaluated by the woman using her post-meal glucose value for that meal and the following day, the dosage for that meal will be adjusted up or down in order to achieve the desired values. Since at meals, occasionally, even the "best" patient may change her food from the recommended meal plan, it is often appropriate to wait for 2 abnormal values before increasing the dose, however only one value lower than the desired goal **requires that the dose be reduced the following day.** Allowing the woman to be responsible for the gradual and persistent adjustments of insulin dose regularly seen in GDM as the placenta continues to grow and her insulin needs rise can facilitate her care. Occasional additional tests in relation to snacks or prior to meals may be necessary to determine glucose control is always good (Montaner, Ripolles, Pamies, & Corcoy, 2011). Visits may be further apart because the woman is making the appropriate adjustments, thus the medical team does not need to. Use of colour-coding has been useful in women whose understanding of the language may be limited so that even women not easily able to read and write have been able to make use of this protocol (Figure 3c). Occasionally, there are women who feel much too insecure to adjust, or simply cannot seem to understand the algorithm. In cases like these, the medical team (diabetes nurse educator and physician) will, of necessity, need to make the adjustments and thus, likely require more frequent visits. This is the exception rather than the rule.

Thus, the patient can continue to adjust her insulin appropriately, gradually increasing the insulin doses until between 34-37 weeks, where some decrease in insulin requirements is often seen as the baby is now bigger and eats more, so siphons off glucose most obviously overnight when the patient is not eating but the baby still is. In addition, the placenta is no longer growing and may be aging, so the placental hormones which have been increasing insulin resistance are gradually decreasing. In fact, an early or dramatic fall in insulin requirements may be an early manifestation of a placental problem and may help alert the health professionals.

HYPERGLYCEMIA	INSULIN to GIVE	INSULIN ADJUSTMENT
Fasting PG remains > 5.0 mmol/L	Intermediate- acting neutral protamine Hagedorn insulin (NPH) – human or pork; Potentially insulin glargine or detemir might be used	Adjustments to the **bedtime insulin dose** to be made **tonight** if glucose monitoring result is: <4.2 **reduce bedtime dose by 2 units** 4.3 - 4.9 maintain present bedtime dose 5.0 – 5.3 increase bedtime dose 1 unit 5.4 - 6.0 – increase bedtime dose 2 units 6.1 – 8.0 - increase bedtime dose by 4 units > 8.0 – increase bedtime dose by 6 units
Postmeal PG remains > 7.8 mmol/L	BEFORE MEALS: Regular Rapid-acting (aspart, lispro)	Adjustments to **tomorrow's pre-meal insulin dose** if today's 1h-post-meal result for that meal is: <5.5 - **decrease pre-meal dose by 2 units** 5.6 – 7.2 - maintain present pre-meal dose 7.2-10.0 - increase pre-meal dose by 1 unit >10.0 – increase pre-meal dose by 2 units for the following day's doses

Fig. 3.

6. Approaching the finish line – what to do for labour and delivery

There are few papers determining the effectiveness of specific protocols for use in labour where the protocols specifics are detailed (Palmer & Inturissi, 1992; Ramanathan, Khoo, & Arismendy, 1991; Leparcq, et al., 2008; Jovanovic & Petersen, 1983; Hawkins & Casey, 2007). In 1983, using a Biostator®, Jovanovic and Peterson determined that the average hourly need for glucose to cover the needs of labour was 2.55 mg/kg/min (Jovanovic & Petersen, 1983). When translated into the approximate hourly rate for a 70kg woman, this would mean 9.45g/hour as an infusion rate. This would require very large amounts of fluids or perhaps a central line to provide such glucose-intense amounts in a normal clinical setting. The majority of the recommended and detailed protocols have been used in type 1 diabetic patients. In the diabetes and pregnancy clinics today, many of the patients have type 2 diabetes with significantly more insulin resistance and a high total daily dose (TDD). Additionally, many women with gestational diabetes picked up in pregnancy may have glucose abnormalities outside of pregnancy and significant underlying insulin resistance. The majority of protocols presume that the hourly needs for insulin are always the same in labour; however, it may be more appropriate to use a gradually adjusting protocol based on insulin need in patients with type 2 or gestational diabetes.

For these reasons, we have developed a protocol based on the patient's total daily dose to provide the initial insulin infusion rate. As a compromise for fluid use, not only for glucose provision, but potentially for oxytocin induction or other fluids needed for obstetric reasons, the protocol developed provides 5g/h of glucose in the form of dextrose 10% at 50 ml/hour beginning on the morning of induction or Caesarean section, or when the patient arrives in labour. Since labour is a significant activity, the obstetricians are encouraged to provide a consistent amount of at least 5g of glucose to be delivered per hour to avoid fatigue and ketosis. If the glucose value exceeds 4.5mmol/L (81mg/dl), an insulin infusion is begun. For women with gestational diabetes, an insulin infusion protocol is not provided if the total daily dose is less than 30 units per day. If above 30 units, the total number of units taken in the day is divided in half (since about half of the insulin she takes will be to cover meals) and the remaining insulin dose is divided by 24 to permit the determination of a starting dose in units per hour.

The insulin dose is adjusted hourly keeping the amount glucose infused stable and realizing that insulin requirements usually fall in labour. If there is a fall of glucose to under 4.0mmol/L (72mg/dl), the dose is reduced quickly, below 3.5mmol/L (63mg/dl)…even more and at 3.0mmol/L, the insulin is stopped - glucose in the form of 50% dextrose is given to provide 10 gm of immediate glucose (i.e. 20 ml.) and repeated every 10 minutes until the glucose rises above 4.5mmol/L (81mg/dl). If the glucose rises, the dose is increased incrementally until a steady state is reached. In our hospital protocol, we aim for a glucose between 4.0 - 5.5mmol/L (72 - 100 mg/dl) during labour using this protocol, with success and minimal hypoglycaemia, however this is due to intensive in-house review of the protocol on a regular basis and consistency over 20 years. The entire protocol is pre-printed in the clinic prior to labour using dosages at about 36-37 weeks and the women is given a copy to present on arrival in the delivery room.

As part of a quality assessment program, we retrospectively evaluated the effectiveness of this protocol for labour and delivery in use 20 years in our institution for glucose control in women with type 1, type 2 and gestational diabetes. Ethical approval of the assessment and chart review was obtained from the McGill University Health Center Ethics Board. Women who delivered for the years 2004-2006 and were treated with an insulin dose ≥ 30units/day prior to labour and managed with an intra-partum protocol were included. Patients were excluded if they did not receive the insulin protocol due to precipitated labor of urgent CS or if the chart was missing vital maternal or neonatal data.

The protocol includes a glucose infusion of 5g/h as 10% dextrose in water and an insulin infusion using ½ of the TDD/24 as the initial hourly rate was begun if CBGM was ≥4.5mmol/L and adjusted to maintain glucose between 4.5-5.5mmol/L. At placental delivery, insulin is held and glucose increased to 10g/h until glucose goes above 5.5mmol/L. A total of 80 women were evaluated in 86 pregnancies. Of those, 31(39%) had type 1 DM with mean BMI 21.7, 9 with microvascular complications, mean duration of DM 14.6 years, 43% had Caesarian sections. The mean A1C by trimester was: T1 6.3%, T2 5.5%,

T3 5.3%. The mean FPG by trimester of T1 7.0, 6.0, 5.6 mmol/L respectively; mean 1hPC T1 7.3 T2 6.2 T3 6.0 mmol/L and insulin was administered in 90% of labours. The 49(61%) women with type 2 DM had a mean BMI of 33kg/m^2, a mean duration of DM of 3.3years, 2 with microvascular complications, and 76% had Caesarian sections. The mean A1C by trimester was T1 8.5%, T2 7% and T3 6.7%. The mean FPG by trimester was: T1 7.7, T2 6.3, T3 5.5mmol/L, and the mean 1hPC T1 9.6, T2 7.0, T3 7.2 mmol/L and insulin infusion was used in 72% of cases.

ORDERS FOR DELIVERY: Joan of Arc Hospital number: 000-00-00

Discontinue subcutaneous insulin and p.o. intake Initiate IV D10W at 50 ml/hr (i.e. 5 gm/hr)

Measure capillary blood glucose (CBG) each hour, urine ketones every 2 - 4 h.

Start insulin if glucose > 4.5 mmol./l with the following insulin infusion:

Total Daily Dose	**< 60 units/d**	**> 60units/d**
Regular human insulin by IV infusion pump in 250 ml of normal saline	**Low dose** 10 units (1unit/5ml)	**High dose** 25 units (1unit/2ml)
Initial dose = Total Daily Dose/2 = ½ dose because not eating, then divided by 24 = hourly infusion rate to start with		
Initial dose of insulin = ________unit(s)/h		
ADJUSTMENT OF INSULIN INFUSION	**Low dose**	**High dose**
CBG > 8.0 mmol/l, increase by 0.4 units/h	↑10 ml/h	↑4ml/h
CBG 5.6 - 7.9 - increase by 0.2 units/h	↑5 ml/h	↑2ml/h
CBG 4.5 - 5.5 - maintain present dose		
CBG 4.0 - 4.4 - decrease by 0.2 units/h	↓5 ml/h	↓2ml/h
CBG 3.5 - 3.9 - decrease by 0.4 units/h	↓10 ml/h	↓4ml/h
CBG < 3.5, - discontinue insulin and give 20 ml of D50W, recheck CBG q 10 min and repeat D50W until above 4.5 mmol/L. Resume insulin infusion at 1/2 previous dose (N.B. if less than 0.4 units/h - stop insulin)		
N.B. Once cervical dilatation is 4-5 cm, insulin needs may drop dramatically		

ONCE PLACENTA DELIVERED → STOP INSULIN

Increase D10W to 100 ml/h until CBG > 5.5mmol/L (100 mg/dl) or 2 hr has passed . . . then, decrease D10W to 50 ml/h - can discontinue intravenous glucose once CBG > 5.5 mmol/L (100 mg/dl) for at least 4 hr and able to eat at least full fluids. Plan to start SC insulin regimen, only if needed.

Check and document glucose fasting and 1h post-meals X 48 hours and call Endocrine service if abnormal.

If GDM, book post-partum OGTT for 6 – 8 weeks later.

Fig. 4.

Mean insulin dose in labour was 1.73units/h for DM1, 2.2unit/h in DM2. Maternal hypoglycemia (CBG <3.3 mmol/L) occurred in 16% of labour occurring equally in DM1 or DM2, however there were only 4 episodes of maternal hypoglycemia <2.5mmol/L. Mean glucose achieved overall was 5.8mmol/L (6.1mmol/L for DM1; 5.6mmol/L for DM2). Of the 863 CBG readings, there were 31% between 4.5-5.5mmol/L, 24% lower, and 43% higher with 9% ≥7mmol/l (See Figure 5). Neonatal hypoglycaemic events (BS ≤2.2mmol/L occurred in 32 neonates (37% - 46% in DM1 offspring, 40% in DM2 offspring (p=0.047) and 4(12%) in babies whose mother did not receive maternal IV insulin. No significant relationship was seen between glucose control in labour, nor in any trimester in labour and neonatal hypoglycemia. The results of the glucose control can be seen in Figure 6. The findings suggest that this relatively simple protocol which can be prepared by house-staff based on total daily dose was able to safely control both DM1 and DM2 /gestational diabetic women with minimal hypo or hyper-glycemic risk for mother or offspring. The degree of glucose control in labour did not appear to relate to the risk of hypoglycemia in the neonate in this sample size. (Figure 5)

Once the baby has been delivered, the needs for insulin fall faster than the insulin is metabolized, so the women is at risk of hypoglycaemia in the first 1-2 hours after delivery. Thus, the protocol emphasizes stopping the insulin at delivery and increasing the glucose infusion to 10g/hour immediately after the delivery of the baby and for the next 2 hours. If the glucose remains above 5.5mmol/L, the infusion rate can be reduced to 5g an hour again or discontinued and the woman would be allowed to eat if she underwent a vaginal delivery. As most women with gestational diabetes have normal glucose post-partum, this can be checked with capillary blood glucose monitoring (CBGM) the following day pre and post breakfast. If there is evidence of abnormal glucose intolerance (particularly in someone who may have had type 2 diabetes only diagnosed in pregnancy) in the initial post-partum period, depending on its severity, the woman may be instructed to continue with medical nutrition therapy and testing and re-assess in 1 month, or she may require some form of therapy with oral agents or insulin on leaving the hospital.

If her glucose appears normal prior to discharge, she should undergo an OGTT at 6 weeks to 6 months post-partum (or before she next conceives) to verify her glucose tolerance status – the actual timing varies related to guidelines established in various countries and related to the ethnic risks present in that country (Canadian Diabetes Association Clinical Practice Guidelines Expert Committee, 2008; Reinblatt, Morin, & Meltzer, 2006; McClean, Farrar, Kelly, Tuffnell, & Whitelaw, 2010). Initial post-partum testing within the first year is most effective if an oral glucose tolerance test is done; however, of those with any abnormality, further regular follow-up is likely adequate with a fasting plasma glucose and potentially an A1C (Lee, Mak, Lao, & Chung, 2011; Kim, Herman, & Vijan, 2007). Many women with GDM will have evidence of some form of dysglycemia or impaired glucose tolerance which would be amenable to preventive therapy. Additionally, even for women who tested normal, they must be reminded that their long term risks of developing diabetes remain elevated as does their cardiovascular risks (Egeland & Meltzer, 2010; Bellamy, Casas, Hingorani, & Williams, 2009; Ratnakaran, Qi, Connelly, Sermer, Hanley, & Zinman, 2010). It should not be forgotten that the presence of gestational diabetes in the mother appears to confer future risk for the offspring in terms of obesity and glucose intolerance (Nolan, Damm, & Prentki, 2011; Deierlein, Siega-Riz, Chantala, & Herring, 2011).

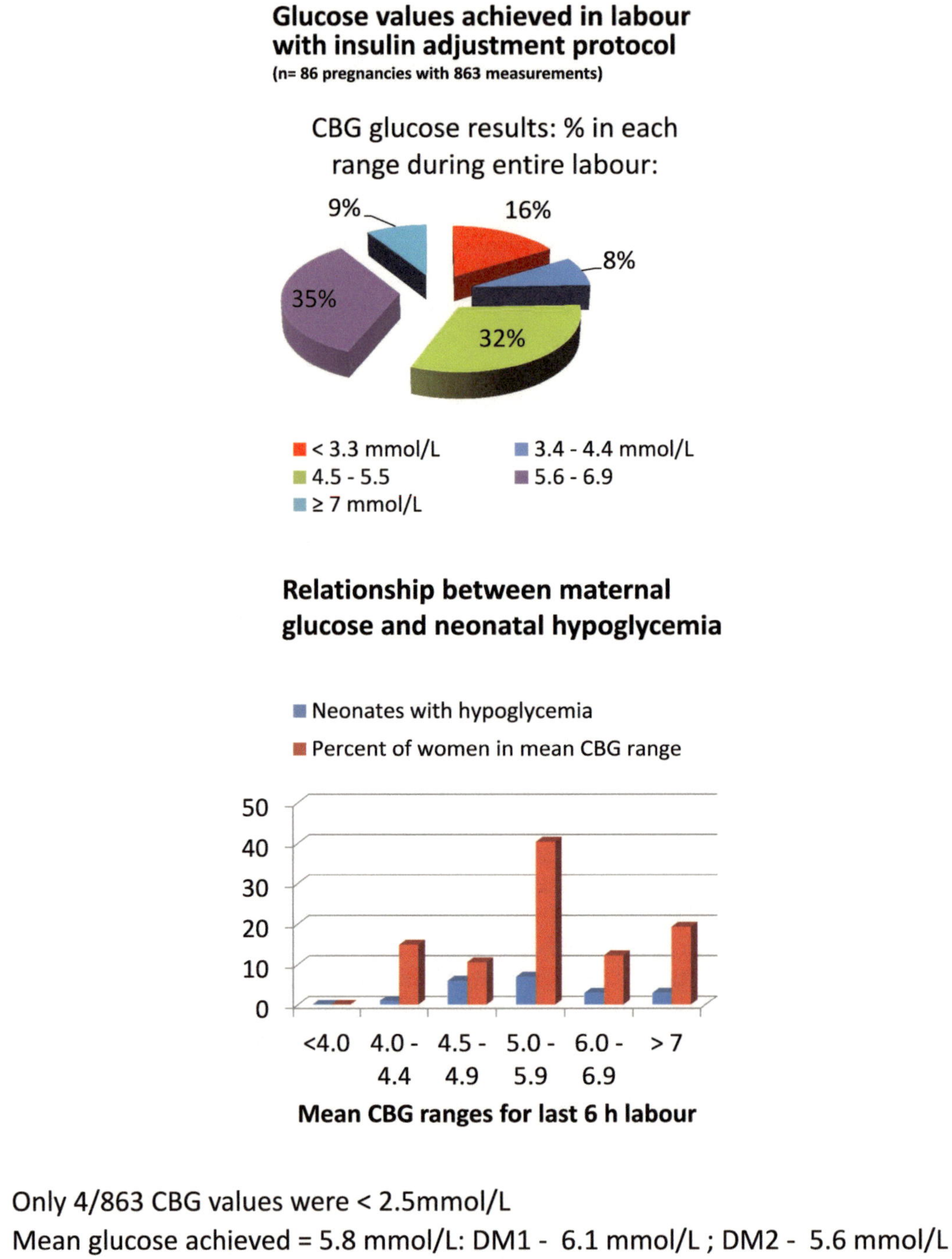

Fig. 5. Glucose values achieved in labour with insulin adjustment protocol and incidence of neonatal hypoglycemia.

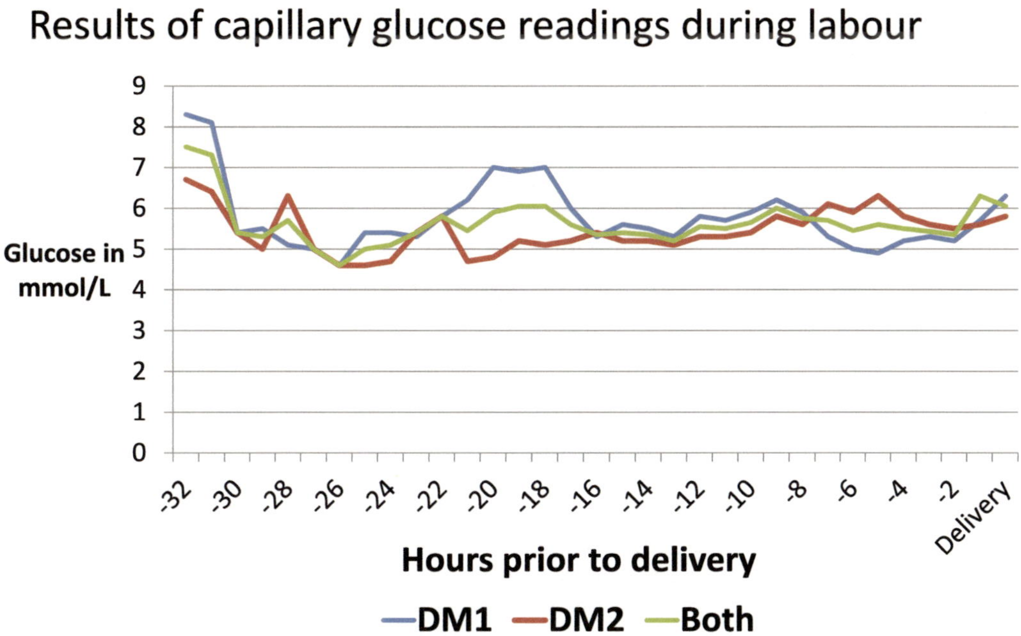

Fig. 6. Mean capillary blood glucose in labour in women with type 1 or type 2 DM

In the appendix there are copies of the insulin adjustment algorithm, document sheets for management in English and French and in-hospital insulin algorithms for day by day management and for insulin in labour protocol.

7. Conclusion

Management of gestational diabetes can be very rewarding. This chapter has tried to raise the important issue that implication of the woman enthusiastically in her own self-care can facilitate care and become a tool to sensitize her to her future role in the family lifestyle choices.

8. Acknowledgements

The authors would like to acknowledge the health care team members that have been integral in development and implementation of the protocols in our clinical care - in particular: A. Benjamin, MD, FRCPS; Lucie Morin, MD, FRCPS, Louise Bastien, RN, and Jennifer Snyder, PtD. MSc. As well, we would like to signal our appreciations to our patients who have taught us much of this information.

9. Appendix 1

Insulin adjustment protocol in English

Appendix 1

Gestational Diabetes How to adjust your insulin dose using today's glucose values

How much long-acting insulin (NPH) **to take at bedtime today?**
If glucose before breakfast is:

> 8.0	Add 6 units to the NPH dose taken yesterday at bedtime
6.1 – 8.0	Add 4 units to the NPH dose taken yesterday at bedtime
5.4 - 6.0	Add 2 units to the NPH dose taken yesterday at bedtime
4.8 - 5.3	Add 1 unit to the NPH dose taken yesterday at bedtime
4.3 - 4.7	**Take the same NPH dose taken yesterday at bedtime**
< 4.3 or night reaction	Reduce by 2 units the NPH dose taken yesterday at bedtime

How much short-acting insulin to take before tomorrow's meals?
(Regular/Humalog®/Novorapid® = R/H/NR)

If glucose after breakfast is:

> 10.0	Add 2 units to R/H/NR dose taken today at breakfast
7.3 - 10.0	Add 1 unit to R/H/NR dose taken today at breakfast
5.5 - 7.2	**Take the same R/H/NR dose tomorrow as you took today at breakfast**
< 5.5 or morning reaction	Reduce by 2 units the R/H/NR dose taken today at breakfast

If glucose after lunch is:

> 10.0	Add 2 units R/H/NR dose taken today at lunch
7.3 - 10.0	Add 1 unit R/H/NR dose taken today at lunch
5.5 - 7.2	**Take the same R/H/NR dose tomorrow as you took today at lunch**
< 5.5 or afternoon reaction	Reduce by 2 units the R/H/NR dose taken today at lunch

If glucose after supper is:

> 10.0	Add 2 units R/H/NR dose taken today at supper
7.3 - 10.0	Add 1 unit R/H/NR dose taken today at supper
5.5 - 7.2	**Take the same R/H/NR dose tomorrow as you took today at supper**
< 5.5 or evening reaction	Reduce by 2 units the R/H/NR dose taken today at supper

- **Calculate your insulin dose** as soon as you have your glucose result
- **Insulin dose will increase** as baby grows and may decrease closer to your due date.
- **Reactions (low blood sugar or hypoglycemia):** could be due to changes in activity or food
  - P **If you know the cause** - take the same dose and correct the cause
  - P **If you do NOT know the cause** - **reduce the dose**, even if next morning glucose is high due to extra food for treating reaction
- **Symbols:** < means less than, and > means more than

10. Appendix 2

Appendix 2

Diabète gestationnel / Gestational Diabetes
Dossier d'autosurveillance / Self-care diary

Nom:
Name:

Questions? Appelez/Call

Pendant la Grossesse... / During Pregnancy ...

Glycémie ideale / Ideal glucose
Avant déjeuner / Before breakfast 4.3 -4.7 mmol/L
Après les repas / After meals 5.5 – 7.2 mmol/L

Initiation de l'insuline / Start insulin . . .
Avant déjeuner / Before breakfast ≥ 5.1 mmol/L
1 à 2h après les repas / 1-2h after meals ≥ 7.8

Date	Déjeuner /Breakfast			Dîner / Lunch			Souper / Supper			Coucher / Bed			
	Avant Before	Insulin	Après After	Avant Before	Insulin	Après After	Avant Before	Insulin	Après After	Avant Before	Insulin	Nuit Night	
KETONES													

June 2010

Documentation sheet for capillary blood glucose and insulin adjustment in English and French

11. Appendix 3

Insulin adjustment protocol for use in hospital

Appendix 3

La Mission Santé de la Femme
Women's Health Mission

Ordonnances pour l'ajustement d'insuline pour le diabete gestationel
Insulin adjustment orders for Gestational Diabetes
ALLERGIES : ______________________ **Poids** / *Weight* (kg):

Initiales du médecin Pour chaque ordonnance *Physician's initial for each order*	**ORDONNANCE DU MÉDECIN** / *PHYSICIAN'S ORDERS*	**Initiales de l'infirmier(ère) notées** *Nurse's initial noted*
	Patient should be on a **diabetic diet** adjusted by the dietitian	
	Capillary blood glucose testing for 2 days AC/ 1h PC meals and HS, then routinely AC breakfast and 1 hour after completing the meal for breakfast, lunch and supper.	
	If glucose <u>before</u> breakfast is: > 8.0 mmol/L Add 6 units to the NPH dose given yesterday at bedtime 6.1 – 8.0 Add 4 units to the NPH dose given yesterday at bedtime 5.3 - 6.0 Add 2 units to the NPH dose given yesterday at bedtime 4.8 - 5.2 Add 1 unit to the NPH dose given yesterday at bedtime **4.3 - 4.7 Give the same NPH dose as given yesterday at bedtime** < 4.3 <u>or</u> night reaction Reduce by 2 units the NPH dose given yesterday at bedtime	
	If glucose <u>after</u> breakfast is: > 10.0 Add 2 units to R/H/NR dose given today at tomorrow's breakfast 7.3 - 10.0 Add 1 unit to R/H/NR dose given today at tomorrow's breakfast **5.5 - 7.2 Give the same R/H/NR dose as given today at tomorrow's breakfast** < 5.5 <u>or</u> morning reaction Reduce by 2 units the R/H/NR dose given today at tomorrow's breakfast	
	If glucose <u>after</u> lunch is: > 10.0 Add 2 units to R/H/NR dose given today at tomorrow's lunch 7.3 - 10.0 Add 1 unit to R/H/NR dose given today at tomorrow's lunch **5.5 - 7.2 Give the same R/H/NR dose as given today at tomorrow 's lunch** < 5.5 <u>or</u> afternoon reaction Reduce by 2 units the R/H/NR dose given today at tomorrow's lunch	
	If glucose <u>after</u> supper is: > 10.0 Add 2 units to R/H/NR dose given today at tomorrow's supper 7.3 - 10.0 Add 1 unit to R/H/NR dose given today at tomorrow's supper **5.5 - 7.2 Give the same R/H/NR dose as given today at tomorrow's supper** < 5.5 <u>or</u> evening reaction Reduce by 2 units the R/H/NR dose given today at tomorrow's supper	

R/H/NR = Humulin R or Novolin Toronto / Humalog(H)/NovoRapid(NR) –to use whatever insulin patient normally takes

	Lettres moulées *Name in print*	**Signature**	**N° Permis** *N° License*	**Heure** *Time* 00:00	**Date** AAYY/MM/JD
Médecin *Physician*					

	Nom en lettres moulées et/ou Numéro de permis *Name in print and/or License Number*	**Parapher** / *Initial*	**Heure** *Time* 00:00	**Date** AAYY/MM/JD
Infirmier(ère) *Nurse*				
Pharmacien(enne) *Pharmacist*				

12. Appendix 4

Insulin orders for vaginal or caesarean delivery of women with Gestational Diabetes / Ordonnances d'insuline autour d'accouchement vaginal ou césarienne pour le diabète de grossesse

***Allergies** (specify type of reaction):

Physician initials	***Admit patient to_________ (unit) under care of Dr _______________________***	Nurse initials
GLUCOSE INFUSION AND MONITORING:		
	Discontinue PO intake	
	Intravenous fluids Initiate IV D10W at 50 ml/hr (to provide 5 g glucose/hr) or an equivalent amount of glucose in IV running.	
	Prior to and at initiation of insulin infusion: Measure capillary blood glucose (CBG) q 1h for 4h; if stable *[not > 1.5 mmol variation and within range]* then q 2h for 2 h, and then if CBG continues to be stable q 4-6h. Monitor urinary ketones q 2h, if positive, inform MD.	
INSULIN INFUSION:		
	Discontinue subcutaneous insulin	
	If glucose > 4.5 mmol/L start IV insulin according to the following guide:	
	Initial infusion dose calculation Since patient NPO, calculate half of total daily insulin dose divided by 24 = initial units/hour dose **Initial insulin dose to start at:_____units/hour** **Insulin infusion concentration**: ***(check one)*** ☐ **Low** dose = 10 units Humulin R in 250ml NS (1unit = 25 ml) ☐ **High** dose = 25 units Humulin R in 250ml NS (1unit = 10ml) ☐ Other solution ___units Humulin R in _____ml NS **(as per *Endo consult service only)***	
	Adjust insulin infusion rate as follows: (see table below)	
	NOTE: Once cervical dilatation is 4-5 cm, insulin needs may drop dramatically	
	Once baby and placenta delivered: **STOP insulin and increase D10W to 100 ml/hr** until CBG > 5.5 or for 2 h; then decrease D10W to 50ml/h. Discontinue IV glucose once CBG > 5.5 mmol/L for at least 4 h and able to eat.	
POST PARTUM		
	1. **Diet –** order postpartum diabetic diet 2. **Check AC/PC breakfast blood sugar** with glucometer daily until discharge home; 3. **Verify OGTT booked at 6- 8 wk postpartum** ____________________ *Insert date and place or phone number*	

CBG (mmol/l)	Adjustment	☐ **Low** dose	☐ **High** dose
> 8.0	increase by 0.4units/h	10 ml/hr	4 ml/h
5.6 - 7.9	increase by 0.2 units/h	5 ml/h	2 ml/h
4.5 - 5.5	**maintain present dose**	--	--
4.0 - 4.4	decrease by 0.2 units/h	5 ml/h	2 ml/h
3.3 - 3.9	decrease by 0.4 units/h	10 ml/h	5 ml/h
< 3.3	**infuse D50W 20ml**; recheck CBG q 10 min and repeat D50W until CBG > 4.5 mmol/L. Resume insulin infusion at 1/2 previous dose; if less than 0.4 units/hr - stop insulin, and continue to monitor; Re-start @ ½ previous dose if CBG > 5.3 mmol/L.		

Physician signature:__________________________ **License no. :**__________

Print name:__________________________ **Date:** YYYY / MM / DD **Time:** 00:00 AM PM

Noted by (Nurse):________________________ **Date:** YYYY / MM / DD **Time:** 00:00 AM PM

Verified by (pharmacist):

Copie blanche / *White copy* – Archives médicales / *Medical Records* Copie jaune /*yellow copy* – Département / *department*

00-00-0000000 P&T Approved date ***(Obtenez un numéro et inscrivez-le ici avec la date de révision** – obtain number and insert here with revision date)*

13. References

ACOG Committee Opinion. (2002). Exercise during pregnancy and the postpartum. *Obstet Gynecol., 99*(1), 171-173.

Alippi, C., Mottarella, A., & Vanini, G. (2005). A RF map-based localization algorithm for indoor environments. *IEEE International Symposium on Circuits and Systems, 2005. ISCAS 2005.* (S. 652-655). IEEE CNF.

American Diabetes Association. (Jan 2011). Standards of medical care in diabetes - 2011. *Diabetes Care, 34*(Supplement 1), S11 - S61.

Artal, R., Lockwood, C., & Brown, H. (2010). Weight gain recommendations in pregnancy and the obesity epidemic. *Obstet Gynecol., 115*(1), 152-155.

Bellamy, L., Casas, J., Hingorani, A., & Williams, D. (2009). Type 2 diabetes mellitus after gestational diabetes: a systematic review and meta-analysis. *Lancet, 373,* 1773-1779.

Ben-Haroush, A., Yogev, Y., Chen, R., Rosenn, B., Hod, M., & Langer, O. (Aug 2004). The postprandial glucose profile in the diabetic pregnancy. *Am J Obstet Gynecol, 191*(2), 576-581.

Buchanan, T. A., Kjos, S. L., Schafer, U., Peters, R. K., Xiang, A., Byrne, J., et al. (Aug. 1998). Utility of fetal measurements in the management of gestational diabetes mellitus. *Diabetes Care. 1998 Aug;21 Suppl 2:B99-106, 21*(Suppl 2.), B99-106.

Bung, P., Artal, R., Khodiguian, N., & Kjos, S. (1991). Exercise in gestational diabetes. An optional therapeutic approach. *Diabetes., 40*(Suppl 2), 182-185.

Burke, L. E., Wang, J., & Sevick, M. A. (Jan 2011). Self-monitoring in weight loss: a systematic review of the literature. *J Am Diet Assoc, 111,* 92-102.

Bush, N. C., Chandler-Laney, P. C., Rouse, D. J., Granger, W. M., Oster, R. A., & Gower, B. A. (Epub 2011 Feb 23. May 2011). Higher maternal gestational glucose concentration is associated with lower offspring insulin sensitivity and altered beta-cell function. *J Clin Endocrinol Metab, 96*(5), E803-809.

Canadian Diabetes Association Clinical Practice Guidelines Expert Committee. (2008). 2008 Guidelines for the Prevention and Management of Diabetes in Canada. *Canadian Journal of Diabetes, 34*(Supplement 1), S168.

Catalano, P. M., Kirwan, J. P., Haugel-de Mouzon, S., & King, J. (2003). Gestational diabetes and insulin resistance: role in short- and long-term implications for mother and fetus. *J. Nutr., 133,* S1674-S1683.

Dabalea, D., Hanson, R. L., Lindsay, R. S., Pettitt, D. J., Imperatore, G., Gabir, M. M., et al. (2000). Intrauterine exposure to diabetes conveys risks for type 2 diabetes and obesity: a study of discordant sibships. *Diabetes, 49*(12), 2208-2211.

Deierlein, A. L., Siega-Riz, A. M., Chantala, K., & Herring, A. H. (Epub 2011 Jan 7. Feb 2011). The association between maternal glucose concentration and child BMI at age 3 years. *Diabetes Care, 34*(2), 480-484.

DeVeciana, M., Major, C. A., Morgan, M. A., Asrat, T., Toohey, J. S., Lien, J. M., et al. (1995). Postprandial versus preprandial blood glucose monitoring in women with gestational diabetes mellitus requiring insulin therapy. *New England Journal of Medicine, 333*(19), 1237-1231.

Diabetes Prevention Program Research Group. (14. Nov 2009). 10-year follow-up of diabetes incidence and weight loss in the Diabetes Prevention Program Outcomes Study. *The Lancet, 374*(9702), 1677-1686.

Division of Nutrition PA, and Obesity, Centers for Disease Control. (kein Datum). *2008 Physical Activity Guidelines for Healthy Pregnant and Postpartum women.* Centres for Disease Control.

Egeland, G. M., & Meltzer, S. J. (Mar. 2010). Following in mother's footsteps? Mother-daughter risks for insulin resistance and cardiovascular disease 15 years after gestational diabetes. *Diabet Med., 27*(3), 257-265.

Gillmer, M. D., Beard, R. W., Brooke, F. M., & Oakley, N. W. (1975). Carbohydrate Metabolism in Pregnancy: Part I - Diurnal Plasma Glucose Profile in Normal and Diabetic Women. Part II - Relation between Maternal Glucose Tolerance and Glucose Metabolism in the Newborn. *BMJ*(3), 399-404.

Grant, S. M., Wolever, T. M., O'Connor, D. L., Nissenbaum, R., & Josse, R. G. (Jan 2011). Effect of a low glycemic index diet on blood glucose in women with gestational diabetes. *Diabetes Research and Clinical Practice, 91*(Jan), 15-22.

HAPO Study Cooperative Research Group, Metger BE; Lowe LR; Dyer AR et al. (8. May 2008). Hyperglycemia and adverse pregnancy outcome study: neonatal glycemia. *N Engl J Med., 358*(19), 1991-2002.

HAPO Study Cooperative Research Group. (2009). Hyperglycemia and Pregnancy Outcome Study: Associations with neonatal anthropometrics. *Diabetes., 58(2),* 453-459.

Harter, A., Hopper, A., Steggles, P., Ward, A., & Webster, P. (1999). The Anatomy of a Context-Aware Application. *Proceedings of the 5th Annual ACM/IEEE International Conference on Mobile Computing and Networking* (S. 59-68). Seattle: ACM/IEEE.

Hawkins, J. S., Casey, B. M., Lo, J. Y., Moss, K., McIntyre, D. D., & Leveno, K. J. (Jun 2009). Weekly compared with daily blood glucose monitoring in women with diet-treated gestational diabetes. *Obstet Gynecol., 113*(6), 1307-1312.

Hawkins, J., & Casey, B. (2007). Labor and Delivery Management for Women With Diabetes. *Obstet Gynecol Clin N Am, 34,* 323-334.

Hightower, J., Borriello, G., & Want, R. (2000). *SpotON: An Indoor 3D Location Sensing Technology Based on RF Signal Strength.* University of Washington.

Hutcheon, J. A., Platt, R. W., Meltzer, S. J., & Egeland, G. M. (Aug 2006). Is birth weight modified during pregnancy? Using sibling differences to understand the impact of blood glucose, obesity, and maternal weight gain in gestational diabetes. *Am J of Obstet Gynecology, 195*(2), 488-494.

Institute of Medicine and National Research Council Committee to Re-examine IOM Pregnancy Weight Guidelines. (2009). *Weight Gain During Pregnancy: Re-examining the guidelines.* Washington, DC, U.S.A.: National Academies Press.

International Diabetes Federation Writing Group. (2009). *Global Guideline on Pregnancy and Diabetes.* Brussels, Belgium: International Diabetes Federation.

Jacqueminet S, J.-L. M. (Dec 2010). Therapeutic management of gestational diabetes. *Diabetes Metab., 36*(6 Pt 2), 658-671.

Jovanovic, L. G. (Mar 2008). Using meal-based self-monitoring of blood glucose as a tool to improve outcomes in pregnancy complicated by diabetes. *Endocr Practice, 14*(2), 239-247.

Jovanovic, L., & Petersen, C. (Oct 1983). Insulin and Glucose Requirements during the First Stage of Labor in Insulin-Dependent Diabetic Women. *Am J. Med, 75, 607-612.*

Kim, C. (Oct 2010). Gestational diabetes: risks, management, and treatment options. (.. 2. 7, & 2:339-51, Hrsg.) *Int J Womens Health, 7*(2), 339-351.

Kim, C., Herman, W. H., & Vijan, S. (May 2007). Efficacy and cost of postpartum screening strategies for diabetes among women with histories of gestational diabetes mellitus. *Diabetes Care, 30*(5), 1102-1106.

Kjos S, B. T. (1999). Gestational Diabetes Mellitus. *N Engl J Med., 341*(23), 1749-1756.

Langer, O., Berkus, M., Brustman, L., Anyaegbunum, A., & Mazze, R. (1991). Rationale for insulin treatment in gestational diabetes. *Diabetes, 40*(Suppl 2), 186-190.

Langer, O., Conway, D., Berkis, M., Xenakis, E., & Gonzales, O. (2000). A comparison of glyburide and insulin in women with gestational diabetes mellitus. *N Engl J Med., 343*(16), 1134-1138.

Langer, O., Yogev, Y., Xenakis, E. M., & Brustman, L. (2005). Overweight and obese in gestational diabetes: The impact on pregnancy outcome Oded Langer, Yogev et al. *Amer Journal of Obstetrics and Gynecology, 192*, 1768-1776.

Lee, K., Mak, M., Lao, K., & Chung, H. (2011). Risk of Developing Diabetes Mellitus in Chinese Women with Persistently Impaired Glucose Tolerance after Gestational Diabetes. *Hong Kong Med J, 17*, 195-201.

Leparcq, J., Abbou, H., Agostini, C., Toubas, F., Francoual, C., Velho, G., et al. (2008). A standardized protocol to achieve normoglycaemia during labour and delivery in women with type 1 diabetes. *Diabetes & Metabolism 34 (2008) 33–37, 34*, 33-37.

McClean, S., Farrar, D., Kelly, C. A., Tuffnell, D. J., & Whitelaw, D. C. (Jun 2010). The importance of postpartum glucose tolerance testing after pregnancies complicated by gestational diabetes. *Diabet Med., 27*(6), 650-654.

Meltzer, S. J. (2010). Prepregnancy care: a shared responsibility. *Diabetes Care*, 2713-2715.

Meltzer, S. J., Snyder, J., Penrod, J. R., Nudi, M., & Morin, L. (Epub 2010 Jan 26. Mar 2010). Gestational diabetes mellitus screening and diagnosis: a prospective randomised controlled trial comparing costs of one-step and two-step methods. *BJOG., 117*(4), 407-415.

Montaner, P., Ripolles, J., Pamies, C., & Corcoy, R. (Epub 2011 Mar 6. Jul 2011). Measurement of fasting ketonuria and capillary blood glucose after main meals in women with gestational diabetes mellitus: How well is the metabolic picture captured? *J Obstet Gynaecol Res, 37*(7), 722-728.

Moore, D., Leonard, J., Rus, D., & Teller, S. (2004). Robust distributed network localization with noisy range measurements. *SenSys '04: Proceedings of the 2nd international conference on Embedded networked sensor systems* (S. 50-61). Baltimore: ACM Press.

Murphy, H., Roland, J., Skinner, T., Simmons, D., Gurnell, E., Morrish, N., et al. (12 2010). Effectiveness of a regional prepregnancy care program in women with type 1 and type 2 diabetes: benefits beyond glycemic control. *Diabetes Care, 33*(12), 2514-2520.

Ni, L. M., Liu, Y., Lau, Y. C., & Patil, A. P. (2003). LANDMARC: Indoor Location Sensing Using Active RFID. *Proceedings of the First IEEE International Conference on Pervasive Computing and Communications, 2003. (PerCom 2003).* Dallas-Fort Worth: IEEE CNF.

Nolan, C. J., Damm, P., & Prentki, M. (24. June 2011). Type 2 diabetes across generations: from pathophysiology to prevention and management. *The Lancet, 378*, 169-181.

Ornoy, A. (2011). Prenatal origin of obesity and their complications: Gestational diabetes, maternal overweight and the paradoxical effects of fetal growth restriction and macrosomia. *Reproductive Toxicology.*

Palmer, D. G., & Inturissi, M. (1992). Intravenous insulin infusion therapy in the intrapartum period. *J Perinatal Neonatol Nursing, 6*(1), 25-36.

Parretti, E., Mecacci, F., Papini, M., Cioni, R., Carignani, L., Mignosa, M., et al. (2001). Third-trimester maternal glucose levles from diurnal profiles in nondiabetic pregnancies: correlaion with sonographic parameters of fetal growth. *Diabetes Care, 24*, 1319-1323.

Patwari, N. (2005). Location Estimation in Sensor Networks. *Ph.D. Dissertation*. Michigan, USA: Electrical Engineering, University of Michigan.

Patwari, N., & Hero, A. (2003). Using proximity and quantized RSS for sensor localization in wireless networks. *Proceedings of the 2nd ACM international conference on Wireless sensor networks and applications* . San Diego: ACM Press.

Pennartz, C., Schenker, N., Menge, B. A., Schmidt, W. E., Nauck, M. A., & Meier, J. J. (20. July 2011). Chronic Reduction of Fasting Glycemia With Insulin Glargine Improves First- and Second-Phase Insulin Secretion in Patients With Type 2 Diabetes. *Diabetes Care*, on line first.

Pettitt, D. J., Ospina, P., Kolaczynski, J. W., & Jovanovic, L. (Jan 2003). Comparison of an insulin analog, insulin aspart, and regular human insulin with no insulin in gestational diabetes mellitus. *Diabetes Care., 26*(1), 183-186.

Priyantha, N. (January 2001). Providing Precise Indoor Location Information to Mobile Devices. *Master's thesis*. Massachusettes, USA: Massachusetts Institute of Technology.

Priyantha, N. B., Chakraborty, A., & Balakrishnan, H. (2000). The Cricket location-support system. *MobiCom '00: Proceedings of the 6th annual international conference on Mobile computing and networking* (S. 32-43). Boston: ACM Press.

Radesky, J. S., Oken, E., Rifas-Shirman, S. L., Kleinman, K. P., Rich-Edwards, J. W., & Gillman, M. W. (Jan 2008). Diet during early pregnancy and development of gestational diabetes. *Paediatr Perinat Epidemiol, 22*(1), 47-59.

Ramanathan, S., Khoo, P., & Arismendy, J. (1991). Perioperative Maternal and Neonatal Acid-Base Status and Glucose Metabolism in Patients With Insulin-Dependent Diabetes Mellitus. *Anesth Analg, 73*, 105-111.

Ratnakaran, R., Qi, Y., Connelly, P. W., Sermer, M., Hanley, A. J., & Zinman, B. (Oct 2010). Risk of early progression to prediabetes or diabetes in women with recent gestational dysglycaemia but normal glucose tolerance at 3-months postpartum. *Clin Endocrinol (Oxf). 2010 Oct;73(4):476-83, 73*(4), 476-483.

Ratner, R., Christophi, C., Metzger, B., Dabalea, D., Bennett, P. H., Pi-Sunyer, X., et al. (2008). Prevention of diabetes in women with a history of gestational diabetes; effects of metformin and lifestyle interventions. *J Clin Endocrinol Metab, 93*(12), 4774-4779.

Reinblatt, S. L., Morin, L., & Meltzer, S. J. (2006). The Importance of a Postpartum 75 g Oral Glucose Tolerance Test in Women With Gestational Diabetes. *J Obstet Gynaecol Can, 28*(8), 690-694.

Reusens, B., & Remacle, C. (Oct 2001). Intergenerational effect of an adverse intrauterine environment on perturbation of glucose metabolism. *Twin Res, 4*(5), 406-411.

Rowan, J. A., Gao, W., Hague, W. M., & McIntyre, H. D. (1 2010). Glycemia and its relationship to outcomes in the MiG trial. *Diabetes Care, 33*(01), 9-16.

Rowan, J. A., Hague, W. M., Gao, W., Battin, M. R., Moore, M. P., & and MiG Trial Investigators. (2008). Metformin versus insulin for the treatment of gestational diabetes. *N Engl J Med. 2008 May 8;358(19):2003-15., 358*(19), 2003-2015.

Sanz, C., Gautier, J. F., & Hanaire, H. (Epub 2010 Aug 2. Nov 2010). Physical exercise for the prevention and treatment of type 2 diabetes. *Diabetes Metab., 36*(5), 346-351.

Shareef, A., Zhu, Y., & Musavi, M. (2008). Comparison of Neural Networks for Localization in Wireless Sensor Networks. Proceedings of ACM First International Conference on Mobile Wireless Middleware, Operating Systems, and Applications (Mobileware'08). Innsbruck: ICST.

Snyder, J., Gray-Donald, K., & Koski, K. (1994). Predictors of birthweight in gestational diabetes. *Am J Clin Nutrition*, 1409-1414.

Standl, E., Schnell, O., & Ceriello, A. (2011). Postprandial Hyperglycemia and Glycemic Variability - Should we care? *Diabetes CAre, Supplement 2*, S120-S127.

Thomas D, E. E. (2009). Low glycaemic index, or low glycaemic load, diets for diabetes mellitus. *Cochrane Database Syst Rev., 21*(1), CD006296.

Tuomilehto, J., Lindstrom, J., Eriksson, J. G., Valle, T. T., Hamaiainen, H., Ilanne-Parikka, P., et al. (2001). Prevention of type 2 diabetes mellitus by changes in lifestyle among subjects with impaired glucose tolerance. *N Engl J Med, 344*, 1343-1350.

Tzanetakou, I. P., Mikhailidis, D. P., & Perrea, D. N. (2011). Nutrition During Pregnancy and the Effect of Carbohydrates on the Offspring's Metabolic Profile: In search of the "Perfect Maternal Diet". *Open Cardiovascular Medicine Journal, 5*, 103-109.

Verier-Mine, O. (Dec 2010). Outcomes in women with a history of gestational diabetes. Screening and prevention of type 2 diabetes. Literature review. *Diabetes Metab., 36*((6 Pt2) Review.), 595-616.

Yogev, Y., Ben-Haroush, A., Chen, R., Rosenn, B., Hod, M., & Langer, O. (Sep 2004). Diurnal glycemic profile in obese and normal weight nondiabetic pregnant women. *Am J Obstet Gynecol., 191*(3), 949-953.

18

Treatment Considerations for Gestational Diabetes Mellitus and Long-Term Postpartum Options

Miroslav Radenković
Department of Pharmacology, Clinical Pharmacology and Toxicology School of Medicine – University of Belgrade Serbia

1. Introduction

Gestational diabetes mellitus is commonly defined as hyperglycemia with onset or first recognition during pregnancy. However, this definition of gestational diabetes does not exclude pregnant women with undiagnosed pre-existing diabetes that now accounts around 1% of diabetes mellitus cases in pregnancy. Prompt identification of pre-existing diabetes, if compared with women with gestational diabetes mellitus, is essential, for the reason that women with pre-existing diabetes are at risk of giving birth to infants with serious malformations, and adverse pregnancy outcomes are increased in this cluster, too. These include serious injury at birth, increased probability of cesarean delivery, and increased incidence of newborn admission in intensive care unit.

The incidence of gestational diabetes is unfortunately increasing, it accounts for 90% of cases of diabetes mellitus in pregnancy, and it has strong association with adverse pregnancy outcomes. Risk factors connected to gestational diabetes mellitus include older age, family history and previous history of gestational diabetes mellitus, obesity, polycystic ovary syndrome and high blood pressure (American Diabetes Association, 2009; Hedderson and Ferrara, 2008). If untreated, it may lead to diverse complications, such as fetal hyperinsulinemia, increased weight at birth, higher rates of cesarian deliveries, shoulder dystocia, more neonatal hypoglycemia, and is associated with concomitant preeclampsia in pregnant women. Therefore, given that gestational diabetes may have long-term pathological consequences for both mother and the child, it is important that it is recognized and correctly managed.

Treatment of gestational diabetes is aimed to maintain euglycemia and it involves regular glucose monitoring, dietary modification, life style changes, exercise, and, when necessary, pharmacotherapy. Insulin therapy is the first choice of treatment, although glyburide and metformin may be indicated, too. In women receiving pharmacotherapy scheduled monitoring of fetal well-being with antenatal tests should be pursued.

2. Non-pharmacological treatment

Self-monitoring of blood glucose is considered to be essential during pregnancy. This is supported, for example by the fact, that self-monitoring of blood glucose in women with mild gestational diabetes positively correlates with reduced rate of fetal overgrowth and gestational weight gain (Hawkins, 2010). Moreover, taking into account that excessive gestational weight gain correlates with postpartum weight retention, regular monitoring of blood glucose during pregnancy might certainly have long-term benefits (Siega-Riz et al., 2009). Common fasting, preprandial and postprandial glucose tests are all recommended in order to attain adequate glycemic targets and reduce overall rate of large-for-gestational-age infant births (Aschwald et al., 2009; Jovanovic, 2008; Riskin-Mashiah et al., 2009). The frequency and timing of home glucose monitoring for gaining and maintaining target glucose levels should be individualized. Generally, the monitoring of blood glucose level is performed in the fasting state, and 1–2 hours after meals, too. Taking into account the increased risk of nocturnal hypoglycemia that may be present during the course of pregnancy; in pregnant women receiving insulin night testing or even continuous glucose monitoring might be suggested (McLachlan et al., 2007).

It is recommended that women diagnosed with gestational diabetes should have expert dietitian counseling to ensure that medical nutrition therapy supports euglycemia, adequate nutritional intake and controlled weight gain. Dietary recommendations should be individualized for each patient. Moderate carbohydrate restriction and proper distribution of daily meals should be emphasized. Namely, six meals per day are recommendable, including three major meals and three smaller ones - snacks. As a result, it has been shown that restriction of carbohydrates to 35–40% will decrease maternal glucose levels and improve maternal and fetal outcomes (Major et al., 1998). For pregnant women with body mass index >30 kg/m^2, a 30–33% calorie restriction is expected to reduce hyperglycemia and plasma triglycerides (Moore, 2010). Moreover, fetal-based strategy to govern maternal glucose control may notably improve outcomes for the fetus given that increased fetal abdominal circumference on an ultrasound (conducted between 28-34 weeks) has been found to be connected to increased insulin in amniotic fluid, thus directly revealing poor maternal glycemic control. Assessing the fetal response to maternal gestational diabetes mellitus by ultrasound measurement of fetal abdominal circumference starting in the second and early third trimesters and repeated every 2– 4 weeks can provide useful information (in combination with maternal self-monitoring of blood glucose levels) to guide management decisions (Metzger et al., 2007).

Individually adjusted physical activity should be promoted, especially in overweight or obese women who are often insulin resistant and at risk for preeclampsia. Thus, the amount of physical activity consisting of 20 minutes aerobic training three days weekly for six weeks, has been shown to result in lower fasting glucose levels, lower glucose responses to a glucose challenge, and a lower glycated hemoglobin - Hb_{A1c} (Jovanovic-Peterson et al., 1989). Avery et al. (1997) have also observed improved glucose levels in women who exercised 30 minutes 3-4 times per week. The delay in requirement of insulin was reported in another study involving resistance training three times per week (Brankston et al., 2004). Exercises may not be advisable if obstetrical contraindications exist, or in cases in which physical activity actually worsens glycemic control.

3. Pharmacological treatment

Insulin is the first-line pharmacological intervention for gestational diabetes and it should be initiated in women diagnosed with gestational diabetes or impaired glucose tolerance who did not achieve glycemic control within two weeks by the sole application of individualized nutrition plan. During pregnancy, the main objective of insulin therapy will be to attain glucose levels similar to those before pregnancy. If indicated, at the beginning small doses of insulin are to be administered, and then insulin doses should be gradually increased. This should be accompanied by the appropriate administration intervals until target glucose levels are attained. Taking into account that insulin resistance rises during the whole pregnancy period, the insulin regimens must be continuously monitored, reviewed and modified. This is particularly significant during the third trimester of pregnancy when the required dosage of insulin usually increases. Hypoglycemia prevention measurements should be clearly explained to all pregnant women on insulin therapy. Sill, insulin therapy is considered to be effective and safe, and it is regarded as the gold standard of pharmacotherapy for gestational diabetes. It has been well determined that the use of insulin to achieve glycemic targets reduces fetal and maternal morbidities. In this way, daily glucose control and diet that were associated with insulin treatment and additional obstetric interventions have been confirmed to reduce the incidence of shoulder dystocia and macrosomia (Horvath et al., 2010).

A diversity of protocols can be used, but multiple injections are considered to be the most effective. The majority insulin protocols include intermediate-acting insulins, such as isophane, and short-acting insulins, such as regular recombinant, as well the insulin analogues aspart and lispro. Although isophane is the intermediate-acting insulin of the first choice for women with gestational diabetes, evidences also support the use of short-acting insulin analogues in women who require pharmacological treatment of gestational diabetes. Moreover, the use of insulin analogs in pregnancy presents the potential benefits of more closely mimicking biological pancreatic insulin secretion compared to regular insulin (Klieger et al., 2008).

Insulin lispro is insulin analog with fast absorption rate and a short duration of action that improves postprandial glucose levels and reduces hypoglycemic episodes when injected immediately prior to meals (Anderson et al., 1997). In the study conducted by Jovanovic et al., (1999) it was of interest to compare the immunologic response to insulin lispro with that to regular human insulin, thereby assuring its safety for use in women with gestational diabetes, and to verify that it is effective. Anti-insulin antibody levels were similar in the two groups. Insulin lispro was not detectable in the cord blood. During a meal test, areas under the curve for glucose, insulin, and C-peptide were significantly lower in the lispro group. Mean fasting and postprandial glucose concentrations and end point Hb_{A1c} were similar in the two groups but the lispro group demonstrated fewer hypoglycemic episodes. Accordingly, in women with gestational diabetes mellitus, the use of insulin lispro enabled the attainment of near-normal glucose levels at the one hour post-prandial time point and was associated with normal anthropometric characteristics; whereas use of regular insulin was not able to blunt the one hour peak post-prandial response to a near-normal extent and resulted in infants with a tendency toward the disproportionate growth (Mecacci et al., 2003). Bhattacharyya et al. (2001) reported no increase in adverse outcome using lispro insulin in diabetic pregnancies, in either gestational or pre-gestational diabetes. Likewise, there was no difference in respect to congenital anomalies of gestational diabetic groups, which used either insulin lispro or regular human insulin (Aydin et al., 2008).

In consideration to insulin aspart use, it has been demonstrated that effective postprandial glycemic control in women with gestational diabetes mellitus who required insulin was brought about by insulin aspart through higher insulin peak and lower demand on endogenous insulin secretion (Pettitt et al., 2003). In particular, the peak insulin concentration was higher and the peak glucose and C-peptide concentrations were lower with both insulin preparations than with no exogenous insulin. Moreover, glucose areas under the curve above baseline were significantly lower with insulin aspart, but not with regular insulin, than with no insulin. In another randomized, parallel, open-label, controlled, multicenter and multinational study of type 1 diabetes pregnancy the fetal outcome using insulin aspart was comparable with human insulin, with a tendency toward fewer fetal losses and preterm deliveries (Hod at al., 2008). In another study, insulin aspart was more effective than regular human isulin in decreasing postprandial glucose concentrations (Pettitt et al., 2007). The authors of this investigation found out that duration of insulin aspart injection 5 min before a meal rather than 30 min prior to meals offered a more convenient therapy for subjects with gestational diabetes mellitus. Moreover, overall safety and effectiveness of insulin aspart were comparable to regular human insulin in pregnant women with gestational diabetes mellitus.

Glyburide and metformin are oral antidiabetics that may be considered as second line agents in cases of gestational diabetes with poor glycemic control with insulin, or in women who refuse insulin. This is supported by the fact that when compared with insulin, administration of oral hypoglycemic agents was not associated with risk of neonatal hypoglycemia, caesarean section, or large-for-gestational-age babies births (Dhulkotia et al., 2010). No significant differences were found in maternal fasting or postprandial glycemic control, too. It appears that glyburide may be preferred, as metformin use is more likely to need supplemental insulin for glycemic control and in addition metformin crosses the placenta with possible long-term effects. It has been estimated that fetal levels of metformin may reach approximately half of maternal levels (Vanky et al., 2005).

The sulfonylurea glyburide is safe and effective at controlling glucose levels in majority of pregnant women with gestational diabetes mellitus. The study of Langer et al. (2005) was aimed to investigate the association between glyburide dose, degree of severity in gestational diabetes mellitus, level of glycemic control, and pregnancy outcome in insulin- and glyburide-treated patients. It has been reported that glyburide and insulin were equally efficient for treatment of gestational diabetes mellitus in all levels of disease severity. In earlier investigation it was also demonstrated that there were no significant differences between the glyburide and insulin groups in the percentage of infants who were large for gestational age, who had macrosomia, who had lung complications, who had hypoglycemia, who were admitted to a neonatal intensive care unit; or who had fetal anomalies (Langer et al., 2000). Glyburide is regarded as a pharmacologically active substance that minimally crosses placenta, as supported by different *in vitro* and *in vivo* investigations that demonstrated very low transplacental transport of glyburide to the fetal circulation. This is due to high plasma protein binding, short half-life, as well as its active transport from the fetus to the mother (Bertini et al., 2005; Koren 2001; Kraemer et al., 2006). In the study aimed to identify placental transporters potentially involved in limiting the transplacental transfer of glyburide to the fetus it was demonstrated that glyburide is preferentially transported by the breast cancer resistance protein pump and multidrug resistance-associated protein 3, that are highly expressed in placental tissues and limit the passage of therapeutic or toxic xenobiotics to the fetus (Gedeon et al., 2006). Unfortunately, poor clinical response to glyburide has been reported in women with higher fasting and postprandial glucose values on their oral glucose tolerance test or in the group of diabetic women on diet therapy. Other identified predictors of glyburide treatment failure were advanced maternal age, earlier diagnosis of gestational diabetes mellitus, higher gravidity or higher parity (Kahn et al., 2006). Otherwise, glyburide can be recommended for women in whom insulin cannot be used. In that way, it has been confirmed that this oral hypoglycemic can be used safely and effectively during the second and the third trimester of pregnancy without increasing maternal or fetal complications when compared with insulin (Langer et al., 2000). Glyburide has been shown to be safe in breastfeeding, too (Feig et al., 2005). However, it has to be emphasized that in some investigations a glyburide-related increased risk of preeclampsia, macrosomia, neonatal hypoglycemia, admission to a neonatal intensive care unit; as well a need for phototherapy have been reported (Jacobson et al., 2005; Ramos et al., 2007).

The second oral antidiabetic drug used in gestational diabetes mellitus, as a monotherapy or with supplemental insulin, is metformin, a biguanide. It lowers blood glucose levels by decreasing hepatic gluconeogenesis, increasing peripheral glucose disposal and reducing intestinal glucose absorption (Hundal & Inzucchi, 2003). In average, up to half the women using metformin may require supplemental insulin. It has been demonstrated that women requiring supplemental insulin had a higher body mass index and had higher baseline glucose levels (Rowan et al. 2008). If compared to insulin, metformin was not associated with increased perinatal complications except of higher incidence of perinatal mortality if administered during the third trimester (Hellmuth et al., 2000). Although it may appear that metformin is safe alternative to insulin therapy, it does cross the placenta (Vanky et al., 2005) and scientific data are still not conclusive enough to recommend the standard use of metformin during pregnancy beyond the first trimester. Data that are more recent suggested that in women with gestational diabetes mellitus, not controlled with diet and exercise, who were then randomized to the metformin or the insulin arm, metformin has been shown to be an effective alternative to insulin in the treatment of gestational diabetes mellitus (Moore et al., 2007). This was substantiated by findings showing that difference in the rate of cesarean delivery was not statistically significant between the two groups, neither the neonatal statistics involving birth weight, Apgar score at 5 minutes, respiratory distress syndrome, hyperbilirubinemia, neonatal hypoglycemia or neonatal intensive care unit admission. Likewise, in investigation of Rowan et al. (2008) women with gestational diabetes mellitus at 20 to 33 weeks of gestation were randomly assigned to open treatment with metformin (with supplemental insulin if required) or insulin. The primary outcome was a composite of neonatal hypoglycemia, respiratory distress, need for phototherapy, birth trauma, 5-minute Apgar score less than 7, or prematurity. The rate of the primary composite outcome was comparable between the group assigned to metformin and the insulin group, suggesting that in women with gestational diabetes mellitus, metformin (alone or with supplemental insulin) was not associated with increased perinatal complications as compared with insulin. The retrospective data of Tertti et al. (2008) have been also indicative for the assumption that metformin was effective in controlling gestational diabetes and was not associated with a higher risk of maternal or neonatal complications compared with insulin. Namely, there were no differences between the metformin-treated group and the other two investigated groups (women treated with insulin and women with no pharmacological treatment) in terms of maternal outcomes (total weight gain during pregnancy or after the diagnosis of gestational diabetes mellitus, pre-pregnancy hypertension, pregnancy induced hypertension, pre-eclampsia etc.). In this investigation, no differences between the metformin-treated group and the other two groups were observed in relation to mean birth weights, prevalence of macrosomia, or gestational weeks at delivery. Finally, there were no differences between the groups in relation to other neonatal outcomes (small for gestational age, Apgar scores, umbilical artery pH or base excess, etc.). This drug is contraindicated in the case of preeclampsia, intrauterine growth restriction or placental insufficiency. Moreover, given that metformin crosses placenta, it could increase insulin sensitivity in the fetus, thus probably affecting growth and fetal hepatic glucose production.

4. Postpartum considerations

After delivery, it is fundamental that women receive the appropriate postpartum counseling, testing, and follow-up. In a long-term view, most women with gestational diabetes do not require insulin therapy following delivery. Nevertheless, glucose levels should be regularly checked after discharge, since it has been confirmed that the progression of gestational diabetes mellitus to type 2 diabetes increased steeply within the first 5 years after delivery and appeared to plateau after 10 years (Kim et al., 2002). It has been determined that progressive beta-cell failure to compensate for the ongoing insulin resistance correlates with progression from gestational diabetes mellitus to type 2 diabetes. Insulin resistance that presents as a high serum insulin concentrations in association with blood glucose concentrations that are normal or high, results from defects in insulin responsiveness in muscle, fat and liver. Therefore, screening for diabetes at regular intervals should be of paramount importance. In addition, among women with a family history of type 2 diabetes, those with prior gestational diabetes mellitus were even more likely not only to have cardiovascular disease risk factors, including metabolic syndrome and type 2 diabetes, but also to have experienced cardiovascular disease events, which occurred at a younger age (Carr et al., 2006). Moreover, the development of metabolic syndrome in children with increasing age is known to be related to maternal gestational diabetes mellitus, maternal glycemia in the third trimester, maternal obesity, neonatal macrosomia, and childhood obesity (Vohr & Boney, 2008). Consequently, post partum evaluation and management of reversible cardiovascular risk factors such as smoking, obesity, hypertension, and hyperlipidemia should be undertaken (Cheung, 2009).

It is confirmed that a good predictor of early postpartum development of diabetes is elevated fasting plasma glucose during pregnancy and, in women having positive tests to specific autoantibodies [anti-glutamic acid decarboxylase (anti-GAD); anti-protein tyrosine phosphatase ICA 512 (anti–IA-2)], higher incidence of diabetes by six months postpartum has been shown, too. In addition, it should be pointed out that some women with gestational diabetes mellitus, especially lean ones under 30 years of age who required insulin during pregnancy, could progress to type 1 diabetes. Therefore, women diagnosed with gestational diabetes should be screened for diabetes 6 to 12 weeks postpartum and should have subsequent screening for the development of diabetes or prediabetes (American Diabetes Association, 2009). An oral glucose tolerance test at three-year intervals has been also shown to be a beneficial approach for screening.

All women with gestational diabetes should be encouraged on a healthy lifestyle and in order to prevent diabetes and cardiovascular complications education on lifestyle modification should start in pregnancy and continue postpartum. In that way, usual recommendations to promote postpartum weight adjustments and decrease the incidence of type 2 diabetes include breastfeeding, exercising at a moderate intensity, and modifications of nutrition for specific weight-loss objectives (National Collaborating Centre for Women's and Children's Health, 2008). It has been determined that breastfeeding itself promotes weight loss for the mother, decreases possibility of maternal progression to type 2 diabetes, reduces insulin resistance in mothers and decreases likelihood of obesity in the child. Children born to mothers who had poor glycemic control should undergo regular evaluations of height, weight and blood glucose concentration, as well as monitoring for appropriate physical activity and diet to minimize the likelihood of obesity (Elchalal, 2004).

5. Conclusion

The incidence of gestational diabetes is increasing and this pathological condition has strong association with adverse pregnancy outcomes. If untreated, gestational diabetes may lead to diverse complications, such as fetal hyperinsulinemia, increased weight at birth, higher rates of cesarian deliveries, shoulder dystocia, neonatal hypoglycemia, and it is also associated with concomitant preeclampsia in pregnant women. Therefore, given that gestational diabetes may have long-term pathological consequences for both mother and the child, it is important that it is recognized and correctly managed. Moreover, preconceptional screening and medical informing of women with diabetes type 1 or 2 would be significant in order to reduce risk to the fetus and mother connected to gestational diabetes. Treatment of gestational diabetes is aimed to maintain euglycemia and it should involve regular glucose monitoring, dietary modification, life style changes, exercise, and, when necessary, pharmacotherapy. Insulin therapy is the first choice of treatment, although glyburide and metformin could be indicated, too. In a long-term view, in order to prevent development of diabetes later in life, as well as different cardiovascular complications, an adequate education on lifestyle modifications should start in pregnancy and continue postpartum.

6. References

American Diabetes Association. (2009). Standards of medical care in diabetes. *Diabetes Care*, Vol. 32, Suppl 1, pp. S13 -S61, ISSN 0149-5992.

Anderson, JH Jr.; Brunelle, R.L.; Koivisto, V.A.; Pfutzner, A.; Trautmann, M.E.; Vignati, L. & DiMarchi, R. (1997). Reduction of postprandial hyperglycemia and frequency of hypoglycemia in IDDM patients on insulin-analog treatment. *Diabetes*, Vol. 46, No. 2, pp. 265–270, ISSN. 0012-1797

Aschwald, C.L.; Catanzaro, R.B., Weiss, E.P Gavard, JA; Steitz, KA; Mostello, D.J. (2009). Large-for-gestationalage infants of type 1 diabetic mothers: an effect of preprandial hyperglycemia? *Gynecological Endocrinology*, Vol. 25, pp.653–660, ISSN. 0951-3590

Avery, M.D.; Leon, A.S. & Kopher, R.A. (1997). Effects of a partially home-based exercise program for women with gestational diabetes. *Obstetrics and Gynecology*, Vol.89, pp.10–15. ISSN 0029-7844

Aydin, Y.; Berker, D.; Direktör, N.; Ustün, I.; Tütüncü, Y.A.; Işik, S.; Delibaşi, T. & Guler, S. (2008). Is insulin lispro safe in pregnant women: Does it cause any adverse outcomes on infants or mothers? *Diabetes Research and Clinical Practice*, Vol.80, No.3, pp. 444-448, ISSN. 0168-8227

Bhattacharyya, A.; Brown, S.; Hughes, S.; Vice, P.A. (2001). Insulin lispro and regular insulin in pregnancy. *QJM: An International Journal of Medicine / Quarterly Journal of Medicine*, Vol.94, pp.255–260, ISSN. 1460-2725

Bertini, A.M.; Silva, J.C.; Taborda, W.; Becker, F.; Lemos Bebber, F.R.; Zucco Viesi, J.M.; Aquim, G.; Engel Ribeiro, T. (2005). Perinatal outcomes and the use of oral hypoglycemic agents. *Journal of Perinatal Medicine*, Vol.33, No.6, pp.519-523, ISSN. 0300-5577

Brankston, G.N.; Mitchell, B.F. & Ryan, E.A. (2004). Resistance exercise decreases the need for insulin in overweight women with gestational diabetes mellitus. *American Journal of Obstetrics and Gynecology*, Vol. 190, pp.188–193, ISSN. 0002-9378

Carr, D.B.; Utzschneider, K.M.; Hull, R.L.; Tong, J.; Wallace, T.M.; Kodama, K.; Shofer, J.B.; Heckbert, S.R.; Boyko, E.J.; Fujimoto, W.Y.; Kahn, S.E. (2006). Gestational diabetes mellitus increases the risk of cardiovascular disease in women with a family history of type 2 diabetes. *Diabetes Care*, Vol.29, No.9, pp.2078-2083. ISSN 0149-5992.

Cheung, N.W. (2009).The management of gestational diabetes. *Vascular Health and Risk Management*, Vol.5, No.1, pp.153-164. ISSN 1176-6344.

Dhulkotia, J.S.; Ola, B.; Fraser, R.; Farrell, T. (2010). Oral hypoglycemic agents vs insulin in management of gestational diabetes: a systematic review and metaanalysis. *American Journal of Obstetrics and Gynecology*. Vol.203, No.5, pp.457.e1-9. ISSN. 0002-9378

Elchalal, U. (2004). Gestational diabetes mellitus: what else is new? *Israel Medical Association Journal / IMAJ*. Vol.6, No.5, pp.268-270. ISSN 1565-1088

Feig, D.S.; Briggs, G.G.; Kraemer, J.M.; Ambrose, P.J.; Moskovitz, D.N.; Nageotte, M.; Donat, D.J.; Padilla, G.; Wan, S.; Klein, J.; Koren, G. (2005). Transfer of glyburide and glipizide into breast milk. *Diabetes Care*, Vol. 28, pp. 1851–1855. ISSN 0149-5992.

Gedeon, C.; Behravan, J.; Koren, G.; Piquette-Miller, M. (2006). Transport of glyburide by placental ABC transporters: Implications in fetal drug exposure. *Placenta*, Vol.27, No.11- 12, pp.1096–1102. ISSN 0143-4004

Hawkins, J.S. (2010). Glucose monitoring during pregnancy. *Current Diabetes Reports*, Vol.10, No.3, pp.229-234. ISSN 1534-4827

Hellmuth, E.; Damm, P.; Mølsted-Pedersen, L. (2000). Oral hypoglycaemic agents in 118 diabetic pregnancies. *Diabetic Medicine*, Vol.17, No.7, pp.507-511. ISSN 0742-3071

Hedderson, M.M.; Ferrara, A. (2008). High blood pressure before and during early pregnancy is associated with an increased risk of gestational diabetes mellitus. *Diabetes Care*, Vol.31, pp.2362–2367. ISSN 0149-5992.

Hod, M.; Damm, P.; Kaaja, R.; Visser, G.H.; Dunne, F.; Demidova, I.; Hansen, A.S.; Mersebach, H.; Insulin Aspart Pregnancy Study Group. (2008). Fetal and perinatal outcomes in type 1 diabetes pregnancy: a randomized study comparing insulin aspart with human insulin in 322 subjects. *American Journal of Obstetrics and Gynecology*, Vol.198, No.2, pp.186.e1-7. ISSN. 0002-9378

Horvath, K.; Koch, K.; Jeitler, K.; Matyas, E.; Bender, R.; Bastian, H.; Lange, S.; Siebenhofer, A. (2010). Effects of treatment in women with gestational diabetes mellitus: systematic review and meta-analysis. *British Medical Journal*, Vol.340, pp.c1395. ISSN 0959-535X

Hundal, R.S.; Inzucchi, S.E. (2003). Metformin: New understandings, new uses. *Drugs*, Vol.63, No.18, pp.1879–1894. ISSN 0012-6667

Jacobson, G.F.; Ramos, G.A.; Ching, J.Y.; Kirby, R.S.; Ferrara, A.; Field, D.R. (2005). Comparison of glyburide and insulin for the management of gestational diabetes in a large managed care organization. *American Journal of Obstetrics and Gynecology,* Vol.193, No.1, pp.118-124. ISSN. 0002-9378

Jovanovic, L.; Ilic, S.; Pettitt ,D.J.; Hugo, K.; Gutierrez, M.; Bowsher, R.R.; Bastyr, E.J. 3rd. (1999). Metabolic and immunologic effects of insulin lispro in gestational diabetes. *Diabetes Care* , Vol.22, No.9, pp.1422–1427. ISSN 0149-5992.

Jovanovic, L.G. (2008). Using meal-based self-monitoring of blood glucose as a tool to improve outcomes in pregnancy complicated by diabetes. *Endocrine Practice,* Vol.14, No.239–247. ISSN 1530-891X

Kahn, B.F.; Davies, J.K.; Lynch, A.M.; Reynolds, R.M.; Barbour, L.A. (2006). Predictors of glyburide failure in the treatment of gestational diabetes. *Obstetrics and Gynecology,* Vol.107, No.6, pp.1303-1309. ISSN 0029-7844

Kim, C.; Newton, K.M.; Knopp, R.H. (2002). Gestational diabetes and the incidence of type 2 diabetes: a systematic review. *Diabetes Care,* Vol.25, No.10, pp.1862-1868. ISSN 0149-5992.

Klieger, C.; Pollex, E.; Koren, G. (2008). Treating the mother--protecting the unborn: the safety of hypoglycemic drugs in pregnancy. *Journal of Maternal-Fetal and Neonatal Medicine,* Vol.21, No.3, pp.191-196. ISSN 1476-7058

Koren, G. (2001). Glyburide and fetal safety; trans-placental pharmacokinetic considerations. *Reproductive Toxicology,* Vol.15, 227–229. ISSN 0890-6238

Kraemer, J.; Klein, J.; Lubetsky, A.; Koren, G. (2006). Perfusion studies of glyburide transfer across the human placenta: implications for fetal safety. *American Journal of Obstetrics and Gynecology,* Vol.195, No.1, pp.270-274. ISSN. 0002-9378

Langer, O.; Conway, D.L.; Berkus, M.D.; Xenakis, E.M.; Gonzales, O. (2000). A comparison of glyburide and insulin in women with gestational diabetes mellitus. *New England Journal of Medicine,* vol.343, No.16, pp.1134-1138. ISSN 0028-4793

Langer, O.; Yogev, Y.; Xenakis, E.M.; Rosenn, B. (2005). Insulin and glyburide therapy: dosage, severity level of gestational diabetes, and pregnancy outcome. *American Journal of Obstetrics and Gynecology,* Vol.192, No.1, pp.134-139. ISSN. 0002-9378

Major CA, Henry MJ, De Veciana M, Morgan MA. The effects of carbohydrate restriction in patients with diet-controlled gestational diabetes. Obstetrics and Gynecology. Apr 1998;91(4):600-4. ISSN 0029-7844

McLachlan, K.; Jenkins, A.; O'Neal, D. (2007) .The role of continuous glucose monitoring in clinical decision-making in diabetes in pregnancy. *Australian and New Zealand Journal of Obstetrics and Gynaecology,* Vol.47, pp.186–190. ISSN 0004-8666

Mecacci, F.; Carignani, L.; Cioni, R.; Bartoli, E.; Parretti, E.; La Torre, P; Scarselli, G.; Mello G. (2003). Maternal metabolic control and perinatal outcome in women with gestational diabetes treated with regular or lispro insulin: comparison with non-diabetic pregnant women. *European Journal of Obstetrics Gynecology and Reproductive Biology,* Vol.111, No.1, pp. 19-24. ISSN 0301-2115

Metzger, B.E.; Buchanan, T.A.; Coustan, D.R.; de Leiva, A.; Dunger, D.B.; Hadden, D.R.; Hod, M.; Kitzmiller, J.L.; Kjos, SL; Oats, JN; Pettitt, DJ; Sacks, DA; Zoupas, C. (2007). Summary and recommendations of the Fifth International Workshop-Conference on Gestational Diabetes Mellitus. *Diabetes Care,* Vol.30, Suppl 2, pp.S251-S260. ISSN 0149-5992.

Moore, L.E.; Briery, C.M.; Clokey, D.; Martin, R.W; Williford, NJ; Bofill, JA; Morrison, J.C. (2007). Metformin and insulin in the management of gestational diabetes mellitus: preliminary results of a comparison. *Journal of Reproductive Medicine*, Vol.52, No. 11, pp.1011-1015. ISSN 0024-7758

Moore, T.R. (2010). Diabetes mellitus and pregnancy. http://emedicine.medscape.com/article/127547.

National Collaborating Centre for Women's and Children's Health (2008). Postnatal care. In: *Diabetes in pregnancy*. Welsh, A (Ed.), pp. 143-152, RCOG Press at the Royal College of Obstetricians and Gynaecologists, ISBN 978-1-904752-47-9, London.

Pettitt, D.J.; Ospina, P.; Kolaczynski, J.W.; Jovanovic, L. (2003). Comparison of an insulin analog, insulin aspart, and regular human insulin with no insulin in gestational diabetes mellitus. *Diabetes Care*, Vol.26, No.1, pp.183-186. ISSN 0149-5992.

Pettitt, D.J.; Ospina, P.; Howard, C.; Zisser, H.; Jovanovic, L. (2007). Efficacy, safety and lack of immunogenicity of insulin aspart compared with regular human insulin for women with gestational diabetes mellitus. *Diabetic Medicine*, Vol.24, No.10, pp.1129-1135. ISSN 0742-3071

Ramos, G.A.; Jacobson, G.F.; Kirby, R.S.; Ching, J.Y.; Field, D.R. (2007). Comparison of glyburide and insulin for the management of gestational diabetics with markedly elevated oral glucose challenge test and fasting hyperglycemia. *Journal of Perinatology*, Vol.27, No.5, pp.262-267. ISSN 0743-8346

Riskin-Mashiah, S.; Younes, G.; Damti, A.; Auslender, R. (2009). First trimester fasting hyperglycemia and adverse pregnancy outcomes. *Diabetes Care*, Vol.32, pp.1639–1643. ISSN 0149-5992.

Rowan, J.A.; Hague, W.M.; Gao, W.; Battin, M.R.; Moore, M.P.; MiG Trial Investigators. (2008). Metformin versus insulin for the treatment of gestational diabetes. *New England Journal of Medicine*, Vol.358, No.19, pp.2003-2015. ISSN 0028-4793

Siega-Riz, A.M.; Viswanathan, M.; Moos, M.K.; Deierlein, A.; Mumford, S.; Knaack, J.; Thieda, P.; Lux, L.J.; Lohr, K.N. (2009). A systematic review of outcomes of maternal weight gain according to the Institute of Medicine recommendations: birthweight, fetal growth, and postpartum weight retention. *American Journal of Obstetrics and Gynecology* , Vol.201, pp.339.e1–339.e14. ISSN. 0002-9378

Vanky, E.; Zahlsen, K.; Spigset, O., Carlsen, S.M. (2005). Placental passage of metformin in women with polycystic ovary syndrome. *Fertility and Sterility*, Vol.83, No.5, pp.1575-1578. ISSN 0015-0282

Vohr, B.R.; Boney, C.M. (2008). Gestational diabetes: the forerunner for the development of maternal and childhood obesity and metabolic syndrome? *Journal of Maternal-Fetal and Neonatal Medicine*, Vol.21, No.3, pp.149-157. ISSN 1476-7058.

19

Glyburide Disposition During Pregnancy

Diana L. Shuster[1], Mary F. Hebert[2] and Qingcheng Mao[1]
[1]Department of Pharmaceutics,
[2]Department of Pharmacy School of Pharmacy,
University of Washington
United States of America

1. Introduction

During pregnancy, 5-14% of women are diagnosed with gestational diabetes mellitus (GDM) and the incidence has been increasing (Jovanovic & Pettitt, 2001; Paglia & Coustan, 2011). While insulin treatment is still the "gold standard" therapy for controlling maternal glycemia, the increasing use of oral anti-diabetic agents such as glyburide and metformin has begun to change standard care (Maymone et al., 2011). Anti-diabetic drugs are often titrated over a prolonged period of time to achieve glycemic control. Prolonged hyperglycemia increases the likelihood of adverse fetal/neonatal and maternal outcomes. Thus, quickly achieving glycemic control during pregnancy can significantly reduce the occurrence of certain adverse perinatal and maternal outcomes (Karakash & Einstein, 2011).

Glyburide is a second generation oral sulfonylurea (Feldman, 1985). Glyburide lowers blood sugar levels by stimulating the pancreas to secrete insulin and by helping the body use insulin efficiently. Considerable data in the literature suggest that glyburide may be a safe alternative to insulin for the treatment of GDM due to its similar efficacy to insulin and its low fetal distribution (Nicholson & Baptiste-Roberts, 2011; Maymone et al., 2011). Physiological and biochemical changes that occur during pregnancy alter the pharmacokinetics of glyburide, thus affecting the safety and efficacy of the drug for both the mother and the fetus. Understanding pregnancy-induced changes in the disposition of glyburide (including fetal exposure) will be important for optimizing dosage guidelines during pregnancy. In this chapter, current knowledge on the safety and efficacy of glyburide for the treatment of GDM, pregnancy-related effects on maternal disposition as well as placental transport and metabolism of the drug will be summarized.

2. Gestational diabetes mellitus and treatment options

The American College of Obstetricians and Gynecologists (ACOG) committee on practice defines GDM as "carbohydrate intolerance that begins or is first recognized during pregnancy" (2001). Similar to type II diabetes mellitus, GDM is the result of an inability to compensate for the degree of insulin resistance. Insulin resistance is normal to some extent during pregnancy as a means of ensuring that glucose is freely available to the developing fetus; however, in women predisposed to diabetes, the degree of insulin resistance can be so high that treatment is necessary to maintain euglycemia.

Properly treating GDM is of great concern as the condition complicates 5-14% of pregnancies. If untreated, GDM presents a danger to both the mother and baby, particularly the risk of hypertension, preeclampsia, urinary tract infections, cesarean delivery and development of type II diabetes mellitus later in life in mothers, as well as macrosomia, neonatal hypoglycemia, childhood obesity and type II diabetes mellitus in the offspring (2002; 2009; 2010; Paglia & Coustan, 2011). Diet therapy is the first line of treatment for GDM and is adequate for controlling glucose concentrations in the majority of patients. Those failing diet therapy are managed with the addition of pharmacotherapy (Landon et al., 2007). The American Diabetes Association (ADA) suggests that women with GDM should seek nutritional counseling by a dietician in order to individualize diet therapy by patient height and weight (2001). To prevent ketonuria, which can hinder the cognitive development of children ages 3 – 9, the ACOG recommends caloric restrictions that are not to exceed 33% of current diet (2001).

There are two general options of pharmacotherapy for the treatment of GDM. Traditionally, insulin therapy has been the "gold standard" for the management of GDM, when diet therapy and exercise fail to achieve maternal glycemic control. Pregnant women have difficulty adhering to insulin therapy regimens because of the challenges with route of administration and schedule. Therefore, oral hypoglycemic agents such as glyburide and metformin are being increasingly used to treat GDM, and have been shown to have similar efficacy and safety as insulin, as well as lower cost and easier route of administration (Maymone et al., 2011; Nicholson & Baptiste-Roberts, 2011). The safety of insulin for use in pregnancy has been well established without the risk of transfer across the placenta. The FDA has not approved the use of glyburide or metformin for the treatment of women with GDM. This chapter will focus its discussion on glyburide.

3. Glyburide and its clinical pharmacokinetics

Glyburide is a second generation oral sulfonylurea, and its chemical structure is shown in Figure 1. Glyburide is indicated as an adjunct to diet therapy and serves to lower blood glucose levels in patients with type II diabetes mellitus (Feldman, 1985). Glyburide exerts its pharmacological effect by stimulating insulin secretion from pancreatic β-islet cells. It inhibits ATP-sensitive potassium channels on the surface of pancreatic β-islet cells, leading to cellular membrane depolarization. Depolarization at the cellular membrane prompts voltage-gated calcium channels to open, increasing the intracellular calcium concentration, which stimulates the release of insulin into the portal vein. Glyburide is administered in 1.25, 2.5 or 5 mg tablets. The FDA approved dosage range is 1.25 mg up to 20 mg per day. When higher dosages of glyburide are required, patients are typically switched to insulin.

Glyburide is a small lipophilic molecule (LogP = 4.8, MW = 494 Da) that is highly bound to plasma proteins (99.8% plasma protein binding). Glyburide is well absorbed with an oral bioavailability of approximately 95% for micronized tablets (Jonsson et al., 1994). It exhibits biphasic elimination kinetics with an initial distribution half-life ($T_{1/2\alpha}$) of roughly 30 min and a terminal elimination half-life ($T_{1/2\beta}$) of approximately 10 hours (Feldman, 1985; Jonsson et al., 1994). Thus, the overall elimination half-life of glyburide is approximately 4 hours. Glyburide has a small volume of distribution (0.2 L/kg), despite its lipophilic nature, and has negligible renal clearance.

Glyburide is extensively metabolized in the liver with a low hepatic extraction ratio. One enzyme involved in glyburide metabolism is CYP2C9, which is highly polymorphic. The CYP2C9 variant, CYP2C9*3, exhibits lower catalytic activity than wild-type CYP2C9*1 (Cavallari & Limdi, 2009). Kirchheriner et al. showed that the oral clearance of glyburide in the CYP2C9*3/*3 subjects (n = 3) was ~40% of that in CYP2C9*1/*1 subjects (n = 4) (Kirchheiner et al., 2002). Niemi et al. reported that the area under plasma concentration-time curve (plasma AUC) of glyburide in subjects heterozygous for CYP2C9*3 (CYP2C9*1/*3 or CYP2C9*2/*3, n = 2) was 280% of that in the CYP2C9*1/*1 subjects (n = 5) (Niemi et al., 2002). Yin et al. demonstrated that the oral plasma AUC of glyburide in CYP2C9*1/*3 subjects (n = 6) of the Chinese population was higher by ~100% as compared with that in the CYP2C9*1/*1 subjects (n = 12) (Yin et al., 2005). These clinical studies appear to suggest that CYP2C9 contributes significantly to glyburide metabolism *in vivo*.

On the other hand, *in vitro* studies using human liver microsomes have shown that CYP3A4 contributes greater than 50% of glyburide metabolism, while CYP2C9 contributes a much smaller percentage (Naritomi et al., 2004; Zharikova et al., 2009; Zhou et al., 2010a). Additionally, Lilja et al. showed that oral administration of clarithromycin, an inhibitor of CYP3A but not CYP2C9, significantly increased C_{max} and the plasma AUC of glyburide (Lilja et al., 2007). The epidemiological study (Schelleman et al., 2010) and case reports (Bussing & Gende, 2002; Leiba et al., 2004) all indicated that the concomitant use of glyburide with clarithromycin was associated with severe hypoglycemia. Thus, CYP3A also appears to contribute to glyburide metabolism *in vivo*. It is possible that glyburide is metabolized *in vivo* through the joint actions of hepatic CYP3A and CYP2C9.

In vitro metabolism studies using human liver microsomes or recombinant systems revealed that, besides CYP3A4 and CYP2C9, glyburide was also metabolized by other cytochrome P450 enzymes such as CYP3A5, CYP2C8 and CYP2C19, but to a much lesser extent (Naritomi et al., 2004; Zharikova et al., 2009; Zhou et al., 2010a). Zharikova et al. determined five metabolites of glyburide formed in human liver microsomes: M1 (4-*trans*-hydrocyclohexyl glyburide), M2a (4-*cis*-hydrocyclohexyl glyburide), M2b (3-*cis*-hydrocyclohexyl glyburide), M3 (3-*trans*-hydrocyclohexyl glyburide), M4 (2-*trans*-hydrocyclohexyl glyburide) and M5 (ethylene-hydroxylated glyburide) (Zharikova et al., 2009; Zharikova et al., 2007). The chemical structures of these glyburide metabolites are shown in Figure 1. CYP3A4 catalyzes the formation of M1-M5. CYP2C9 catalyzes the formation of M1-M3. CYP2C8 catalyzes the formation of M1, M2b, M3 and M4. CYP2C19 catalyzes the formation of M2a, M2b and M3 (Zharikova et al., 2009; Zharikova et al., 2007). The two major metabolites of glyburide, M1 and M2b, which account for approximately half of all the metabolites formed *in vitro* by human liver microsomes (Zharikova et al., 2007), are excreted into the bile and urine (~50% each) (Feldman, 1985). M1 and M2b are not likely to contribute significantly to hypoglycemic action in humans since they are only weakly active ($1/400^{th}$ and $1/40^{th}$ as active, respectively, as glyburide in preclinical models, as described in the FDA labeling). However, there were also studies indicating that M1 and M2b retain 75% and 50%, respectively, of the hypoglycemic activity of glyburide in humans (Rydberg et al., 1994). The systemic exposure of M1 is only 2 - 4% of that of glyburide (Zheng et al., 2009). The pharmacological activity of other glyburide metabolites is currently not known.

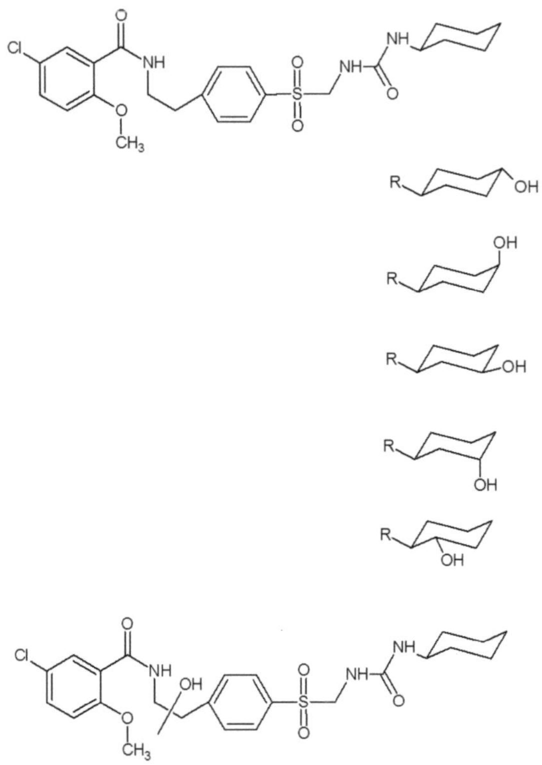

Glyburide

M1

M2a

M2b

M3

M4

M5

Fig. 1. The chemical structures of glyburide and its metabolites. M1, 4-*trans*-hydrocyclohexyl glyburide; M2a, 4-*cis*-hydrocyclohexyl glyburide; M2b, 3-*cis*-hydrocyclohexyl glyburide; M3, 3-*trans*-hydrocyclohexyl glyburide; M4, 2-*trans*-hydrocyclohexyl glyburide; and M5, ethylene-hydroxylated glyburide.

4. The efficacy and safety of glyburide during pregnancy

Although glyburide is not currently approved by the FDA to treat GDM, the pathophysiology of GDM is similar to type II diabetes mellitus and consequently, glyburide has been increasingly prescribed to women with GDM. There are obvious benefits to using oral hypoglycemic agents such as glyburide and metformin rather than insulin. Oral agents are less expensive, easier to administer and demonstrate improved patient compliance as compared to insulin. Clinical studies have been conducted to compare the efficacy and safety of such oral agents with those of insulin for the treatment of GDM. In this section, the results of clinical studies comparing the efficacy and safety of glyburide versus insulin will be summarized.

4.1 Clinical efficacy during pregnancy

There are several randomized controlled clinical trials that examined the efficacy of glyburide during pregnancy (Langer et al., 2000; Anjalakshi et al., 2007; Bertini et al., 2005; Ogunyemi et al., 2007). Langer et al. performed the largest clinical study that compared the efficacy of glyburide to insulin for the treatment of GDM (Langer et al., 2000). This group randomly assigned 404 women with GDM into two treatment groups (insulin or glyburide), and showed no statistically significant difference in fasting, preprandial, 2-hour postprandial and mean blood glucose concentrations between the glyburide and insulin groups (~106 mg/dL, 105 mg/dL, 130 mg/dL, and 115 mg/dL, respectively). Langer concluded that glyburide was as effective as insulin for the treatment of GDM and therefore can be used as a clinically effective alternative to insulin therapy. These authors reported eight women in the glyburide group (4%) who required insulin therapy. These authors also performed a subsequent analysis of the data from this clinical study to determine if the severity of GDM was linked to the dosage of glyburide required to achieve adequate glycemic control (Langer et al., 2000). It was found that glyburide doses were increased and the success rate of glyburide therapy decreased as disease severity increased. At each level of disease severity, there was no difference in maternal and neonatal outcomes between the insulin and glyburide groups.

Two smaller clinical studies also compared the efficacy of glyburide and insulin in the treatment of GDM, and no difference was observed in fasting and 2-hour postprandial blood glucose concentrations (Anjalakshi et al., 2007; Bertini et al., 2005). In contrast, Ogunyemi et al. reported significantly higher fasting and 2-hour postprandial blood glucose concentrations in patients receiving glyburide than in patients receiving insulin (Ogunyemi et al., 2007). Bertini et al. found that glucose control was not achieved in 5 patients in the glyburide group (20.8% failure rate) who had to switch to insulin therapy, despite similarities in maternal demographics across groups (age, weight and parity) (Bertini et al., 2005). Since the sample size of this randomized-controlled trial was relatively small, this may not accurately reflect the true failure rate of glyburide therapy.

In addition, retrospective studies have been conducted to assess the efficacy of glyburide. Jacobson et al. performed a retrospective study of 584 women with GDM who had failed diet therapy and were treated with glyburide or insulin between the years of 1999-2002 (Jacobson et al., 2005). Patients from both groups were similar in age and nulliparity; however, women in the insulin group weighed more on average and had a higher mean fasting blood glucose level (105.4 versus 102.4 mg/dL). Women in the glyburide group had significantly lower post-treatment fasting and postprandial blood glucose levels. The failure rate of glyburide was reported to be 12%. The glyburide group did experience a higher rate of preeclampsia (12% versus 6%), despite controlling for body mass index and ethnicity. Jacobson et al. observed no statistical difference in neonatal outcomes such as birth weight and macrosomia, as well as incidence of cesarean delivery between groups. Ramos et al. retrospectively examined the effectiveness of glyburide (n = 44) versus insulin (n = 78) in women with GDM who had a 50 g 3-hour oral glucose challenge test of ≥200 mg/dL and a pretreatment fasting plasma glucose level of ≥105 mg/dL (Ramos et al., 2007). There were no significant differences between the two groups with respect to blood glucose levels. The failure rate of glyburide was 16%. There were no significant differences in fetal outcomes between the two treatment groups; however, the incidence of neonatal hypoglycemia was higher in glyburide-treated women (34% versus 15%, respectively) (Ramos et al., 2007). It is worth noting that retrospective studies were often not adequately powered and were without adequate controls. Therefore, making general conclusions regarding the efficacy of glyburide is difficult.

To predict the treatment failure rate for glyburide in women with GDM, Kahn et al. conducted a prospective cohort study (n = 75) which demonstrated that fasting blood glucose levels ≥ 110 mg/dL, in women with GDM, were associated with higher glyburide failure rates (Kahn et al., 2006). The authors also reported that women who were older, had more than one child and were diagnosed with GDM earlier in their pregnancy were more likely to fail glyburide therapy. On the other hand, Rochon et al. suggested that only higher mean blood glucose levels (≥ 200 mg/dL in the 50 g 1-hour oral glucose challenge test) were indicators of glyburide failure (Rochon et al., 2006).

4.2 Maternal and neonatal safety

Several studies have been conducted to investigate the adverse effects of glyburide versus insulin (Anjalakshi et al., 2007; Bertini et al., 2005; Langer et al., 2000; Ogunyemi et al., 2007; Yogev et al., 2004). Among these studies, Langer et al. conducted the largest randomized controlled trial with 404 pregnant women to receive glyburide or insulin, and found a significantly higher percentage of women with a blood glucose level <40 mg/dL in the insulin group compared with the glyburide group (20% versus 4%) (Langer et al., 2000). Yogev et al. demonstrated that 19 of 30 insulin-treated patients with GDM (63%) experienced asymptomatic hypoglycemia versus 7 of 25 (28%) glyburide-treated patients (Yogev et al., 2004). On the other hand, in the study with 97 pregnant women, Ogunyemi et al. did not report a significant difference in hypoglycemia between the insulin and glyburide groups (31% verse 38%, respectively) (Ogunyemi et al., 2007). Other studies reported no hypoglycemic events (Anjalakshi et al., 2007; Bertini et al., 2005). Although the results varied, possibly due to difference in definition of hypoglycemia, these studies appear to support the notion that glyburide therapy generally causes fewer hypoglycemic events than insulin therapy. Langer et al. also showed no difference in the incidence of preeclampsia among women treated with insulin or glyburide (Langer et al., 2000). Bertini et al. found no significant difference in changes in maternal weight of women treated with insulin as compared to glyburide (Bertini et al., 2005). Likewise, no significant differences were reported in the percentage of women with cesarean delivery in the insulin group compared with the glyburide group (Anjalakshi et al., 2007; Bertini et al., 2005; Langer et al., 2000; Ogunyemi et al., 2007).

Various clinical studies have also analyzed the effects of glyburide and insulin on neonatal adverse outcomes. In an earlier study, Coetzee and Jackson treated over 600 pregnant women suffering from GDM or type II diabetes mellitus with glyburide/metformin combination therapy (Coetzee and Jackson, 1985). Patients were classified as new diabetics, known diabetics or untreated diabetics. The untreated diabetic group was made up of pregnant women with type II diabetes mellitus or GDM who were not seen in the clinic until term. Each class of patients was further organized into four treatment groups: (1) diet therapy, (2) diet plus metformin therapy, (3) diet plus glyburide therapy, (4) diet plus metformin/glyburide combination therapy, and (5) treatment group (4) with the addition of insulin therapy due to inadequate glucose control (Coetzee and Jackson, 1985). Metformin therapy appeared to be the safest (0 still births, 1 neonatal death, and 33 per 1,000 perinatal morbidities, i.e. large for gestational age, low birthweight, hypoglycemia, jaundice and congenital abnormalities), followed by glyburide (1 still birth, 0 neonatal deaths, and 43 per 1,000 perinatal morbidities) and the emergency insulin group (1 still birth, 4 neonatal deaths, and 59 per 1,000 perinatal morbidities). In women with newly diagnosed GDM, insulin therapy appeared to be the safest (no adverse birth outcomes), followed by metformin (1 neonatal death and 16 per 1,000 perinatal morbidities) and glyburide (1 still birth and 42 per 1,000 perinatal morbidities). The authors also reported a decrease in perinatal morbidities among the glyburide group compared with the diet therapy group as well as zero cases of serious neonatal hypoglycemia.

Bertini et al. found just the opposite to be true in a clinical study with 70 patients diagnosed with GDM (Bertini et al., 2005). Patients were placed on insulin therapy (n = 27), glyburide therapy (n = 24) or acarbose therapy (n = 19). The authors reported that neonatal hypoglycemia was observed in 8 newborns, 6 of which were from the glyburide group. Likewise, in the study with 97 women (n = 49 in the insulin group and n = 48 in the glyburide group), Ogunyemi et al. reported that 28% of infants in the glyburide group experienced an episode of hypoglycemia versus 13% in the insulin group, and the difference was statistically significant (Ogunyemi et al., 2007). In contrast, Langer et al. showed no difference in the incidence rate of hypoglycemia for infants between the insulin and glyburide treatment groups (Langer et al., 2000). Bertini et al. also demonstrated that a significantly higher percentage of fetuses were large for gestational age (LGA) infants in the glyburide group compared with the insulin group (25% versus 3.7%, respectively) (Bertini et al., 2005); however, Langer et al. reported comparable incidence rates of LGA between the two groups (n = 404) (Langer et al., 2000). All the clinical studies consistently reported higher average infant birth weights in the glyburide group than the insulin group, but the difference was small (an average of ~100 g) and not statistically significant (Anjalakshi et al., 2007; Bertini et al., 2005; Langer et al., 2000; Ogunyemi et al., 2007). Few congenital malformations or anomalies were reported in either group. It is worth noting that the study by Langer et al. investigated significantly more subjects than any other study, and hence the results obtained could be more adequately powered and reliable.

Overall, in women with GDM, glyburide achieved similar efficacy of glycemic control as insulin therapy. The maternal and neonatal safety of glyburide does not substantially differ from insulin therapy. However, it should be noted that, at present, there is no long-term safety data for infants whose mothers were treated with glyburide. Thus, further studies are needed to assess the long-term effects of maternal glyburide administration on child and adolescent development (neurologic and behavioral) as well as the incidence rate of type II diabetes mellitus and obesity.

5. Pregnancy-induced pharmacokinetic changes of glyburide

Physiological and biochemical changes that occur in pregnancy may affect the pharmacokinetics of drugs, namely absorption, distribution, metabolism and elimination (Anderson, 2005; Klieger et al., 2009; Loebstein et al., 1997). Such changes include, among others, changes in volume of distribution of drugs and plasma protein binding (Loebstein et al., 1997; Mendenhall, 1970), induction or down-regulation of cytochrome P450 enzyme expression and activity (Hebert et al., 2008; Tracy et al., 2005), and increase in renal blood flow and glomerular filtration (Dunlop & Davison, 1987). The effects of such pregnancy-induced pharmacokinetic changes may be such that a dosage adjustment is required to accommodate increased potency of a drug or decreased efficacy. However, the balance of treating the mother and protecting the fetus may likely present challenges specifically for drug compounds that require increased dosages in order to be effective during pregnancy. Glyburide is such a case.

5.1 Clinical pharmacokinetic studies

To evaluate pregnancy-induced changes in the pharmacokinetics of glyburide, Hebert et al. compared parameter estimates for steady-state pharmacokinetics of glyburide in pregnant women with GDM (n = 40) and non-pregnant women with type II diabetes mellitus (n = 26)

(Hebert et al., 2009). Dose-normalized steady-state plasma concentrations of glyburide were approximately one-half in pregnant women with GDM as compared with those in non-pregnant women with type II diabetes mellitus, consistent with a 2-fold increase in apparent oral clearance of glyburide during pregnancy. Modeling and simulations of this data demonstrate that pregnant women with GDM require much higher dosages of glyburide to achieve comparable concentrations as non-pregnant women. Whether higher dosages will be required during pregnancy to achieve glycemic control still needs further study.

5.2 *In vivo* animal studies

In vivo pharmacokinetic studies in pregnant mice have been performed to investigate the mechanism of pregnancy-induced increase in the apparent oral clearance of glyburide (Zhou et al., 2010b). Several groups have shown that CYP3A is a major enzyme responsible for the *in vitro* metabolism of glyburide (Naritomi et al., 2004; Zharikova et al., 2009; Zhou et al., 2010a). It has also been well established that hepatic CYP3A activity is significantly induced by pregnancy (Hebert et al., 2008; Tracy et al., 2005). Therefore, it has been hypothesized that pregnancy induces the activity of hepatic CYP3A, resulting in an increase in the oral clearance of glyburide (Zhou et al., 2010b). Since it has been shown that the levels of hepatic Cyp3a content in pregnant mice and its activity measured using testosterone as the probe substrate are significantly increased compared with those in non-pregnant mouse controls (Mathias et al., 2006; Zhang et al., 2008), the pregnant mouse was used as the animal model to test this hypothesis (Zhou et al., 2010b). Upon characterization, the pharmacokinetics of glyburide indeed demonstrated a two-fold increase in its hepatic clearance in pregnant mice on gestation day 15 compared to non-pregnant mice, a magnitude of change similar to that observed in the human clinical study, but with no changes in plasma protein binding (Zhou et al., 2010b).

To investigate the mechanism of this pharmacokinetic change in pregnant mice, Zhou et al. further determined glyburide depletion in mouse hepatic S-9 fractions and found the half-life of glyburide depletion to be markedly shorter in S-9 fractions from pregnant mice compared to non-pregnant mice. Glyburide depletion was also inhibited to a large extent by the Cyp3a inhibitor, ketoconazole, suggesting that the increase in hepatic clearance of glyburide during pregnancy may be due to an increase in the activity of hepatic Cyp3a (Zhou et al., 2010b). These studies support the notion that CYP3A plays a significant role in the clearance of glyburide in pregnancy. This finding has significant clinical implications. For example, significant drug-drug interactions may occur with glyburide and CYP3A inducers or inhibitors (Lilja et al., 2007).

5.3 Placental transport of glyburide

Hebert et al. have also shown that glyburide concentrations are measurable in umbilical cord blood at the time of delivery, suggesting that glyburide crosses the placenta and thus may pose adverse effects on the developing fetus (Hebert et al., 2009). The average umbilical cord to maternal plasma concentration ratio of glyburide was 0.7 ± 0.4 (Hebert et al., 2009). This less than unity ratio indicates that glyburide does not cross the placental barrier entirely by passive diffusion, even though it is highly lipophilic (LogP = 4.8). Many ATP-binding cassette (ABC) efflux transporters such as P-glycoprotein (P-gp), breast cancer resistance protein (BCRP), and multidrug resistance proteins (MRPs) are highly expressed on the apical membrane of placental syncytiotrophoblasts facing maternal blood, where they protect the fetus by expelling drugs, xenobiotics, and metabolites from the fetal compartment to the maternal circulation (Behravan & Piquette-Miller, 2007; Ceckova-Novotna et al., 2006; Mao, 2008; Ni & Mao, 2010). Glyburide has been shown to be a substrate of such ABC efflux transporters. Thus, it is likely that ABC efflux transporters in the placenta play an important role in limiting fetal exposure to glyburide.

To test this hypothesis, Gedeon et al. examined the role of P-gp, BCRP and MRPs in the efflux of glyburide using stable cell lines expressing these transporters in the presence or absence of selective inhibitors (Gedeon et al., 2006). Their results suggested that glyburide was preferentially transported by BCRP and MRP3, but not by P-gp, MRP1 or MRP2. Likewise, Gedeon et al. demonstrated that inhibition of P-gp or MRP1 did not affect accumulation of [^{3}H]-glyburide in inside-out brush border human placental membrane vesicles; however, inhibition of BCRP did (Gedeon et al., 2008b). Using the dually perfused human placental cotyledon model, Gedeon et al. further showed that the rate of transfer of glyburide across the placenta in the presence of indomethacin (an inhibitor of MRP1, MRP2 or MRP3) was not different from the rate of transfer in the absence of inhibitor (Gedeon et al., 2008a), suggesting that MRP1, 2, or 3 may be only minimally involved in the transport of glyburide across the human placenta. On the other hand, the role of BCRP in the transfer of glyburide across the human placenta was confirmed in a similar human placental perfusion study (Pollex et al., 2008). In contrast, Hemauer et al showed that MRP1 appears to play a greater role in the efflux of glyburide than P-gp or BCRP (Hemauer et al., 2010). Using inside-out brush border membrane vesicles isolated from human term placentas in the presence or absence of selective inhibitors (verapamil for P-gp, Ko143 for BCRP, and indomethacin for MRP1), Hemauer et al. determined the relative contribution of P-gp, BCRP, and MRP1 to the uptake of glyburide into the inside-out membrane vesicles to be 9 ± 5%, 25 ± 5%, and 43 ± 4%, respectively (Hemauer et al., 2010).

Zhou et al. confirmed that glyburide is a substrate for human BCRP and mouse Bcrp1 using Madin Darby canine kidney (MDCK) cell transwell transport experiments (Zhou et al., 2008). Zhou et al. also characterized glyburide disposition in wild-type and Bcrp1$^{-/-}$ pregnant mice to elucidate the role of Bcrp1 in limiting glyburide transfer across the placenta to the fetal compartment. The results showed that the maternal plasma concentration-time profiles remained the same between wild-type and knockout mice; however, the fetal area under the concentration-time curve (AUC) of glyburide in Bcrp1$^{-/-}$ pregnant mice was two times greater than that in wild-type mice (Zhou et al., 2008). It is worth noting that the amount of glyburide entering the fetus only accounts for a small fraction of the total amount of glyburide in the body (Zhou et al., 2008). These results confirm that BCRP and Bcrp1 are important determinants of fetal exposure to glyburide (Zhou et al., 2008). All these *in vitro, ex vivo,* and *in vivo* studies suggest that ABC efflux transporters, particularly BCRP, are important in protecting the fetus from exposure to glyburide. Thus, if a drug known to be a BCRP inhibitor is co-administered with glyburide, fetal exposure to glyburide may be increased through inhibition of placental BCRP.

5.4 Placental metabolism of glyburide

The placenta may also protect the fetus by metabolizing drugs or xenobiotics ingested by the mother. Human term placentas have been used in several studies to characterize placental metabolism of glyburide (Jain et al., 2008; Zharikova et al., 2009; Zharikova et al., 2007). Zharikova et al. reported that placental microsomes converted ~87% of glyburide to the M5 metabolite (ethylene-hydroxylated glyburide), and the rest to other metabolites (Zharikova et al., 2007). When compared to human liver microsomes; however, the total V_{max} for all metabolites was much lower for placental microsomes (13 ± 0.8 pmol/min/mg protein) than human liver microsomes (213 ± 37 pmol/min/mg protein). Although the relative contribution of placental drug-metabolizing enzymes to the overall disposition of glyburide may in fact be minimal, the formation of M5 in such close proximity to the fetus could have clinical implications for fetal metabolite exposure. However, at this time, the pharmacological activity of M5 is unknown. Zharikova et al. further identified CYP19 to be the major drug-metabolizing enzyme responsible for the biotransformation of glyburide to M5 in the human placenta (Zharikova et al., 2009). The intrinsic clearance of CYP19 for glyburide was 0.02 μL/min/pmol CYP and only represented 1.8% of the overall intrinsic clearance of human liver microsomes for glyburide.

Jain et al. studied glyburide metabolism using placental microsomes isolated from human term placentas from women with uncomplicated pregnancies, women with GDM on diet therapy, or women with GDM on glyburide (Jain et al., 2008). They found that placental microsomes from uncomplicated pregnancies showed higher M1 and M2 metabolite formation rates compared to placentas from women with GDM on diet therapy or on diet therapy plus glyburide. However, there was no difference in glyburide metabolism between placentas from diet therapy and diet therapy plus glyburide (Jain et al., 2008). The differences in placental microsomal metabolite formation may reflect the effects of GDM on the placenta. Histologic abnormalities in the placenta are more common in women with GDM than non-diabetic controls (Daskalakis et al., 2008).

Based upon the results obtained so far, the placenta appears to play a very minor role in determining maternal disposition of glyburide, but may play a significant role in controlling fetal exposure to the drug and metabolites. Very limited data is available in this regard, and the role of placental metabolism in controlling fetal drug exposure warrants further investigation.

6. Conclusions

Although insulin therapy has been the "gold standard" for the treatment of GDM, the increasing use of oral anti-diabetic agents such as glyburide and metformin has begun to change the standard of care. Glyburide is a second generation sulfonylurea. Clinical studies demonstrate that glyburide is a safe alternative to insulin therapy for the treatment of GDM due to its similar efficacy to insulin, relatively low fetal exposure, lower cost and ease of administration. The pharmacokinetic properties of glyburide resulting in low fetal exposure include: high plasma protein binding, a relatively short elimination half-life, and efflux transport by ABC transporters such as BCRP in the placenta. Glyburide is also metabolized in the placenta by CYP19, which may limit fetal exposure to the parent compound but simultaneously expose the fetus to metabolites. However, it is reassuring that the currently used glyburide dosage range for pregnant women with GDM has comparable maternal, fetal and neonatal outcomes as insulin therapy.

In addition to the concern of fetal exposure, physiological changes that occur during pregnancy may alter the pharmacokinetics of glyburide, thus affecting the safety and efficacy of the drug for both the mother and the fetus. Indeed, a recent clinical study has demonstrated that the apparent oral clearance of glyburide is increased two-fold in pregnant women with gestational diabetes as compared to non-pregnant women with type II diabetes mellitus (Hebert et al., 2009). This finding implies the need for further evaluation and dosage optimization for glyburide during pregnancy. The mechanism of such a change in glyburide disposition during pregnancy has not been fully understood, but is likely related to increased expression and activity of cytochrome P450 enzymes in the liver, such as CYP2C9 and CYP3A.

In summary, glyburide has been increasingly used for the treatment of GDM with similar safety and efficacy to insulin therapy. The mechanistic understanding of pregnancy-induced changes in the disposition of this drug (including fetal exposure) will be important for optimizing dosage guidelines for glyburide during pregnancy.

7. References

(2001) ACOG Practice Bulletin. Clinical management guidelines for obstetrician-gynecologists. Number 30, September 2001 (replaces Technical Bulletin Number 200, December 1994). Gestational diabetes. *Obstet Gynecol* 98(3):525-538.

(2002) The Hyperglycemia and Adverse Pregnancy Outcome (HAPO) Study. *Int J Gynaecol Obstet* 78(1):69-77.

(2009) Hyperglycemia and Adverse Pregnancy Outcome (HAPO) Study: associations with neonatal anthropometrics. *Diabetes* 58(2):453-459.

(2010) Hyperglycaemia and Adverse Pregnancy Outcome (HAPO) Study: associations with maternal body mass index. *BJOG* 117(5):575-584.

Anderson GD (2005) Pregnancy-induced changes in pharmacokinetics: a mechanistic-based approach. *Clin Pharmacokinet* 44(10):989-1008.

Anjalakshi C, Balaji V, Balaji MS and Seshiah V (2007) A prospective study comparing insulin and glibenclamide in gestational diabetes mellitus in Asian Indian women. *Diabetes Res Clin Pract* 76(3):474-475.

Behravan J and Piquette-Miller M (2007) Drug transport across the placenta, role of the ABC drug efflux transporters. *Expert Opin Drug Metab Toxicol* 3(6):819-830.

Bertini AM, Silva JC, Taborda W, Becker F, Lemos Bebber FR, Zucco Viesi JM, Aquim G and Engel Ribeiro T (2005) Perinatal outcomes and the use of oral hypoglycemic agents. *J Perinat Med* 33(6):519-523.

Bussing R and Gende A (2002) Severe hypoglycemia from clarithromycin-sulfonylurea drug interaction. *Diabetes Care* 25(9):1659-1661.

Cavallari LH and Limdi NA (2009) Warfarin pharmacogenomics. *Curr Opin Mol Ther* 11(3):243-251.

Ceckova-Novotna M, Pavek P and Staud F (2006) P-glycoprotein in the placenta: expression, localization, regulation and function. *Reprod Toxicol* 22(3):400-410.

Coetzee EJ and Jackson WP (1985) The management of non-insulin-dependent diabetes during pregnancy. *Diabetes Res Clin Pract* 1(5):281-287.

Daskalakis G, Marinopoulos S, Krielesi V, Papapanagiotou A, Papantoniou N, Mesogitis S and Antsaklis A (2008) Placental pathology in women with gestational diabetes. *Acta Obstet Gynecol Scand* 87(4):403-407.

Dunlop W and Davison JM (1987) Renal haemodynamics and tubular function in human pregnancy. *Baillieres Clin Obstet Gynaeco l*1(4):769-787.

Feldman JM (1985) Glyburide: a second-generation sulfonylurea hypoglycemic agent. History, chemistry, metabolism, pharmacokinetics, clinical use and adverse effects. *Pharmacotherapy* 5(2):43-62.

Gedeon C, Anger G, Lubetsky A, Miller MP and Koren G (2008a) Investigating the potential role of multi-drug resistance protein (MRP) transporters in fetal to maternal glyburide efflux in the human placenta. *J Obstet Gynaecol* 28(5):485-489.

Gedeon C, Anger G, Piquette-Miller M and Koren G (2008b) Breast cancer resistance protein: mediating the trans-placental transfer of glyburide across the human placenta. *Placenta* 29(1):39-43.

Gedeon C, Behravan J, Koren G and Piquette-Miller M (2006) Transport of glyburide by placental ABC transporters: implications in fetal drug exposure. *Placenta* 27(11-12):1096-1102.

Hebert MF, Easterling TR, Kirby B, Carr DB, Buchanan ML, Rutherford T, Thummel KE, Fishbein DP and Unadkat JD (2008) Effects of pregnancy on CYP3A and P-glycoprotein activities as measured by disposition of midazolam and digoxin: a University of Washington specialized center of research study. *Clin Pharmacol Ther* 84(2):248-253.

Hebert MF, Ma X, Naraharisetti SB, Krudys KM, Umans JG, Hankins GD, Caritis SN, Miodovnik M, Mattison DR, Unadkat JD, Kelly EJ, Blough D, Cobelli C, Ahmed MS, Snodgrass WR, Carr DB, Easterling TR and Vicini P (2009) Are we optimizing gestational diabetes treatment with glyburide? The pharmacologic basis for better clinical practice. *Clin Pharmacol Ther* 85(6):607-614.

Hemauer SJ, Patrikeeva SL, Nanovskaya TN, Hankins GD and Ahmed MS (2010) Role of human placental apical membrane transporters in the efflux of glyburide, rosiglitazone, and metformin. *Am J Obstet Gynecol* 202(4):383 e381-387.

Jacobson GF, Ramos GA, Ching JY, Kirby RS, Ferrara A and Field DR (2005) Comparison of glyburide and insulin for the management of gestational diabetes in a large managed care organization. *Am J Obstet Gynecol* 193(1):118-124.

Jain S, Zharikova OL, Ravindran S, Nanovskya TN, Mattison DR, Hankins GD and Ahmed MS (2008) Glyburide metabolism by placentas of healthy and gestational diabetics. *Am J Perinatol* 25(3):169-174.

Jonsson A, Rydberg T, Ekberg G, Hallengren B and Melander A (1994) Slow elimination of glyburide in NIDDM subjects. *Diabetes Care* 17(2):142-145.

Jovanovic L and Pettitt DJ (2001) Gestational diabetes mellitus. *JAMA* 286(20):2516-2518.

Kahn BF, Davies JK, Lynch AM, Reynolds RM and Barbour LA (2006) Predictors of glyburide failure in the treatment of gestational diabetes. *Obstet Gynecol* 107(6):1303-1309.

Karakash SD and Einstein FH (2011) Diabetes in pregnancy: glycemia control guidelines and rationale. *Curr Opin Endocrinol Diabetes Obes* 18:99-103.

Kirchheiner J, Brockmoller J, Meineke I, Bauer S, Rohde W, Meisel C and Roots I (2002) Impact of CYP2C9 amino acid polymorphisms on glyburide kinetics and on the insulin and glucose response in healthy volunteers. *Clin Pharmacol Ther* 71(4):286-296.

Klieger C, Pollex E, Kazmin A and Koren G (2009) Hypoglycemics: pharmacokinetic considerations during pregnancy. *Ther Drug Monit* 31(5):533-541.

Landon MB, Catalano PM, Gabbe SG (2007) Diabetes mellitus complicating pregnancy. Chapter 37, In: Gabbe SG, Niebyl JR, Simpson JL ed., *Obstetrics - Normal and Problem Pregnancies (5)*, Elsevier Churchill Livingstone, Philadelphia, PA.

Langer O, Conway DL, Berkus MD, Xenakis EM and Gonzales O (2000) A comparison of glyburide and insulin in women with gestational diabetes mellitus. *N Engl J Med* 343(16):1134-1138.

Leiba A, Leibowitz A and Grossman E (2004) An unusual case of hypoglycemia in a diabetic patient. *Ann Emerg Med* 44(4):427-428.

Lilja JJ, Niemi M, Fredrikson H and Neuvonen PJ (2007) Effects of clarithromycin and grapefruit juice on the pharmacokinetics of glibenclamide. *Br J Clin Pharmacol* 63(6):732-740.

Loebstein R, Lalkin A and Koren G (1997) Pharmacokinetic changes during pregnancy and their clinical relevance. *Clin Pharmacokinet* 33(5):328-343.

Mao Q (2008) BCRP/ABCG2 in the placenta: expression, function and regulation. *Pharm Res* 25(6):1244-1255.

Mathias AA, Maggio-Price L, Lai Y, Gupta A and Unadkat JD (2006) Changes in pharmacokinetics of anti-HIV protease inhibitors during pregnancy: the role of CYP3A and P-glycoprotein. *J Pharmacol Exp Ther* 316(3):1202-1209.

Maymone AC, Baillargeon JP, Menard J and Ardilouze JL (2011) Oral hypoglycemic agents for gestational diabetes mellitus? *Expert Opin Drug Saf* 10(2):227-238.

Mendenhall HW (1970) Serum protein concentrations in pregnancy. I. Concentrations in maternal serum. *Am J Obstet Gynecol* 106(3):388-399.

Naritomi Y, Terashita S and Kagayama A (2004) Identification and relative contributions of human cytochrome P450 isoforms involved in the metabolism of glibenclamide and lansoprazole: evaluation of an approach based on the in vitro substrate disappearance rate. *Xenobiotica* 34(5):415-427.

Ni Z and Mao Q (2010) ATP-binding Cassette Efflux Transporters in Human Placenta. *Curr Pharm Biotechnol* 12(4):674-685.

Nicholson W and Baptiste-Roberts K (2011) Oral hypoglycaemic agents during pregnancy: The evidence for effectiveness and safety. *Best Pract Res Clin Obstet Gynaecol* 25(1):51-63.

Niemi M, Cascorbi I, Timm R, Kroemer HK, Neuvonen PJ and Kivisto KT (2002) Glyburide and glimepiride pharmacokinetics in subjects with different CYP2C9 genotypes. *Clin Pharmacol Ther* 72(3):326-332.

Ogunyemi D, Jesse M and Davidson M (2007) Comparison of glyburide versus insulin in management of gestational diabetes mellitus. *Endocr Pract*13(4):427-428.

Paglia MJ and Coustan DR (2011) Gestational diabetes: evolving diagnostic criteria. *Curr Opin Obstet Gynecol* 23(2):72-75.

Pollex E, Lubetsky A and Koren G (2008) The role of placental breast cancer resistance protein in the efflux of glyburide across the human placenta. *Placenta* 29(8):743-747.

Ramos GA, Jacobson GF, Kirby RS, Ching JY and Field DR (2007) Comparison of glyburide and insulin for the management of gestational diabetics with markedly elevated oral glucose challenge test and fasting hyperglycemia. *J Perinatol* 27(5):262-267.

Rochon M, Rand L, Roth L and Gaddipati S (2006) Glyburide for the management of gestational diabetes: risk factors predictive of failure and associated pregnancy outcomes. *Am J Obstet Gynecol* 195(4):1090-1094.

Rydberg T, Jonsson A, Roder M and Melander A (1994) Hypoglycemic activity of glyburide (glibenclamide) metabolites in humans. *Diabetes Care* 17(9):1026-1030.

Schelleman H, Bilker WB, Brensinger CM, Wan F and Hennessy S (2010) Anti-infectives and the risk of severe hypoglycemia in users of glipizide or glyburide. *Clin Pharmacol Ther* 88(2):214-222.

Tracy TS, Venkataramanan R, Glover DD and Caritis SN (2005) Temporal changes in drug metabolism (CYP1A2, CYP2D6 and CYP3A Activity) during pregnancy. *Am J Obstet Gynecol* 192(2):633-639.

Yin OQ, Tomlinson B and Chow MS (2005) CYP2C9, but not CYP2C19, polymorphisms affect the pharmacokinetics and pharmacodynamics of glyburide in Chinese subjects. *Clin Pharmacol Ther* 78(4):370-377.

Yogev Y, Ben-Haroush A, Chen R, Rosenn B, Hod M and Langer O (2004) Undiagnosed asymptomatic hypoglycemia: diet, insulin, and glyburide for gestational diabetic pregnancy. *Obstet Gynecol* 104(1):88-93.

Zhang H, Wu X, Wang H, Mikheev AM, Mao Q and Unadkat JD (2008) Effect of pregnancy on cytochrome P450 3a and P-glycoprotein expression and activity in the mouse: mechanisms, tissue specificity, and time course. *Mol Pharmacol* 74(3):714-723.

Zharikova OL, Fokina VM, Nanovskaya TN, Hill RA, Mattison DR, Hankins GD and Ahmed MS (2009) Identification of the major human hepatic and placental enzymes responsible for the biotransformation of glyburide. *Biochem Pharmacol* 78(12):1483-1490.

Zharikova OL, Ravindran S, Nanovskaya TN, Hill RA, Hankins GD and Ahmed MS (2007) Kinetics of glyburide metabolism by hepatic and placental microsomes of human and baboon. *Biochem Pharmacol* 73(12):2012-2019.

Zheng HX, Huang Y, Frassetto LA and Benet LZ (2009) Elucidating rifampin's inducing and inhibiting effects on glyburide pharmacokinetics and blood glucose in healthy volunteers: unmasking the differential effects of enzyme induction and transporter inhibition for a drug and its primary metabolite. *Clin Pharmacol Ther* 85(1):78-85.

Zhou L, Naraharisetti SB, Liu L, Wang H, Lin YS, Isoherranen N, Unadkat JD, Hebert MF and Mao Q (2010a) Contributions of human cytochrome P450 enzymes to glyburide metabolism. *Biopharm Drug Dispos* 31(4):228-242.

Zhou L, Naraharisetti SB, Wang H, Unadkat JD, Hebert MF and Mao Q (2008) The breast cancer resistance protein (Bcrp1/Abcg2) limits fetal distribution of glyburide in the pregnant mouse: an Obstetric-Fetal Pharmacology Research Unit Network and University of Washington Specialized Center of Research Study. *Mol Pharmacol* 73(3):949-959.

Zhou L, Zhang Y, Hebert MF, Unadkat JD and Mao Q (2010b) Increased glyburide clearance in the pregnant mouse model. *Drug Metab Dispos* 38(9):1403-1406.

20

Exercise Guidelines for Women with Gestational Diabetes

Michelle F. Mottola and Stephanie-May Ruchat
University of Western Ontario, London,Ontario
Canada

1. Introduction

1.1 Obesity and type 2 diabetes prevalence are increasing among women of child-bearing age

There has been a significant increase over the past few decades in the the prevalence of women of child-bearing age who are overweight (body mass index, BMI ≥ 25 kg/m^2) or obese (BMI ≥ 30 kg/m^2). Women of childbearing age are at an increased risk for obesity (Villamor & Cnattingius, 2006) and type 2 diabetes (Lipscombe & Hux, 2007) because of excessive weight gain during pregnancy and weight retention after delivery (Rooney et al., 2005). Data from the 2007-2008 "National Health and Nutrition Examination Survey" (NHANES) showed that 60% and 34% of American women aged 20-39 years were overweight or obese, respectively (Flegal et al., 2010). Abdominal obesity (i.e. waist circumference ≥ 88 cm; (Lean et al., 1995)), a risk factor for many chronic diseases (Després, 2001) also increased and reached 51.3% in 2007-2008 (Ford et al., 2010). Data from the "Pregnancy Risk Assessment Monitoring System" in nine states indicated that pre-pregnancy obesity increased from 13% to 22% between 1993 and 2002 (Kim et al., 2007). Worldwide population estimates of pre-pregnancy overweight is approximately 34% (Callaway et al., 2006; LaCoursiere et al., 2005) and that of pre-pregnancy obesity is 25% (Chu et al., 2009), which may be an underestimation. This escalating problem may contribute to the obesity and diabetes epidemics, as overweight women who gain 10% or more of their pre-pregnancy body mass are at higher risk for complications such as gestational diabetes mellitus (GDM; (Carducci et al., 1999)) and pregnancy-induced hypertension (Pole & Dodds, 1999). Additionally, higher recurrence of GDM has been associated with greater pre-pregnancy weight, BMI and excessive pregnancy weight gain (Foster-Powell & Cheung, 1998).

1.2 Women of child-bearing age are inactive, particularly overweight and obese women

Low levels of physical activity may be contributing to the obesity and type 2 diabetes epidemics in women of child-bearing age. Physical activity levels may be evaluated using different tools but pedometers and accelerometers provide an accurate and objective method of measuring walking and other ambulatory activities. Physical activity levels based on step counts have been defined: <5,000 steps per day = sedentary, 5,000-7,499 steps per day = low active, 7,500-9,999 steps per day = somewhat active, 10,000-12,499 = active and ≥

12,500= highly active (Tudor-Locke et al., 2008). Pedometer data from the "American On the Move" study showed that women aged 18-39 years took approximately 5500 steps per day (Bassett et al., 2010). Similar results were found by Tudor-Locke et al. using accelerometer data from the 2005-2006 NHANES (Tudor-Locke et al., 2010). They reported that women took approximately 5,800 steps per day (Tudor-Locke et al., 2010). Interestingly, the authors also reported that normal weight women took more steps per day compared to overweight and obese women (6,486, 5,069 and 5,782, respectively). In Canada, accelerometer results from the 2007-2008 "Canadian Health Measures Survey" showed that women aged 20-39 years took nearly 9,000 steps per day. Again, obese women were less active compared to normal weight women. Noteworthy, studies conducted on populations that have a lower prevalence of overweight and obesity, like Japan and Australia, reported higher steps per day (Inoue et al., 2006; McCormack et al., 2003). Achievement of public health recommendation (i.e ≥ 30 minutes of moderate-to-vigorous physical activity per day, accumulated in bouts lasting at least 10 minutes, on at least 5 out of 7 days (Canadian Society for Exercise Physiology & ParticipACTION, 2010; WHO, 2010)) were also examined using accelerometers. Results showed that less than 5% of women of child-bearing age meet these recommendations (Colley et al., 2011; Troiano et al., 2008; Tudor-Locke et al., 2010). Taken together, these findings showed that women of child-bearing age are inactive and suggested that being sedentary, and the prevalence of physical inactivity, may be contributing to the obesity and diabetes epidemics.

1.3 Maternal obesity is associated with impaired glucose metabolism

Entering pregnancy overweight or obese are closely linked to numerous unfavourable pregnancy outcomes, such as the development of impaired glucose tolerance (IGT) or GDM (Catalano & Ehrenberg, 2006; Chu et al., 2007; Davies et al., 2010; Nelson et al., 2009). Women who are obese prior to pregnancy are more likely to develop IGT as compared to normal weight women (Saldana et al., 2006; Tovar et al., 2009). Similarly, the risk of developing GDM has been shown to increase with increasing BMI: overweight and obese women have 2.14 (95% CI 1.82-2.53) and 3.56 (95% CI 3.05-4.21) times the risk of developing GDM compared to normal weight women (Chu et al., 2007). GDM prevalence rates are 0.7% in normal weight, 2.3% in overweight, 4.8% in obese and 5.5% in extremely obese (BMI ≥ 35 kg/m^2) women (Kim et al., 2010). More than 70% of women with GDM have a BMI of 25 kg/m^2 or higher (Kim et al., 2010). Similarly, maternal abdominal adiposity in early pregnancy has been associated with a positive glucose challenge test (i.e. glucose levels ≥ 7.8 mmol/L) and an increased risk of GDM (Brisson et al., 2010; Martin et al., 2009).

1.4 Excessive gestational weight gain is associated with impaired glucose metabolism

Another risk factor for developing IGT and GDM is excessive gestational weight gain (GWG). A cohort study revealed a positive relationship between weight gain in excess of the Institute of Medicine (IOM) guidelines (IOM, 1990) and the development of IGT, although these findings were limited to Hispanic women with a pre-pregnancy BMI ≥ 35 kg/m^2 (Tovar et al., 2009). Saldana et al. found in the "Pregnancy, Infection and Nutrition" (PIN) cohort a two-fold increased risk of IGT among overweight women who gained excessive weight up to the end of the second trimester (Saldana et al., 2006). Data from the "Project Viva" showed similar findings, with women in the highest quartile of GWG (i.e. 12.9 kg to

29.1 kg) being at increased risk for IGT, compared to those women in the lowest quartile of GWG (i.e -9.4 kg to 7.9 kg), independent of pre-pregnancy BMI (Herring et al., 2009). Finally, Kieffer et al. showed an estimated 2% increase in risk of GDM associated with each pound of maternal weight gained after adjusting for pre-pregnancy BMI (Kieffer et al., 2001). Excessive GWG, especially during the first trimester of pregnancy, has been found to be associated with an increased risk of GDM (Hedderson et al., 2010; Morisset et al., 2011), suggesting that timing of excessive GWG may be important and may be related to different patterns of metabolic change affecting glucose metabolism regulation.

Data from the 2006 "Maternity Experiences Survey", conducted in Canada, showed that 52% of Canadian women gained more than the recommended weight in pregnancy (Lowell & Miller, 2010). Moreover, the survey showed that women with a higher pre-pregnancy BMI were more likely than normal weight and underweight women to gain more weight than recommended. Fifty-five percent of overweight and obese women gained more weight than recommended, compared with 41% of those who were in the normal range and 26% of those who were underweight (Lowell & Miller, 2010). Previous studies reported similar findings, that is, overweight and obese women are more likely to exceed their target weight gain (Caulfield et al., 1996; Tovar et al., 2009; Saldana et al., 2006; Stuebe et al., 2009). Avoidance of excessive GWG may therefore constitute an opportunity for the prevention of impaired glucose metabolism during pregnancy.

1.5 Insulin resistance, the link between overweight/obesity, excessive gestational weight gain and impaired glucose metabolism

The underlying mechanism linking pre-pregnancy overweight/obesity to IGT or GDM is insulin resistance, coupled with an inadequate insulin response due to pancreatic beta-cell dysfunction (Buchanan & Xiang, 2005). Althought overweight and obese women present a similar 50% decrease in insulin sensitivity over the period of gestation, they are more insulin resistant than normal weight women throughout pregnancy (Catalano, 2010). Positive correlations have been reported between maternal body weight, BMI, fat mass and insulin resistance (Ahlsson et al., 2010). Maternal fat mass explained 36% of the variation in insulin resistance, and insulin resistance accounted for 62% of the variation in glucose production (Ahlsson et al., 2010). Adipose tissue is an active organ that secretes numerous factors involved in the development of insulin resistance, such as free fatty acids, leptin, adiponectin, interleukin-6 (IL-6), plasminogen activator inhibitor-1 (PAI-1), tumor necrosis factor-α (TNF-α), resistin, retinol binding protein 4, visfatin, etc. (Rasouli & Kern, 2008). In obese non-pregnant individuals, adipose tissue releases increased amounts of these factors, except adiponectin, which may explain the link between obesity, insulin resistance and type 2 diabetes (Kahn et al., 2006). In pregnant women, it has been reported that mean levels of adiponectin declined, and PAI-1 increased as BMI increments increased (Lowe et al., 2010). Recent studies have focused on the role of adipokines during normal pregnancy and pregnancy complicated by GDM and showed that the pattern of change in maternal circulating adipokine levels may be involved in the pathophysiology of GDM (Briana & Malamitsi-Puchner, 2009).

Excessive GWG may also further enhance normal pregnancy-induced insulin resistance and be linked to impaired glucose metabolism. Maternal adipose tissue represents 30% of GWG (IOM, 1990) but the proportion of GWG attributed to adipose tissue is more important in early pregnancy (Hedderson et al., 2010). The timing of GWG seems to be important as early excessive GWG has been associated with GDM risk (Hedderson et al., 2010; Morisset et al., 2011). It is therefore possible that rapid GWG in early pregnancy results in an increased release of "diabetogenic" factors, exacerbating earlier pregnancy-induced insulin resistance and thereby leading to IGT or GDM in women having beta-cell defects.

In summary, an increased number of women of child-bearing age are overweight or obese and physically inactive and these women will likely start their pregnancy overweight or obese and sedentary. These factors have been associated with an increased risk for excessive GWG, a deterioration in insulin resistance beyond that induced by pregnancy and impaired glucose metabolism. Therefore, any intervention that helps to limit excessive gestational weight gain and attenuate pregnancy-induced insulin resistance may be successful in preventing impaired glucose metabolism.

2. Physical activity is part of a healthy pregnancy

A minimal amount of physical activity must be maintained to achieve health benefits during pregnancy. Physical inactivity and a sedentary lifestyle may put the mother and fetus at risk for disease through altered maternal pregnancy adaptations (Mottola 2008). In fact, women who were the most active before pregnancy (Chu et al. 2007) and throughout pregnancy (Dye et al. 1997), had the lowest prevelence of GDM. If GDM and IGT can be prevented, overall rates of obesity and type 2 diabetes, especially in at risk population groups may also be decreased.

2.1 Maternal physical activity is associated with reduced risk of impaired glucose metabolism

Pregnancy-induced insulin resistance develops at the skeletal muscle level (Buchanan & Xiang, 2005). Investigators have demonstrated that exercise increases the rate of glucose uptake into the skeletal muscle, a process that is regulated by the translocation of the glucose transport protein GLUT-4 (Goodyear & Kahn, 1998; Hayashi et al., 1997; Ryder et al., 2001). Regular exercise in non pregnant individuals results in numerous beneficial adaptations in skeletal muscle, including increases in GLUT-4 expression, which contributes to an increased responsiveness of muscle glucose uptake to insulin (i.e. increased muscle insulin sensitivity) (Goodyear & Kahn, 1998; Hayashi et al., 1997; Ryder et al., 2001). This may explain the observed link between level of physical activity and improvement in glucose homeostasis and insulin sensitivity (Goodyear & Kahn, 1998; Koivisto et al., 1986), and a risk reduction of 50% for type 2 diabetes mellitus (T2DM) in at risk individuals (Madden et al., 2008; Yates et al., 2007). These physiological and molecular mechanisms underlying the beneficial effects of exercise may also be present in pregnant women since successful reduction in the risk of developing IGT and GDM have been reported in women who were active either before and/or during pregnancy (Tobias et al., 2010).

In the "Nurse Health Study II", women in the highest quintile of physical activity before pregnancy, specifically vigorous activity, had a 20% risk reduction for the development of GDM compared with inactive women (Zhang et al., 2006). In women not performing vigorous activity, brisk walking was also significantly associated with a reduced risk. Similarly, physical activity before pregnancy, particularly vigorous activity, was associated with a 44% risk reduction of GDM and a 24% risk reduction of any antepartum IGT in women participating in "Project Viva" (Oken et al., 2006). Women who reported physical activity both before and during pregnancy presented a greater risk reduction in both GDM and IGT (51% and 30%, respectively) compared with women reporting no activities in both time periods (Oken et al., 2006). Dempsey et al. reported that women who participated in any physical activity during the year before getting pregnant experienced a 56% risk reduction in GDM compared with inactive women, but those who engaged in physical activity during both time periods experienced a 69% reduced risk (Dempsey et al., 2004b). It has also been shown that pre-gravid physical activity (vigorous activity) was associated with a reduced risk of IGT in pregnancy, an effect likely mediated by enhanced insulin sensitivity (Retnakaran et al., 2009).

Similar results were found when investigating the effect of physical activity during pregnancy. Dye et al. reported that exercise during pregnancy (i.e. 30 minutes of exercise once or more per week) was associated with reduced rates of GDM, but only among women with a pre-pregnancy BMI>33 kg/m^2 (Dye et al., 1997). A study including only Latina women showed that those in the lowest quartile of sports or exercise in mid-pregnancy had a two-fold increased risk of IGT as compared with women in the highest quartile (Gollenberg et al., 2010). Similar association was found with total sedentary behaviours (a composite score of TV watching, sitting at work and sport or exercise reverse scores) (Gollenberg et al., 2010). A case-control study reported that women who participated in any recreational physical activity during the first 20 weeks of pregnancy experienced a 48% reduction in GDM risk, as compared with inactive women (Dempsey et al., 2004a). It has also been shown that women who were previously inactive but became active during pregnancy had a 57% risk reduction in GDM compared to those who remained inactive (Liu et al., 2008). Finally, a prospective study reported that increased physical activity during pregnancy was associated with decreased fasting insulin concentrations (Liu et al., 2010), suggesting that being active during pregnancy may prevent impaired glucose metabolism through attenuation of pregnancy-induced insulin resistance.

2.2 Maternal physical activity is associated with preventing excessive gestational weight gain

Another mechanism through which physical activity may prevent impaired glucose metabolism is by limiting excessive GWG. Prospective data from the "Project Viva" showed that 30 minutes per day of walking, vigorous physical activity or total physical activity during pregnancy were inversely associated with the risk of excessive GWG (Stuebe et al., 2009). Similar findings were found by Olson et al. who found that decreased physical activity was associated with excessive GWG (Olson & Strawderman, 2003). Lifestyle intervention studies also showed successful results with respect to the prevention of excessive GWG. Two reports using meta-analyses of intervention trials showed that exercise programs, combined with or without nutrition counselling, helps to limit GWG (Streuling et al., 2010a; Streuling et al., 2010b). Interventions that combined exercise and dietary counseling were found to be more successful in limiting GWG, with an average reduction of GWG of 1.2 kg (p=0.01) found in the intervention groups compared to the control groups (Streuling et al., 2010b). Three studies found significant lower GWG in the exercise plus nutrition intervention group compared with the control groups (Asbee et al., 2009; Claesson et al., 2008; Shirazian et al., 2010), 3 studies found a non significant trend in lower GWG in the intervention group compared with the control group (Gray-Donald et al., 2000; Guelinckx et al., 2010; Olson et al., 2004) and three found no significant results (Hui et al., 2006; Kinnunen et al., 2007; Polley et al., 2002). Findings from intervention studies using only exercise were less consistent than findings from intervention studies combining exercise and nutrition. Seven trials reported a trend for less GWG in the exercise group (Barakat et al., 2009; Cavalcante et al., 2009; Clapp et al., 2000; Ong et al., 2009; Santos et al., 2005; Sedaghati et al., 2007; Yeo, 2009) which was significant in only one of these trials (Sedaghati et al., 2007). Five trials reported that women in the exercise group did not gain significantly less weight than women in the control group (Collings et al., 1983; Garshasbi & Faghih Zadeh, 2005; Hopkins et al., 2010; Marquez-Sterling et al., 2000; Prevedel et al., 2003). An average reduction in GWG of 0.6 kg ($p=0.03$) was found in the exercise intervention groups compared to the control groups (Streuling et al., 2010a). A single arm intervention study, combining exercise and diet, reported that 56% of obese women kept their GWG to ≤ 6 kg (study weight goal) and no cases of reduced glucose tolerance were observed (Lindholm et al., 2010). Finally, a recent study conducted in our laboratory showed that excessive GWG was prevented in 80% of overweight and obese women using a Nutrition and Exercise Lifestyle Intervention Program (NELIP) (Mottola et al., 2010).

In summary, the prevailing literature clearly indicates that physical activity before and/or during pregnancy has a protective effect against excessive GWG and impaired glucose metabolism. Results from intervention studies suggest that in order to be the most successful in limiting GWG, and thus in helping to prevent impaired glucose metabolism, lifestyle interventions should promote both regular physical activity and healthy eating habits. Promoting a healthy lifestyle during pregnancy, especially in overweight and obese women, becomes increasingly important in the context of the prevention of impaired glucose metabolism.

2.3 Guidelines for physical activity during pregnancy

Active promotion of physical activity for pregnant women is strongly recommended by professionnal societies, such as the American College of Obstetricians and Gynecologists (ACOG, 2002), the Royal College of Obstetricians and Gynaecologists (RCOG, 2006), the Society of Obstetricians and Gynaecologists of Canada (SOGC) and the Canadian Society of Exercise Physiologists (CSEP) (Davies et al., 2003). The ACOG suggested that "in the absence of either medical or obstetric contraindications, 30 minutes or more of moderate exercise a day on most, if not all, days of the week is recommended for pregnant women" (ACOG, 2002). The recent opinion statement from the SOGC (Davies et al., 2010) on obesity during pregnancy strongly suggests that regular exercise during pregnancy may help to reduce the risk of medical complications associated with maternal obesity. However, all pregnant women should be medically prescreened and consult their health care provider before engaging in an exercise program. In 2008, the Unites States government released physical activity guidelines for Americans, including recommendations specifically for pregnant women to attain at least 150 minutes of moderate intensity aerobic activity per week if not already highly active or doing vigorous intensity activity. Healthy pregnant women who engaged in vigorous aerobic activity or are highly active prior to pregnancy are encouraged to continue physical activity (U.S Department of Health and Human Services 2008). Finally, the joint SOGC/CSEP Clinical Practice Guidelines encourage women to exercise if they have no contraindications (Davies et al., 2003). The SOGC/CSEP Clinical Practice Guidelines provide detailed recommendations about the frequency, intensity, time and type of exercise, following the FITT principle for exercise prescription. Women should exercise 3 to 4 times per week, starting with 15 minutes of aerobic activity at a target heart rate intensity and increasing time slowly to a maximum of 30 minutes per exercise session. All aerobic activity should be preceded by 10- to 15-minutes of warm-up and followed by 10- to 15-minutes of cool-down. Appropriate exercise intensity may be monitored by using target heart-rate zones, the Borg-scale (rating of perceived exertion, RPE) or the "talk test" (Davies et al., 2003). Heart-rate zones that are provided in the guidelines correspond to moderate-intensity exercise (i.e. 60-80% of maximal aerobic capacity, $VO_{2\ max}$). Aerobic exercise in which large muscle groups are used, including walking, stationary cycling, aqua exercise, or low-impact aerobics are recommended for low risk pregnant women (Davies et al. 2003).

Overweight and obese women can participate in exercise, if they have no contraindications to being physically active. Twenty medically pre-screened obese and 20 normal weight pregnant women participated in a graded treadmill exercise test to volitional fatigue to examine the impact of obesity on the ventilatory response to weight-bearing exercise during pregnancy (Davenport et al., 2009). We concluded that exercise ventilatory response is increased during pregnancy but is not affected further by obesity during graded treadmill exercise (Davenport et al., 2009). This is important in that there is no apparent ventilatory limitation to submaximal weight-bearing exercise representing daily living activities such as walking, in pregnant obese women, which lends support to the feasibility of exercise prescription in this population group (Mottola, 2009). Target heart rate zones developed for normal weight pregnant women may be too difficult for overweight and obese women to obtain, and thus we developed and validated target heart rate zones for medically pre-screened overweight and obese women at a much lower intensity but high enough to achieve aerobic benefits (Davenport et al. 2008a). The intensity is approximately 20-39% heart rate reserve (HRR), and at a normal walking pace which may help with compliance in this population group.

Currently, there are no step recommendations for pregnant women but those that have been defined for adults (Tudor-Locke et al., 2008) may be used for pregnant women. As walking is the most reported activity during pregnancy (Evenson et al., 2004; Evenson & Wen, 2010; Mottola & Campbell, 2003; Petersen et al., 2005), providing step recommendations to pregnant women may encourage them to be more active. Previous studies conducted in our laboratory showed that pregnant women took more than 10,000 steps per day when a 40-minute walk was added to their usual daily activities (Davenport et al., 2008b; Mottola et al., 2010).

2.4 Are pregnant women meeting the physical activity guidelines?

Although maternal physical activity has clear health benefits on pregnancy outcomes, and professional societies strongly recommend active promotion of physical activity for pregnant women, most women remain inactive during pregnancy. In Canada, only 30% of pregnant women meet the adult step recommendations of 10,000 steps per day (Cohen et al., 2010). Data from large cohort studies, such as the "Behavioral Risk Factor Surveillance System" (BRFSS), NHANES and PIN showed that the majority of women do not meet the recommendations for physical activity during pregnancy, based on information collected by interviews or questionnaires (Borodulin et al., 2008; Evenson et al., 2004; Evenson & Wen, 2010; Petersen et al., 2005). The guidelines from the ACOG and from the Center for Controlled Disease (CDC)/American College of Sports Medicine (ACSM) both suggest 30 minutes or more of moderate-intensity activity on most of the days of the week, but differ on the type of activity, as guidelines for ACOG include only exercise and guidelines from CDC/ACSM include any type of physical activity. If the recommendations for physical activity were based on the ACOG guidelines, only 3% of pregnant women meet the recommendations (Borodulin et al., 2008). If the recommendations for physical activity were based on the CDC/ACSM guidelines, approximately 15% of pregnant women meet the recommendations (Borodulin et al., 2008; Evenson et al., 2004; Evenson & Wen, 2010; Petersen et al., 2005). In Spain, 20% of women comply with ACOG criteria whereas 70% comply with CDC/ACSM criteria (Amezcua-Prieto et al., 2010).

In summary, most women are physically inactive during pregnancy. This may be contributing to excessive GWG given that women who are meeting the recommendations for exercise during pregnancy are more likely to achieve appropriate GWG (Cohen et al., 2010). Moreover, given the clear association between physical inactivity during the perinatal period and risk for impaired glucose metabolism, physical inactivity may be contributing to the 10 to 100% increase in GDM prevalence observed in several race/ethnic groups during the past 20 years (Dabelea et al., 2005; Ferrara, 2007; Getahun et al., 2008).

3. Exercise as an adjunctive therapy for gestational diabetes mellitus management

3.1 Conventional management of gestational diabetes mellitus

The primary management for women with GDM is control of energy intake, usually referred to as medical nutrition therapy (MNT) (Metzger, 2006). As a dietary intervention, the goals of MNT are to provide adequate nutrition for the mother and fetus, provide sufficient calories for appropriate maternal weight gain, maintain normoglycemia, and avoid ketosis (Franz et al., 2002). The dietary plan suggested by a registered dietitian usually includes eating smaller meals more often, more choices of complex carbohydrates with a low glycemic index, and the elimination of high glycemic foods, including carbonated beverages, sweets, and cake (CDA, 2008). Self-capillary glucose monitoring using a glucometer may be recommended up to seven times per day. The goal of monitoring is to maintain glucose concentrations in acceptable ranges. The Canadian Diabetes Association (CDA) recommends maintaining the following capillary blood glucose values: pre-prandial glucose < 5.3 mmol/L, 1-hour post-prandial glucose < 7.8 mmol/L, and 2-hour post-prandial glucose < 6.7 mmol/L. The Fifth International Workshop-Conference on Gestational Diabetes Mellitus guidelines are the same (Metzger et al., 2007). If after 2 weeks of MNT, failure to control capillary glucose concentrations will progress to management of glycemia by insulin injections. It is imperative that maternal blood glucose be maintained below these values, either with MNT plus insulin injections or MNT and lifestyle changes. The type and amount of insulin injected is beyond the scope of this article but depends on medical intervention and management (Metzger et al., 2007).

3.2 Exercise/lifestyle management for women with gestational diabetes mellitus

Exercise has long been accepted as an adjunctive intervention in the management of diabetes in non pregnant individuals (ADA, 2011; CDA, 2008; Colberg et al., 2010). In type 2 diabetic individuals, exercise has been reported to improve insulin sensitivity and insulin-stimulated muscle glucose uptake (Kennedy et al., 1999), to have a positive effect on glycemic control and to decrease cardiovascular risk (Kavookjian et al., 2007). However, there is still controversy regarding the benefits of exercise in improving glycemic control in GDM women, despite endorsements by professionnal organisations. The ACOG (ACOG, 2001) suggests that "women with GDM who lead an active lifestyle should be encouraged to continue a program of exercise approved for pregnancy." The American Diabetes Association (ADA) (ADA, 2004) suggests that "women without medical or obstetrical contraindications be encouraged to start or continue a program of moderate exercise as part of treatment for GDM." The CDA (CDA, 2008) suggests that "physical activity should be encouraged, with the frequency, type, duration and intensity tailored to individual obstetric risk." The recommendation from the Fifth International Workshop-Conference on GDM suggests "planned physical activity of 30 minutes/day is recommended ... Advising GDM patients to walk briskly or do arm exercises while seated in a chair for at least 10 minutes after each meal accomplishes this goal" (Metzger et al., 2007).

Evidence-based studies determining the frequency, intensity, time, and type of activity are needed to provide the best possible outcomes for women with GDM. When exercise was evaluated for controlling blood glucose concentrations or for delaying or preventing insulin therapy, the results were discordant. In the recent ACSM/ADA joint position statement, level of evidence concerning the effect of physical activity to control GDM was non-existent for the ADA, and weak for the ACSM (Colberg et al., 2010). These mixed results could be due to the non-randomization of the subject pool, the different anthropometric characteristics of the women, small sample sizes, lack of well-controlled or reported exercise intensity, the differences in exercise modalities, or questionable compliance to the exercise program. Consequently, because of lack of consistent evidence regarding the benefits of exercise in improving glycemic control in GDM women, exercise remains an adjunctive therapy.

The acute effect of exercise on glucose excursion has been evaluated by several authors (Table 1). Avery and Walker (2001) reported that a single 30-minute bout of exercise on a cycle ergometer at 35% or 55% of maximum oxygen consumption ($VO_{2\ max}$) improved glucose excursion compared with rest in women with GDM (Avery & Walker, 2001). Garcia-Patterson et al. found similar results, showing that light postprandial walking at 2.5 km/h decreased glucose excursion in GDM women (Garcia-Patterson et al., 2001). Lesser et al. (1996) determined the effects of a single bout of stationary cycling for 30 minutes at 60% $VO_{2\ max}$, comparing six GDM women to five normal glycemic pregnant women. The effects of a mixed meal 14 hours after the exercise bout were examined. In contrast to the above studies, no improvement in glucose excursion due to the exercise was found in the GDM women. This could be due to a mixed meal being used in the acute experiment and because measurements occurred 14 hours after the exercise bout.

The chronic effect of exercise for controlling blood glucose concentrations has also been investigated (Table 2). A 6-week arm ergometry exercise program was successful in normalizing fasted and 1-h plasma glucose concentrations and glycosylated hemoglobin (HbA1c) in GDM women randomized to diet therapy plus exercise compared with diet therapy alone (Jovanovic-Peterson et al., 1991). The exercise program consisted of 20 minutes of arm ergometry, three times per week, at an intensity less than or equal to 50% $VO_{2\ max}$. The results of this study gave rise to the recommendation of arm exercise for GDM women mentioned above. In contrast to the above studies, Bung et al. (Bung et al., 1991) randomized GDM women into a group with diet and insulin therapy or diet and exercise. The exercise program consisted of stationary cycle ergometry (50% $VO_{2\ max}$) for 45 minutes (three 15-minute bouts with two rests), three times per week. Because no differences in

References	Population	Intervention program	Gestational age	Main findings
(Lesser et al., 1996)	N=11: 6 GDM, 5 NGT Ethnicity: na Pre-pregnancy BMI (kg/m²): NGT=24.3±0.9 GDM=25.9±1.8 Age (years): NGT=23.7±20 GDM=27.6±2.8	Control situation Standardized breakfast, followed by blood samples. Exercise situation Intensity: 60% $VO_{2\,max}$ Duration: 30 min Type: stationary cycle. Exercise performed 14 h before standardized breakfast, followed by blood samples.	28-38 w of gestation	Similar mean values for fasting glucose, peak glucose, area under the glycemic curve with vs without exercise. Similarly, plasma insulin levels did not differ between protocols for either group of subjects. Not successful
(Avery & Walker, 2001)	N=13, GDM Ethnicity: na Pre-pregnancy BMI (kg/m²): 29.0±7.4 Age (years): 31.9±3.6	Control situation Remained seated for 2h30 Exercise situation Intensity: 35% and 55% $VO_{2\,max}$ Duration: 30 min Type: stationary cycle. The women exercised at the two intensities for 30 min and rested for 2 h after each session.	30-34 w of gestation	Blood glucose levels were significantly different after 30 min of rest, low- and moderate-intensity exercise: Rest: 5.2 mmol/L Low: 4.3mmol/L Mod: 3.9 mmol/L. Successful
(Garcia-Patterson et al., 2001)	N=20, GDM Ethnicity: na Pre-pregnancy BMI: na Age (years): 33.5±4.6	Control situation remained seated for 2h after a standard breakfast. Exercise situation walked self-paced (2.5 km/h) in the 1st hour after breakfast and remained seated during the 2nd hour.	30.7±5.5 w of gestation	During control situation, higher 1-h postprandial blood glucose (p=0.001) and 1-h blood glucose excursion (p=0.001) compared to exercise situaton. Successful

NGT – normal glycemia; BMI – body mass index.

Table 1. Summary of studies using acute exercise to change blood glucose concentrations in women with gestational diabetes mellitus (GDM).

glycemic control were found between groups, the authors suggested that exercise may provide avoidance of insulin therapy through an increase in insulin sensitivity. In another study, GDM women were randomized to a partial home-based exercise program (70% of estimated maximal heart rate) and compared with GDM women with no structured exercise program (Avery et al., 1997). Although the exercise program improved the cardiorespiratory fitness of the GDM women, glucose excursion was not different compared with the women with no structured exercise program (Avery et al., 1997). More recently, Artal et al. (2007) randomized obese GDM women into MNT plus exercise (60% $VO_{2\ max}$) or MNT alone. Results showed that the MNT plus exercise group limited GWG and had no adverse pregnancy outcomes. The authors concluded that placing obese women with GDM on a lifestyle intervention strategy of weight gain restriction may optimize pregnancy outcomes and impact future weight management behaviors. Using a different exercise modality, de Barros et al. (de Barros et al., 2010) randomized GDM women into a resistance exercise program (elastic band) group or MNT alone group. A reduction in the number of patients who required insulin was obseved in the exercise group compared with the MNT group. Furthermore, the percentage of time spent within the proposed target glucose range was higher in the exercise group compared with the MNT group.

In a 2004 retrospective chart review from London, Canada, assessing conventional management of women diagnosed with GDM, Davenport et al. (2005) showed that by 30 weeks of pregnancy, 62% of these women required insulin therapy (after trying conventional management for 2 weeks after diagnoses). Of this cohort, women with a pre-pregnancy BMI of 25 kg/m^2 or greater were 2.6 times more likely to require insulin therapy than those women with a BMI below 25 kg/m^2 . The average pre-pregnancy BMI of women requiring insulin therapy was 30.6 ± 6.4 kg/m^2. This high incidence of insulin therapy in women with a BMI of 25 kg/m^2 or greater may indicate the need for intensive therapy to delay or prevent insulin usage. In women with an early GDM diagnosis (at 16 to 20 weeks of gestation) who followed a structured walking program (30% HRR), 3-4 times per week in addition to conventional management, only 50% required insulin therapy (Davenport et al., 2005). In another study evaluating 30 GDM women, 10 following conventional management plus a low-intensity walking program (30% HRR, 3-4 times per week) matched by insulin useage to 20 women following conventional management alone, we reported lower mean capillary glucose concentrations at the end of pregnancy (fasting and 1h after meals) in the exercising group (Davenport et al., 2008b). The lower glucose concentrations were achieved while requiring fewer units of insulin per kg per day. Using a different exercise modality, Brankston et al. (Brankston et al., 2004) randomized GDM women to a group with diet alone or a group of diet plus circuit-type resistance training. The number of women requiring insulin was not different between groups. However, they found that within the diet plus exercise group, 30% of the women who exercised 2-3 times per week were prescribed insulin therapy compared to 67% of those who exercised <2 per week. Moreover, a subgroup analysis that examined only overweight and obese women showed a lower incidence of insulin use, a lower prescription of insulin and a longer delay from diagnosis to the initiation of insulin therapy in the diet plus exercise group.

Taken together, the above results are very encouraging. However, future lifestyle intervention programs are required to confirm these promising results and to determine the frequency, intensity, time, and type of activity that are needed to provide the best possible outcomes for women with GDM.

References	Study type	Population	Intervention program	Length of program	Main findings
(Jovanovic-Peterson et al., 1991)	Randomization: diet (D) vs diet+exercise (D+EX) group	N=19: D=9, D+EX=10 Ethnicity: na Pre-pregnancy BMI (kg/m²): na Age (years): D=31.1±2.8 D+EX=29.5±2.5	Diet 24 to 30 kcal/kg/24 h; 40% CHO, 20% P, 40% F Exercise Freq: 3/week Intensity: 50% VO_2max Duration: 20 min Type: arm ergometry	6 weeks	Lower HbA1C, fasting and 1-hour plasma glucose concentrations in D+EX group compared to D group ($p<0.001$ for all). Successful
(Bung et al., 1991)	Randomization: diet+exercise (D+EX) vs diet+insulin (D+I) group	N=34: D+EX=17, D+I=17 Ethnicity: Hispanic Pre-pregnancy BMI (kg/m²): na Age (years): D+EX=31.0±4.5 D+I=32.0±5.7	Diet 30 kcal/kg/day Exercise Freq: 3/week Intensity: 50% $VO2_{max}$ Duration: 45 min (3x15 min) Type: stationary cycle	From diagnosis (30±2 w of gestation) to delivery	No differences in glycemic control between D+EX and D+I groups. Similar maternal and neonatal outcomes between groups. Successful
(Avery et al., 1997)	Randomization: exercise (EX) vs control (CON) groups	N=29: EX=15, CON=14 Ethnicity: Caucasian Pre-pregnancy BMI (kg/m²): EX=28.4±7.6 CON=25.5±5.5 Age (years): EX=32.2±4.9 CON=30.4±5.1	Exercise Freq: 3-4/week (2 supervised) Intensity: 70% (220-age) Duration: 30 min (including 5 min warm-up and cool-down) Type: stationary cycle or walking	From <34 w of gestation to delivery	No difference in HbA1C and insulin usage among EX and CON groups. Similar infant birth weight and incidence of hypoglycemia between groups. Not successful
(Brankston et al., 2004)	Randomization: diet (D) vs diet+exercise (D+EX) group	N=32: D=16, D+EX=16 Ethnicity: na, from Canada Pre-pregnancy BMI (kg/m²): D=28.0±5.7 D+EX=25.9±3.4 Age (years): D=31.3±5.0 D+EX=30.5±4.4	Diet 40% CHO, 20% P, 40% F. 3 meals and 3 snacks. Exercise Freq: 3/week Intensity: <140bpm Type: Circuit-type resistance training.	From 26-32 w of gestation to delivery	Within D+EX group, 30% of the women who exercised 2-3 per week were prescribed insulin therapy compared to 67% of those who exercised <2 per week. In overweight women only, lower incidence of insulin use, lower prescription of insulin and longer delay from diagnosis to the initiation of insulin therapy in D+EX vs D group ($p<0.05$). Successful

References	Study type	Population	Intervention program	Length of program	Main findings
(Artal et al., 2007)	Self-enrollement in diet (D) vs diet+exercise (D+EX) groups	N=96: D=57, D+EX=39 Ethnicity: 55-60% caucasian from the US Pre-pregnancy BMI (kg/m^2): ≥ 30 Age (years): D=30.6±5.5 D+EX=32.4±5.3	Diet CHO 40%-45% Exercise Freq: 1/week in lab, unsupervised ex. session at home Intensity: 60% $VO_{2\,peak}$ Duration: 20 min Type: treadmill or stationary cycle	<33 w of gestation until delivery	Lower GWG per week in D+EX group than in D group (0.1±0.4 kg vs 0.3±0.4 kg, p <0.05). Similar pregnancy outcomes between the groups. Successful
(Davenport et al., 2008b)	Exercise (EX) vs conventional management (CM) group -matched by BMI, insulin use -2 CM/EX	N=30: EX=10, CM=20 Ethnicity: na, from Canada Pre-pregnancy BMI (kg/m^2): ≥ 25 Age (years): EX=33.4±3.3 CON=33.3±5.3	Exercise Freq: 3-4/week, Intensity: 30% HRR mild Duration: 25-40 min Type: treadmill	Minimum 6 weeks (from diagnosis to delivery)	Lower mean capillary glucose levels at the end of pregnancy (fasting and 1h after meals) in EX group but not in CM group (p <0.05). Ex group needed less insulin than CM group. Successful
(de Barros et al., 2010)	Randomization: exercise (EX) vs control (CON) group	N=64: EX=32, CON=32 Ethnicity: na, from Brasil Pre-pregnancy BMI (kg/m^2): EX=25.34±4.16 CON=25.39±3.81 Age (years): EX=31.8±4.87 CON=32.40±5.40	Exercise Freq: 3/week (2 at home) Intensity: "somewhat heavy" exercise perception. Duration: 30-40 min Type: resistance training circuit (elastic band)	24-34 w of gestation to delivery	Reduction in the number of patients who required insulin in the EX (7/32) compared with the CON group (18/32) (p=0.005). The % of time spent within the proposed target glucose range was higher in EX group compared with CON group (p=0.006). Successful

BMI - body mass index; Freq - frequency; CHO - carbohydrate; P - protein; F - fat; na - not given; HRR - heart rate reserve.

Table 2. Summary of studies using the chronic effect of exercise to control blood glucose concentration, to delay or prevent insulin usage in women with gestational diabetes mellitus (GDM).

3.3 Exercise guidelines for women with gestational diabetes mellitus

In 2003, Artal proposed guidelines to develop exercise programs for pregnant women with GDM (Artal, 2003). He suggested 3 to 4 exercise sessions per week, at 50% $VO_{2\,max}$ for three

15-minute bouts with 5-minute rests between each, for a total of 45 minutes. The joint SOGC/CSEP Clinical Practice Guidelines (Davies et al., 2003) provides detailed recommendations regarding frequency, intensity, time, and type of activity for healthy pregnant women. The same recommendations may be used for pregnant women with GDM, except that the intensity of exercise might be adapted and that precaution should be taken, especially for women using insulin. The SOGC/CSEP Clinical Practice Guidelines provides heart-rate zones corresponding to exercise of moderate intensity (i.e. 60-80% of $VO_{2\ max}$). However, this intensity may be too high for pregnant women with GDM who are overweight or obese and possibly sedentary. The ACSM suggested that previously sedentary overweight and obese pregnant women should initiate an aerobic exercise program at an intensity equivalent to 20% to 39% of reserve aerobic capacity ($VO_{2\ reserve}$) (ACSM, 2005). These developed and validated target heart-rate zones based on age, equivalent to 20% to 39% $VO_{2\ reserve}$ are 102 to 124 beats per minute (bpm) for overweight and obese women 20 to 29 years of age and 101 to 120 bpm for those aged 30 to 39 years (Davenport et al., 2008a).

Interestingly, lower-intensity aerobic exercise seems to be more efficient in term of glycemic control than moderate-intensity exercise for pregnant women. Indeed, all intervention studies that used lower-intensity aerobic exercise (i.e. ≤60% $VO_{2\ max}$) were successful in controlling blood glucose concentrations and/or limiting/preventing insulin therapy (Artal et al., 2007; Bung et al., 1991; Davenport et al., 2008b; Jovanovic-Peterson et al., 1991) whereas the only study that used moderate-intensity aerobic exercise (i.e. 70% $VO_{2\ max}$) was not succesfull (Avery et al., 1997). Mottola et al. (1998b) investigated low-risk pregnant women and showed that mild exercise (30% HRR) on a stationary bike was better at promoting glucose tolerance in response to an oral glucose load after exercise than moderate intensity exercise (70% HRR) in late gestational women. Biopsies of the vastus lateralis muscle in these late pregnant women showed that total GLUT4 (glucose transporters sensitive to insulin) was elevated in the mild exercise–trained women (starting at 16–20 weeks gestation until delivery) compared with moderately trained women (Mottola et al., 1998a). Subsequently, when nutritional intake was controlled during pregnancy (to ~ 8350 kJ/day, with 200 g of carbohydrate/day), the combination of nutritional control and mild exercise (30% HRR on a stair climber) was better than mild exercise alone in controlling blood glucose concentrations and preventing excessive weight gain during pregnancy. This effect remained at 2 months postpartum (Mottola et al., 1999).

The above studies provided groundwork for development of a Nutrition and Exercise Lifestyle Intervention Program (NELIP), in which a mild walking program (30% HRR) was combined with nutritional control (8350 kJ/day; 200 g of carbohydrate/day) for women at risk for GDM (Sopper et al., 2004). Preliminary results are encouraging, in that women at risk for GDM did not develop this disease while on NELIP (N = 23), excessive weight gain was prevented, and normal glucose tolerance remained at 2 months postpartum (Batada et al., 2003). In addition, pregnant women at risk for GDM on NELIP maintained an insulin sensitivity index similar to those at low risk for GDM, and none developed GDM (Mottola et al., 2005b). It is suggested that overweight women at risk for GDM can be given a NELIP at 16 weeks of pregnancy to maintain insulin sensitivity and glucose excursion and to prevent excessive weight gain and GDM. Assessment of HbA 1c in these women also showed values well below the diabetic range (Mottola et al., 2005a). Studies conducted by our lab suggest that mild exercise, regardless of modality (bike, stair climber, or walking), may be a key factor—in combination with nutritional control—in helping women at risk for GDM and those women diagnosed with GDM, regulate blood glucose concentrations and prevent excessive weight gain during pregnancy.

4. Summary and recommendations

Obesity and type 2 diabetes are reaching epidemic proportions in society today and women of childbearing age are at risk for developing these diseases because of excessive weight gain during pregnancy and weight retention after birth. If modifiable risk factors for developing diabetes during pregnancy, such as preventing excessive weight gain and preserving glucose tolerance, can be reduced by incorporating physical activity, then exercise can be used as a powerful tool to reduce the diabetes and obesity epidemics in successive generations. Unfortuately, researchers have not be able to suggest an evidence-based program with guidelines for frequency, intensity, time and type of activity (FITT principal for exercise presciption) that would produce the best possible outcomes for women with GDM. Although preliminary results are encouraging, exercise is still considered an adjunctive therapy, and the true effectiveness of a specific exercise program in controlling glucose excursion and reducing the incidence of insulin therapy remains untapped.

Based on the literature reviewed, it is suggested that in using the FITT principal of exercise prescription, women who are at risk for or who have been diagnosed with GDM, should engage in activity at a frequency of 3-4 times per week, for at least 25 minutes each session, at a mild intensity (walking pace), building to 40 minutes, would be sufficient to provide health benefits. In addition, it is suggested that if pedometers are available, 10,000 steps per day may also regulate glucose metabolism. If women with GDM are overweight or obese, a target heart rate of 102-124 beats per minute (20 to 29 years of age) and 101 to 120 beats per minute (30 to 39 years of age) may also be used to monitor intensity. Continuing research is necessary in this important field especially if new stringent cut-offs for diagnoses of GDM are adopted as guidelines, as they will cause a higher prevalance of GDM, increasing the cost of medical care. Prevention of GDM by adoption of a healthy lifestyle and active living may be key.

5. Acknowledgements

The authors acknowledge funding sources: Canadian Institute of Health Research and the Rx & D Health Research Foundation of Canada, the Lawson Foundation, and the MollyTowell Research Foundation. Dr. Ruchat is funded by a Canadian Diabetes Association Postdoctoral Fellowship Award.

6. References

American College of Obstetricians and Gynecologists (ACOG). 2001. Practice Bulletin. Clinical management guidelines for obstetrician-gynecologists. Number 30, September. Gestational diabetes. *Obstet Gynecol*. 98:525-38.

American College of Obstetricians and Gynecologists (ACOG). 2002. Exercise during pregnancy and the postpartum period. *Obstet Gynecol.* 99:171-3.

American College of Sports Medicine (ACSM). 2005. *Guidelines for exercise testing and exercise prescription.* 7th edition. Lippincott Williams & Wilkins, Philadelphia.

American Diabetes Association (ADA). 2004. Gestational diabetes mellitus. *Diabetes Care.* 27 Suppl 1:S88-90.

American Diabetes Association (ADA). 2011. Standards of medical care in diabetes--2011. *Diabetes Care.* 34 Suppl 1:S11-61.

Ahlsson, F., Diderholm, B., Jonsson, B., Nordén-Lindberg, S., Olsson, R., Ewald, U., Forslund, A., Stridsberg, M., and Gustafsson, J. 2010. Insulin resistance, a link between maternal overweight and fetal macrosomia in nondiabetic pregnancies. *Horm Res Paediatr.* 74:267-74.

Amezcua-Prieto, C., Lardelli-Claret, P., Olmedo-Requena, R., Mozas-Moreno, J., Bueno-Cavanillas, A., and Jimenez-Moleon, J.J. 2010. Compliance with leisure-time physical activity recommendations in pregnant women. *Acta Obstet Gynecol Scand.* Dec 7.

Artal, R. 2003. Exercise: the alternative therapeutic intervention for gestational diabetes. *Clin Obstet Gynecol.* 46:479-87.

Artal, R., Catanzaro, R.B., Gavard, J.A., Mostello, D.J., and Friganza, J.C. 2007. A lifestyle intervention of weight-gain restriction: diet and exercise in obese women with gestational diabetes mellitus. *Appl Physiol Nutr Metab.* 32:596-601.

Asbee, S., Jenkins, T., Butler, J., White, J., Elliot, m., and Rutledge, A. 2009. Preventing excessive weight gain during pregnancy through dietary and lifestyle counseling: a rondomized controlled trial. *Obstet Gynecol.* 113:305-12.

Avery, M.D., Leon, A.S., and Kopher, R.A. 1997. Effects of a partially home-based exercise program for women with gestational diabetes. *Obstet Gynecol.* 89:10-5.

Avery, M.D., and Walker, A.J. 2001. Acute effect of exercise on blood glucose and insulin levels in women with gestational diabetes. *J Matern Fetal Med.* 10:52-8.

Barakat, R., Lucia, A., and Ruiz, J.R. 2009. Resistance exercise training during pregnancy and newborn's birth size: a randomised controlled trial. *Int J Obes (Lond).* 33:1048-57.

Bassett, D.R., Jr., Wyatt, H.R., Thompson, H., Peters, J.C., and Hill, J.O. 2010. Pedometer-measured physical activity and health behaviors in U.S. adults. *Med Sci Sports Exerc.* 42:1819-25.

Batada, A., Mottola, M.F., Brun, C., Giroux, I., Hammond, J.M.S., McManus, R., and Lebrun, C. 2003. Effects of a Nutrition, Exercise and Lifestyle Intervention Program (NELIP) on women at risk for gestational diabetes (GDM). *Can J Appl Physiol.* 28:S29.

Borodulin, K.M., Evenson, K.R., Wen, F., Herring, A.H., and Benson, A.M. 2008. Physical activity patterns during pregnancy. *Med Sci Sports Exerc.* 40:1901-8.

Brankston, G.N., Mitchell, B.F., Ryan, E.A., and Okun, N.B. 2004. Resistance exercise decreases the need for insulin in overweight women with gestational diabetes mellitus. *Am J Obstet Gynecol.* 190:188-93.

Briana, D.D., and Malamitsi-Puchner, A. 2009. Reviews: adipocytokines in normal and complicated pregnancies. *Reprod Sci.* 16:921-37.

Brisson, D., Perron, P., Guay, S.P., Gaudet, D., and Bouchard, L. 2010. The "hypertriglyceridemic waist" phenotype and glucose intolerance in pregnancy. *Cmaj.* 182:E722-5.

Buchanan, T.A., and Xiang, A.H. 2005. Gestational diabetes mellitus. *J Clin Invest*. 115:485-91.
Bung, P., Artal, R., Khodiguian, N., and Kjos, S. 1991. Exercise in gestational diabetes. An optional therapeutic approach? *Diabetes*. 40 Suppl 2:182-5.
Callaway, L.K., Prins, J.B., Chang, A.M., and McIntyre, H.D. 2006. The prevalence and impact of overweight and obesity in an Australian obstetric population. *Med J Aust*. 184:56-9.
Carducci Artenisio, A., Corrado, F., Sobbrio, G., Bruno, L., Todisco, L., Galletta, M.G., Galletta, M.R., Campisi, R., and Mancuso, A. 1999. Glucose tolerance and insulin secretion in pregnancy. *Diabetes Nutr Metab*. 12:264-70.
Catalano, P.M. 2010. Obesity, insulin resistance, and pregnancy outcome. *Reproduction*. 140:365-71.
Catalano, P.M., and Ehrenberg, H.M. 2006. The short- and long-term implications of maternal obesity on the mother and her offspring. *Bjog*. 113:1126-33.
Caulfield, L., Witter, F., and Stoltzfus, R. 1996. Determinants of gestational weight gain outside the recommended ranges among black and white women. *Obstet Gynecol*. 87:760-6.
Cavalcante, S.R., Cecatti, J.G., Pereira, R.I., Baciuk, E.P., Bernardo, A.L., and Silveira, C. 2009. Water aerobics II: maternal body composition and perinatal outcomes after a program for low risk pregnant women. *Reprod Health*. 6:1.
Canadian Diabetes Association (CDA) : 2008 Clinical Practice Guidelines for the Prevention and Management of Diabetes in Canada. *Canadian Journal of Diabetes*. 32:S1-S201.
Chu, S.Y., Callaghan, W.M., Kim, S.Y., Schmid, C.H., Lau, J., England, L.J., and Dietz, P.M. 2007. Maternal obesity and risk of gestational diabetes mellitus. *Diabetes Care*. 30:2070-6.
Chu, S.Y., Kim, S.Y., and Bish, C.L. 2009. Prepregnancy obesity prevalence in the United States, 2004-2005. *Matern Child Health J*. 13:614-20.
Claesson, I.M., Sydsjo, G., Brynhildsen, J., Cedergren, M., Jeppsson, A., Nystrom, F., Sydsjo, A., and Josefsson, A. 2008. Weight gain restriction for obese pregnant women: a case-control intervention study. *Bjog*. 115:44-50.
Clapp, J.F., 3rd, Kim, H., Burciu, B., and Lopez, B. 2000. Beginning regular exercise in early pregnancy: effect on fetoplacental growth. *Am J Obstet Gynecol*. 183:1484-8.
Cohen, T.R., Plourde, H., and Koski, K.G. 2010. Are Canadian women achieving a fit pregnancy? A pilot study. *Can J Public Health*. 101:87-91.
Colberg, S.R., Sigal, R.J., Fernhall, B., Regensteiner, J.G., Blissmer, B.J., Rubin, R.R., Chasan-Taber, L., Albright, A.L., and Braun, B. 2010. Exercise and type 2 diabetes: the American College of Sports Medicine and the American Diabetes Association: joint position statement executive summary. *Diabetes Care*. 33:2692-6.
Colley, R.C., Garriguet, D., Janssen, I., Craig, C.L., Clarke, J., and Tremblay, M.S. 2011. Physical activity of Canadian adults: Accelerometer results from the 2007 to 2009 Canadian Health Measures Survey. *Health Reports*. 22.
Collings, C.A., Curet, L.B., and Mullin, J.P. 1983. Maternal and fetal responses to a maternal aerobic exercise program. *Am J Obstet Gynecol*. 145:702-7.
Canadian Society for Exercise Physiology and ParticipACTION. 2010. The Canadian Society for Exercise Physiology and ParticipACTION share new research to inform Canadians of physical activity levels required. Available at: www.csep.ca; www.participaction.com.

Dabelea, D., Snell-Bergeon, J.K., Hartsfield, C.L., Bischoff, K.J., Hamman, R.F., and McDuffie, R.S. 2005. Increasing prevalence of gestational diabetes mellitus (GDM) over time and by birth cohort: Kaiser Permanente of Colorado GDM Screening Program. *Diabetes Care*. 28:579-84.

Davenport, M., Yakubchuk, H., McManus, R., and Mottola, M. 2005. The need for an alternative lifestyle treatment for gestational diabetes. *Can J Appl Physiol*. 30.

Davenport, M.H., Charlesworth, S., Vanderspank, D., Sopper, M.M., and Mottola, M.F. 2008a. Development and validation of exercise target heart rate zones for overweight and obese pregnant women. *Appl Physiol Nutr Metab*. 33:984-9.

Davenport, M.H., Mottola, M.F., McManus, R., and Gratton, R. 2008b. A walking intervention improves capillary glucose control in women with gestational diabetes mellitus: a pilot study. *Appl Physiol Nutr Metab*. 33:511-7.

Davenport, M.H., Steinback, C.D., and Mottola, M.F. 2009. Impact of pregnancy and obesity on cardiorespiratory responses during weight-bearing exercise. *Resp Physiol Neurobiol*. 167:341-347.

Davies, G.A., Maxwell, C., McLeod, L., Gagnon, R., Basso, M., Bos, H., Delisle, M.F., Farine, D., Hudon, L., Menticoglou, S., Mundle, W., Murphy-Kaulbeck, L., Ouellet, A., Pressey, T., Roggensack, A., Leduc, D., Ballerman, C., Biringer, A., Duperron, L., Jones, D., Lee, L.S., Shepherd, D., and Wilson, K. 2010. Obesity in pregnancy. *J Obstet Gynaecol Can*. 32:165-73.

Davies, G.A., Wolfe, L.A., Mottola, M.F., and MacKinnon, C. 2003. Joint SOGC/CSEP clinical practice guideline: exercise in pregnancy and the postpartum period. *Can J Appl Physiol*. 28:330-41.

de Barros, M.C., Lopes, M.A., Francisco, R.P., Sapienza, A.D., and Zugaib, M. 2010. Resistance exercise and glycemic control in women with gestational diabetes mellitus. *Am J Obstet Gynecol*. 203:556 e1-6.

Dempsey, J.C., Butler, C.L., Sorensen, T.K., Lee, I.M., Thompson, M.L., Miller, R.S., Frederick, I.O., and Williams, M.A. 2004a. A case-control study of maternal recreational physical activity and risk of gestational diabetes mellitus. *Diabetes Res Clin Pract*. 66:203-15.

Dempsey, J.C., Sorensen, T.K., Williams, M.A., Lee, I.M., Miller, R.S., Dashow, E.E., and Luthy, D.A. 2004b. Prospective study of gestational diabetes mellitus risk in relation to maternal recreational physical activity before and during pregnancy. *Am J Epidemiol*. 159:663-70.

Després, J.P. 2001. Health consequences of visceral obesity. *Ann Med*. 33:534-41.

Dye, T.D., Knox, K.L., Artal, R., Aubry, R.H., and Wojtowycz, M.A. 1997. Physical activity, obesity, and diabetes in pregnancy. *Am J Epidemiol*. 146:961-5.

Evenson, K.R., Savitz, D.A., and Huston, S.L. 2004. Leisure-time physical activity among pregnant women in the US. *Paediatr Perinat Epidemiol*. 18:400-7.

Evenson, K.R., and Wen, F. 2010. National trends in self-reported physical activity and sedentary behaviors among pregnant women: NHANES 1999-2006. *Prev Med*. 50:123-8.

Ferrara, A. 2007. Increasing prevalence of gestational diabetes mellitus: a public health perspective. *Diabetes Care*. 30 Suppl 2:S141-6.

Flegal, K.M., Carroll, M.D., Ogden, C.L., and Curtin, L.R. 2010. Prevalence and trends in obesity among US adults, 1999-2008. *Jama*. 303:235-41.

Ford, E.S., Li, C., Zhao, G., and Tsai, J. 2010. Trends in obesity and abdominal obesity among adults in the United States from 1999-2008. *Int J Obes (Lond)*. 35:736-43.

Foster-Powell, K.A., and Cheung, N.W. 1998. Recurrence of gestational diabetes. *Aust N Z J Obstet Gynaecol*. 38:384-7.

Franz, M.J., Bantle, J.P., Beebe, C.A., Brunzell, J.D., Chiasson, J.L., Garg, A., Holzmeister, L.A., Hoogwerf, B., Mayer-Davis, E., Mooradian, A.D., Purnell, J.Q., and Wheeler, M. 2002. Evidence-based nutrition principles and recommendations for the treatment and prevention of diabetes and related complications. *Diabetes Care*. 25:148-98.

Garcia-Patterson, A., Martin, E., Ubeda, J., Maria, M.A., de Leiva, A., and Corcoy, R. 2001. Evaluation of light exercise in the treatment of gestational diabetes. *Diabetes Care*. 24:2006-7.

Garshasbi, A., and Faghih Zadeh, S. 2005. The effect of exercise on the intensity of low back pain in pregnant women. *Int J Gynaecol Obstet*. 88:271-5.

Getahun, D., Nath, C., Ananth, C.V., Chavez, M.R., and Smulian, J.C. 2008. Gestational diabetes in the United States: temporal trends 1989 through 2004. *Am J Obstet Gynecol*. 198:525 e1-5.

Gollenberg, A.L., Pekow, P., Bertone-Johnson, E.R., Freedson, P.S., Markenson, G., and Chasan-Taber, L. 2010. Sedentary behaviors and abnormal glucose tolerance among pregnant Latina women. *Med Sci Sports Exerc*. 42:1079-85.

Goodyear, L.J., and Kahn, B.B. 1998. Exercise, glucose transport, and insulin sensitivity. *Annu Rev Med*. 49:235-61.

Gray-Donald, K., Robinson, E., Collier, A., David, K., Renaud, L., and Rodrigues, S. 2000. Intervening to reduce weight gain in pregnancy and gestational diabetes mellitus in Cree communities: an evaluation. *Cmaj*. 163:1247-51.

Guelinckx, I., Devlieger, R., Mullie, P., and Vansant, G. 2010. Effect of lifestyle intervention on dietary habits, physical activity, and gestational weight gain in obese pregnant women: a randomized controlled trial. *Am J Clin Nutr*. 91:373-80.

Hayashi, T., Wojtaszewski, J.F., and Goodyear, L.J. 1997. Exercise regulation of glucose transport in skeletal muscle. *Am J Physiol*. 273:E1039-51.

Hedderson, M.M., Gunderson, E.P., and Ferrara, A. 2010. Gestational weight gain and risk of gestational diabetes mellitus. *Obstet Gynecol*. 115:597-604.

Herring, S.J., Oken, E., Rifas-Shiman, S.L., Rich-Edwards, J.W., Stuebe, A.M., Kleinman, K.P., and Gillman, M.W. 2009. Weight gain in pregnancy and risk of maternal hyperglycemia. *Am J Obstet Gynecol*. 201:61 e1-7.

Hopkins, S.A., Baldi, J.C., Cutfield, W.S., McCowan, L., and Hofman, P.L. 2010. Exercise training in pregnancy reduces offspring size without changes in maternal insulin sensitivity. *J Clin Endocrinol Metab*. 95:2080-8.

Hui, A.L., Ludwig, S.M., Gardiner, P., Sevenhuysen, G., Murray, R., Morris, M., and Shen, G.X. 2006. Community-based exercise and dietary intervention during pregnancy: a pilote study. *Canadian Journal of Diabetes*. 30:169-175.

Inoue, S., Takamiya, T., Yoshiike, N., and Shimomitsu, T. 2006. Physical activity among the Japanese: results of the National Health and Nutrition Survey. In *Proceedings of the International Congress on Physical Activity and Public Health*. US Department of Health and Human Services, Atlanta (GA).

Institute of Medicine (IOM). 1990. *Nutrition During Pregnancy. Part I, Weight Gain.* Washington, DC: National Academy Press.

Jovanovic-Peterson, L., Peterson, C.M., Reed, G.F., Metzger, B.E., Mills, J.L., Knopp, R.H., and Aarons, J.H. 1991. Maternal postprandial glucose levels and infant birth weight: the Diabetes in Early Pregnancy Study. The National Institute of Child Health and Human Development--Diabetes in Early Pregnancy Study. *Am J Obstet Gynecol.* 164:103-11.

Kahn, S.E., Hull, R.L., and Utzschneider, K.M. 2006. Mechanisms linking obesity to insulin resistance and type 2 diabetes. *Nature.* 444:840-6.

Kavookjian, J., Elswick, B.M., and Whetsel, T. 2007. Interventions for being active among individuals with diabetes: a systematic review of the literature. *Diabetes Educ.* 33:962-88; discussion 989-90.

Kennedy, J.W., Hirshman, M.F., Gervino, E.V., Ocel, J.V., Forse, R.A., Hoenig, S.J., Aronson, D., Goodyear, L.J., and Horton, E.S. 1999. Acute exercise induces GLUT4 translocation in skeletal muscle of normal human subjects and subjects with type 2 diabetes. *Diabetes.* 48:1192-7.

Kieffer, E., Carman, W., Gillespie, B., Nolan, G., Worley, S., and Guzman, J. 2001. Obesity and gestational diabetes among African-American women and Latinas in Detroit: implications for disparities in women's health. *J Am Med Women Assoc.* 56:181-7.

Kim, S., Dietz, P., England, L., Morrow, B., and Callaghan, W. 2007. Trends in pre-pregnancy obesity in nine states, 1993-2003. *Obesity (Silver Spring).* 15:986-93.

Kim, S.Y., England, L., Wilson, H.G., Bish, C., Satten, G.A., and Dietz, P. 2010. Percentage of gestational diabetes mellitus attributable to overweight and obesity. *Am J Public Health.* 100:1047-52.

Kinnunen, T.I., Pasanen, M., Aittasalo, M., Fogelholm, M., Hilakivi-Clarke, L., Weiderpass, E., and Luoto, R. 2007. Preventing excessive weight gain during pregnancy - a controlled trial in primary health care. *Eur J Clin Nutr.* 61:884-91.

Koivisto, V.A., Yki-Jarvinen, H., and DeFronzo, R.A. 1986. Physical training and insulin sensitivity. *Diabetes Metab Rev.* 1:445-81.

LaCoursiere, D.Y., Bloebaum, L., Duncan, J.D., and Varner, M.W. 2005. Population-based trends and correlates of maternal overweight and obesity, Utah 1991-2001. *Am J Obstet Gynecol.* 192:832-9.

Lean, M.E., Han, T.S., and Morrison, C.E. 1995. Waist circumference as a measure for indicating need for weight management. *Bmj.* 311:158-61.

Lesser, K.B., Gruppuso, P.A., Terry, R.B., and Carpenter, M.W. 1996. Exercise fails to improve postprandial glycemic excursion in women with gestational diabetes. *J Matern Fetal Med.* 5:211-7.

Lindholm, E.S., Norman, M., Kilander, C.P., and Altman, D. 2010. Weight control program for obese pregnant women. *Acta Obstet Gynecol Scand.* 89:840-3.

Lipscombe, L.L., and Hux, J.E. 2007. Trends in diabetes prevalence, incidence, and mortality in Ontario, Canada 1995-2005: a population-based study. *Lancet.* 369:750-6.

Liu, J.H., Laditka, J.N., Mayer-Davis, E.J., and Pate, R.R. 2008. Does physical activity during pregnancy reduce the risk of gestational diabetes among previously inactive women? *Birth.* 35:188-95.

Liu, J.H., Mayer-Davis, E.J., Pate, R.R., Gallagher, A.E., and Bacon, J.L. 2010. Physical activity during pregnancy is associated with reduced fasting insulin--the Pilot Pregnancy and Active Living Study. *J Matern Fetal Neonatal Med.* 23:1249-52.

Lowe, L.P., Metzger, B.E., Lowe, W.L., Jr., Dyer, A.R., McDade, T.W., and McIntyre, H.D. 2010. Inflammatory mediators and glucose in pregnancy: results from a subset of the Hyperglycemia and Adverse Pregnancy Outcome (HAPO) Study. *J Clin Endocrinol Metab.* 95:5427-34.

Lowell, H., and Miller, D. 2010. Weight gain during pregnancy: Adherence to Health Canada's guidelines. Statistics Canada. Health Reports, Vol. 21, no. 2.

Madden, S.G., Loeb, S.J., and Smith, C.A. 2008. An integrative literature review of lifestyle interventions for the prevention of type II diabetes mellitus. *J Clin Nurs.* 17:2243-56.

Marquez-Sterling, S., Perry, A.C., Kaplan, T.A., Halberstein, R.A., and Signorile, J.F. 2000. Physical and psychological changes with vigorous exercise in sedentary primigravidae. *Med Sci Sports Exerc.* 32:58-62.

Martin, A.M., Berger, H., Nisenbaum, R., Lausman, A.Y., MacGarvie, S., Crerar, C., and Ray, J.G. 2009. Abdominal visceral adiposity in the first trimester predicts glucose intolerance in later pregnancy. *Diabetes Care.* 32:1308-10.

McCormack, G., Milligan, R., Giles-Corti, B., and Clarkson, J. 2003. Physical Activity Levels of Western Australian Adults: Results from the Adult Physical Activity Survey and pedometer Study, Pert, Western Australia. p. 112. Available from http://www.patf.dpc/wa.gov.au.

Metzger, B.E. 2006. Diet and medical therapy in the optimal management of gestational diabetes mellitus. *Nestle Nutr Workshop Ser Clin Perform Programme.* 11:155-65; discussion 165-9.

Metzger, B.E., Buchanan, T.A., Coustan, D.R., de Leiva, A., Dunger, D.B., Hadden, D.R., Hod, M., Kitzmiller, J.L., Kjos, S.L., Oats, J.N., Pettitt, D.J., Sacks, D.A., and Zoupas, C. 2007. Summary and recommendations of the Fifth International Workshop-Conference on Gestational Diabetes Mellitus. *Diabetes Care.* 30 Suppl 2:S251-60.

Morisset, A.S., Tchernof, A., Dube, M.C., Veillette, J., Weisnagel, S.J., and Robitaille, J. 2011. Weight Gain Measures in Women with Gestational Diabetes Mellitus. *J Womens Health.* 20:375-80.

Mottola, M.F. 2008. The role of exercise in the prevention and treatment of gestational diabetes mellitus. *Curr Diabet Reports. 8:299-304.*

Mottola, M.F. 2009. Exercise prescription for overweight and obese women: pregnancy and postpartum. *Obstet Gynecol Clin N Am.* 36:301-16.

Mottola, M.F, Hammond, J., and McManus, R. 1999. Effects of a controlled nutrition and mild exercise program on glucose metabolism in healthy pregnant women. *Can J Appl Physiol.* 24:468.

Mottola, M.F., and Campbell, M.K. 2003. Activity patterns during pregnancy. *Can J Appl Physiol.* 28:642-53.

Mottola, M.F., Giroux, I., Gratton, R., Hammond, J.A., Hanley, A., Harris, S., McManus, R., Davenport, M.H., and Sopper, M.M. 2010. Nutrition and exercise prevent excess weight gain in overweight pregnant women. *Med Sci Sports Exerc.* 42:265-72.

Mottola, M.F., Lander, S., Giroux, I., Hammond, J.M.S., Lebrun, C., McManus, R., and Sopper, M.M. 2005a. Glucose and insulin responses in women at risk for gestational diabetes mellitus before and after a Nutrition and Exercise Lifestyle Intervention Program (NELIP). *Med Sci Sports Exerc.* 37:S309- S310.

Mottola, M.F., Sopper, M.M., and Vanderspank, D. 2005b. Insulin sensitivity is maintained in late pregnancy among overweight women at risk for gestational diabetes participating in a Nutrition and Exercise Lifestyle Intervention Program (NELIP). *Proceedings of the 48th Annual Meeting of the Canadian Federation of Biological Societies.* 62.

Mottola, M.F., Weis, C.A., Hammond, J.M.S., Bartha, C., Schachter, C.L., and Bonen, A. 1998a. Effects of mild vs. moderate maternal exercise training on GLUT4. *Can J Appl Physiol.* 23:496.

Mottola, M.F., Weis, C.A., Lewis, N.T., Hammond, J.M.S., Bartha, C., Schachter, C.L., Sloboda, D.M., Sirna, K., and Petrik, J. 1998b. Effects of mild vs. moderate maternal exercise on glucose metabolism. *Med Sci Sports Exerc.* 30:S:259.

Nelson, S.M., Matthews, P., and Poston, L. 2009. Maternal metabolism and obesity: modifiable determinants of pregnancy outcome. *Hum Reprod Update.* 16:255-75.

Oken, E., Ning, Y., Rifas-Shiman, S.L., Radesky, J.S., Rich-Edwards, J.W., and Gillman, M.W. 2006. Associations of physical activity and inactivity before and during pregnancy with glucose tolerance. *Obstet Gynecol.* 108:1200-7.

Olson, C.M., and Strawderman, M.S. 2003. Modifiable behavioral factors in a biopsychosocial model predict inadequate and excessive gestational weight gain. *J Am Diet Assoc.* 103:48-54.

Olson, C.M., Strawderman, M.S., and Reed, R.G. 2004. Efficacy of an intervention to prevent excessive gestational weight gain. *Am J Obstet Gynecol.* 191:530-6.

Ong, M.J., Guelfi, K.J., Hunter, T., Wallman, K.E., Fournier, P.A., and Newnham, J.P. 2009. Supervised home-based exercise may attenuate the decline of glucose tolerance in obese pregnant women. *Diabetes Metab.* 35:418-21.

Petersen, A.M., Leet, T.L., and Brownson, R.C. 2005. Correlates of physical activity among pregnant women in the United States. *Med Sci Sports Exerc.* 37:1748-53.

Pole, J.D., and Dodds, L.A. 1999. Maternal outcomes associated with weight change between pregnancies. *Can J Public Health.* 90:233-6.

Polley, B.A., Wing, R.R., and Sims, C.J. 2002. Randomized controlled trial to prevent excessive weight gain in pregnant women. *Int J Obes Relat Metab Disord.* 26:1494-502.

Prevedel, T., Calderon, I., De Conti, M., Consonni, E., and Rudge, M. 2003. Maternal and perinatal effects of hydrotherapy in pregnancy. *RBGO.* 25:53-9.

Rasouli, N., and Kern, P.A. 2008. Adipocytokines and the metabolic complications of obesity. *J Clin Endocrinol Metab.* 93:S64-73.

Royal College of Obstetricians and Gynaecologists (RCOG). 2006. *Exercise in pregnancy.* RCOG Statement No. 4. January 2006, 1-7.

Retnakaran, R., Qi, Y., Sermer, M., Connelly, P.W., Zinman, B., and Hanley, A.J. 2009. Pre-gravid physical activity and reduced risk of glucose intolerance in pregnancy: the role of insulin sensitivity. *Clin Endocrinol (Oxf).* 70:615-22.

Rooney, B.L., Schauberger, C.W., and Mathiason, M.A. 2005. Impact of perinatal weight change on long-term obesity and obesity-related illnesses. *Obstet Gynecol.* 106:1349-56.

Ryder, J.W., Chibalin, A.V., and Zierath, J.R. 2001. Intracellular mechanisms underlying increases in glucose uptake in response to insulin or exercise in skeletal muscle. *Acta Physiol Scand.* 171:249-57.

Saldana, T.M., Siega-Riz, A.M., Adair, L.S., and Suchindran, C. 2006. The relationship between pregnancy weight gain and glucose tolerance status among black and white women in central North Carolina. *Am J Obstet Gynecol.* 195:1629-35.

Santos, I.A., Stein, R., Fuchs, S.C., Duncan, B.B., Ribeiro, J.P., Kroeff, L.R., Carballo, M.T., and Schmidt, M.I. 2005. Aerobic exercise and submaximal functional capacity in overweight pregnant women: a randomized trial. *Obstet Gynecol.* 106:243-9.

Sedaghati, P., Ziaee, V., and Ardjmand, A. 2007. The effect of an ergometric training program on pregnants weight gain and low back pain. *Gazz Med Ital- Arch Sci Med.* 166:209-13.

Shirazian, T., Monteith, S., Friedman, F., and Rebarber, A. 2010. Lifestyle modification program decreases pregnancy weight gain in obese women. *Am J Perinatol.* 27:411-4.

Sopper, M.M., Hammond, J.M.S., Giroux, I., McManus, R., and Mottola, M.F. 2004. Genesis of NELIP: a Nutrition, Exercise and Lifestyle Intervention Program to help prevent excess weight gain and gestational diabetes mellitus in high-risk women. *Can J Diabetes.* 28:296.

Streuling, I., Beyerlein, A., Rosenfeld, E., Hofmann, H., Schulz, T., and von Kries, R. 2010a. Physical activity and gestational weight gain: a meta-analysis of intervention trials. *Bjog.* 118:278-84.

Streuling, I., Beyerlein, A., and von Kries, R. 2010b. Can gestational weight gain be modified by increasing physical activity and diet counseling? A meta-analysis of interventional trials. *Am J Clin Nutr.* 92:678-87.

Stuebe, A., Oken, E., and Gillman, M. 2009. Associations of diet and physical activity during pregnancy with risk for excessive gestational weight gain. *Am J of Obstet Gynecol.* 201:e1-8.

Tobias, D.K., Zhang, C., van Dam, R.M., Bowers, K., and Hu, F.B. 2010. Physical activity before and during pregnancy and risk of gestational diabetes mellitus: a meta-analysis. *Diabetes Care.* 34:223-9.

Tovar, A., Must, A., Bermudez, O.I., Hyatt, R.R., and Chasan-Taber, L. 2009. The impact of gestational weight gain and diet on abnormal glucose tolerance during pregnancy in Hispanic women. *Matern Child Health J.* 13:520-30.

Troiano, R.P., Berrigan, D., Dodd, K.W., Masse, L.C., Tilert, T., and McDowell, M. 2008. Physical activity in the United States measured by accelerometer. *Med Sci Sports Exerc.* 40:181-8.

Tudor-Locke, C., Brashear, M.M., Johnson, W.D., and Katzmarzyk, P.T. 2010. Accelerometer profiles of physical activity and inactivity in normal weight, overweight, and obese U.S. men and women. *Int J Behav Nutr Phys Act.* 7:60.

Tudor-Locke, C., Hatano, Y., Pangrazi, R.P., and Kang, M. 2008. Revisiting "how many steps are enough?" *Med Sci Sports Exerc.* 40:S537-43.

U.S Department of Health and Human Services. 2008. *Physical Activity Guidelines for Americans.* Available at : www.health.gov/paguidelines.

Villamor, E., and Cnattingius, S. 2006. Interpregnancy weight change and risk of adverse pregnancy outcomes: a population-based study. *Lancet.* 368:1164-70.

World health Organisation (WHO). 2010. *Global Recommandations on Physical Activity for Health.* W.H.O. Geneva.

Yates, T., Khunti, K., Bull, F., Gorely, T., and Davies, M.J. 2007. The role of physical activity in the management of impaired glucose tolerance: a systematic review. *Diabetologia*. 50:1116-26.

Yeo, S. 2009. Adherence to walking or stretching, and risk of preeclampsia in sedentary pregnant women. *Res Nurs Health*. 32:379-90.

Zhang, C., Solomon, C.G., Manson, J.E., and Hu, F.B. 2006. A prospective study of pregravid physical activity and sedentary behaviors in relation to the risk for gestational diabetes mellitus. *Arch Intern Med*. 166:543-8.

21

Gestational Diabetes Mellitus After Delivery

Aleida M. Rivas
Diabetes and Pregnancy Unit,
University of Carabobo - Dr. Enrique Tejera Hospital, Valencia
Venezuela

1. Introduction

Gestational Diabetes Mellitus (GDM) bring repercussions not only during pregnancy and delivery, but also in the future, with implications for Public Health. Nonetheless, after delivery, there is a tendency of the health team and medical institutions to relax the care given to women with GDM, probably due to the fact that their blood glucose values usually return rapidly to their normal level, wasting in this way the opportunity of preserving the health status of these relatively young group of women with a high risk of cardiovascular events, greatly due to the subsequent development of type 2 diabetes (Bentley-Lewis, 2009; Shah et al., 2008). In recent years an increase in the prevalence of GDM in different populations and ethnic groups has been observed (Dabelea et al., 2005; Hunt & Schuller, 2007). Being GDM, very frequently, a diabetes precursor, a large number of fertile women will be increasingly subjected to a higher risk of developing it in a variable time, generally during middle age. This implies a long period of potential risk for chronic micro and macroangiophatic complications, with implied high social and economical costs.

Women with GDM constitute an excellent target for applying diabetes preventive measures and its comorbidities. In this sense, a continuous and prolonged post-partum follow-up is recommended with two main objectives: to implement non-pharmacological and pharmacological preventive measures, whose efficiency has been shown in some studies (Buchanan et al., 2002; Ratner et al., 2008), and also to carry out early detection of diabetes and other cardiovascular risk factors by guidelines that unfortunately, vary from one organization to another (Asociación Latinoamericana de Diabetes (ALAD), 2008: Metzger et al., 2007: National Institute for Health and Clinical Excellence (NICE), 2008), partly explaining low compliance rates and short duration of follow-ups, even in developed countries (Blatt et al., 2011; Dinh et al., 2003; Ferrara et al., 2009; Kim et al., 2007a). Moreover, maternal breastfeeding stimulus and the most adequate contraceptive method are included (Kim, 2009, 2010; Kitzmiller et al., 2007). More recently, the association between GDM with periodontal disease has been demonstrated, therefore it was considered pertinent to include oral health measures (Friedlander et al., 2007; Novak et al., 2006).

During pregnancy, women with GDM require education under the premise that glucose intolerance is not always transitory, but that at any time after delivery it can become permanent, in order to increase awareness of the importance of postpartum follow-up, during which educational strategies aimed at correcting knowledge deficits on healthy life-styles are studied in-depth (Rivas et al., 2010a); moreover, to overcome difficulties found in substituting inadequate habits in practice (Smith et al., 2005; Stage et al., 2004). To do so, it

seems essential to incorporate profound changes in the quality of life of the population that favor individual life-style changes. However, for a postpartum follow-up program to be successful, it is also important to amend existing weaknesses regarding knowledge and motivation of the interdisciplinary team responsible for health care in this area (Almario et al., 2008; Clark et al., 2003), and also, to provide health care services with easy access for all women with previous GDM (Kim et al., 2007a).
This chapter will expound on focusing the future risks of women with GDM, as well as the basic aspects regarding early detection and prevention of diabetes and other cardiovascular risk factors.

2. Maternal risks

Maternal GDM repercussions in the future include an increased risk of developing GDM in subsequent pregnancies (Moses, 1997a), type 2 diabetes (Kim et al., 2002) and other cardiovascular risk factors such as obesity (Yun et al., 2007), dyslipidemia (Meyer-Seifer, 1996) and hypertension (Gonçalves et al., 2005), which show up isolated or grouped in the Metabolic Syndrome (Madarász et al., 2008). Generally, they are accompanied by some degree of vascular, fibrinolytic and inflammatory dysfunction (Farhan et al., 2006¸ Heitritter, 2005). Furthermore, the risk of other clinical conditions like polycystic ovary (PCO) (Kousta et al., 2000), periodontal disease (Xiong et al., 2006) and depression (34 Kozhimannil et al., 2009) is increased (Table 1).

- GDM in subsequent pregnancies
- Type 1 diabetes
- Type 2 diabetes
- Metabolic Syndrome
- Vascular abnormalities
- Cardiovascular Disease
- Polycystic ovaries
- Periodontal Disease
- Depression

Table 1. Maternal Risks in women with Previous GDM

2.1 GDM in subsequent pregnancies

GDM recurrence occurs due to an abnormal glucose tolerance state that aggravates primarily due to physiological demands and hormonal changes of pregnancy itself, but may also show the presence of type 2 diabetes, that was not diagnosed between pregnancies, since a postpartum diabetes screening was not carried out.
GDM recurrence rates in subsequent pregnancies show contradictory results, varying in different studies according to the population studied, GDM diagnostic criteria used, diabetes postpartum screenings and the exclusion or not of the preexisting diabetes proportion. In a review, it was found that they ranged from 30 and 84%, being White women rates <40% and in other ethnic groups that include African-American, Latin-American an Asian women >50%, constituting ethnic group different from Caucasian, the most consistent predictor of GDM recurrence (Kim et al., 2007b).Other associations have been reported with GDM recurrence such as fat intake (Moses et al., 1997b), pre-pregnancy

maternal weight (Macneill et al., 2001) and the presence of impaired fasting glucose (IFG) or impaired glucose tolerance (IGT) in two-month postpartum screenings (Kwak et al., 2008).
GDM risk in a second pregnancy has been found nearly ten-folds higher among women with previous GDM than in women without this family history, 41.3% and 4.2%, respectively. The risk increases with the number of previous GDM episodes and thus, with the third pregnancy, GDM recurrence was more marked when GDM had been diagnosed during the two previous pregnancies (Getahun et al., 2010).
A new GDM pregnancy is not associated itself to a risk increase of type 2 diabetes in women with GDM history (Russel et al., 2008). Nonetheless, the absence of recurrent GDM in a subsequent pregnancy may show a decrease in the risk of developing type 2 diabetes (Retnakaran et al., 2011).

2.2 Diabetes

There is strong evidence proving that women with GDM show a high risk of developing diabetes through their lives (Damm et al., 2003). Even though the highest frequency corresponds to type 2 diabetes, type 1 diabetes may also occur, whose proportion will vary depending on the population studied (Järvelä et al., 2006).

2.2.1 Type 1 diabetes

For many decades GDM has been acknowledged as a heterogeneous alteration, where autoimmunity against beta cells constitutes the pathogenic basis in a small group of patients, who show a higher risk of developing type 1 diabetes during pregnancy or after delivery (Mauricio et al., 1996).
In women with GDM, the determination of different specific antibodies against pancreatic beta cells, like antibodies to islet cells (ICA), glutamic acid decarboxilase antibodies (GADA), tyrosine phosphatase tyrosine (IA-2A), and most recently, GAD 65, proven pre-clinical markers of type 1 diabetes (Mitchell et al., 2000; Murgia et al., 2008), has allowed to know that autoimmune GDM corresponds to 10% of GDM cases in Caucasian women and contributes to a peculiar and complex pre-diabetic state, with a high risk for progressing to type 1 diabetes and to a latent autoimmune diabetes of adulthood (LADA) (de Leiva et al., 2007; Lapolla et al., 2009). The risk increases with the number of antibodies present (Füchtenbusch et al., 1997), and is higher during the first postpartum years (Nilsson et al., 2007). In studies carried out on women with GDM that show positive antibodies, it was found that they were younger, showed lower body mass index (BMI), less proportion of family members with diabetes, less abdominal circumference, and lower levels of plasmatic insulin than in those women without antibodies. Moreover, they had gained less weight during pregnancy and had required insulin treatment in a higher proportion (Bo et al., 2003). Non-Caucasian women with GDM have been less studied looking for autoimmune markers, being found in some cases, similar GADA incidence than in Caucasian women (Kousta et al., 2001), while in other studies, lower incidences have been obtained, but resulting likewise, the presence of antibodies against beta cells, an indicator of future type 1 diabetes, even at early stages after delivery (Yu et al, 2009).
The presence of antibodies in women with GDM shows immune-mediated pancreas destruction that causes a deficit in insulin secretion and development of type 1 diabetes. Therefore, the importance of making a type 1 diabetes diagnose as soon as possible, to apply therapeutic measures that allow preserving the endogenous insulin secretion and to reach

an adequate metabolic control that lowers the risk of poor pregnancy results (Wucher et al., 2011) and of micro-vascular maternal complications in the future. Thus, in high risk populations of women with GDM, type 1 diabetes screenings must be carried out, looking for antibodies against beta cells.

2.2.2 Type 2 diabetes

Numerous epidemiological data suggest an association between GDM and type 2 diabetes, showing correspondence in both prevalences in a given population. These two disorders share metabolic aspects, risk factors and genetic susceptibility (Ben-Haroush et al., 2004).

Physiopathological changes that occur in GDM, insulin resistance and the relative insulin deficiency due to the pancreatic beta cells deterioration, are similar to processes that occur in other pre-diabetic states of type 2 diabetes (Harlev & Wiznitzer, 2010) and they persist after pregnancy (Kousta et al., 2003). GDM and type 2 diabetes also have in common risk factors like BMI increase, family history of diabetes, increased age, Asian and African ethnic origin (Kim et al., 2002). Likewise, evidence has been gathered regarding that GDM susceptibility, as well as type 2 diabetes, has a genetic component where pregnancy could act as an environmental stressor that catalyses progression to a diabetic state in women with genetic predisposition. It is possible that both conditions are multigenic diseases in whose etiology interact variations of multiple genes with environmental factors, but no definite conclusions can yet be established, since the study on GDM genetics is on its initial stages and also because most researches have been carried out on a small group of White ethnic women (Robitaille & Grant, 2008), finding in some of them, that alleles associated to an increase of developing type 2 diabetes, are elevated in women with previous GDM (Lauenborg et al., 2009).

Cumulative incidence of type 2 diabetes varies widely in different reports, with a range of 2.6 to 70% in studies that examined women between 6 weeks postpartum to 28 years postpartum (Kim et al., 2002. During the first months, glucose tolerance abnormalities in women with previous GDM were already found, showing diabetes prevalence rates < 10% in White ethnic women (Pallardo et al., 1999; Feig et al., 2008) and ~10%, or higher in other ethnic groups (Kjos et al., 1990; Lin et al., 2005; Rivas et al., 2007). These rates most probably include women with type 2 diabetes, whose diagnosis had been unnoticed before pregnancy, being impossible to exclude them, due to the GDM definition used worldwide.

Progress to diabetes is strong during the first years after delivery, with an annual rate of 5-10%, reaching ~50% in five years, followed by a slower progression, and appearing a plateau after ten years (Kim et al., 2002; Wollitzer & Jovanovic, 2007). However, more recent studies show that postpartum risk of diabetes in women with DGM increases linearly through the follow-up period, without indication of decrease after five years or plateau evidence of the incidence at ten years postpartum (Feig et al., 2008; Chodick et al.,2010).

It has been estimated that in women with GDM, the risk of developing type 2 diabetes along their lives is almost eight-fold higher than in those women who have not developed it (Chodick et al., 2010; Bellamy et al., 2009). In the well-known study Diabetes Prevention Program (DPP), women with GDM history showed a 74% increased hazard for developing diabetes than women without this history (17.1%/year compared to 9.8%/year, respectively) (Ratner et al., 2008) and, in Australia, it was found that 20-30% of women with type 2 diabetes refer previous GDM (Cheung & Byth, 2003).

Several maternal risk factors have been associated to the conversion rate to diabetes, resulting highly predictive at short and long-term the oral glucose tolerance test (OGTT) values during pregnancy, mainly, fasting plasma glucose (FPG) (Kim et al., 2002; Golden et al., 2009) and in lower proportion, 2-hour glucose values (Golden et al., 2009; Åberg et al., 2002), area under OGTT curve (Golden et al., 2009; Weijers et al., 2006) and the number of OGTT abnormal values (Chodick et al., 2010). It has also been found that insulin therapy during pregnancy predicts future maternal diabetes (Chodick et al., 2010; Catalano et al., 1991) and it is known that weight gain before, during and after pregnancy increases and accelerates the development of type 2 diabetes in women with previous GDM (Metzger et al,. 1993; Baptiste-Roberts et al., 2009; Xiang et al 2010).

Other risk factors of type 2 diabetes in women with DGM have been reported, among them, age, non-Caucasian ethnicity, early GDM onset (Sinha et al,. 2003), length of postpartum period, deterioration of beta cell function and use of progestin-only contraception (Xiang et al 2010, Xiang et al 2006a). A series of modifiable factors like low physical activity, low fruit and vegetable consumption, tobacco habits, low educational instruction, and low family income have also been found associated to the risk of type 2 diabetes in women with GDM history (Yun S et al., 2007). There is less knowledge on other risk factors of diabetes described in recent years in women with GDM, such as alteration of some inflammatory and fibrinolytic dysfunction markers, among them adiponectin decrease (Retnakaran et al. 2010), increase in C-reactive protein (CRP) (Di Benedetto et al., 2005), homocysteine (Cho et al., 2005) and plasminogen activator inhibitor type 1 (PAI-1) (Morimitsu et al., 2007), among others.

2.3 Metabolic syndrome and its components

GDM is a marker for future development of type 2 diabetes and Metabolic Syndrome in the mother, currently acknowledging pregnancy as a window that reveals future metabolic and cardiovascular risks for the mother (Sattar & Greer 2002).

Glucose tolerance abnormalities in postpartum have been associated to other components of the Metabolic Syndrome. General obesity (Vohr & Boney, 2008), visceral obesity (Albareda et al,. 2005) and increases in body fat content, particularly visceral fat (Lim et al., 2007), are more frequent in women with GDM history compared to those in control groups. Also there is a higher risk of high blood pressure (Gonçalves et al., 2005; Wender-Ozegowska et al., 2007) and impairment of lipid profile like high triglycerides and LDL-cholesterol values and low HDL-cholesterol values, even though some results are not always consistent (Wender-Ozegowska et al., 2007; Meyers-Seifer & Vohr, 1996; Rivas et al., 2010b). Frequently, varying abnormalities are found both in insulin sensitivity as well as in the secretion function of pancreatic beta cells (Tura et al., 2008).

The prevalence of the Metabolic Syndrome, regardless of the diagnostic criteria used, is three-fold higher in women with previous GDM than in women without this history and increases seven-fold in obese women (Lauenborg et al., 2005). Pre-pregnancy obesity, OGTT fasting plasma glucose during index pregnancy and postpartum weight gain are predictors of developing Metabolic Syndrome (Akinci et al., 2010).

2.4 Vascular abnormalities

As in other high risk type 2 diabetes groups, in women with previous GDM, apart from abdominal obesity and insulin resistance, vascular abnormalities including impaired vascular reactivity, increased levels of some markers of endothelial activation, fibrinolysis/coagulation and low grade subclinical inflammation have been found (Caballero, 2005).

Among the reported vascular abnormalities are increase of peripheral vascular resistance (Heitritter et al., 2005) and impaired endothelium-dependent vasodilation, assessed at the brachial artery by high resolution ultrasound (Anastasiou etal., 1998), but this finding was not found in another study (Hannemann et al., 2002). On the other hand, serum adiponectin levels, an adipokine with known vascular effects, have been found to be lower in women with GDM during pregnancy and postpartum (Heitritter et al., 2005; Vitoratos et al., 2008a; Costacou et al., 2008). On the contrary, PAI-1 has been found elevated, considered as an expression of fibrinolytic dysfunction (Farhan et al., 2006), and of markers of low-grade sub-clinical inflammation, Interleukin-1beta (IL-1β) has also been found elevated (Vitoratos et al., 2008b), whereas CRP shows contradictory results, since in some studies higher values have been obtained in women with previous GDM than in women with normoglycemic pregnancies (Heitritter et al., 2005; Di Cianni et al., 2007), no differences have been shown in other studies (Thomann et al., 2008) and in some, it is only significant the increase of CRP when diabetes has already been developed (Kim et al., 2008).

2.5 Cardiovascular disease (CVD)

As it has been described previously, women with previous GDM show in higher proportion, compared to women in control groups, numerous cardiovascular risk factors such as abdominal obesity, insulin resistance, abnormal glucose tolerance, dyslipidemia, high blood pressure values, Metabolic Syndrome, impairments of endothelial dysfunction and inflammation markers. For this reason, it has been proposed that these women have higher long-term probabilities of developing CVD (Bentley-Lewis, 2009), showing in an incidence research review that GDM history increases the risk of CVD about 1.7 folds (Verier-Mine, 2010). This topic is of vital importance since CVD, and particularly, coronary artery disease, constitute one of the main causes of mortality and disability in different countries, thus its prevention and early identification in this group of young women may contribute to improve health indicators.

2.6 Polycystic ovaries

The prevalence of PCO has been found elevated in women with previous GDM, showing that both pathologies have common associations like obesity and insulin resistance (Kousta et al., 2000; Koivunen et al., 2001).

2.7 Periodontal disease

Women with GDM have shown higher frequency and severity of periodontal disease during pregnancy and postpartum than women without GDM, after controlling for age, income, smoking, dental calculus (Novak et al., 2006). The prevalence of periodontal disease in women with previous GDM is lower than in non-pregnant women with type 1 and 2 diabetes, but higher than in non-diabetic women and without GDM family history (Xiong et al., 2006). A higher risk of dental caries also seems to exist (Friedlander et al., 2007).

2.8 Stress, anxiety and depression

Pregnancy generally represents an increase in stress and anxiety in all women, therefore, when GDM develops, considered as a high risk pregnancy demanding comprehensive treatment measures and monitoring of metabolic control, stress levels may increase even more (York et al., 1996). However, there are very few studies on this topic. On the other hand, an association between diabetes during pregnancy and prenatal depression in low-income women has been found (Kozhimannil et al., 2009), showing the importance of psycho-social aspects.

3. Detection and prevention of diabetes and other cardiovascular risk factors

Care for women with GDM is extended after delivery in order to assess at an early stage their new metabolic status, and more importantly, to take individual and collective measures that contribute to prevent or at least, retard the progression to diabetes and other cardiovascular risk factors. Thus, it is necessary that health services provide postpartum follow-up programs and motivate women with GDM to attend the activities programmed. Moreover, it is fundamental that the environment surrounding such women promotes life-style changes that not only favor them, but also their family and the rest of the population.

3.1 Postpartum follow-up of women with GDM

For many years the importance of postpartum follow-up of women with GDM has been emphasized (Beischer et al., 1997). More recent findings suggest that it should be extended to women with any abnormal glucose homeostasis level during pregnancy (Retnakaran et al., 2008). Such a follow-up includes the aspects shown in Table 2.

- Diabetes screening
- Detection of cardiovascular risk factors
- Education
- Incentive and facilities for breastfeeding
- Appropriate family planning and contraception
- Oral health measures
- Life-style changes
- **Pharmacologic intervention**

Table 2. Postpartum Follow-up of women with GDM

3.1.1 Diabetes screening

During the immediate post-partum period of patients with GDM, glucose tests are run to detect those few cases where hyperglycemia persists, which mainly correspond to women whose type 2 diabetes had not been detected before pregnancy. The diabetes diagnose is confirmed if FPG is $\geq$ 126 mg/dl (7.0 mmol/l) or if hyperglycemia symptoms and a random plasma glucose $\geq$ 200 mg/dl (11.1 mmol/l) are present (American Diabetes Association (ADA), 2011).

All those women not diagnosed with diabetes are programmed for a diabetes screening between weeks six and twelve of postpartum, due to a high incidence of glucose tolerance abnormalities already detected at that time and also because these results allow identifying women with high risks of developing diabetes during the next fifteen years (Kjos et al., 1995). If diabetes screening is not possible at this time, it must be emphasized in the following weeks. Diabetes screening is carried out with a 75g- 2h- OGTT, of higher sensitivity and less expensive per diabetes case detected than FPG (Ferrara et al., 2009; Kim et al., 2007b). If the results are not compatible with diabetes diagnose, whether they are normal or indicators of IGT, or IFG, the test is repeated the following year and then, annually or every three years, according to the different international scientific associations since regarding periodicity of screening, no current criteria uniformity exists (Metzger et al., 2007, American College of Obstetricians and Gynecologists (ACOG), 2009, Asociación Latinoamericana de Diabetes (ALAD), 2008). It is possible that HbA_{1c} will be recommended in the future for postpartum diabetes screening in women with GDM, but studies on this test have not yet been published.

3.1.2 Detection and treatment of cardiovascular risk factors

Every time diabetes screenings are carried out, for detecting hypertension, obesity and dyslipidemias, women with previous GDM are determined for blood pressure, abdominal circumference, body mass index and triglyceride plasma levels, cholesterol, HDL-c and LDL-c. Determination of insulin levels, insulin-sensitivity indices, markers of endothelial activation, fibrinolysis/coagulation and low grade subclinical inflammation, and other specialized tests are optional in the clinical practice and are reserved in most cases, for research purposes. If the presence of any cardiovascular risk factor is confirmed, the corresponding therapeutic measures are prescribed.

3.1.3 Education

Education, initiated during pregnancy, constitutes the basis for GDM management. It is imparted in theoretical-practical sessions individually or in groups, whose content and strategies take into account the socio-economical and cultural characteristics of the enrolled women. At the postpartum stage, it is directed basically to imparting knowledge on future maternal risks and on their off-spring, as well as to the life-style changes that contribute to prevent or retard diabetes development and its co-morbidities. It has been found that knowledge on these topics is limited in women with GDM, but increases after participating in an educational program imparted by specialized health personnel (Rivas et al., 2010a).

3.1.4 Breastfeeding incentive and facilities

As other women, women with GDM must be actively stimulated for exclusively breastfeeding for the longest period during the first year of their child (Metzger et al., 2007). But in this case, it is paramount to contribute in reducing subsequent risks of obesity and glucose tolerance abnormalities. Even though there is currently no definite conclusion on this (Gouveri et al., 2011), many studies show beneficial results of breastfeeding in women with GDM (Kjos et al., 1993; Gunderson et al., 2010).

3.1.5 Appropriate family planning and contraception

In women with GDM postpartum contraception is recommended (Metzger et al., 2007) in order to prevent a future unplanned pregnancy, with a high risk of developing once more GDM and where teratogenic effects of non-diagnosed diabetes may also be present. There is a wide option of contraceptive methods (Kim, 2009; Kim, 2010; Damm et al., 2007) that in general differ little from the ones used by other women. However, it is important to choose a contraceptive method that does not increase maternal risk of glucose intolerance, metabolic syndrome and CVD, as it occurs with barrier methods, the lactation amenorrhea method during the first six months and intrauterine devices (IUD), both copper and levonorgestrel-releasing IUD, which possess known advantages and limitations. Low-dose combination oral contraceptives, with ethinyl estradiol and a progestin, may also be used, but they are not recommended for women that have other cardiovascular risk factors like hypertension. Even though family history of GDM does not mean contraindication of any method, progestin-only pills should be avoided in women who are breastfeeding, since in a study carried out on Latin-women it was found that it was associated to an increase of diabetes risk, assuming that breastfeeding may be a relatively progestagenic state (Kjos et al., 1998). Neither long-acting progestin methods like depot medroxyprogesterone acetate nor medroxyprogesterone, may be suggested as a first option since they may have major effects on the hydrocarbonated metabolism, as it was proven in Navajo women (Kim et al., 2001). In parous women refraining from another pregnancy, surgical sterilization is a good option, particularly in those delivering by cesarean section, since sterilization may be practiced during surgical procedures.

3.1.6 Oral health measures

It is important that oral health measures proposed to the population in general for prevention of caries and periodontal disease, are rigorously adopted by women with previous GDM, who moreover, should visit at least annually the dentist in order to carry out an early diagnose of these complications when they arise and to apply the required therapeutic measures. The dentist will be on the alert to detect if progression to diabetes has occurred, contributing with this pathology screening (Friedlander et al., 2007).

3.1.7 Life-style changes

Childbearing years constitute one of the stages in the life of a woman more prone to weight gain. Thus, life-style changes make up the building blocks for the prevention of diabetes and other cardiovascular risk factors in women with GDM. Providing preventive care leading to reach and maintain an adequate weight, that include strategies on the aspects shown on Table 3, would result extremely beneficial for the health of this vulnerable population group and also cost-effective (Kapustin, 2008). Even though specific studies on this aspect are scarce and show limitations, it has been found that intensive intervention on life-style changes in women with previous GDM, reduced to a 50% diabetes incidence (Ratner et al., 2008). Undoubtedly, there is a need to study in depth this topic.

- Healthy nutrition
- Physical activity
- Non-smoking
- Low to Moderate alcohol consume
- Adequate stress management

Table 3. Life-style changes in women with previous GDM

3.1.7.1 Healthy nutrition

In general, nutritional recommendations for women with a high risk of developing type 2 diabetes tend to reduce the consumption of processed foods with high content of sugars, salt and trans fats, favoring the consumption of fresh foods like whole grains, legumes, vegetables, fruits, nuts, seeds, low-fat dairy, skinless poultry, and fish to provide omega-3 fatty acids; in other words, foods with low levels of cholesterol and saturated fats but rich in fiber, micronutrients and antioxidants (Melanson, 2008). Daily calorie intake is tailored by nutritionists, according to the characteristics of each woman, so they guarantee weight loss if recommended and at the same time, an adequate nutrition. It is fundamental to provide education on calorie count, food portions, food selection and preparation, reading and interpreting labels, since self-monitoring of intake may help them to incorporate the food plan in their life-styles and adopt these new behavior patterns (Case et al., 2006). Uniform nutritional recommendations in women with a GDM history are needed.

3.1.7.2 Physical activity

Increasing physical activity is paramount in the daily routine of women with previous GDM, if there is no contraindication for this after a thorough medical evaluation. The goal is to reach a program of aerobic exercises like walking, swimming, dancing, bike riding for 30 minutes five or more days a week, beginning gradually from 5-10 minutes daily in sedentary women. Before and after exercising, stretching exercises must be done for 5-10 minutes. If this is complemented with strength training using light weights or elastic bands, weight loss is increased and muscle tone is improved, having a favorable effect on the glucose metabolism (Case et al., 2006).

3.1.7.3 Non-smoking

Quitting smoking is recommended in women with previous GDM (Verier-Mine, 2010), in spite of the lack of studies assessing the effects of tobacco in this group with a high risk of diabetes and cardiovascular disease. Nonetheless, it has been found that smoking increases the risk of diabetes in women, without discerning if they have this family history or not (Rimm et al., 1993).

3.1.7.4 Light to moderate alcohol consumption

Light to moderate alcohol consumption has been found associated with a minor risk of developing type 2 diabetes in middle-aged women and this benefit does not seem to persist when alcohol consumption increases (Wannamethee et al., 2003). It is not known if this result may be generalized to women with previous GDM, but it results sensible to avoid a high level of alcohol consumption due to the possible weight gain and the potential increase of type 2 diabetes risk.

3.1.7.5 Adequate stress management

Learning and the use of periodic tools to allow managing stress adequately may contribute to the goal of keeping healthy women with GDM history. The presence of symptoms of depression or excessive anxiety is an indication for assessment and treatment by specialized Mental Health professionals, according to each case.

3.1.8 Pharmacologic intervention

The use of pharmacologic agents has been explored for preventing or retarding diabetes in women with previous GDM. Studies with troglitazone (Buchanan et al., 2002) and pioglitazone (Xiang et al., 2006b) have been carried out, demonstrating effectiveness in both cases in overweight women. Nonetheless, the former has been discontinued for its hepatotoxic effects, and the use of the latter is limited since its prescription is not authorized for prevention, due to its safety profile regarding future cardiovascular and osteoporosis disease, and its cost (Verier-Mine, 2010; Kim, 2009: Kim, 2010). When metphormine was used in a study, the risk of type 2 diabetes was half reduced in women with overweight and obesity (Ratner et al., 2008). Therefore, further research will provide more insight for its prescription in clinical practice in combination with a healthy life-style, particularly in obese women with glucose intolerance after a GDM pregnancy.

As shown, an adequate postpartum follow-up program for women with GDM comprises a wide range of health-care, clinical-metabolic, gynecological, nutritional, educational, psycho-social, physical training, and odontological activities, among others, carried out by an interdisciplinary team, in order to prevent or retard progression to diabetes and other cardiovascular risk factors, and if this is not attained, to confirm its diagnose as soon as possible.

Unfortunately worldwide, postpartum follow-ups of women with GDM are low. In the United States during the first postpartum months, FPG measurements were ordered on 60.5% women and only completed by 34% (Dinh et al., 2003). In a long cohort of women with GDM, 42% were not tested for FPG, the test was not ordered in 21% of them and none were tested for OGTT (Dietz et al., 2008). Only 37% were tested for FPG or OGTT with a mean of ~ 14 months of postpartum (Smirmakis et al., 2005). In Canada, it has been shown that physicians do not order postpartum OGTT, in spite of counting on a publication with guidelines based on expert opinions on the subject (Clark et al., 2003). At a Venezuelan hospital, in a follow-up program, a 66.19% OGTT adherence after a postpartum period of 4.04 years $\pm$ 2.68 was met, with only 17.98% attendance to all basic education sessions (Rivas et al., 2010c). Achieving favorable changes in life-styles of women with GDM has resulted even more difficult to attain (Stage et al., 2004; Smith et al., 2005), and progression to diabetes continues increasing.

3.2 Changes in quality of life of the population

Individual approach directed to inform women with GDM on the need of reclassifying their metabolic status after delivery, results insufficient for making possible the prevention of diabetes and other cardiovascular risk factors. The need to reinforce knowledge and motivation in the health care team is evident, as well as the access to health care in this area. Moreover, there is a need for stronger research and confrontation on the social determinants that make difficult for GDM women, adherence to postpartum follow-up and the adoption of healthy life-styles (Hjaltested & Conroy, 2010). Structural measures targeted to the population in general, like the ones shown in Table 4, would undoubtedly result in greater benefit.

- Increasing production, distribution and marketing of fresh foods
- Promoting the creation and use of public transportation, bicycle lanes, walking lanes
- Promoting the creation and use of public sport courts and parks
- Promoting and protecting breastfeeding
- Regulating production, distribution and marketing of processed foods rich in trans fats, saturated fats, salt and refined sugars
- Regulating publicity through communication media of this kind of foods
- Promoting smoke-free environments

Table 4. Changes in quality of life of the population

4. Conclusion

After delivery, women with GDM have a high risk of developing diabetes, metabolic syndrome, CVD and other clinical disorders that imply a decrease in the quality of life and high health-care costs. Thus, over several decades early detection of diabetes and other cardiovascular risk factors has been emphasized. For those women who do not show this, it is very important to apply strategies directed towards primary prevention like healthy life-style changes and possible pharmacological intervention, even though further research on these results is needed. To meet both objectives, it is paramount to carry out, on one hand, life-long postpartum follow-up in women with GDM, and also, to research social determinants that affect compliance to these preventive programs and to put into practice collective measures that create favorable conditions for its adherence.

5. References

Åberg, A.; Jönsson, E. & Eskilsson, I. (2002). Predictive factors of developing diabetes mellitus in women with gestational diabetes. *Acta Obstet Gynecol Scand,* Vol. 81, N° 1, (Jan 2002) pp. 11–16

Akinci, B.; Celtik, A. & Yener, S. (2010). Prediction of developing metabolic syndrome after gestational diabetes mellitus. *Fertil Steril,* Vol. 93, N° 4, (Mar 2010), pp. 1248-1254

Albareda, M.; Caballero, A. & Badell, G. (2005). Metabolic syndrome at follow-up in women with and without gestational diabetes mellitus in index pregnancy. *Metabolism,* Vol. 54, N° 8, (Aug 2005), pp. 1115-1121

Almario, C.; Ecker, T. & Moroz, L. (2008). Obstetricians seldom provide postpartum diabetes screening for women with gestational diabetes. *Am J Obstet Gynecol,* Vol. 198, N° 5, (May 2008) pp. 528.e1-5

American College of Obstetricians and Gynecologists (ACOG). (2009). Postpartum Screening for Abnormal Glucose Tolerance in Women Who Had Gestational Diabetes Mellitus. *Obstet Gynecol*, Vol. 113, N° 6, (Jun 2009), pp. 1419-1421

American Diabetes Association (ADA). (2011). Diagnosis and Classification of Diabetes. *Diab. Care,* Vol. 34, Suppl 1, (Jan 2011), pp. S62-S69

Anastasiou, E.; Leakakis, J. & Alevizaki, M. (1998). Impaired endothelium-dependent vasodilatation in women with previous gestational diabetes. *Diab. Care,* Vol. 21, N° 12, (DEC 1998), pp. 2111–2115

Asociación Latinoamericana de Diabetes (ALAD). (2008). Latin America Consensus on Diabetes and Pregnancy. *Rev Asoc Latinoam Diabetes,* Vol. XVI, N° 2, (Jun 2008), pp. 55-69

Baptiste-Roberts, K.; Barone, B. & Gary, T. (2009). Risk factors for type 2 diabetes among women with gestational diabetes: a systematic review. *Am J Med.,* Vol. 122, N° 3, (Mar 2009), pp. 207-214

Beischer, N.; Wein, P. & Sheedy, M. (1997). A Follow-up Program for Women with Previous Gestational Diabetes Mellitus. *MJA,* Vol. 166, N° 7, (Apr 1997), pp. 353-357

Bellamy, L.; Casas, J & Hingorani, A. Type 2 diabetes mellitus after gestational diabetes: a systematic review and meta-analysis. *Lancet,* Vol. 373, N° 9677, (May 2009), pp. 1773–1779

Ben-Haroush, A.; Yogev, Y. & Hod, M. (2004). Epidemiology of gestational diabetes mellitus and its association with type 2 diabetes. *Diabetes Med,* Vol. 21, N° 2, (Feb 2004), pp. 103-113

Bentley-Lewis, R. (2009). Late cardiovascular consequences of Gestational Diabetes Mellitus. *Sem Reprod Med,* Vol. 27, N° 4, (Jul 2009), pp. 322-329

Blatt, A.; Nakamoto, J. & Kaufman, H. (2011). Gaps in Diabetes Screening During Pregnancy and Postpartum. *Obstet Gynecol,* Vol. 117, N° 1, (Jan 2011), pp. 61–68

Bo, S.; Menato, G. & Pinach S. (2003). Clinical characteristics and outcome of pregnancy in women with gestational hyperglycaemia with and without antibodies to beta-cell antigens. *Diabet Med,* Vol. 20, N°1, (Jan 2003), pp. 64-68

Buchanan, T.; Xiang, A. & Peters, R. (2002). Preservation of pancreatic beta cell function and prevention of type 2 diabetes by pharmacological treatment of insulin resistance in high-risk Hispanic women. *Diabetes,* Vol. 51, N° 9, (Sep 2002), pp. 2796-2803

Caballero, E. (2005). Metabolic and vascular abnormalities in subjects at risk for type 2 diabetes: The early start of a dangerous situation. *Arch Med Res.,* Vol. 36, N° 3, (May-Jun 2005), pp. 241-249

Case, J.; Willoughby D. & Haley-Zitlin V. (2006). Preventing type 2 diabetes after gestational diabetes. *Diabetes Educ,* Vol. 32, N° 6, (Nov-Dec 2006), pp. 877-886

Catalano, P.; Vargo, K. & Bersntein, I. (1991). Incidence and risk factors associated with abnormal postpartum glucose tolerance in women with gestational diabetes. *AM J Obstet Gynecol,* Vol. 165, N° 4, (Oct 1991), pp. 914-919

Clark, H.; Walraven, C. & Code, C. (2003). Did publication of a clinical Practice Giideline Recommendation to Screen for type 2 Diabetes in Women With Gestational Diabetes Change Practice?. *Diab. Care,* Vol. 26, N° 2, (Feb 2003), pp. 265-268

Cheung, N. & Byth, K. (2003). Population health significance of gestational diabetes. *Diab. Care,* Vol. 26, N° 7, (Jul 2003), pp. 2005- 2009

Cho, N.; Lim, S. & Jang, H. (2005). Elevated homocysteine as a risk factor for the development of diabetes in women with a previous history of gestational diabetes mellitus: a 4-year prospective study. *Diab. Care,* Vol. 28, N° 11, (Nov 2005), pp. 2750-2755

Chodick, G.; Elchalal, U. & Sella, T. (2010). The risk of overt diabetes mellitus among women with gestational diabetes: a population-based study. *Diabet.Med,* Vol. 27, N° 7, (Jul 2010), pp. 779–785

Costacou, T.; Bosnyak, Z. & Harger, G. (2008). Postpartum Adiponectin Concentration, Insulin Resistance and Metabolic Abnormalities Among Women With Pregnancy-Induced Disturbances. *Prev Cardiol,* Vol. 11, N° 2, (Spring 2008), pp. 106–115

Dabelea, D.; Snell-Bergeon, J. & Hartsfield, C. (2005). Increasing prevalence of Gestational Diabetes Mellitus (GDM) over time and by birth cohort. *Diab. Care,* Vol. 28, N° 3, (Mar 2005), pp. 579–584

Damm, P. (2003). Diabetes following gestational diabetes mellitus. In: *Diabetes and Pregnancy,* Hod M, Jovanovic L, Di Renzo, GC, de Leiva A, Langer O, pp. (191–200), Martin Dunitz, ISBN 1 84184 110 2, London

Damm, P.; Mathiesen, E. & Petersen, K. (2007). Contraception after Gestational Diabetes, *Diab. Care,* Vol. 30, Suppl 2, (Jul 2007), pp. S236-S241 de Leiva, A.; Mauricio, D. & Corcoy, R. (2007). Diabetes-Related Autoantibodies and Gestational Diabetes. *Diab. Care,* Vol. 30, Suppl 2, (Jul 2007), pp. S127-S133

Di Benedetto, A.; Russo, G. & Corrado, F. (2005). Inflammatory markers in women with a recent history of gestational diabetes mellitus. *J Endocrinol Invest,* Vol. 28, N° 1, (Jan 2005), pp. 34-38

Di Cianni, G.; Lencioni, C. & Volpe, L. (2007). C-reactive protein and metabolic syndrome in women with previous gestational diabetes. *Diabetes Metab Res Rev,* Vol. 23, N° 2, (Feb 2007), pp.135–140

Dietz, P.; Vesco, K. & Callaghan, W. (2008). Postpartum screening for diabetes after a gestational diabetes Mellitus affected pregnancy. *Obstet Gynecol,* Vol. 112, N° 4, (Oct 2008), pp. 868-874

Dinh, D.; Musser, B. & Bayliss, P. (2003). Does postpartum diabetic testing occur in gestational diabetes?. *Prim Care Update Ob Gyn,* Vol. 10, (Oct 2010), pp. 182-185

Farhan, S.; Winzer, C. & Tura, A. (2006). Fibrinolytic dysfunction in insulin-resistant women with previous gestational diabetes. *Eur J Clin Invest,* Vol. 36, N° 5, (May 2006), pp. 345–352

Feig, D.; Zinman, B. & Wang, X. (2008). Risk of development of diabetes mellitus after diagnosis of gestational diabetes. *CMAJ,* Vol. 179, N° 3, (Jul 2008), pp. 229-234

Ferrara, A.; Tiffany, P. & Kim, C. (2009). Trends in postpartum diabetes screening and subsequent diabetes and impaired fasting glucose among women with histories of gestational diabetes mellitus. *Diab. Care,* Vol. 32, N° 2, (Feb 2009), pp. 269-274

Friedlander, A.; Chaudhuri, G. & Altman, L. (2007). A past medical history of gestational diabetes: its medical significance and its dental implications. *Oral Surg Oral Med Oral Pathol Oral Radiol Endod,* Vol. 103, N° 2, (Feb 2007), pp. 157-163

Füchtenbusch, M.; Ferber, K. & Standl, E. (1997). Prediction of type 1 diabetes postpartum in patients with gestational diabetes mellitus by combined islet cell autoantibody screening: a prospective multicenter study. *Diabetes,* Vol. 46, N° 9, (Sep 1997), pp. 1459-67

Getahun, D.; Fassett, M. & Jacobsen, S. (2010). Gestational diabetes: risk of recurrence in subsequent pregnancies. *Am J Obstet Gynecol,* Vol. 203, N° 5, (Nov 2010), pp. 467.e1-6.

Golden, S.; Bennett, W. & Baptist-Roberts, K. (2009). Antepartum glucose tolerance test results as predictors of type 2 diabetes mellitus in women with a history of gestational diabetes mellitus: a systematic review. *Gend Med,* Vol.6, Suppl 1, (Jan 2009), pp. 109-122

Gonçalves, L.; Gabaldi, M. & Peraçoli, J. (2005). Hypertension After Gestational Hyperglycemia. *Arq Bras Endocrinol Metab,* Vol. 49, N° 2, (Apr 2005), pp. 265-270

Gouveri, E.; Papanas, N. & Hatzitolios, A. (2011). Breastfeeding and diabetes. *Curr Diabetes Rev,* Vol. 7, N° 2, (Mar 2011), pp. 135-142

Gunderson, E.; Jacobs Jr., D. & Chiang, V. (2010). Duration of Lactation and Incidence of the Metabolic Syndrome in Women of Reproductive Age According to Gestational Diabetes Mellitus Status: A 20-Year Prospective Study in CARDIA (Coronary Artery Risk Development in Young Adults). *Diabetes,* Vol. 59, N° 2, (Feb 2010), pp. 495–504

Hannemann, M.; Liddell, W. & Shore, A. (2002). Vascular function in women with previous gestational diabetes. *J Vasc Res,* Vol. 39, N° 4, (Jul-Aug 2002), pp. 311–319

Harlev, A. & Wiznitzer, A. (2010). New Insights on Glucose Pathophysiology in Gestational Diabetes and Insulin Resistance. *Curr Diab Rep, V*ol. 10, N° 3, (Jul 2010), pp. 242–247

Heitritter, S.; Solomon, C. & Mitchell, G. (2005). Subclinical inflammation and vascular dysfunction in women with previous gestational diabetes mellitus. *J Clin Endocrinol Metab,* Vol. 90, N° 7, (Jul 2005), pp. 3983-3988

Hjaltested, L. & Conroy, S. (2010). Development of Macrosomia Resulting From Gestational Diabetes Mellitus. Physiology and Social Determinants of Health. *Adv Neonatal Care,* Vol. 10, N° 1, (Feb 2010), pp. 7-12

Hunt, K. & Schuller, K. (2007). The increasing prevalence of diabetes in pregnancy. *Obstet Gynecol Clin North Am,* Vol. 34, N° 2, (Jun 2007), pp. 173–199

Järvelä, I.; Juutinen, J. & Koskela, P. Gestational Diabetes Identifies Women at Risk for Permanent Type 1 and Type 2 Diabetes in Fertile Age. *Diab. Care,* Vol. 29, N° 3, (Mar 2006), pp. 607-612

Kapustin, J. (2008). Postpartum management for gestational diabetes mellitus: Policy and practice implications. *J Am Acad Nurse Pract,* Vol. 20, N° 11, (Nov 2008), pp. 547-554

Kim, C.; Seidel, K. & Begier, E. (2001). Diabetes and depot medroxyprogesterone contraception in Navajo women. *Arch Intern Med,* Vol. 161, N° 14, (Jul 2001), pp.1766–1771

Kim, C.; Newton, K. & Knoop, R. (2002). Gestational diabetes and the incidence of Type 2 Diabetes. A systematic review. *Diab. Care,* Vol. 25, N° 10, (Oct 2002), pp. 862-1868

Kim, C.; Berger, D. & Chamany, S. (2007). Recurrence of Gestational Diabetes Mellitus. A systematic review. *Diab. Care,* Vol. 30, N° 5, (May 2007), pp. 1314–1319

Kim, C.; Herman, W. & Vijan, S. (2007). Efficacy and cost of postpartum screening strategies for diabetes among women with histories of gestational diabetes mellitus. *Diab. Care,* Vol. 30, N° 5, (May 2007), pp. 1102- 1106

Kim, C.; Cheng, Y. & Beckles, G. (2008). Inflammation Among Women With a History of Gestational Diabetes Mellitus and Diagnosed Diabetes in the Third National Health and Nutrition Examination Survey. *Diab. Care,* Vol. 31, N° 7 (Jul 2008), pp. 1386–1388

Kim, C. (2009). Postpartum Management of Gestational Diabetes Mellitus. *Postgraduate Obstetric & Gynecologic,* Vol. 29, N° 3, (Feb 2009), pp. 1-6

Kim, C. (2010). Managing women with gestational diabetes mellitus in the postnatal period. *Diabetes, Obes Metab.,* Vol. 12, N° 1 (Jan 2010), pp. 20–25

Kitzmiller, J.; Dang-Kilduff, L. & Taslimi, M. (2007). Gestational Diabetes After Delivery. Short-term management and long-term risks. *Diab. Care,* Vol. 30, Suppl 2, (Jul 2007), pp. S225- S235

Koivunen, R.; Juutinen, J. & Vauhkonen, I. (2001). Metabolic and Steroidogenic Alterations Related to Increased Frequency of Polycystic Ovaries in Women with a History of Gestational Diabetes. *J Clin Endocrinol Metab,* Vol. 86, N° 6, (Jun 2001), pp. 2591–2599

Kjos, S.; Buchanan, T. & Greenspoon, J. (1990). Diabetes Mellitus: the prevalence of glucose intolerance and diabetes mellitus in the first two months postparto. *AM J Obstet Gynecol*, Vol. 163, N° 1 (Jul 1990), pp: 93-98

Kjos, S.; Henry, O. & Lee, R. (1993). The effect of lactation on glucose and lipid metabolism in women with recent gestational diabetes. *Obstet Gynecol*, Vol. 82, N° 3, (Sep 1993), pp. 451–455

Kjos, S.; Peters, R. & Xiang, A. (1995). Predicting future diabetes in Latino women with gestational diabetes. Utility of early post-partum glucose tolerance testing. *Diabetes*, Vol. 44, N° 5, (May 1995), pp. 586 – 591

Kjos, S.; Peters, R. & Xiang, A. (1998). Contraception and the Risk of Type 2 Diabetes Mellitus in Latina Women With Prior Gestational Diabetes Mellitus. *JAM*, Vol. 280, N° 6, (Aug 1998), pp. 533-538

Kousta, E.; Cela, E. & Lawrence, N. (2000). The prevalence of polycystic ovaries in women with a history of gestational diabetes. *Clin Endocrinol (Oxf)*, Vol. 53, N° 4, (Oct 2000), pp. 501-507

Kousta, E.; Lawrence, N. & Anyaoku, V. (2001). Prevalence and features of pancreatic islet cell autoimmunity in women with gestational diabetes from different ethnic groups. *BJOG*, Vol. 108, N° 7, (Oct 2001), pp. 716-720

Kousta, E.; Lawrence, N. & Godsland, I. (2003). Insulin resistance and beta-cell dysfunction in normoglycaemic European women with a history of gestational diabetes. *Clin Endocrinol (Oxf)*, Vol. 59, N° 3, Sep 2003), pp. 289-297

Kozhimannil, K.; Pereira, M. & Harlow, B. (2009). L Association Between Diabetes and Perinatal Depression Among Low-Income Mothers. *JAMA*, Vol. 301, N° 8, (Feb 2009), pp. 842-847

Kwak, S.; Kim, H. & Choi, S. (2008). Subsequent Pregnancy After Gestational Diabetes Mellitus. Frequency and risk factors for recurrence in Korean women. *Diab. Care*, Vol. 31, N° 9, (Sep 2008), pp.1867–1871

Lapolla, A.; Dalfrà, M. & Fedele, D. (2009). Diabetes related autoimmunity in gestational diabetes mellitus: is it important?. *Nutr Metab Cardiovasc Dis.*, Vol. 19, N° 9, (Nov 2009), pp. 674-682

Lauenborg, J.; Mathiesen, E. & Hansen, T. (2005). The Prevalence of the Metabolic Syndrome in a Danish Population of Women with Previous Gestational Diabetes Mellitus Is Three-Fold Higher than in the General Population. *J Clin Endocrinol Metab*, Vol. 90, N° 7, (Jul 2005), pp. 4004–4010

Lauenborg, J.; Grarup, N. & Damm, P. (2009). Common Type 2 Diabetes Risk Gene Variants Associate with Gestational Diabetes. *J Clin Endocrinol Metab*, Vol. 94, N° 1 (Jan 2009), pp. 145–150

Lim, S.; Choi, S. & Park, Y. (2007). Visceral fatness and insulin sensitivity in women with a previous history of gestational diabetes mellitus. *Diab. Care*, Vol. 30, N° 2, (Feb 2007), pp. 348-353

Lin, C.; Wen, S. & Wu, Y. (2005). The Postpartum Metabolic Outcome of Women with Previous Gestational Diabetes Mellitus. *Chang Gung Med J*, Vol. 28, N° 11, (Nov 2005), pp. 794-800

Mauricio, D.; Balsells, M. & Morales, J. (1996). Islet cell autoinmunity in women with gestational diabetes and risk of progression to insulin-dependent diabetes Mellitus. *Diabetes Metab Rev*, Vol. 12, N° 4, (Dec 1996), pp. 275-285

Macneill, S.; Hamilton, D. & Armson, A. (2001). Rates and Risk Factors for Recurrence of Gestational Diabetes. *Diab. Care*, Vol. 24, N° 4, (Apr 2001), pp. 659–662

Melanson, K. (2008). Nutrition for Women in the Prevention and Treatment of Type 2 Diabetes and Cardiovascular Diseases. *AJLM*, Vol. 2, N° 3, (May-Jun 2008), pp. 214-218

Metzger, B.; Cho, N. & Roston, S. (1993). Prepregnancy weight and antepartum insulin secretion predict glucose tolerance five years after gestational diabetes mellitus. *Diab. Care*, Vol. 16, N° 12, (Dec 1993), pp. 1598-60

Metzger, B.; Buchanan, T. & Coustan, D. (2007). Summary and Recommendations of the Fifth International Workshop - Conference on Gestational Diabetes Mellitus. *Diab. Care*, Vol. 30, Suppl 2, (Jul 2007), pp. S251-S260

Meyer-Seifer, C.; Vohr, B. (1996). Lipid levels in former gestational diabetic mothers. *Diab. Care*, Vol. 19, N° 12, (Dec 1996), pp. 1351–1355

Mitchell, M.; Hermos, R. & Larson, C. (2000). Prevalence of GAD Autoantibodies in Women With Gestational Diabetes. *Diab. Care*, Vol. 23, N° 11, (Nov 2000), pp. 1705-1706

Morimitsu, L.; Fusaro, A. & Sanchez, V. (2007). Fibrinolytic dysfunction after gestation is associated to components of insulin resistance and early type 2 diabetes in latino women with previous gestational diabetes. *Diabetes Res Clin Pract*, Vol. 78, N° 3, (Dec 2007), pp. 340-348

Moses, R. (1997). The recurrence rate of gestational diabetes in subsequent pregnancies. *Diab. Care*, Vol. 20, N° 12, (Dec 1996), pp. 1647–1650

Moses, R.; Shand, J. & Tapsell, L. (1997). The recurrence of gestational diabetes: could dietary differences in fat intake be an explanation?. *Diab. Care*, Vol. 20, N° 11, (Nov 1997), pp.1635-1637

Murgia, C.; Orrù, M. & Portoghese, E. (2008). Autoimmunity in gestational diabetes mellitus in Sardinia: a preliminary case-control report. *Reprod Biol and Endocrinol*, Vol. 6, (Jun 2008), pp.24

National Institute for Health and Clinical Excellence (NICE). (2008). Diabetes in Pregnancy: Management of Diabetes and its Complications from Preconception to the Postnatal Period. London: National Collaborating Centre for Women's and Children's Health. *Diabet Med.*, Vol 25, N° 9, (Sep 2008), pp.1025- 1027

Nilsson, C.; Ursing, D. & T¨orn, C. (2007). Presence of GAD Antibodies During Gestational Diabetes Mellitus Predicts Type 1 Diabetes. *Diab. Care*, Vol. 30, N° 8, (Aug 2007), pp. 1968-1971

Novak, K.; Taylor, G. & Dawson, D. (2006). Periodontitis and gestational diabetes mellitus: exploring the link in NHANES III. *J Public Health Dent*, Vol. 66, N° 3, (Summer 2006), pp. 163-16

Pallardo, F.; Herranz, L. & Garcia-Ingelmo, T. (1999). Early Postpartum Metabolic Assessment in Women With Prior Gestational Diabetes. *Diab. Care*, Vol. 22, N° 7, (Jul 1999), pp. 1053–1058

Ratner, R.; Christophi, C. & Metzger, B. (2008). Prevention of diabetes in women with a history of gestational diabetes: Effects of metformin and lifestyle interventions. *J Clin Endoc Metab*, Vol. 93, N° 12, (Dec 2008), pp. 4774-4779

Retnakaran, R.; Qi, Y. & Sermer, M. (2008). Glucose intolerance in pregnancy and future risk of prediabetes or diabetes. *Diab. Care,* Vol. 31, N° 10 (Oct 2008), pp. 2026-2031

Retnakaran, R.; Qi, Y. & Connelly, P. (2010). Low Adiponectin Concentration in Pregnancy Predicts Postpartum Insulin Resistance, Beta-cell Dysfunction, and Fasting Glycaemia. *Diabetologia*, Vol. 53, N° 2, (Feb 2010), pp. 268–276

Retnakaran, R.; Austin, P. & Shah, B. (2011). Effect of subsequent pregnancies on the risk of developing diabetes following a first pregnancy complicated by gestational diabetes: a population-based study. *Diabet. Med*, Vol. 28, N° 3, (Mar 2011), pp. 287–292

Rimm, E.; Manson, J. & Stampfer, M. (1993). Cigarette smoking and the risk of diabetes in women. *Am J Public Health*, Vol. 83, N° 2 (Feb 1993), pp. 211–214

Rivas, A.; Gonzalez, N. & Gonzalez, J. (2007). High Frequency of Diabetes in Early Post-Partum Assessment of Women with Gestational Diabetes Mellitus. *Diab Metab Syn Clin Res Rev*, Vol. 1, N° 3, (Sep 2007), pp. 159-165

Rivas, A.; Landon, M. & Gaillard, T. (2010). Awareness of Risk Factors for Type 2 Diabetes in Women with Current and Former Gestational Diabetes Mellitus: Implications for future primary diabetes prevention. *Diab Metab Syn Clin Res Rev*, Vol. 4, N° 2, (Apr-Jun 2010), pp. 89–94

Rivas, A.; González, J. & Guevara, M. (2010). Clinical and metabolic disorders in women with previous gestational diabetes. *Rev Obstet Ginecol Venez*, Vol. 70, N° 1 (Mar 2010), pp. 18-23

Rivas, A.; Guerra, C. & Gonzalez, J. (2010). Women with Previous Gestational Diabetes Included in the Postpartum Follow-up Program. *Rev Asoc Latinoam Diabetes,* Vol. XVIII, N° 1 (Mar 2010), pp. 16-23

Robitaille, J.; Grant, A. (2008). The genetics of gestational diabetes mellitus: evidence for relationship with type 2 diabetes Mellitus. *Genet Med*, Vol. 10, N° 4, (Apr 2008), pp. 240–250

Russell, C.; Dodds, L. & Armson, B. (2008). Diabetes mellitus following gestational diabetes: role of subsequent pregnancy. BJOG, Vol. 115, N° 2, (Jan 2008), pp. 253-259

Sattar, V. & Greer, I. (2002). Pregnancy complications and maternal cardiovascular risk: Opportunities for intervention and screening? *BMJ,* Vol. 325, N° 7356, (Jul 2002), pp. 157-160

Shah, B.; Retnakaran, R. & Booth, G. (2008). Increased risk of cardiovascular disease in young women following Gestational Diabetes Mellitus. *Diab. Care*, Vol. 31, N° 8, (Aug 2008), pp. 1668-1669

Smith, B.; Cheung, N. & Bauman, A. (2005). Postpartum psychosocial factors among women with recent gestational diabetes mellitus. *Diab. Care,* Vol. 28, N° 11, (Nov 2005), pp. 2650-2654

Stage, E.; Ronneby, H. & Damm, P. (2004). Lifestyle change after gestational diabetes. *Diabetes Res Clin Pract*, Vol. 63, N° 1, (Jan 2004), pp. 67-22

Sinha, B.; Brydon, P. & Taylor, R. (2003). Maternal antenatal parameters as predictors of persistent postnatal glucose intolerance: a comparative study between Afro-Caribbeans, Asians and Caucasians. *Diabet Med*, Vol. 20, N° 5, (May 2003), pp. 382-386

Smirmakis, K.; Chasan-Taber, L. & Wolf, M. (2005). Postpartum diabetes screening in women with a history of gestational diabetes. *Obstet Gynecol*, Vol. 106, N° 6, (Dec 2005), pp. 1297-1303

Thomann, R.; Rossinelli, N. & Keller, U. (2008). Differences in low-grade chronic inflammation and insulin resistance in women with previous gestational diabetes mellitus and women with polycystic ovary syndrome. *Gynecol Endocrinol*. Vol. 24, N° 4, (Apr 2008), pp.199-206

Tura, A.; Mari, A. & Prikoszovich, T. (2008). Value of the intravenous and oral glucose tolerance tests for detecting subtle impairments in insulin sensitivity and beta-cell function in former gestational diabetes. *Clinical Endocrinology*, Vol. 69, N° 2, (Aug 2008), pp. 237–243

Verier-Mine, O. (2010). Outcomes in women with a history of gestational diabetes. Screening and preventiion of type 2 diabetes. Literature review. *Diabetes Metab*, Vol. 36, N° 6, (Dec 2010), pp. 595-616

Vitoratos, N; Deliveliotou, A. & Vlahos, N. (2008). Serum adiponectin during pregnancy and postpartum in women with gestational diabetes and normal controls. *Gynecological Endocrinology*, Vol. 24, N° 11, (Nov 2008), pp. 614–619

Vitoratos, N.; Valsamakis, G. & Mastorakos, G. (2008). Pre- and early post-partum adiponectin and Interleukin-1beta levels in women with and without gestational diabetes. *Hormones*, Vol. 7, N° 3, (Jul-Sep 2008), pp. 230-236

Vohr, B. & Boney, C. (2008). Gestational diabetes: the forerunner for the development of maternal and childhood obesity and metabolic syndrome?. *J Matern Fetal Neonatal Med*, Vol. 21, N° 3, Mar 2008), pp.149-157

Wannamethee, S.; Camargo, C. & Manson, J. (2003). Alcohol Drinking Patterns and Risk of Type 2 Diabetes Mellitus Among Younger Women. *Arch Intern Med*, Vol. 163, N° 11, (Jun 2003), pp. 1329-1336

Weijers, R.; Bekedam, D. & Goldschmidt, H. (2006). The clinical usefulness of glucose tolerance testing in gestational diabetes to predict early postpartum diabetes mellitus. *Clin Chem Lab Med*, Vol. 44, N° 1, (Jan 2006), pp. 99–104

Wender-Ozegowska, E.; Sporna, M. & Zawiejska, A. (2007). Components of metabolic syndrome in women after Gestational Diabetes. *Pol Arch Med Wewnetrznej*, Vol. 117, N° 10, (Oct 2007), pp. 457-461

Wollitzer, A. & Jovanovic, L. (2007). 10 years later......Diabetes Mellitus and Pregnancy. *The Endocrinologist*, Vol.17, N° 1 (Feb 2007), pp. 30-34

Wucher, H.; Lepercq, J. & Carette, C. (2011). Poor prognosis of pregnancy in women with autoimmune type 1 diabetes mellitus masquerading as gestational diabetes, Vol. 37, N° 1, (Feb 2011), pp. 47-51

Xiang, A.; Kawakubo, M. & Kjos, S. (2006). Long-Acting Injectable Progestin Contraception and Risk of Type 2 Diabetes in Latino Women With Prior Gestational Diabetes Mellitus. *Diab. Care*, Vol. 29, N° 3, (Mar 2006), pp. 613–617

Xiang, A.; Peters, R. & Kjos, S. (2006). Effect of Pioglitazone on Pancreatic β-Cell Function and Diabetes Risk in Hispanic Women With Prior Gestational Diabetes. *Diabetes*, Vol. 55, N° 2, (Feb 2006), pp. 517–522

Xiang, A.; Kjos, S. & Takayanagi, M. (2010). Detailed physiological Characterization of the Development of Type 2 Diabetes in Hispanic Women With Prior Gestational Diabetes Mellitus. *Diabetes*, Vol. 59, N° 10, (Oct 2010), pp. 2625-2630.

Xiong, X.; Buekens, P. & Vastardis, S. (2006). Periodontal disease and gestational diabetes mellitus. *Am J Obstet Gynecol*, Vol. 195, N° 4, (Oct 2006), pp. 1086-1089

York, R.; Brown, L. & Armstrong-Persily, C. (1996). Affect in diabetic women during pregnancy and postpartum. *Nurs Res*, Vol. 45, N° 1, (Jan-Feb 1996), pp. 54-56

Yu, S.; Park, S. & Kim, H. (2009). The prevalence of GAD antibodies in Korean women with gestational diabetes mellitus and their clinical characteristics during and after pregnancy. *Diabetes Metab Res Rev*, Vol. 25, N° 4, (May 2009), pp. 329–334

Yun, S.; Kabeer, N. & Zhu, B. (2007). Modifiable Risk Factors for Developing Diabetes Among Women With Previous Gestational Diabetes. *Prev Chronic Dis*, Vol. 4, N° 1, (Jan 2007), pp. 1-6